THE

# SPECIAL SYMPTOMATOLOGY

OF

## THE NEW REMEDIES.

# MATERIA MEDICA

AND

# SPECIAL THERAPEUTICS

OF THE

# NEW REMEDIES.

BY EDWIN M. HALE, M. D.,

PROFESSOR OF MATERIA MEDICA AND THERAPEUTICS OF THE NEW REMEDIES IN HAHN
EMANN MEDICAL COLLEGE, CHICAGO: AUTHOR OF "LECTURES ON DISEASES
OF THE HEART," "CHARACTERISTICS OF NEW REMEDIES," ETC.

FIFTH EDITION—WITH APPENDIX.

IN TWO VOLUMES.

VOL. I.

# SPECIAL SYMPTOMATOLOGY,

WITH NEW BOTANICAL AND PHARMACOLOGICAL NOTES.

## B. JAIN PUBLISHERS PVT. LTD.
## NEW DELHI - 110 055

*Price* : Rs. 300.00 (2 Vols)

**Reprint Edition 1995**

© Copyright with Publishers

*Publishers by :*
**B. Jain Publishers Pvt. LTD.**
7, Wazir Pur, Printing Press Complex,
Ring Road, Delhi-110 052 (INDIA)

*Printed in India by :*
**J.J. Offset Printers**
7, Wazirpur, Delhi-110 052

ISBN 81-7021-597-8

ISBN 81-7021-598-6

*BOOK CODE B-3651*

TO THE

# HOMŒOPATHIC PHYSICIANS

OF

## AMERICA AND ENGLAND,

**THIS VOLUME IS RESPECTFULLY DEDICATED,**

BY

*THE AUTHOR.*

# EXPLANATION OF SYMBOLS.

Symptoms without a symbol prefixed, are simply pathogenetic; if in *italics*, they may be considersd *important*, or of constant appearance in the provings.

The * signifies that the symptom is pathogenetic, and has been verified by *cures*.

The ° signifies that clinical experience has proven the medicine to be curative for that symptom or condition.

In a few cases the letter (v) has been used to indicate a *verification*. The letters (p) and (s) have been used to designate *primary* and *secondary* symptoms.

# PREFACE TO THE FOURTH EDITION.

IN my preface to the *first* edition of NEW REMEDIES, written in 1864, I used the following language:

"The object in the preparation of this work has been to furnish the physicians and students of the homœopathic school of medicine with full and accurate information relative to a class of remedies, mostly indigenous, but few of which have had any place in the published Homœopathic Materia Medica. Some of the provings have been incorporated into the Symptomen Codex (*Phytolacca, Podophyllum and Sanguinaria*), others have been published in the various journals of our School (*Rumex, Cimicifuga, Cornus c., etc.*), but the great majority have never been proven until now, and the only mention of them has been in occasional clinical or empirical suggestions. To the first and second classes I have added many pathogenetic symptoms gleaned from various sources, re-provings, poisonings, etc., and added also all the clinical observations that could be collected from reliable sources. The latter class may be divided into two others, namely: (1) those which have been proven; and (2) those of which we have only empirical data upon which to base clinical use and suggestive or theoretical deductions.

"As we gather experience in the use of these remedies, and institute accurate provings, the necessity for these suggestions and theoretical deductions will be done away with. Each physician should consider himself bound to collect all the symptoms which are really pathogenetic, and note down all reliable curative experience belonging to these medicines, and faithfully report the same to our journals.

"The causes which led me to investigate the properties and virtues of the remedies mentioned in the following pages, will be patent to every progressive mind. After using for many years those invaluable remedies found in our standard Materia Medica, most of which were handed down to us by Hahnemann and his colleagues, I found that although their curative scope was very wide, it did not apparently include many symptoms and diseases. I was led to investigate the field of *indigenous* remedies for

(7)

these reasons: (1) the suggestion of TESTE, that plants are adapted to cure the diseases which infest the same localities; and (2) the many cures which had come under my observation, made by these remedies in the hands of eclectic and domestic practitioners, (some of the cases will be mentioned in the body of this work). These reasons, together with a natural ambition to enlarge the sphere of Homœopathic Materia Medica, induced me to throw away all prejudice, and devote my energies to the task of introducing, by *provings* and clinical experience, the indigenous medicines which so largely abound in the United States. A few others had started before me, and Cimicifuga, Cornus, Podophyllum and Sanguinaria had been proven, and their pathogeneses published. But from some cause they had not attracted the attention which they deserved. After several years spent in the investigation and study of the new remedies, publishing from time to time items from my experience with them, I was induced to attempt the work of collecting all that had been published concerning the indigenous plants of this country, and to add to such all the knowledge, clinical and theoretical, which could be gleaned from my colleagues, together with my own.

"To this I have taken the liberty of adding the testimony and empirical experience of physicians of the allopathic and eclectic schools, relative to the medicines under consideration. If any object to this method, I would refer them to the writings of Hahnemann and his colleagues — Dudgeon, Hughes, Madden and Drysdale, of England; Teste and Roth, of France; and Hering, Joslin, Marcy, Hempel, and others, of this country. I contend that the experience of others, besides members of the Homœopathic School, is often useful in building up our pathogeneses, and adding to trustworthy clinical knowledge.

" I shall not be held responsible for the opinions of any writer quoted in the following pages. Let each be judged upon his own merits. I do not claim that this work is in any way *complete*. Indeed, I shall be satisfied if it is only pronounced by the profession as eminently *suggestive*. Many of the provings are very imperfect, and some of the clinical remarks open to criticism. Let the wheat be separated from the chaff by the inexorable test of honest trial."

In my preface to the *second* edition, which appeared in 1867, I gave the following reasons for rewriting and enlarging the work.

" The favorable reception which the first edition of this work received, from the homœopathic physicians of this country and England, induced me to prepare a second edition.

"Another reason which impelled me to rewrite the work, was, that the first edition met with such rapid sale that at the expiration of two years from its issue, not a copy was for sale in the United States. This fact was as much an encouragement to the publisher as to myself, and it will doubtless result in an improvement in the style and appearance of the second edition.

"Not only was I encouraged by the above, but by other inducements, namely: the prompt and courteous response of many of my professional colleagues to my request for new provings and clinical reports. It would be invidious to mention any names of physicians, when so many have contributed to swell our knowledge of the pathogenetic and curative powers of these medicines. I cannot, however, in justice, omit to record my acknowledgments of the valuable aid received from the members of the North-Western Provers' Association, who have enriched this edition with several excellent provings.

"Pharmacological observations of a practical character are made concerning each remedy. The officinal preparations are also designated. These practical additions will do away with the necessity felt for a pharmacopœia of the new remedies, until a complete Homœopathic Dispensatory shall be published.

"Of some of the medicines added to this edition no provings have been made, and the clinical experience is almost entirely wanting. This was the case with several of the medicines in the former issue; but their appearance called attention to them, provings were instituted, they were used in practice, and are now valuable additions to our Materia Medica. This, I believe, will be the case with the unproven medicines in this edition."

In answer to some criticisms on this, as well as the first edition, I thus defended the quotations taken from allopathic authorities:

"Since the first appearance of this work, various critics in our school have expressed doubts as to the propriety of introducing clinical testimony drawn from allopathic and eclectic sources. These objections were fully answered through the columns of the *American Homœopathic Observer*, ano *Medical Investigator*. That my views in this matter, which I consider to be logical and scientific, may be known to my colleagues, I herewith again present them for consideration.

"'In my private correspondence I am frequently asked the question, 'Why do you quote allopathic authorities in your New Remedies and other writings?' In some of the periodicals of our school I find the same question asked. In other words, the questioners ask: 'Can allopathic authority, or allopathic cures, become of value to the homœopathist?'

"'I answer, 'Their bald *dictum* cannot, but their *cures* can.' I propose to state the reasons for this belief. But first, I would ask the reader to glance over the pages of the 'Introduction' to that immortal work of Hahnemann, the 'Organon.' He will there find page after page occupied with a concise narration of allopathic cures. He makes such testimony contribute to the proof of the homœopathic law, and intimates, in the strongest language, that *all* the cures were homœopathic. I have only fol lowed, humbly I admit, in the footsteps of our great Master.

"'It is true that in writing of new and unproven remedies, I have quoted all medical authors, but not as *authority*, except in certain cases. I mention their alleged cures for the purpose of drawing attention to the successful uses of the medicines in certain diseases. I mention their theoretical deductions and even their crude recommendations, thinking that perhaps we may get a little grain out of the great amount of such chaff. It must be recollected that I have had little or no homœopathic experience to draw from, and had to use such material as I could find. That such mention of allopathic and eclectic experience was not productive of injury, the contents of the second edition will prove. The valuable use of Caulophyllum, Dioscorea, and many other medicines, first came to us from that source, yet our school has since verified the reality of their cures — and more; they have proved that such cures were made homœopathically, because the medicines are capable of causing similar affections.

"'It seems strange to some of our school that because Allopathists use such massive doses, they can make any cures at all. But *a cure is a fact.* We can not explain it away. The testimony of a physician of one school is as good as that of another, provided his alleged cure was made with *one medicine given singly.*

"'No proposition is more generally accepted in our school than, that a dose, to be homœopathic, need not be a high potency dose. The true definition of a homœopathic dose is, *any quantity of medicine capable of effecting a cure.* If we do not admit this, we must admit that allopathists cure by virtue of the law of *contraria*, and if we do this, we give them vantage ground at once. *All cures are Homœopathic cures*, whether made with the 200th, or with grain doses of the crude drug. For example, Hahnemann cured a severe case of *colicodynia* with *Veratrum album*— 'four powders, each containing four grains' of the crude powdered root. Although the patient took two powders a day, instead of one, and aggravated the pain temporarily, yet it was as brilliant a cure as ever Hahnemann made with the 30th potency.

"'The remarkable cures made by Eclectics with *Caulophyllum* and *Dioscorea*, were made with material doses. Are such cures to be denied and pronounced worthless? If so, then Hahnemann's cure with *Veratrum* must be placed in the same list. I do not say that such material doses are necessary to the cure; but if they remove suffering, or prevent dangerous conditions, let us, instead of ignoring them, claim the remedies as gifts of Providence, and by experience show that they really cure according to our *law.*

"'If an eclectic cures a cough of long standing and grave character with crude doses of *Rumex* or *Sanguinaria*, is not the cure as good, as homœopathic, as though made by Joslin or Hering, with the 30th or 200th dilution of the same remedies?

"'Those who are familiar with my theory of the action of medicines, and the law of dose deduced therefrom, need not be told that I would consider that where an allopathist does not use a drug in a certain disease, for fear of aggravations, that the drug is *primarily* homœopathic to such dis ease, and must be used in a high dilution; also, that when the opposite school cure a disease or condition with *material* doses, as, for instance, uterine inertia, with *Ergot* or *Caulophyllum*, paralysis with *Nux vomica*, etc., the drug must be *secondarily* homœopathic to the condition, and will generally act better in the lower dilutions.

"'Our course, as consistent homœopathicians, is, to CLAIM ALL CURES AS MADE BY THE LAW OF SIMILIA, AND PROVE THEM TO BE SUCH, as did Hahnemann. The law discovered by our great master is all-embracing, universal, and the sooner his followers adopt this proposition, the better it will be for the honor and influence of our school.'"

In the preface to the *third* edition I explained that owing to the great bulk to which the second edition had attained, and the impracticability of increasing the size of the work, I had changed the plan. I say:

"In writing this third edition, I have, after due consideration, omitted the descriptions, history, etc., of the remedies, as well as the voluminous provings and reports of cases, and have given only those symptoms which I believe to be peculiar and characteristic, or have been verified by new provings, or clinical experience. I have also added over *eighty* medicines to those contained in the second edition, and have treated them in the same manner as I have the older remedies, namely: condensed the provings, clinical experience, etc., into the smallest compass compatible with their value. The former editions contained only indigenous vegetable remedies. This contains agents from all parts of the world, and from the animal, vegetable and mineral kingdoms. I have attempted to bring our information of these agents up to the present date; if I have failed it has not been from any negligence in the matter, but from my inability to find any further material and experience."

In this, *fourth,* edition, the botanical, chemical, and pharmacological notes have been reinstated in a condensed form. This was done in deference to the wishes of a large majority of the profession. This portion of the work was placed in the hands of my colleague, DR. DELAMATER, who occupied the position of Lecturer on the above topics in the Hahnemann Medical College, of Chicago.

Nearly every pathogenesis found in the *third* edition has been revised and rewritten; new and important symptoms added, and also additional clinical indications.

I have added many *new* indigenous and foreign vegetable remedies, as well as many from the animal and mineral kingdoms. Instead of mingling clinical notes and experience with the characteristic symptoms of each remedy, I have given only brief "curative symptoms."

In the second volume, however, of this work, I have given the *therapeutics* of each medicine, based mainly upon my own experience. It is made up mainly from my lectures delivered before the Hahnemann Medical College, of Chicago, during the sessions of 1873 and 1874. I have also drawn largely upon that of my professional colleagues in all schools of medicine.

I have been conscientious and careful in my recommendations of these new remedies, and have not advised their use in disease from mere theoretical grounds, but from my actual observation of their effects on the sick. When speaking of those medicines which I have not used in my own practice, I have given only those authorities whom I consider to be honest and trustworthy.

**E. M. HALE.**

CHICAGO, April, 1875.

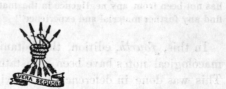

# PREFACE

## BY THE

## BOTANICAL AND PHARMACOLOGICAL EDITOR.

Prof. Hale, in his Preface to the third edition of "The New Remedies,' writes as follows:

"In writing the first and second editions of this work, it seemed to me necessary, or at least important, that all that was known relative to the medicines therein mentioned should be given, because the homœopathic school at that time was quite unacquainted with nearly all of them.

"I therefore gave the botanical description, natural history, medical history, chemical analysis, and method of preparation of each remedy, together with many other observations. In writing this third edition, I have, after due consideration, omitted the descriptions, history, etc., of the remedies."

After the publication of this, the fourth edition of the "Materia Medica of the New Remedies," had been fully decided upon, and the arrangements completed, the author and the publishers, after weighing the matter very carefully, thought best to add, or rather to *reinstate*, in this edition, botanical descriptions, chemical characters, physical properties, and pharmacological notes on each remedy, and to have them carefully revised, and made to correspond with the teachings of to-day, for the following reasons: *First*, That many entirely *new* remedies have been inserted which are nearly unknown, and have never been treated of in any work on Homœopathic Pharmacology. *Second*, That in some instances there has been a clashing of opinion as to which of two or more species of certain plants is officinal. *Third*, The younger members of the profession have left their *alma mater* with their diplomas in their hands, without having received a word of instruction as to the botany or pharmacology of any of the remedies, not even of the older ones. This knowledge, so far as many of the New Remedies are concerned, could not be obtained from any of the textbooks. *Fourth*, From the criticisms on the third edition, in the various journals, and in private letters of many prominent members of the profession, it seemed to be demanded that this department be included in the present edition.

Having determined to meet this demand, Prof. Hale united with the publishers in requesting me to accept the editorship of this department. I have endeavored to make it as complete as possible in the space and the short time allotted me for this work. So far as the remedies mentioned in former editions are concerned, I have simply revised them, making such alterations only as seemed necessary. The *newer* remedies I have written up in accordance with the very latest authorities.

With a few exceptions, namely, those medicines which in the established preparations do not seem to be reliable, from not containing all the curative powers of the drug, I have given as officinal the established formulæ.

The new preparations recommended are the result of many thorough and careful experiments made by myself, and verified by the reports of many of our most prominent physicians, who have done me the favor to compare their relative certainty and promptness of action.

TINCTURES.—I recognize four fundamental rules in the preparation of tinctures: *First*, A tincture should contain all of the medicinal properties of its drug, and, in order to accomplish this, the drug must be entirely exhausted. *Second*, Alcohol is not a universal solvent of the medicinal properties of plants. *Third*, Some drugs require, for the extraction of all their dynamic or medicinal properties, not simply water and alcohol, but *hot* water or alcohol. *Fourth*, That where it is possible, a tincture should be made from the fresh plant. This last rule, I have no doubt, is followed by many of our pharmacists, certainly by the well-known house of Boericke & Tafel. It is our deliberate opinion that in no case should tinctures be made from the dried plants and roots, except when it is impossible to procure the fresh. It is equally important that these plants should be gathered at the proper time, *i. e.*, the season in which their medicinal qualities exist in their greatest potency. We know that Messrs. Boericke & Tafel have been particularly careful in carrying out this recommendation.

In making a tincture from a fresh plant, we can nearly always succeed in exhausting it by simple maceration in alcohol of 94 to 98 per cent. proof. Where it is necessary to use the dried plant, the alcohol should be diluted by an amount of distilled water equal to the amount of water lost during the process of drying. In those plants where we have no table showing the loss of water, it will be necessary to estimate, from the general appearance, etc., the proportion of water lost in drying, thus following out the plan so vigorously enforced by the " British Homœopathic Pharmacopœia " —making all tinctures as near the standard of a fresh plant tincture as possible.

DECOCTION TINCTURE.—I have recommended in some few instances an entirely new preparation or tincture, which may be termed a permanent infusion, permanent decoction, or *decoction tincture*. There are a few plants which, in the ordinary tincture, have always disappointed us, but, when used in the form of infusion or decoction, act with promptness and certainty. In such cases I have made officinal this new tincture, prepared as follows : Take of the powdered or bruised drug one part, prepared as for ordinary tinctures, pour upon it seven parts distilled water at about 200° F. ; allow to stand, tightly covered, for from six to twelve hours ; add three parts 96 per cent. alcohol, and allow to stand six hours ; filter slowly, and then add to the residue left in the filter two parts more of alcohol ; allow to percolate slowly, and until the substance is dry. This tincture will be found to possess all the promptness and certainty of action of the infusion or decoction, and also have all the advantages of any tincture. Each ounce represents one-tenth of an ounce of the crude drug, about two parts of the liquid being lost by evaporation, etc., during the process of manufacture.

I wish to call particular attention also to the tincture-trituration recommended by Prof. HALE in the second edition, where he says there are several drugs which, when diluted, no matter with what proportion of alcohol or water, will throw down a sediment, which sediment, in many instances, is the most active part of the drug. In order to attenuate the drug, and at the same time save this part, he recommends that to nine parts *coarse* sugar of milk, add one part mother tincture, and triturate for one hour. After the 1st x , he advises the use of *fine* sugar of milk.

As to other pharmaceutical processes peculiar to our school, I need not say anything, as the subject is fully taught in the different pharmacopœias.

As stated by the author in his Preface, this edition contains many new indigenous foreign and other remedies. An enumeration will show their number and importance. They are : *Amyl Nitrite, Apomorphia, Aranea diadema, Arsenite of Iron, Arsenite of Quinia, Berberina, Caffeine, Cedron, Chionanthus, Clematis Virginiana, Coccus cacti, Croton chloral, Digitaline, Ergotine, Eucalyptus globulus, Euphorbia hypericifolia, Fagopyrum esculentum, Ferro-cyanuret of Potassium, Gallic acid, Hecla lava, Hydrophyllum, Ilex opaca, Iodide of Barium, Juniperus communis, Kaolin, Kino, Lapis albus, Lobelia cardinalis, Œnanthe crocata, Oleum Cajuputi, Oleum Jecoris Aselli, Oleum Ricinus communis, Opuntia vulgaris, Pancreatine, Passiflora incarnata, Pepsin, Protosulphide of Mercury, Ricinus communis, Solanum nigrum, Strychnia, Tanacetum vulgare, Thaspium aureum, Valerianate of Ammonia, Viscum album;* 44 in all. Of these, *nineteen* have been subjected to physiological experimentation on the healthy, sufficient to enable us to fix upon certain symptoms which may be relied upon as *characteristic.* Of the others we have only fragmentary provings, or clinical experience.

All these will be fully treated of in the second volume, where the author will give their sphere of action, therapeutics, and the experience of himself and others in their use in disease.

N. D. DELAMATER, M.D.

CHICAGO, April, 1875.

# SYMPTOMATOLOGY

#### OF THE

# NEW REMEDIES.

## ABIES CANADENSIS.

### (Hemlock-Spruce.)

DESCRIPTION.—A large tree, evergreen. When young the most graceful of the spruces, with a light, spreading spray, and delicate foliage, bright green above and silvery underneath. Very common northward.

OFFICINAL PREPARATIONS.—Tincture of the bark and buds, dilutions.

ANALOGUES.—*Æsculus, Copaiva, Terebinth, Nux, Ignatia, Lithium.*

### Mind.

Mind careless, quiet, but easily fretted, and irritable.

### Head.

Feels light-headed, a tipsy feeling, a swimming in the head.

Top of the head feels congested, a faint, drunken feeling.

Sweating about the head, at night.

### Eyes.

A feeling as of a stye, on the outer canthus of the left eyelid.

### Gastric Symptoms.

Dryness of the mouth, with thirst.

Gnawing, hungry, faint feeling at the epigastrium.

A bloated feeling in the stomach, with burning.

* Craving for meat, pickles, and other coarse food. (*Gatchell.*)

A tendency to eat far beyond the capacity for digestion.

Great appetite, with rumbling in the bowels after eating.

° Canine hunger, with torpid fever. (*Gatchell.*)

° Dyspepsia, with very weak digestion. (*Beckwith.*)

2　　　　(17)

### Abdomen.

Rumbling in the bowels after eating, with great appetite.

Irritable feeling in the region of the *spleen*.

A feeling in the *liver* as if it was small and hard, and as if the bile was deficient.

Burning in the *rectum*, with constipation.

### Urine.

Urination very frequent, day and night; urine profuse and straw colored.

Increased nocturnal, involuntary urination.

### Uterus.

She thinks the womb feels soft and "feeble."

A sore feeling in the fundus of the uterus, relieved by pressing.

"Pregnant ewes lose their lambs from gnawing the bark."

### Generalities.

Skin clammy, hands cold and shrunken.

Pain behind the right shoulder-blade.

Increased action of the heart, with distension of stomach.

Great restlessness at night, with tossing from side to side; he lies with the knees drawn up.

Wants to lie down all the time, with weakness in the sacral regions; gaping and drowsiness.

Chills down the back; cold, shivering all over, as if the blood turned to ice-water.

Twitching of the muscles.

---

# ACALYPHA INDICA.

### (*Indian Acalypha.*)

A plant found in the East Indies. Proved by Dr. Tonnere, of Calcutta. An indigenious species grows in the south, the A. Virginiana, used by the people in asthma and croup.

BOTANICAL DESCRIPTION.—We have three American species, homely weeds, growing in fields and open places, found in flower in July and September; one or two feet high, stems thick or rather hairy, often turning purplish in autumn.

OFFICINAL PREPARATIONS.—Tincture of the plant with alcohol by maceration; dilutions.

ANALOGUES.—*Arnica*(?) *Hamamelis*(?) *Ipecacaanha*(?) *Calcarea carbon-ica*(?) *Millefolium*(?)

### Respiratory Organs.

* Dry cough, followed by spitting of blood.

° *Hæmoptysis.* The patient had tuberculous affection of the upper portion of the left lung, with expectoration of blood; in the *morning*, pure blood; in *evening*, dark lumps of clotted blood; the fits of coughing were very violent at night. In this case the hæmoptysis did not return. (*Dr. Tonnere.*)

° *Hæmoptysis* in three cases of consumption, in the last stage. (*Ib.*)

° Hæmoptysis, with loss of voice; the bleeding stopped, but the disease progressed. (*Thomas.*)

° Hæmorrhage from the lungs, a severe case, after other remedies had failed. (*Holcombe.*)

[Used in the above cases in the 6th, 7th and 10th dilutions.]

° Leucorrhœa, sometimes thick, sometimes watery, in a consumptive patient. (*Neidhard.*)

---

# ÆSCULUS GLABRA.
### (*Ohio Buckeye.*)

BOTANICAL DESCRIPTION.—This is a large tree, growing abundantly in the rich alluvial bottom lands of Ohio, and other States watered by the Ohio river. The *bark* exhales an unpleasant odor, as in the rest of the genus. Flowers small, not showy, stamens curved, much longer than the corolla, which is of a pale yellow, and consists of four upright petals. Fruit prickly when young. Leaves opposite, pointing out. Leaflets fine, with a serrate or toothed edge and straight veins, like a chestnut leaf. This species belongs to the Æsculus proper, differing from the "Pavia," in having *the fruit covered with prickles when young.* The fruit contains the most active poisonous qualities, The rind of the fruit, the bark and leaves also possess toxical powers.

OFFICINAL PREPARATIONS.—Triturations of the dried fruit. Tincture from the bark and whole fruit, made by maceration with dilute alcohol.

SPHERE OF ACTION.—An irritant of the cerebro-spinal system; affects the intestinal canal, and probably the liver.

ANALOGUES.—*Æsculus hippocastanum, Aloes, Collinsonia, Cocculus, Gymnocladus, Ignatia, Nux Vomica.*

### Mental Sphere.

Confusion of mind, always attended by vertigo, and generally followed by stupefaction and coma.

### Head.

Vertigo, with staggering, reeling and unconsciousness.
Vertigo, with fullness and heaviness of the head, dimness of
    sight, thickness of speech, nausea and vomiting.

### Eyes.

Dimness of sight, even loss of sight.
Eyes fixed and expressionless.

### Mouth.

Thickness of speech, from paralysis of the tongue.

### Stomach and Abdomen.

Great tympanetic distension of the stomach and abdomen.
Nausea, with loathing of food and vomiting, with cramp-like
    pain in the stomach.

### Stool and Anus.

* Obstinate constipation; hard, knotty stools.
* Hemorrhoidal tumors, dark purple, with lameness and
    weakness of the back. (*B. L. Hill.*)

### Back and Neck.

Wry neck (spasmodic).   Opithotomus.

### Extremities.

Great lameness and weakness of the back.
Paralysis of the hinder extremities of animals.
Trembling of the lower limbs, with spasmodic contraction.

### Sleep.

Stupefaction, with confusion of ideas, followed by coma. state.

### Generalities.

Spasms and convulsions, followed by paralysis.

---

# ÆSCULUS HIPPOCASTANUM.

### (*Horse Chestnut.*)

The beauty of the horse chestnut consists chiefly in its inflorescence—
surpassing that of almost all our native trees; the huge clusters of gay
blossoms, which every spring are distributed with such luxuriance and
profusion over the surface of the foliage, and at the extremity of the
branches, give the whole tree the aspect of some monster flower, than of
an ordinary tree of the largest size.  Early in June this beautiful tree puts

forth large pyramidal racemes or thyrses of flowers, of pink and white, mottled with red and yellow—finely contrasting with the dark green of its foliage, which has great grandeur and richness in its depth of hue and massiveness of outline.

HISTORY.—The horse-chestnut is a highly ornamental tree, and is greatly admired for its majestic proportions, and for the beauty of its flowers and foliage. It grows rapidly, and often attains the height of forty or fifty feet. It is a native of middle Asia, but flourishes well in the temperate climates of both hemispheres. Its genus comprises about twelve known species, the genus *Æsculus*, however, is incomparably the finest, and is the only one found in the Northern States, and this, even, is not indigenous in New England.

It was introduced into Europe nearly three centuries ago, by Baron Ungnad, ambassador of the Ottoman Porte, who, in the year 1576, sent the seeds of the common horse-chestnut to Clausius, at Vienna. It is now extensively cultivated as an ornamental tree in Europe as well as in this country.

The name Æsculus was originally applied to a species of oak, also to a tree which bore esculent fruit, and probably is derived from esca—"food." It was transferred to this genus by Linnæus, to the exclusion of the earlier and more appropriate name of "hippocastanum" (*horse-chestnut*), on account of the resemblance of the large seeds to chestnuts, and because the Turks often grind them into a coarse flour, which is mixed with other food, and given to horses which are broken-winded.

In the Southern and Western States there are several species, which bear the name of buck-eye, from a resemblance of the seeds to the eye of that animal.

MEDICINAL PROPERTIES.—The timber is not valuable. The large farinaceous seeds contain a considerable amount of nourishment, which is rendered unavailable, because of the intensely bitter and narcotic principle with which they are charged. Common horse-chestnuts, nevertheless, with some precautions, are largely and advantageously used in Switzerland for fattening sheep. They are also eaten eagerly by deer, horses and oxen. Starch prepared from them is superior to that of wheat, and excels, as an article of diet, that of the potato. Paste prepared from them is preferable to any other, not only because possessing great tenacity, but also from the fact that no moths or vermin will attack anything cemented with it. They have been recommended as a substitute for coffee.

It may seem strange, that while so many persons consider the nuts poisonous, they are fed to animals, and even prepared for man. This is explained by the fact that the poison in the nut is removed by a process of prolonged cooking.

The young leaves are aromatic, and have been used instead of hops in brewing beer.

The roots contain a mucilaginous and saponaceous matter, which is thought to be poisonous. Active and poisonous properties prevail in the root, seeds, bark and foliage.

The bark has little odor, but an astringent and bitter, though not dis agreeable, taste. It contains, among other ingredients, bitter extractive and tannin, and imparts its virtues to boiling water. Its active constituent is supposed to be tannin, hence it has been employed in tanning. It is recommended as a tonic, astringent, narcotic, and antiseptic; in fevers as a febrifuge, for gangrene, and as an errhine. A strong decoction is recommended as a lotion to gangrenous ulcers.

It has attracted much attention in Europe as a substitute for Cinchona, although it certainly cannot be considered comparable to Peruvian Bark in its power over intermittents. It is at present seldom used, and never in this country. The bark of the branches from three to five years old is considered the best. It should be collected in the spring.

The powdered kernel snuffed up the nostrils produces sneezing, and has been used with advantage as a sternutatory in complaints of the head and eyes. In Europe the oil at present is a fashionable remedy for gout and rheumatism.

The bark contains an active principle termed Æsculin—which is prepared from a strong hydro-alcoholic tincture, by distilling off the alcohol and setting the residue in a cool place for some time. It appears as a white powder, which is formed of minute acicular crystals, having a bitter taste; no odor; soluble in 12½ parts water at 212° F., and in 672 parts at 50° F.; partially soluble in alcohol; insoluble in ether. It is colored red and then yellow by hydrochloric acid.

OFFICINAL PREPARATIONS.—Triturations of the meat of the nut, with the rind or shuck. It is usually prepared by grating both. When dry they can easily be reduced to a fine powder.

Tincture from the meat of the nuts and the shuck; made by maceration, in dilute alcohol.

Tincture from the bark, roots and flowers. If dry, by maceration for an hour in a small quantity of hot water; afterwards adding requisite amount of alcohol to the maceration. If fresh, in strong alcohol, one part to ten.

For external use, in glyceroles, salves, cerates, etc.

*As a lotion*, ℥ i of mother tincture, to ℥ 8 of water.

ANALOGUES.—*Æsculus glabra, Aloes, Collinsonia, Ignatia, Nitric acid. Nux vomica, Mercurius, Sulphur, Podophyllum, Iris versicolor, Hydrastis. Rhus.*

SPHERE OF ACTION.—On the spinal cord, the mucous membrane of the alimentary canal, especially the lower portion, the liver and portal system.

## Mental Sphere.

On waking, cannot recognize what she sees; knows not where she is, nor whence come the objects about her.

Inward cheerfulness and placidity of temper.

Feels miserably; cross; sad; disinclination to perform any labor.

Vertigo very annoying all the forenoon.

### Head.

Aching in the forehead; sometimes over the left, sometimes over the right eye; also the right temple.

Heaviness, with dull, stupefying pain in the head.

In the *occiput* dull pain; also a bruised feeling, with heat, extending to the ears.

A sensation of fullness and pressure, rather than of acute pain.

### Eyes.

Sensation of weight and heat of the eyes.

Flickering before the eyes.

° Can read without spectacles, and see at a distance, which she could not do before. (*A prover,*)

### Nose.

Severe fluent coryza, with burning and raw feeling in the nostrils; thin watery discharge, and headache.

### Face.

Flying heat and redness of the left side of the face.

Pale, ill-looking countenance.

### Mouth.

Tongue feels as if it had been scalded, with a constricted sensation in the fauces.

Bitter taste, with yellowish-white coated tongue.

### Throat.

Dryness and a sense of excoriation and constriction.

Pricking and stinging pain in the fauces.

Heat, dryness, smarting, with desire to swallow.

### Stomach and Gastric Symptoms.

Nausea; violent vomiting and retching, with burning in the stomach.

Vomiting of thick, viscid mucus, with eructations.

Pain in the stomach for four or five hours after eating, which continues till food is taken. (*Arnica.*)

A feeling of fullness and tightness in the stomach, with labored breathing.

* Cardialgia; aching, cutting and burning distress in the stomach.

Fluttering sensation, with faintness, in the pit of the stomach

* Congestion of the liver and portal system.

Pain and distress in the stomach and bowels, attended with
a constant desire for stool.

### Abdomen.

Cramp-like and constricted feeling in the bowels.

Pain extends from the bowels to the small of the back.

Tearing pain in the right side, above the hip.

Colicky pains in the bowels, with severe cutting pains in the
rectum.

Dull aching and burning in the umbilical region.

° Hemorrhoidal colic, with pains in the hypogastrium, sacrum
and loins.

Rumbling in the bowels, with distension and bearing down.

### Liver.

Dull aching pains in the right hypochondriac **region and**
region of the gall-bladder.

Pinching pains, stitches and aching in the liver, **extending**
between the shoulders.

White, soft stool.

### Rectum and Stool.

Frequent, loose stool, with constant urging (primary) diarrhœa,
composed of ingesta.

Pressure in the rectum, with constant desire but ineffectual
efforts to stool.

Difficult, hard, scanty stool, followed by burning and constriction in the rectum.

Stool very hard and dry, with colicky pains in the umbilical
region, followed by severe cutting pains in the rectum.

* Very hard, dry, knotted, difficult stool, followed by *prolapsed*
feeling in the rectum.

* Stool very large, hard and difficult, followed by severe pain,
with a sensation as if something was protruding, with
severe pains in the lumbar and sacral regions.

An evacuation, at first black and hard, then white and soft,
(the last four symptoms are secondary).

Dryness and itching in the rectum, with a feeling of stiffness
of the skin and adjacent cellular tissues.

Dryness of the passage for several days, followed by a secretion of moisture.

\* Soreness of the rectum, with a feeling as if something would pass off all the time.

\* Dry, uncomfortable feeling in the rectum, which feels as if it were filled with small sticks.

\* Feeling in the rectum as though folds of the mucous membrane obstructed the passage, and as if, were the effort continued, the rectum would protrude.

Soreness of the rectum, with increased secretion of mucus.

Pressure in the rectum, with inclination to stool, with empty eructations.

\* Copious, soft stool, followed by burning, and a feeling of swelling and constriction of the rectum.

Soreness, aching and fullness of the rectum.

\* Appearance of hemorrhoids, like ground-nuts, of a purple color, very painful, and with a sensation of burning.

\* Hemorrhoids, *blind* and *painful, rarely bleeding.*

\* Prolapsus of the rectum (after Podoph., Nitric acid or Ignatia).

\* Sharp, shooting pains running through the hemorrhoidal tumors, up to the sacrum and along the back.

Fissure of the anus. (?)

Stricture of the sphincter ani. (?)

### Urinary Organs.

Frequent urging to urinate, with scanty, high-colored urine.

### Sexual Organs.

(Men.)   Seminal emissions; diseases of the prostate. (?)

(Women.)   ° Leucorrhœa, always associated with hæmorrhoids.

° During pregnancy, pain about the sacro-iliac symphysis.

° She cannot walk, because that part of her back gives out, compelling her to sit down.

° Uterine congestions with soreness and *throbbing* pains in the hypogastrium.

° Lameness of sacro iliac region, during pregnancy. (*Guernsey.*)

### Larynx.

Short cough, increased by swallowing and breathing deeply.

Tickling in the larynx, and cough, with mucus expectoration.

Dryness in the larynx. (Similar to the dryness in the rectum.)

Pressure in the throat-pit, as if something had stuck there
which required to be expelled.

° Chronic cough, with emaciation. (*Buchner.*)

° Catarrhal laryngitis, laryngeal cough, and perhaps those
coughs dependent on hepatic disorders. (*Hale.*)

### Chest.

Burning and heat in the chest, and raw feeling in the throat
and chest.

Pains in the sternum, as if a piece were torn out of the chest.

Sudden stitches through the chest.

Pain in right scapula and in the left side of the chest, increased
on inspiration.

On the right side of the chest a sensation as if the lung painfully moved up and down at each respiration.

Tightness in the chest.

\* Palpitation of the heart; severe, periodic, frequent, with
great anguish.

Neuralgic pain in region of apex of the heart and stomach.

Severe neuralgic pains in region of the heart, so painful as to
arrest the breathing, lasting ten minutes.

Frequent stitches in region of the heart.

Dull, aching, burning pain in region of heart for half an hour;
pulse 66, soft and regular.

° Functional disorder of the heart from hemorrhoidal com
plaints. (*Hale.*)

### Back and Neck.

Weakness, weariness and lameness in the back of the neck.

Weakness, weariness and lameness in the small of the back.

Heat in the back of the neck and shoulders.

Severe dull aching pain in the lumbar and sacral region, aggravated by walking.

Tearing pain in the small of the back and hips.

\* Constant back ache, affecting the sacrum and hips, aggravated on stooping and rising from seat, but going off on
walking awhile. (*Rhus.*) (*Guernsey.*)

Back ache is attended with aching in the legs and knees.

° Pains attending curvature of the spine. (*Buchner.*)

**Extremeties.**

The arm and hand of the left side become numb, as if p  ralyzed.

The legs and knees ache, with the back ache.

**Sleep.**

Yawning and stupefying sleepiness.

Wakes with dull pressing pain the stomach.

**Fever.**

Chilliness, with rigor.

Flashes of heat in the occipital region, back of the neck and shoulders.

Feverish sensations, with hot and dry hands.

Disposition to stretch and yawn.

Feeling of extreme illness, great weakness, faintness, and tottering gait.

---

# AGAVE AMERICANA.

### (*American Aloe.*)

BOTANICAL DESCRIPTION.—This is an evergreen succulent plant, sometimes called the century plant, and by the natives of Mexico, the *Maguey*. It is found growing in Florida, Mexico, and other parts of tropical America. It bears a strong resemblance to the plants of the genus Aloe, with which it is sometimes confounded.

The root and leaves, when cut, furnish a saccharine juice, which may be converted into syrup and sugar by evaporation, and into a vinous liquor by fermentation. The natives of Mexico manufacture from it their favorite drink—the *Pulque*—which is capable of causing considerable intoxication.

The juice of the Maguey contains a large amount of vegetable and saccharine matter, and is of itself sufficiently nutritious to sustain a person for several days. It delights in a dry sandy soil, and car be cultivated where nothing but the cactus will grow. The cortical portion near the root may be eaten, when cooked by roasting. The white internal portion is the edible part. Dr. Perrin has seen muleteers use it for food, and they seem to be very fond of it. He was informed upon good authority that several tribes of Indians in New Mexico make use of It in the same manner.

The juice, when evaporated to the consistence of a soft extract, forms a lather with water, and is sometimes employed as a substitute for soap. The *fresh* juice is said to be diuretic, laxative and emmenagogue.

So far, only the juice of the roasted leaves has been used as a remedia. agent. The tincture of a fresh root prepared from it, may possess valuable medicinal qualities. The same virtues may exist in the leaves, as it is well known that cooking deprives some plants and roots of their poisonous qualities.

OFFICIAL PREPARATION.—Tincture made by expression and maceration, or by percolation from the fresh leaves and the root.

ANALOGUES.— *Lime juice, Lemon juice, Citric acid, Kali chloratum, Natrum muriaticum.*

### General Symptoms.

° Army scurvy, with pale and dejected countenance.

° Gums swollen, and bleeding, legs covered with dark, purple blotches, swollen, painful, and of stony hardness; pulse small and feeble; appetite poor; bowels constipated.

° Eleven cases rapidly improved under the use of the Maguey after lime juice and lemon juice had failed.

The fermented juice intoxicates.

---

# AILANTUS GLANDULOSA.

### *(Tree of Heaven.)*

The Ailantus (not Ailan*thus*, as many of our prominent physicians and authors spell it) belongs to the natural System Xanthoxylacæ and to the Linnæan system, Monæica Polygamia.

DERIVATIONS.—The word *Ailantus* was given to this genus by Desfontaine, who formed it from the Molucca name *Ailanti.* For a long time this tree was considered as a species of Rhus, whence the French name, *Verne;* Angik or Angika it is said, signifies the Tree of Heaven; hence the American name, and the German name of Gœtterbaum, "Tree of the Gods."

DESCRIPTION.—The Ailantus Glandulosa is a deciduous tree of the first rank, growing to the height of sixty feet and upwards. Its straight, erect, column-like trunk, from two to three feet in diameter, its gigantic boughs and shoots, clothed with large pendulous leaves, give it a noble appearance, and seem to justify the appellation—Tree of Heaven. The leaves are from one-and-a-half to six feet in length, pinnated, with an odd one, and having leaflets with coarse glandulous teeth near the base.

On the first approach of frost, the leaves begin to fall, without having previously shown much change of color, displaying 'n this respect, a striking difference from the leaves of most species of Rhus, to which those of this tree bear a general resemblance.

The flowers, which appear in June and July, occur in rather large compact panicles, of a whitish-green color, and exhale a disagreeable odor.

The keys, or fruit, resemble those of the Ash, but are much smaller and more numerous. In some years the tree is said to bear only male flowers; and L'Heritie states that only twice in ten years it bore male and female blossoms at the same time, in France. In his time it had produced fruit in the Jarden des Plantes, at Paris, and in the botanic garden at Leyden; but in both cases it was immature. It has since, however, produced perfect fruit, from which plants have been raised. It has also ripened seeds at White King's, near Reading, in England. At Philadelphia and New York, the seeds of the tree ripen fully in October, and plants are raised from them in abundance.

The Ailantus is not now grown as extensively as formerly as an ornamental tree in the United States. The odor of the flowers is extremely offensive to most persons; this, together with a belief that the emanations of its flowers is injurious to health, has created a prejudice against it. In some places epidemics of cholera and other unusual disorders have occurred during its flowering. In Washington City and Philadelphia hundreds of fine trees have been cut down in deference to this prejudice. I believe that Drs. Hering and Wells reported some cases of poisoning of children from exposure to the volatile poison of its flowers. *Hale.*

OFFICINAL PREPARATIONS.— Tincture with strong alcohol from the fresh well developed flowers, and of the fresh bark of the young shoots and roots, in equal parts. Tincture of dry bark of branches and roots and of the ripe seeds in equal parts, with dilute alcohol.

ANALOGUES.—*Æthusa, Agaricus, Arum tri, Arsenicum, Belladona, Baptisia, Hyoscymus, Lachesis, Phosphorus, Rhus* [*tox. rad. and ver.*] *Stramonium, Solanum, Veratrum alb.*

## Mind.

Continual sighing, with depression of spirits.

Stoical indifference to whatever happens.

Restlessness, with great anxiety.

Inability to concentrate mental effort; compelled to read a subject several times to get even a misty understanding of it.

Confusion of intellect; found it almost impossible to add columns of figures correctly; had to go over it several times to get it right.

Loss of memory.

*Mental* alienation.

## Head.

Vertigo, especially when stooping.

Dizziness and confusion of the head.

Staggering dizziness when rising or moving.

A sensation of giddiness with nausea and sickness at the stomach.

Tottering gait, with an inclination to stagger, requires extra effort to walk straight.

Giddiness, nausea, with retching and some vomiting.

Slight headache, accompanied with nausea and giddiness.

The figures on the ledger began to dance up and down the columns, my head grew dizzy.

Pain in the occiput, with dizziness and ringing pain in the forehead.

A fullness and somewhat of an intoxicated sensation in the brain.

A fullness and burning on the brain.

Apoplectic fullness of the head.

Thick, heavy feeling in the head, figures and letters look blurred.

Electrical thrill starting from the brain and extending to the extremities.

Feeling as if an electrical current were passing through the left side of the head.

Headache with confusion of intellect.

Dull heavy headache with heavy feeling in the sternal region, and burning in the eyes.

Heaviness of head with pain over the eyes; ameliorated by pressure.

Dull compressed feeling with confusion and pain in the forehead.

Pain in center of the forehead, more to the left.

A peculiar, heavy dull pressing pain in the forehead, of no great severity, but which indisposes to or even incapacitates for intellectual labor. This is always relieved by Aloes, 200th.

Between one and two P. M., a heavy frontal headache with drowsiness; slept two hours.

Severe darting pain through the temples and back part of the head, with confusion of ideas.

Severe pain through the temples on waking.

Tender, bruised feeling over parieto-frontal sutures.

Pain in the occiput, with dizziness and ringing pain in the forehead, and swelling in the left side of the face, below the
eye, and upon the cheek.

Severe pains in the head with chills followed by flushings of
heat.

Tingling sensation of left arm and hand, with dull headache,
no appetite, tongue coated, pasty taste (on waking in A. M.)

Pain in back, head, neck, and numbness extending from under
the left scapula in a band down to the left hip.

### Eyes.

Eyes feel rough and irritated as from wind and dust.

Burning and smarting and aching as from powerful astringents.

Sneezed and experienced a sensation of cold about the eyes,
and a gnawing in the chest.

Light affects the eyes; intolerance of light.

Figures and letters look blurred.

Lachrymation in the open air, or by brilliant light.

Purulent discharge with agglutinated lids in the morning.

Conjunctivitis, with redness and inflammation extending
around the external canthus.

Falling out of the eyebrows.

° Chronic gonorrhœal ophthalmia.

° Eyes suffused and congested; startled look when roused;
pupils *dilated* and *sluggish ;* in scarlet fever. (*Dr. Chalmers.*)

### Nose.

Itching and uneasy feeling around the nose.

Soreness and pain on left side of the nose.

Catarrhal obstruction, as from cold in the head.

Loss of smell.

° Chronic catarrh, discharge thin, watery and excoriating.

° Copious thin ichorous discharge without fetor; discharge of
blood and pus. In scarlet fever. (*Dr. Chalmers.*)

### Face.

Dusky bilious complexion.

Complexion sallow and inactive; dark blue circle around the
eyes.

Irregular spots of capillary congestion, as in the face of a
　　drunkard after a debauch.

Hot, red face.

\* Miliary rash more profuse on the face and forehead — espe-
　　cially the forehead — than upon the rest of the body.

Pain in the occiput with dizziness and ringing pain in the fore-
　　head, and swelling in the left side of the face, soreness
　　and pain on the left side of the nose, puffed erysipelatous
　　face, feels heavy and sleepy, nausea coming on at intervals

On the second evening tearing in the upper and lower teeth
　　of the left side, also in the face and head, aggravated by
　　lying down and forcing him to walk about. External
　　pressure relieves. Improvement only toward morning.

### Tongue.

Tongue coated, pasty taste, in morning.

Tongue thickly covered with a whitish coat, brown in center

° Tongue *dry*, parched and cracked; *moist*, and covered with
　　white fur, tip and edges livid. Under the favorable action
　　of Ailantus the clearing off of the coating revealed prom-
　　inent papillæ. In scarlet fever. (*Dr. Chalmers.*)

### Throat.

Sensation as after applying an astringent to the pharynx.

Thick, œdematous, and dry choky feeling in the throat, con-
　　tinuing in the acute form only a short time and then
　　becoming chronic.

A fullness in the throat just above the sternum, and a desire
　　to hawk up something.

Throat dry, rough and scrapy; more so in the morning.

Irritability of the throat and hawking up of mucus.

She hawks up greenish puruloid matter from the throat.

Constant hawking and efforts to raise lumps of whitish and
　　yellow matter.

Great accumulation of matter, part of which is easily expec-
　　torated, while a portion is with much exertion detached
　　in small flakes.

Croupy choking.

Throat tender, sore on swallowing or on the admission of air.

When deglutition is painful the pain always extends to the ears.

F.2

Redness of the throat with or without pain during deglutition.

The fauces and tonsils are inflamed with spots of incipient ulceration.

Shedding ulcers, feeling as after the application of Nitrate of Silver.

Tenderness and enlargement of the parotid and thyroid glands.

Thickened and swollen feeling of the muscles of the neck.

° The throat is livid and swollen, the tonsils studded with numerous deep, angry-looking ulcerations, from which a scanty fœtid discharge exudes; the neck is very tender and swollen. ° The tonsils are prominent and studded with ulcerated points. In scarlet fever. (*Dr. Chalmers.*)

### Nausea.

Every morning nausea, and during the day a febrile heat. With this nausea (but frequently without it,) a diarrhœa set in, four or five stools daily, with pains in the abdomen Sometimes vomiting with the diarrhœa.

With the nausea an oppression and pain below the hypochondria; in some like a stricture below the short ribs. Some find this symptom very debilitating.

Excessive nausea, but no vomiting, during the headache.

In women nausea similar to that of pregnancy.

Nausea and sickness at the stomach, with sour eructations; nausea and vomiting.

Any food taken was speedily vomited.

### Appetite.

No feeling of hunger, but eats his usual quantity.

No appetite for dinner, everything tasting flat and insipid.

She could take no food; the sight of it made her feel worse.

Appetite capricious; or complete loss of appetite.

Loss of appetite, slight nausea, disgust at food.

During the chill there was great hunger, with a distressing sense of general emptiness.

### Stomach.

Peculiar feeling of emptiness in the stomach.

Inactive condition of the stomach, as though its contractive power was impaired.

2

**Water** tastes brackish and flat; no desire for drinks except when eating.

**Took a** teaspoonful of the tincture. In half an hour began to feel queer and somewhat frightened—a sensation of giddiness, with nausea and sickness at the stomach, came over me; cold perspiration stood out upon the skin; my fingers, in fact my whole body, began to tingle and prick; my limbs felt as, if they were asleep; the figures on the ledger began to dance up and down; my head grew dizzy; I staggered back and fell into my chair almost unconscious. Drank half a tumbler of Bourbon; soon began to vomit and purge, and was very ill for two hours. Two days after was as well as common, excepting some headache and a sort of numbness of the left arm.

### Abdomen and Stool.

Tympanitis.

Burning in the stomach and bowels.

Weak, burning, uneasy feeling in the bowels, as of approaching diarrhœa.

A feeling of "insecurity," as if he would be attacked with diarrhœa any minute.

Bowels moved easier than natural two or three times a day.

Looseness of the bowels appearing more in the large intestine.

Colicky and griping pains in the bowels, with rumbling.

Frequent watery dejections, which are expelled with great force.

Morning nausea with diarrhœa, which is sometimes attended with vomiting.

\* Dysentery, frequent painful stools, little fœcal matter, much bloody mucus, with very little fever. (*Hering.*)

° *Dysentery;* a specific remedy among the Chinese — tested with good results by Dr. Roberts, a navy surgeon.

### Genitals.

A sore appeared on the prepuce of the prover which had the exact appearance of an incipient chancre; it dried up and disappeared in a few days after ceasing Ailantus. [This sore and the rash are similar to those which characterize primary syphilis.]

## Cough.

Cough somewhat oppressed; expectoration muco-purulent, free in the morning, sticky and scanty during the day.

Deep, painful, exhausting cough, with asthmatic expansion of the lungs.

Violent fits of coughing before retiring and on rising; she coughs continually until expectoration becomes free, afterwards is comfortable during the day.

° Dry, constant cough, with oppression, burning, and pains in chest. (*Dr. Alley.*)

° Whooping cough. (*Dr. Alley.*)

° Dry, hacking cough—almost constant—attended with tenderness and soreness of the chest (occurring in measles). (*Dr. Freligh.*)

° Catarrhal cough, attended with dry coryza and heat of the throat and chest. (*Dr. Freligh.*)

## Chest.

Asthmatic oppression in the larger bronchi.

On the second day after suspending the drug, wheezing, asthmatic respiration.

Feeling as though the air-cells were stuck together; inability to completely expand the lungs; can hear the air-cells open (?) as the lungs expand.

Tired feeling in the lungs, rendering it almost an exertion to breathe.

Excessive soreness and tenderness of the lungs, compelling a suspension of the drug.

Soreness of the internal chest, with pain and aching of the lungs.

Soreness and pain of the lungs increased; severe pains in the head, with chills followed by flushes of heat.

Pain and contracted feeling, especially through the centre of the left lung, sternal edge.

Aching in the anterior portion of the left lung, extending to the posterior.

Pain, as from a small blade, two inches at the left of the lower portion of the sternum.

Heated, burning feeling, as from breathing hot steam or air.

Burning in the right lung, and under the left shoulder.

Aching pain directly under the clavicle, sometimes extending to the sternum.

### Back.

Soreness in the glands of the neck, with pain under the left shoulder blade.

Intolerable pain in the back of the neck, upper part of the back, and in the right hip joint.

Pain in the head, neck, back, and numbness under left scapula, extending as a band down to left hip.

Constant aching between the shoulders.

Aching, pressed feeling of the dorsal vertebra.

Shooting, aching pains in the shoulders and hips.

Constant sharp pain through the small of the back and hips.

### Superior Extremities.

Pain in right scapula, deep inside; it prevents motion of the arm—a similar pain in the right foot prevents walking.

Numbness of the left arm, and a sensation as though the fingers were asleep.

Tingling sensation of left arm, hand and fingers on waking in the morning.

The numbness of left arm and hand, with pain in the shoulder, back, and hips, lasted four or five days after ceasing to take the drug.

Electrical thrill, extending to the ends of the fingers.

### Inferior Extremities.

Limbs felt as though they were asleep.

Numbness of the left leg, with tingling, pricking pain in the foot and toes.

Feeling of uneasiness and aching restlessness in the limbs.

Heaviness of the extremities.

Severe pain in left foot, a kind of tension in walking.

### Sleep.

Sleep disturbed and unrefreshing.

Heavy sleep during the night.

Great sleepiness in the morning or forenoon; sleepiness the whole day; but this is not refreshing.

After drinking a glass of wine great sleepiness, with fullness
of the head.

### Fever.

Dry, hot skin, especially in the morning, lasting until the
middle of the day. [This symptom will coexist with
Ailantus pulmonary affections. (*S. A. Jones.*)

Cold perspiration stood out upon the skin. [This will occur
in conjunction with choleraic symptoms rather than as an
integer of the Ailantus febrile *role.* (*Ib.*)

Felt slightly ill on rising in the morning; could take no food;
sight of it made her feel worse; was suddenly seized with
vomiting; severe headache, dizziness, hot, red face; inability to sit up; rapid, small pulse; drowsy, at the same
time very restless; great anxiety. In two hours drowsiness had become insensibility, with constant muttering
delirium; did not recognize the members of her family.
She was now covered, in patches, with an eruption of
miliary rash, all of a dark, almost of a livid, color. The
patches between the points of the eruption were of a
dingy, dull opaque appearance. The eruption was more
profuse on the forehead and face than elsewhere, and
especially on the forehead. The pulse was now small, and
so rapid as hardly to be counted; the surface had become
cold and *dry;* the livid color of the skin when pressed
out returned very slowly; the whole was a most complete
picture of torpor.

The chill was always preceded by a miliary eruption—most
copiously developed on the forehead and face. During
the chill there was great hunger, with a distressing sense
of general emptiness. Any food taken was speedily
vomited. Intolerable pain was felt in the back of the
neck, the upper part of the back, and the right hip-joint.
During the hot stage there was urgent thirst, with
delirium, and a strong desire for brandy.

Pulse weak, sometimes barely perceptible, very frequent and
irregular. In scarlet fever. (*Dr. Chalmers.*)

Eruption, dark colored in many instances, and in some

almost of a violet hue, scanty, patchy, evanescent, and
often long delayed. In scarlet fever. (*Dr. Chalmers.*)

° Large maculæ and bullæ, filled with a claret-colored serum
In scarlet fever. (*Dr. Chalmers.*)

° Petechiæ. In scarlet fever. (*Dr. Chalmers.*)

° The eruption is slow to make its appearance, and never takes
on the genuine scarlet color; it *remains livid.* (*Ib.*)

Ailanthus produces an eruption which has an exact resemblance to ordinary measles; but is attended by no catarrhal symptoms or other concomitants of that exanthem.
(*P P. Wells.*)

### Generalities.

Languor and lassitude on making exertions.

Incapability of standing long at a time.

Tottering gait, with an inclination to stagger; requires extra
effort to walk straight.

All asthmatics who are exposed to the odor feel worse during
the blossoming period. (*Hering.*)

The odor affects women and children more than men, and old
people least of all. (*Ib.*)

If odor gives any indication, Ailantus should prove a good
remedy in malignant puerperal fever. (*Ib.*)

Affects the organism in the following order: throat, lungs,
eyes, head. (*Dr. Alley.*) [In one prover this order of
evolution is exactly reversed..]

After discontinuing the drug the head, throat and chest symptoms lasted for about twenty-four hours, and then gradually died away.

The numbness of (*left*) arm and leg, with pain in shoulder,
back and hips, continued four or five days.

Two days after taking a teaspoonful of the mother tincture, as
well as ever, with the exception of some headache, and a
sort of numbness of the left arm.

The neuralgic pains (facial) force him to walk about.

*Aggravation.* Evening; at night. [In the nervous sphere.] L.
While lying down. L. [Neuralgic pains.]

Morning. During the day. [Chylo-poietic sphere.] (*Hering* )

*Amelioration.* Towards morning. L. [Nervous sphere.]

By walking about. L. [Nervous sphere.]
By pressure. L. [Nervous sphere.]
*Side of Body.* Left.
*Sphere of action.* Most marked on the sympathetic system. Evidently on the par vagum. On the right half of the posterior column of the medulla spinalis. On the fifth nerve (through its connexion with the Pneumagastric?)

**Antidotes.**
Aloes. Nux vomica. Rhus tox. Ars. iod.

---

# ALETRIS FARINOSA.
### (*Star Grass, or False Unicorn.*)

BOTANICAL DESCRIPTION.—*Root,* perennial, small, black outside, brown inside, branched, crooked. *Root leaves,* from six to twelve, spreading on the ground like a star, but all unequal in size, sessile, lanceolate, entire, very smooth, thin and translucent, with many longitudinal veins, very sharp at the end. They are of a pale green or glaucous, and bleach in winter, or by drying. The longest are four inches. *Stem,* from one to two feet high, very simple and upright, scapiform or nearly naked, with remote scales, whitish and pressed, sometimes changing into narrow, sharp-pointed leaves. *Flowers* white, forming a long, slender, scattered spike. Each flower has a minute bract and very short pedicel; shape oblong, spreading into six acute segments like a star, at the top; the outside has a mealy, rugose appearance. Six short *stamina* are inserted near the mouth; anthers heart shaped. *Germ,* one central, (not inferior) pyramidal. *Style,* one separable into three. Capsules triangular, clothed by the calyx, triangular, three valved at the top, three celled and with many central minute seeds.

The genus Aletris takes its name from a Greek word, which signifies "a slave who grinds corn." The name is applied in allusion to the apparent mealiness dusted over the blossoms.

This genus includes two species—the A. farinosa, and A. aurea.

The A. farinosa is the one used in medicine. The name "star-grass" is also applied to several other plants, namely, the Helonias dioica, the Hypoxis, and others. The Aletris far. is designated by many common names, as Blazing-star, Aloe-root, Bettie-grass, Unicorn-root, Ague-root, Ague-grass, Star-root, Devils-bit, etc. But all these names are also applied to the Helonias dioica, (Chamælirium luteum, *Gray.*) and other plants, so that there is no reliance to be placed upon the collections of uneducated plant-gatherers, or the preparations of the druggists. For homœopathic uses, the plants or roots should be examined by a scientific botanist before they are used in our pharmacies.

HISTORY.—This species has a wide range, being found from New England to Georgia, and west to Kentucky and Missouri. The Aletris aurea is limited to a range from New Jersey to the Carolinas. The A. farinosa is abundant at the South, and always confined to dry and poor soil, in sunny glades and fields. It is unknown to the rich limestone soil, and alluvial regions. In the West it is confined to the hilly glades, open prairies, and borders of the knob-hills. It is estival, blossoming in June and July. The *root* is the part employed; and being small, does not afford much hopes to become an article of trade.

*Rafinesque* says the root contains an intensely bitter emulsive resin, soluble in alcohol, somewhat similar to Aloes, but less cathartic. This bitter principle is also partly soluble in water. The tincture is rendered milky by water. *Aletris* is prepared from the root, and is supposed to contain its active medicinal principles, but it is not a reliable preparation.

OFFICINAL PREPARATIONS.—*Tincture* is made from the fresh root by maceration with pure alcohol. Triturations from the dried root.

SPHERE OF ACTION.—On the digestive organs, muscular system, ligamentous tissues, and uterus.

ANALOGUES.—*China, Chelone, Gentiana, Helonias, Populus, Hydrastis, Viburnum, Ferrum.*

### Sensorium.

Vertigo, with vomiting, purging, sleepiness, and even stupefaction.

### Gastric.

Excessive nausea and giddiness, followed by vomiting and purging.

Great increase of appetite.

° Obstinate vomiting during pregnancy.

° Obstinate indigestion, with much debility; nausea, disgust for food; least food caused distress in the stomach; very constipated; frequent attacks of fainting, with vertigo; sleepy all the time, with emaciation. (*Hale.*)

° Flatulent colic, in weak, emaciated persons.

### Female Generative Organs.

Colic in the hypogastrium.

" It is the China of the uterine organs."

* Premature and profuse menses, with labor-like pains.

° Pressure and pain in the region of the uterus.

Heaviness in uterine region.

° Habitual tendency to abortion in feeble persons of lax fibre and anæmic condition.

° Threatened abortion, even after hemorrhage has appeared.

° Prolapsus uteri from muscular atony.

° Anomalous myalgic pains, simulating "false pains," occurring during pregnancy.

### Generalities.

° Debility, general or local, from protracted illness; loss of fluids, defective nutrition and imperfect assimilation.

---

# ALNUS RUBRA.
### (*Tag Alder.*)

BOTANICAL DESCRIPTION.—This is an indigenous shrub, growing by the side of streams, in swamps, wet grounds and marshes. It is the *Alnus serrulata* of Wildenow, and is known by the common name of *Tag Alder*, from the tops, or cones, with which it is covered in winter. It grows in clumps or thickets. *Stems* numerous, from ten to eighteen feet high. It blossoms in March and April, bearing flowers of a reddish-green color. The *bark* is the part used in medicine; it is inodorous, and has a slightly bitter astringent taste. Boiling water and dilute alcohol extract its medicinal properties. *Alnuin* is a dry, powdered extract, said to contain the active principles of this agent.

OFFICIAL PREPARATIONS.—The tincture and dilutions made from the bark; triturations prepared from the *Alnuin;* a decoction.

SPHERE OF ACTION.—An *Antipsoric;* acts principally upon the skin and glandular system.

ANALOGUES.—*Sulphur, Stillingia, Arsenicum, Iodide of Potash, (Hamamelis,) Iodide of Mercury, Phytolacca, Hepar Sulphur.*

### Generalities.

° Cutaneous eruptions, such as *impetigo.* (?)
° Scrofulous eruptions, (?) syphilitic skin diseases. (?)
° Chronic herpes and porrigo. (?)
° Diseases of mucous membrane which arise from or alternate with eruptions of the skin.
° Scrofulous disease of the hip joints.
° Hæmaturia! and other passive hemorrhages. (*No proving.*)

---

# AMPELOPSIS QUINQUEFOLIA.
### (*American Ivy.*)

BOTANICAL DESCRIPTION.—This is a woody vine, with a rooting, climbing stem, and leaves pointed out; leaflets oblong, having a long, projecting and tapering point, having five leaflets on a petal or foot stalk; the edge uneven or dented, smooth, turning crimson in autumn; flowers inconspicuous, greenish, or white, in clusters, regularly divided by pairs, from top to bottom; calyx entire; petals five, distinct, spreading; ovary two-celled, cells two-ovuled; style very short; berries dark blue, acid, smaller than peas, and two-celled; cells one or two-seeded. The American Ivy is a common and familiar shrubby vine, climbing extensively, and, by means of its radicating tendrils, supporting itself firmly upon trees, ascending to the height of fifty feet. In the same manner it ascends and overspreads walls and buildings, its large leaves constituting a luxuriant foliage of dark glossy green. It is found in wild woods and thickets throughout the United States, and blossoms in July, ripening its small blackish berries in October. In various sections it has different names, as *Woodbine, Virginia Creeper, Five Leaves, False Grape, Wild Wood Vine, etc.*

OFFICINAL PREPARATIONS.—The tincture prepared from the fresh bark and young twigs. [Or a permnnent decoction, using one part by weight to four parts by fluid measure of water, and adding six parts absolute alcohol.]

SPHERE OF ACTION.—Antipsoric; affects the skin, mucous membrane and glandular system.

ANALOGUES.—*Alnus, Apocynum, Arsenicum, Calcarea. Dulcamara, Graphites, Iodine, Chimaphilla, Phytolacca, Rumex, Stillingia, Sulphur, Rhus.*

### Generalities.

° Chronic cutaneous eruptions, (?) scrofula.

° Chronic and mercurial rheumatism, (?) indolent ulcers, (?) chronic bronchitis and laryngitis, (?) dropsy. (?)

(No provings.)

## AMYL NITRITE.

*(Nitrite of Amyl.)*

PHARMACOLOGY.—This drug was discovered by the French chemist, Balard, in 1844, and the attention of physiologists was called to it, in 1859, by Guthrie. But it was not until 1865 that Dr. Richardson introduced it to the profession.

It is a yellowish, oily, very volatile liquid, of a very penetrating, persistent, fruity odor; very highly inflammable; is lighter than water, boiling at 182° F. It may be prepared by gently heating Amylic alcohol (*Fusel Oil*) in a retort, with nitric acid, removing the heat as soon as bubbles form, repressing the effervescence, if too strong, by cold water, rectifying from Potassa the distillate passing over under 212° F., and collecting apart the product which distills under 170° F.

OFFICINAL PREPARATION.—Alcoholic dilutions, on the centesimal scale. (Usually inhaled, a few drops at a time.)

ANALOGUES:— *Agaricus,* (?) *Belladonna,* (?) *Ether; Glonoine.*

(See Therapeutics, for symptoms and clinical remarks.)

---

## APOCYNUM ANDROSEMIFOLIUM.

*(Bitter Root.)*

BOTANICAL DESCRIPTION.—This is an indigenous, perennial, herbaceous plant, from three to six feet in height, and abounding in a milky juice, which exudes when any part of the plant is wounded. The stem is smooth and simple below, branched above, usually red on the side exposed to the sun, and covered with a tough, fibrous bark. It grows in all parts of the United States, from Carolina to Canada; is found along fences, wet places, the skirts of woods, and flowers in June and July. The leaves are opposite, having sharp stems, ovate, acute, entire, smooth on both edges, and two or three inches long. The flowers are white, tinged with red, and grow in loose, nodding, terminal or axillary bunches. The peduncles are furnished with very small and acute bracts. The tube of the corolla is larger than the calyx, and its border spreading. The fruit consists of a pair of long, linear, acute follicles, containing numerous imbricated seeds, attached to a central receptacle, and each furnished with a long seed-down. The root, which is the part employed, is large, and like other parts of the plant, contains a milky juice. Its taste is unpleasant and extremely bitter.

"The flowers have a pleasant, honey-like odor, and contain that substance. Bees and other insects collect this honey; but small flies are often caught by inserting their proboscis between the fissues of the anthers, when it is not easy for them to extricate it. They are often seen dead in that confined situation, after unavailing struggles — whence one of the names of the plant, 'catch-fly.' No animals eat it." (*Rafinesque.*)

This plant is known by many common names, illustrative of certain physical qualities which it possesses. The name Apocynum, is from the Greek — meaning dog's bane; alluding, probably, to the poisonous effects of the European genus, when given to the canine species. It is called Milk-weed, Catch-fly, Fly-trap, Bitter-root, Honey-bloom, etc.

The root, when chewed, has an intensely bitter and very unpleasant taste; this taste is perceptible in the whole plant, except the flower. A decoction is of a red color, and very bitter. A tincture with alcohol is colorless but very bitter. It contains, therefore, a bitter principle, soluble in water and alcohol, and a coloring principle, not soluble in alcohol. It also contains a volatile oil. Bigelow says the milk-like juice contains caoutchouc. I would advise homœpathic pharmaceutists to make the tincture with dilute alcohol, and use the fresh, whole plant, collected just after the flowering season, in August.

OFFICINAL PREPARATIONS.— Tincture of the root, or whole plant by maceration with dilute alcohol.

SPHERE OF ACTION.—It appears to have a marked action on the muscular system and joints, and possibly on serrous tissues.

ANALOGUES.—*Aconite, Asclepias tuberosa, Benzoic acid, Bryonia, Caulophyllum, Colchicum, Cimicifuga, Iris versicolor, Podophyllum.*

## Head.
\* Bilious rheumatic and congestive headaches.
\* Rheumatic or neuralgic hemicrania.

## Nose.
Severe sneezing, with great itching and irritation in nostrils.

### Face and Teeth.
Swollen sensation of the face and body.
Violent itching of the body and face.
Itching and burning of the face; twitching of the face.
Pain in all the teeth of the lower jaw, left side.

### Gastric Spmptoms.
Tongue coated white.
Excessive nausea, with violent headache.
Vomiting, severe and long, with retching.
Increased appetite.

### Bowels.
Diarrhœa, with persistent nausea and vomiting.
Copious evacuations in the evening, of soft consistency, brown
    in color, with slight colic.
° Expulsion of worms (ascarides.) (*Eclectic authorities.*)
° Constipation. ° Dyspepsia. (*Eclectic authorities.*)

### Urinary Organs.
Enormous increase of urine. (*Primary effect.*)
Scanty urine with headache. (*Secondary effect.*)
Burning sensation in the urethra when urinating.
° Uræmia. ° Scarlatinal dropsy. ° Anasarca.
° Dropsy from disease of the heart. Recommended by Eclec-
    tics. It is affirmed that it acts in this disease like the
    apoc. cann. (*Hale.*)

### Generative Organs.
(Men.) Tickling sensation at the end of the penis.
Burning in the urethra when urinating.
° Chancres on the glans penis; syphilis. (?)
(Women.) ° Intermitting, bearing down, labor-like pains.
° Dysmenorrhœa, and threatened abortion, with copious flow
    of urine.

### Bronchia, Lungs, etc.
An expectorant in bronchitis and other pulmonary complaints.
° Bronchial irritation, (rheumatic ?)

### Back and Extremities.
° Acute rheumatism, the inflammation confined to the small
    joints, with much pain and swelling. (*Dr. Williams.*)
° Acute rheumatism of the great toe joints. (*Dr. E. M. Mc-
    Affee.*)

° Pains in the limbs, especially the feet.  (*Dr. Henry.*)

### Skin.

Profuse sweating all night, with coldness of the skin.

### Sleep.

Great sleepiness, with profuse sweating.

### Fever.

Heart's action increased; pulse 98, quick, full.

---

# APOCYNUM CANNABINUM.

### (*Indian Hemp.*)

This should not be confounded with A Androsemifolium.  The medical properties of the two are widely different.

BOTANICAL DESCRIPTION.—It is a perennial plant, stems herbaceous, erect, branching, of a brown color, and two or three feet in height; the leaves are opposite, ovate, oblong, acute at both ends, and somewhat downy beneath; the cymes are pedunculate, many-flowered and pubescent; the corolla is small and greenish, with a tube not longer than the calyx, and with an erect border.  The pod, or follicle is from three to five inches long, and resembles the pods of the Asclepias syriaca, or common silk weed, but are much smaller.

The stalk and root abounds in a milky juice which concretes into a sub stance closely resembling caoutchouc.  It is the juice which contains the active principles.

The *root*, which is the officinal part, is horizontal, five or six feet in length, about one-third of an inch thick, dividing near the end into branches, which terminate abruptly, of a yellowish brown color when young, but dark chestnut when old, of a strong odor, and a nauseous, somewhat acrid, and a permanently bitter taste.

It grows in damp places, by marshes and running streams, and is indigenous to nearly every part of the United States.

OFFICINAL PREPARATIONS.—Tincture of the root, made by maceration with dilute alcohol.  Triturations of the root.

(The tincture should be dark red, or light brown, and of an intensely bitter taste.  I have used a tincture made with Spirit. Nitri dulc., with most excellent effects.  The tincture and its dilutions seem to affect the urinary organs, but are not as efficacious in *Dropsy*, etc.  An infusion of one ounce of the fresh root in one quart of water, has been successfully administered and seems to act more promptly in dropsy in teaspoonful doses than any other preparation.  The trituration seems to be most efficacious in affections of pulmonary organs.)

From the fact that in many cases, particularly in dropsical effusions, the most powerful, as well as the most speedy and certain effects, have been obtained from the decoction, and that Hunt's decoction seemed to answer the purpose better than any other preparation ever proposed.  It may be procured through Boericke & Tafel. This formula, which is almost the same as Hunt's, and which will act equally well: Take of the fresh root one part, by weight, add nine parts, by fluid measure, of boiling water, allow to stand six or eight hours, then add one part alcohol, allow to stand six or eight hours more, when it may be filtered and kept as a permanent decoction. Dilutions may be made from this, the first and second, using part water, the third, and higher, all alcohol.

SPHERE OF ACTION.—Mucous surfaces, serous membranes, skin and kidneys; causing increased secretion and elimination (primary,) followed by the opposite condition, (secondary.)

ANALOGUES.—*Asclepias tuberosa and syriaca, Eupatorium purpureum, Helleborus niger, Kali-hydrojod, Benzoate of ammonia.*

### Head.

Heavy, stupid headache, with drowsiness.

° Hydrocephalus acutus, in children, (third stage.)

### Eyes.

Heat, with redness and irritation, as if several sharp grains of sand were in the eyes.

### Nose.

Nostrils and throat filled with thick yellow mucus.

\* Coryza; first dryness, then thin, irritating watery discharge, followed by discharge of thick mucus.

° Infantile coryza, "snuffles."

### Mouth and Tongue.

Dryness, with nausea and thirst.

### Throat.

Throat filled with thick, well concreted yellow mucus in the morning.

Unpleasant degree of heat in the throat.

### Stomach.

Distension of the stomach and bowels after very light meals.

° Sinking at the stomach, with profuse urine and nausea.

Violent vomiting, with prostration and drowsiness.

\* Increases the appetite and digestion.

° Irritable stomach, so bad that the patient could not retain even a draught of water, in dropsy.

### Abdomen.

Decided distension of the abdomen, especially after a moderate dinner.

The upper bowels seem distended,—the lower not at all.

Occasional flatulence, with uneasy sensations of the bowels.

*Ascites* — many cases, from a variety of causes.

## Stools.

Loose but not very copious bilious stools.

\* Evacuations very scanty.

Watery diarrhœa.

## Kidneys and Urine.
### Primary.

\* Dull, aching pain in the region of the kidneys, with increased secretion of straw-colored urine.

Very profuse light-colored urine; several quarts were passed every day.

No sediment in the urine.

### Secondary.

\* Decided scantiness of urine, with slight dyspnœa.

Urine diminished to about one-third the usual amount.

Scanty urine, with little expulsive power in the bladder.

\* Very peculiar *torpid* action of the kidneys.

Urine of a light golden, sherry yellow color.

° Dropsy, complicated with chronic diarrhœa.

\* *Difficult* and *painful urination*, from catarrh of the bladder, disease of the prostate, or morbid irritability. (*Freligh.*)

° Retention of urine, with paralysis of the lower extremities.

° Diabetes insipidus.

° *Dropsy, general* or *local*, and from various causes, but chiefly from lack of eliminating power of the kidneys. (*Hale.*)

In cases of acute idiopathic dropsies, use the dilutions, beginning with the highest, and descending more or less rapidly according to the progress of the disease. (*Ib.*)

In chronic or atonic dropsies (secondary,) use the tincture, or if neccessary, the decoction, in one or two drachm doses. (*Ib.*)

## Sexual Organs.

° Uterine hemorrhage with great irritability of the stomach and vomiting; syncope and failure of the pulse when moved; blood expelled in large clots, sometimes florid. (*Dr. Marsden.*)

° Amenorrhœa in young girls with bloating of the abdomen and extremities. (*Ib.*)

## Larynx, Bronchi and Chest.

Unpleasant sensation of heat about the fauces and larynx.

Irresistible disposition to sigh.

Short, dry cough, and scanty expectoration of white mucus in the morning.

Oppression of the chest on waking.

Sense of oppression about epigastrium and chest.

It was difficult to breathe enough at times.

° Loose, rattling cough, with oppression of the chest. (*p.*)

° Short, dry cough. with scanty expectoration. (*s.*)

° Hydrothorax and hydropericardium. (*?*)

° Hæmoptysis. (?)

### Back and Extremities.

Unusual heaviness of the head, with dull, aching pains in the small of the back and limbs.

No tenderness of the region of the kidneys on pressure, but a slight soreness of the parts when bringing the muscles into action, thus indicating the muscles as the seat of the pains.

Hard aching was felt several times in both knees, sufficiently severe to make me fear that an attack of inflammatory rheumatism was coming on.

° Œdema of the feet and ankles, remaining after typhus, or in dropsy. (*Hale.*)

---

# APOMORPHIA.

An alkaloid of Opium, differing from Morphia only in having one less atom of water. Its chemical composition is expressed $C_{17}H_{17}NO_2HCl$ It may be made by treating Morphia under pressure with strong hydrochloric acid.

Apomorphia differs, in its reactions, from Morphia in giving a blood-red color, in place of an orange-yellow, with Nitric acid, and in giving a dense yellow precipitate with bichromate of potassium, no precipitate being produced by Morphia.

OFFICINAL PREPARATIONS.—Tincture with strong alcohol. Triturations, to the 3c, for higher attenuations.

SPHERE OF ACTION.—Probably the great sympathetic, and reflex nervous system.

ANALOGUES.—*Cocculus*, (?) *Ipecac.* (?)

### Brain and Cord.

Slight deafness, giddiness, singing in the ears.

F.3

Great excitement.

[Epileptiform convulsions, brought on by touching.]

[Tetanic condition, running round and round the room, scaling walls, and turning summersaults.]

[Partial paralysis of the hinder extremities, clawing, natatory movements.]

[Diminution of reflex irritability, continuous workings of the stomach, depression.]

[Uncomfortable sensation in the head.]

The symptoms in brackets were observed in animals.

### Eyes.

Pupils dilated; no action when applied locally in powder.

### Ears.

Dullness of hearing.

### Circulation.

Pulse accelerated, or accelerated and then retarded.

Syncope; lessening of blood pressure.

Fall of bodily temperature.

### Gastric.

\* Qualmishness, nausea, vomiting and retching.

Vomiting in from three to eight minutes.

Convulsive movements of the stomach.

Præcordial pain

Salivation.

Diarrhœa (in cats).

\* A feeling of nausea coming on at intervals, especially after taking food; no pain, clean tongue, and no headache.

\* Sudden vomiting, almost without nausea; vomiting of food, mucus, rarely of bile.

---

# ARANEA DIADEMA.
### (*Diadem Spider.*)

(*Eperia diadema.* Fr. *Araignèe Porte-croix, Araignèe diadema, Araignèe a'croix papule;* Gr. *Kreutz-spinne.*)

This spider is found all over Europe and America, in stables, on old walls, etc. It may be distinguished by its ovoid form of body; often as large as a small nut; a longitudinal line on the back, composed of yellow and white points, and traversed by three other similar lines. This is some-

4

times called the "Geographical Spider," on account of its circular web, with latitudinal and longitudinal lines.

OFFICINAL PREPARATIONS.—Dr. Gross recommends a puncture to be made in the belly of the living insect, and that the serosity which flows out be collected on one hundred grains Sugar of Milk, and the first three triturations be made from it.

(I can see no good reason for such a recommendation. First, we get no certain strength for a starting point, as many circumstances will render the flow of his serosity very uncertain; secondly, it is probable that whatever of poisonous fluid there may be in the insect is not in the belly, but somewhere in the head.)

Dr. Hering recommends that the whole insect be macerated with alcohol for some months, and that then the alcoholic attenuation be prepared from this tincture. I would recommend that one live spider be used for every one hundred minims of absolute alcohol, and macerated for ten or twelve days; dilutions be made from this, or that a trituration be made by triturating the live spider with sugar of milk—one to each one hundred grains.

### Head.

Confusion of the head after eating.

Confusion of the head, with relaxation.

In the evening, while studying, confusion of the head and pressing pain, as if upon the bones of the right temple and upper part of the forehead; relieved by supporting the head with the hand, but returning on removing the hand.

Drawing in the head, extending towards the lower jaw.

* Headache, especially in the forehead; *relieved* by smoking tobacco, but it soon returns.

Continued headache; * *ceases in the open air.*

° Vertigo on rising from a recumbent posture.

Headache, which is ameliorated by smoking, and is entirely relieved by smoking in the open air (in fine fall weather).

The headache lasts until evening; is, however, better after some hours duration, and ceases entirely in the open air.

Headache and confusion of the head; both removed by smoking, but afterwards returning and lasting nearly the whole day.

Headache, with *burning* in the eyes and *heat* in the face.

The headache is less severe while walking than when sitting, and is relieved, without being entirely removed, by smoking.

### Eyes, Face and Mouth.

\* Disagreeable, trembling (glittering) sensation in the eyes while reading or writing, aggravating the headache, and accompanied by heat in the head and eyes.

Heat in the face, and especially in the eyes (ceases after four hours).

\* Sudden violent pains in the teeth of upper and lower jaws, at night, immediately on lying down.

Pinching pains in the right ear and parotid, which, as they ceased here, went over to the left.

Sensitive, cold feeling in right lower incisor, especially on inspiring; returned next day at the same hour.

Sticking (stitches) in roof of mouth and larynx.

° Pinching, pressing pains in upper incisors, with sensitiveness to cold air.

### Gastric.

Nauseous, bitter taste in the mouth, with coated tongue.

An unpleasant taste remains after drinking milk.

Bitter taste; relieved by smoking.

Belly-ache during a thin, fluid stool; relieved by rubbing the abdomen with the hand. Stool only at intervals, accompanied by straining. Half an hour later fermentation in the abdomen.

Heaviness and fullness in the lower abdomen, as if a stone laid there; while in the pit of the stomach is an unpleasant feeling of faintness, together with a griping in the abdomen.

### Stool.

\* Thin fluid stool, with pain in the abdomen.

### Sexual Organs.

\* Periods eight days too early, too strong and too copious.

### Chest.

\* Hæmorrhage from the lungs.

### Catarrhal.

Coryza for three days, with thirst.

### Extremities.

Fibrillar twitching in muscles of left arm (for two and a half hours in the evening).

Early in the morning, in bed, dull, digging pains in the right
humerus, radius, ulna, and tibia; also at intervals
through the day (a three days).
Severe, dull, digging bone-pains in right os calcis for some days,
occurring when the foot is moved after being quiet, but
disappearing on continued moving (first day a second
dose).
At times, dull, digging bone-pains in the extremities.
Bone-pains for four weeks; feverish attacks, mostly consisting
of coldness; abdominal pains, mostly accompanied with
a chill, and generally coming towards evening.
*Eruptions*, pimples here and there.
In the ring and little fingers, of both hands, a feeling as if
they had gone to sleep, and of formication.

### Generalities.

Feeling of heaviness and fullness in lower abdomen, as if a
stone laid there, with qualmishness in the scrobicular
region. At the same time there is a gnawing in the
abdomen, feeling of weight in the legs, so that they can
hardly move, and confusion in the head. These symptoms
return the next day, about the same time, lasting half an
hour.
Weariness, without heaviness, in the feet, relaxation.
* *Restless sleep, with frequent waking, and always with a
feeling as if the arms and forearms were greatly swollen*
(apparently as large again as natural). They also seem so
heavy that he imagines he cannot raise them.
c Ailments from cold and damp, with constant chilliness.
(*Grauvogl.*)

### Fever.

° Tertian and quartan intermittents.
° *Hæmorrhage* from all the openings in the body, and from
*wounds*.
° Violent hæmorrhages from the *lungs*. (*Grauvogl.*)

# ARALIA RACEMOSA.

### (*Spikenard.*)

DESCRIPTION.—This is a large, spreading, shrubby plant, with leaflets, heart-ovate—pointed, double, serrate, slightly downy. Umbels racemose, panicled; styles united below. It has large, spicy, aromatic roots, many feet in length. It has greenish-white flowers in umbels, and a berry-like stone-fruit.

OFFICINAL PREPARATION.—Tincture of the fresh root; dilutions.

The tincture from the fresh root has a yellowish brown color, an insipid, sweetish, aromatic, and slightly bitter taste. That from the dry root is of a dark brown color, and intensely bitter; it has hardly any effect. (*Dr. S. A. Jones.*)

ANALOGUES.—*Asarum canadense, Asarum europæum, Chamomilla, Cimicifuga, Caulophyllum, Eryngium,Trillium.*

### *Provings by Dr. S. A. Jones, of New York.*

At 3 P. M., August 26th, 1870, I took ten drops of the mother tincture in two oz. of water. An interesting book caused me to forget my "dose." The events of the night jogged my memory very effectually. Here are the notes taken on the following morning:

On retiring at 12 P. M. felt as well as ever I did. Had no sooner lain down than I was seized with a fit of asthma. I had lain upon my back when the following symptoms supervened: Dry, wheezing respiration, sense of impending suffocation and rapidly increasing dyspnœa. Very loud musical whistlings during both inspiration and expiration, but *louder during inspiration.* The attack soon reached its acme, and phlegm began to come up. It was scanty, but each expectoration was attended with a sensation that more would soon follow. My wife now observed that my wheezing was so labored as to make the whole bed vibrate. Could not possibly lie down; felt that I would suffocate if I did not sit up. Phlegm began to come freer and more abundantly; had a markedly salty taste, and felt quite warm in the mouth. Right lung appeared to be more oppressed than the left.

When the worst of the attack was over I lay on my right side, and then it seemed as if all the oppression and discomfort was in the right lung. Shortly after, I turned over, and soon it felt as if my left lung was affected, *while the right was entirely relieved.*

It took a long time for me to "come to." Had a constant desire to clear the chest of something, so that I could inspire better. *All the obstruction seemed to be in inspiration.* On making a forcible expiration, in the attempt to clear the chest, had a raw, burning, sore feeling behind the whole length of the sternum, and in each lung—most intense behind the sternum. Slept well all night. After rising in A. M. raised some loose phlegm easily.

I am inclined to asthma, and at first thought this one of its attacks; but as the phenomena was evolved the programme was so different that my drink of *Aralia* flashed into memory.

On the night of the 28th I was literally drenched with perspiration while asleep. Was awakened by a patient, when it passed off and did not recur.

29th. Have been annoyed all day by a dread that my right lung is seriously diseased. Could not shake off the fear. Cough now and then, raising a little phlegm, which is involuntarily swallowed. Took ten drops of the tincture at 1:30 A. M. No symptoms that night. On rising at 8:30, bowels felt as they have done after a large-sized "spree." Faintly defined nausea in throat and stomach, and sensation in intestines as if diarrhœa would set in. At 3:15 P. M. went to closet, expecting, from my feelings, a loose stool. Evacuation was soft, yellow, about a teaspoonful in quantity, and expelled with great difficulty. Mucous membrane of rectum came down like a tumor, (Have had hæmorrhoids.) After stool, and while sitting on the "throne," an aching pain in the rectum, extending upwards and on the left side.

Feel weak, prostrated, half-sick, and filled with a vague nausea..

"It is good to provoke urine, and cureth the pain of the stone in the reins and kidneys." (*Culpepper.*)

° Leucorrhœa, with pressing down pains in the uterus. (*Eclectic.*)

° Leucorrhœa, acrid and offensive. (*Ib.*)

° Suppressed lochia, with tympanitis; excruciating pains in the bowels and uterine region. (*Dr. Rodgers.*)

° Sudden suppression of the menses from a cold. (*Ib.*)

° Dry cough in bronchitis and laryngitis. (*Ib.*)

* *Hay-fever*—many cases. (See therapeutics.) (*Hale.*)

---

# ARCTIUM LAPPA.

### (*Burdock.*)

There are two species of the Burdock, formerly known as the *Lappa Major*, having large leaves; and the *Lappa Minor*, with small leaves. The *Arctium L.* is the one used, having the large leaves.

OFFICINAL PREPARATIONS.—Tincture of the root and seeds.

ANALOGUES.—*Iris, Lycopodium, Calcarea carb., Phytolacca, Graphites, Hepar sulph., Sulphur, Viola tricolor.*

## Head.

* Eruptions of the head, face and neck.

° Headaches from suppressed eruption on the scalp.

° *Tinea capitis*—the head completely covered with a grayish-white crust, and most of the hair gone: the eruption extends to the face; cured rapidly and permanently by a weak infusion of the root, after a long and useless trial of *Sulphur, Iris, Mercurius, Graphites, Calcarea carb.*, and *Lycopodium*. (*Dr. Burt. See U. S. Medical and Surgical Journal, Jan.* 1872.)

° *Crusta lactea*, various forms of eczema. (*Ib.*)

° Chronic erysipelas of years standing. (*Ib.*)

° Moist, bad smelling eruptions on the heads of children.

## Face and Eyes.

° Boils on the face and eyelids.

° Styes, and ulcerations on the edges of the eyelids.

## Urinary Organs.

* Profuse and frequent urination.

° Pain in the bladder after urinating.

° Dropsy from non-malignant renal disease.

## General Symptoms.

° Swelling and suppuration of the axillary glands.

° Boils all over the body, painful and slow to heal.

° Fetid sweat of the axillæ.

# ARUM TRIPHYLLUM.

## (*Indian Turnip.*)

BOTANICAL DESCRIPTION.—The A. Triphyllum of the United States cor-responds closely with the A. Maculatum of Europe; both have very simi-lar effects. Our native species is found throughout North and South America, growing in rich, shady woods and swamps. The *cormus* is an inch or two in diameter, and covered with brown, wrinkled epidermis, and internally white, fleshy and solid. The whole plant, when recent, has a peculiar odor and a violent acrid taste; the root, when chewed, causes an insupportable burning and biting sensation in the mouth and throat, con-tinuing for a long time. This acrid principle is very volatile, and is expelled by heat. Hence they are roasted and eaten by the Indians. The acrid principle is not imparted to water, ether, alcohol, or olive oil. By drying, the root loses all its activity. The medicinal qualities of the root reside principally in this acrid, volatile principle. Owing to its unstable nature, it will be found very difficult to procure any preparation in which it will be retained.

This acrid principle has been called *Aroine* and becomes an inflammable gas, by heat or distillation. Prof. Lee says: "The only way to preserve the active principles of the root is to bury it in dry sand, by which method it may be preserved for a year."

OFFICINAL PREPARATION.—Trituration of the juice of the fresh root with ten parts coarse sugar of milk, made very rapidly. Tincture from fresh roots.

It should be kept in hermetically sealed jars, and protected from light and heat. (*Hale.*)

SPHERE OF ACTION.—Mucous membrane of the mouth, throat, bronchi, etc., and probably some profoundly injurious effect on the blood.

ANALOGUES.—*Arum mac., Ailantus, Arsenicum, Allium cepa, Nitric acid, Phosphorus, Causticum, Phytolacca, Baptisia.*

### Eyes.

Aversion to light, with redness of the eyes.

### Nose.

\* Discharge of a burning ichorous fluid, from the nostrils, exco-riating the mucous membrane, and skin of the upper lip.

Nose stopped up, can only breathe through the mouth.

° Constant picking at the nose, until it is sore and bleeding, (in a child.)

### Face.

Face swollen and red.

Swelling of the sub-maxillary glands.

\* Lips swollen, cracked; corners of the mouth sore, bleeding, cracked.

' The child picks constantly at the lips, cheeks and chin, until they are raw and bleeding (in cases of scarlatina.)

## Mouth.

* The mouth burns, and is so sore that he refuses to drink, and cries when anything is offered.

Intense prickling, stinging pain, felt all over the tongue, mouth, lips and fauces, as if from thousands of needles.

* Tongue swollen, red, sore with raised and irritable looking papillæ.

Excessive salivation, and saliva acrid.

## Throat.

Very severe prickling and stinging in the fauces and throat, all the time; worse when swallowing.

Throat feels constricted, sore, burning, cannot swallow.

° Sudden, severe attacks of tonsillitis; œdema of the glottis; acute catarrhal inflammation of the fauces.

## Stomach.

Burning heat in the œsophagus and stomach, which spreads rapidly all over the body.

## Urine.

Frequent discharge of abundant, pale urine.

## Respiratory Organs.

Great hoarseness—inability to talk.

Voice uncertain, changing continually.

* Accumulation of mucus in the trachea; hawking up of thick, white mucus.

° Hoarseness and sore throat of clergymen, public speakers, and singers.

Dry cough, with dryness, prickling and soreness in the fauces. (*p.*)

Loose rattling cough in children and aged persons, with inability to expectorate.  (*s.*)

° Asthma humida, with mucous rales and difficult expectoration.

## Skin.

Dry, feverish heat of the skin.

* Eruption like scarlet rash, the skin peels off afterwards, with itching.

## Fever.

Excited circulation, followed by hot perspiration, with prickling of the skin.

# ASARUM CANADENSE.

### (Wild-Ginger.)

BOTANICAL DESCRIPTION.—Asarum canadense, likewise called Indian ginger, Colt's foot, or Canada Snakeroot, has a close resemblance to the A. Europæum. The root stalk is long, creeping, fleshy, pointed, yellowish, and furnished with root leaves of a similar color. The stem is very short, dividing before it emerges from the ground, into two long, round, hairy leaf-stalks, each of which bears a broad half formed leaf, are covered with soft short hairs on both sides, light green and shining above, veined and pale, or bluish, below. The flower is solitary, growing from the fork of the stem, upon a pendulous, hairy peduncle, being often concealed by the loose soil, or decayed vegetable matter, around it. The calyx is very wooly, consisting of three broad concave sharp-pointed segments, of a brownish, dull purple or greenish color, on the inside and at top and bottom, depending on the amount of light which the plant enjoys, and terminated by a long, spreading, inflected point, with reflected sides. Corolla wanting. Filaments twelve, unequal in length, inserted upon the ovary, and rise with a slender point above the anthers, which are attached to their sides just below the extremity. Ovary inferior, somewhat hexagonal; style conical, striated and parted at top into six recurved, radiating stigmas. Capsule six-celled, stiff, and crowded with the adhering calyx. The Asarum c. is a native of the United States, growing in woods and shady places, and flowering from April to July. The whole plant has a grateful, aromatic odor, and bitter, but agreeably aromatic taste. The roots are in long, contorted pieces, varying in thickness from a line to four or five inches in diameter, brownish and wrinkled externally, internally hard, brittle and whitish. It contains a light-colored, pungent, and fragrant essential oil, a reddish, bitter, resinous matter, starch, gum, fatty matter, chlorophyll, and salts of potassa, lime and iron.

OFFICINAL PREPARATIONS.—Tincture by maceration from fresh root with alcohol; triturations of the root.

### (NO PROVINGS.)

ANALOGUES.—*Asarum Europæum, Senecio, Tanacetum, Sabina, Arnica, Senega.*

### Head.

° Headache from suppressed nasal catarrh.

### Nose.

Watery, irritating discharge from the nose.

### Generative Organs.

Frequent and profuse menses.

Miscarriage in the early months. (?)

Relieves excessive pain in labor.

(Resembles the Asarum Europæum in its general action.)

# ASCLEPIAS INCARNATA.

### (*Swamp Milkweed.*)

BOTANICAL DESCRIPTION.—This plant is known by various names, as *Swamp Silkweed, Flesh-colored Asclepias, Rose-colored Silkweed, White Indian Hemp*, etc. It has a smooth, erect *stem*, with two downy lines above and on the branches and peduncles, branching above, and about two or three feet high. The *leaves* are opposite, oblong, lance-shaped, acute or pointed, obtuse at the base, on short leaf stems, and slightly downy or woolly. The *flowers* are red or reddish-purple, sweet-scented, and disposed in numerous umbels, which are crowded, erect, mostly terminal, and often in opposite pairs. Hoods of the crown entire, horn, standing out, and awl-shaped. The leaves are four to seven inches long, and from one-half an inch to an inch and a half wide; umbels are from two to six, on a peduncle two inches long, and consists of from ten to twenty small flowers. There are several varieties of this plant: the A. *pulchra*, which is more hairy, with broader and shorter petioled leaves; the A. *glabra*, which is almost destitute of hairs, with two opposite longitudinal hairy lines on the stem, and leaves with rough margins, midrib glandular below; and the A. *alba*, which has white flowers. This plant grows in damp and wet soils throughout the United States, and bears red flowers from June to August. It emits a milky juice on being wounded.

The root is the officinal part; it varies in thickness from one to six lines, and is of a light yellowish or brownish color. It imparts its properties to water and alcohol.

OFFICINAL PREPARATIONS.—Tincture by maceration, and triturations of the root.

ANALOGUES.—*Asclepias tuberosa and Asclepias syriaca, Pulsatilla, Senecio, Copaiva, Sabina.*

° Catarrh of the bronchi. (?)     ° Humid Asthma. (?)

° Mucous diarrhœa. (?)

° Gonorrhœa, with greenish discharge and chordee.

° Amenorrhœa, with cough and catarrh.

° Pleurisy. (?)    ° Dropsy.    ° Rheumatism.

Nausea and vomiting, with papescent diarrhœa.

Profuse discharge of urine, and profuse perspiration.

---

# ASCLEPIAS TUBEROSA.

### (*Pleurisy Root.*)

BOTANICAL DESCRIPTION.—The root of this variety of Asclepias is perennial, and gives origin to numerous stems, which are erect, ascending, or may be trailing, round, hairy, of a green or reddish color, branching at the top, and about eighteen inches in height. (It rarely exceeds this, although it is stated to be *three* feet by some authorities.) The leaves are scattered, oblong, lance-shaped, very hairy, of a deep rich green color on their upper surface, paler beneath, and supported usually on short foot stalks. The flowers are of a beautiful reddish-orange color, and disposed in terminal or lateral umbels, their stems rising along the stalk, but differing in length, so as to make them all nearly on a level. The fruit is an erect, lance-shaped follicle, with flat, egg-shaped seeds, connected to a longitudinal receptacle by long silky hairs. This plant differs from other species of Asclepias in not emitting a milky juice when wounded. It flourishes from Massachusetts to Georgia, and when in full bloom, in the months of June and July, exhibits a splendid appearance. The root is the part used in medicine. This is large, irregularly tuberous, branching, often spindle-shaped, externally brown, internally white and striated, and in the recent state, of a sub-acrid nauseous taste. When dried it is easily pulverized, and has a bitter, but not otherwise unpleasant taste.

This plant, under the common names of Pleurisy-root, White-root, Butterfly-weed, Flux-root, Wind-root, Tuber-root, etc., is one of the oldest in use, and one of the most popular of our indigeneous remedies. It is best known by the name first mentioned, and is indicative of its well-known usefulness in painful affections of the thoracic organs.

OFFICINAL PREPARATIONS.—Tincture of the root. Triturations of the root. (No confidence can be placed in the so-called active principles of this plant. They are impure, and do not represent its medicinal qualities.)

SPHERE OF ACTION.—In acute pains of the thoracic organs, catarrhal affections of the larynx, bronchi and respiratory tract, and to some extent functional derangements of the stomach.

ANALOGUES.—*Antimonium crudum, Asclepias syriaca, Arnica, Apocynum cannabinum, Bryonia, Cimicifuga, Caulophyllum, Dioscorea, Dulcamara, Eryngium, Eupatorium perfoliatum, and Eupatorium purpureum, Ipecacuanha, Iris versicolor, Kali carbonicum, Kali hydrojodicum, Pulsatilla, Senega, Squilla, Tartar emeti:.*

## Mind.

Weakness of memory and concentration.

Mental dejection and gloominess.

At first cheerful, then fretful and peevish.

## Head.

Dull headache in the forehead and vertex, aggravated by motion, and relieved by lying down.

Headache, pressing deeply on the base of the skull; resembling an Ipecacuanha headache.

Swimming of the head, with dullness in the forehead.

* Pain in the forehead from coughing. (*also Bryonia.*)

Dull, gloomy feeling in the head.

### Nose.
* Fluent coryza, with much sneezing
Blowing of blood from one nostril.

### Face.
Pale face, with dejected look, after the diarrhœa.

### Mouth.
Yellow, tough coating on the tongue, and putrid taste.

### Throat.
Transitory constriction and stinging in the throat, extending
    to the larynx.
Soreness and pain in the throat.

### Gastric Symptoms.
Putrid taste in the mouth; also taste of blood.
Nausea and efforts to vomit.
Vomiting, purging, and great prostration.
Nausea, with constipation; bilious vomiting.
° Bilious vomiting, with or without diarrhœa, but with pains
    in the limbs, cramps in the feet, etc.
Burning in the stomach.
Pressive pain in the stomach, with rumbling in the bowels.
Disagreeable feeling of weight in the stomach, with deficient
    appetite.

### Stomach and Bowels.
Flying pains in the stomach; fullness and pain in the right
    side, with feeling as if something would pass the bowels,
    and slight nausea.
Constipation, after diarrhœa.
* Bilious and painful diarrhœa.
Rumbling and uneasiness in the bowels, with a feeling of
    heat in the umbilical region.
Rumbling in the bowels, with sharp, cutting pains.
* Soft, fœtid stool, preceded by rumbling, and followed by
    urging to stool.
Rumbling in the bowels, on waking at 6 p. m., with soreness
    of the abdomen and pain on pressure.
Stool like white of eggs.
Clammy stool, green; smelling like rotten eggs.
° Catarrhal diarrhœa, in children, or in warm weather when
    the nights were cool and damp.

° Dysentary, chiefly catarrhal and autumnal.

° Sub-acute mucous enteritis.

° Anomalous symptoms, supposed to be due to the abuse of
    tobacco; namely: Acute soreness, attended by sharp, grip-
    ing pains in the lower part of the abdomen; so severe
    that at times he was unable to walk or ride in a carriage.
    Five or six stools a day. At times the pain came on
    with great violence at 2 or 3 o'clock in the morning, with
    sudden discharges from the bowels, leaving such soreness
    of the abdomen that he could not walk. (Five drops of
    the tincture, in a wineglass of water, taken at one dose,
    cured this case of twenty-five years standing.) (*Dr
    Martin.*)

### Urinary Organs.

Frequent passing of clear urine. (*p.*)

Dark red, saturated urine. (*s.*)

### Genital Organs.

Profuse menstruation, with violent pressing down pain.

Painful stitches in penis.

Sweat of genitals.

° Primary and secondary syphilis. (?)

### Larynx.

Sensation of constriction of the larynx.

\* Dry cough, with constricted sensation in larynx.

\* Dry, hard cough, with pain in forehead and abdomen.

### Chest, etc.

Want of breath, like asthma, worse after eating.

Warm feeling in chest.

Dull pain at base of both lungs, with tightness of chest.

\* Sharp pains shooting from left nipple downward, with stiff-
    ness of left side of neck.

Pain at base of left lung, with dry and spasmodic cough, mak-
    ing respiration painful, with some dullness on percussion
    there.

\* Sharp cutting pain behind the sternum, aggravated by draw-
    ing a long breath, or moving the arms, by singing or loud
    speaking.

Chest feels weak and sore; without cough.

\* The spaces between the ribs, close to the sternum are sensitive to pressure.

Stitches in the left side, shooting over to the right side and up to left shoulder.

\* Acute pleuritic pain in right side, with dry, hacking cough, and scanty mucus expectoration.

Pain in the chest, low down, on the diaphragm.

The pains in the chest are *relieved by bending forward and aggravated by motion.*

° Sub-acute peri-pneumonia of a catarrhal origin.

° *Pleurisy,* (equals *Bryonia* in some cases.)

° Catarrhal cough, hard, spasmodic, from irritation of the larynx or bronchia.

° Influenza, with pleuritic or myalgic pains.

° Capillary bronchitis in children.

° *Bronchitis,* acute and chronic.

° Humid asthma; dyspnœa in bronchial affections.

### Heart.

\* Pain beneath the left nipple, with palpitation of the heart; pulse rising from 64 to 88.

Pains in the region of the heart, shooting up to left shoulder.

\* Pricking pains in region of the heart.

\* Contractive pain in the heart.

Tenderness on pressure over the region of the heart.

° Acute rheumatic pericarditis (not very severe). (*Hale.*)

° Hard, heavy, forcible beating of the heart, with some dyspnœa. (*Hale.*)

### Back and Extremities.

Severe pains in back of the head, arms, legs, feet, shoulders, and violent pains in all the joints.

Pains in *left* shoulder, shooting from left chest.

Sharp, shooting pains in right shoulder.

Aching pains in knees, and drawing pains in thighs.

Pains in the loins, like lumbago.

Rheumatic pains in all the joints.

° Muscular and articular rheumatism, with stitching pains, dark red urine, and hot, perspiring skin.

### Skin.

Vesicles, pimples and pustules, all over the body, especially on
    arms, legs and face.
Itching of the skin of the thighs and nates, without eruption.
Hot, feverish, but moist skin.

### Sleep.

Uneasy sleep, with frightful dreams.

### Fever.

Pulse rises from 64 to 88, with increased action of the heart.
Chilliness, in a warm room, with cold feet.
* High fever, with hot sweat.
° Rheumatic and catarrhal fevers.
° Bilious fever (?), "marsh fever of the rice plantations."

### Generalities.

Weak, languid, as if he had been sick a long time.

---

# ASCLEPIAS SYRIACA.

### (Silk Weed.)

BOTANICAL DESCRIPTION.—This is the Asclepias cornuti of Gray. (I
retain the name Syriaca given it by Linnæus, as in the first edition.) The
plant is known as *Milkweed* in many parts of the country, has a large,
stout, simple, somewhat branched *stem*, growing from two to five feet high.
The *leaves* are egg-shaped, elliptical, spreading, opposite, with a short but
distinct stem, gradually acute, and downy or hairy beneath. The *flowers*
are fragrant; *umbels* several, axillary, nodding, dense, round, each of
twenty or more flowers. *Calyx segments* lance-shaped. *Corolla* pale or
greenish purple, reflexed, leaving the corona, which is of nearly the same
hue, quite conspicuous. But few of the flowers prove fertile, producing
oblong-pointed pods or follicles, covered with sharp prickles which contain a mass of long silky fibres with seeds attached, and which fibres have
been used for beds, pillows, and in the place of fur in manufacturing hats.

HISTORY.—This herb is indigenous to the United States, inhabiting rich
soil, uncultivated fields, etc., and bearing whitish-purple flowers from
June to September. When wounded it emits a milky fluid which contains
water, wax-like fatty matter, gum, caoutchouc, sugar, various salts, etc.
A crystalline, resinous substance allied to lactucone, has been obtained
from the juice of the *A. cornuti*, to which the name of the *Asclepione* has
been given. It is procurred by boiling and then filtering the juice and
separating the Asclepione from the filtrate by ether, from which it may be
subsequently obtained by evaporation, and purified by several washings
with pure ether. Asclepione thus obtained is a crystaline solid, without

F.4

taste or smell, and is readily dissolved by spirits of turpentine, pure acetic acid, and sulphuric ether.

OFFICINAL PREPARATIONS.—Tincture of the fresh root by maceration with strong alcohol; dilutions. Triturations of the dried root; and tincture by maceration with dilute alcohol.

(Triturations of a solid extract of the milky juice, made by evaporation at a low temperature over a water bath.)

ANALOGUES.—*Asclepias tuberosa, Bryonia, Colchicum, Senega,* and the analogues of *Asclepias tuberosa.*

## Head.

Headache, with scanty urine.

Headache, with vertigo, dullness and stupidity.

❋ Headache, from suppressed perspiration, or from the retention of effete matters in the system.

° Nervous headaches, followed by profuse diuresis.

Violent headache, confined principally between the eyes.

Severe headache, quick, full pulse, and nausea.

A *feeling as if some sharp instrument was thrust through from one temple to the other.*

A sense of constriction across the forehead.

## Mouth and Throat.

Burning and tickling in fauces, with nausea and headache.

Tongue coated with a white fur.

## Stomach.

Excessive nausea, with violent headache.

Slight pain in the stomach, with diuresis and inclination to evacuate the bowels.

Vomiting, severe and long continued, with retching, leaving a sensation of rawness in the stomach, and a slight pain, with cold skin, feeble pulse, and a feeling as if some sharp instrument was thrust through from one temple to the other.

Great appetite, even a few hours after a meal.

Increased appetite, notwithstanding the vomiting and headache, with constipation.

## Abdomen and Stool.

Frequent movements from the bowels.

Diarrhœa, with persistent nausea and vomiting.

Inclination to evacuate the bowels, with nausea and diuresis.

5

Copious evacuations in the evening, soft, brown, with slight colic.

Soft yellow stool at noon, with increase of appetite.

Diarrhœa, with excoriation of the anus.

Copious evacuations without pain or other unpleasant effects.

° Expulsion of worms—(ascarides.)

° Constipation, pain in right side, lower extremities, and loss of appetite.

## Urinary Organs.

Enormous increase of urine, ( *primary*,) from 35 to 128 ounces.

Scanty urine, with headache. (*secondary*.)

Profuse urine after headache.

Pale-colored urine, with lighter specific gravity.

Burning sensation in the urethra when urinating.

° Uræmia, preceded by profuse, then scanty or suppressed urine.

° Post-scarlatinal dropsy.

° Dropsy from suppressed perspiration, or renal disease.

° General dropsy from heart disease.

[This medicine is one of the few like *Colchicum, Bryonia,* and *Cimici-fuga*, that increase notably the *solid* matters in the urine, namely, from 568 grains to 700 grains.—*Hale*.]

## Generative Organs.

(*Female*.)  * Intermitting, bearing-down, labor-like pains, (in a case of dropsy.)

Dysmenorrhœa, accompanied with diuresis.

° Suppression of the menses, in a case of dropsy.

(*Male*.)  Tickling sensation at the end of the penis.

Burning in the urethra when urinating.

## Bronchia, Lungs.

Severe bronchial irritation, with burning and tickling in fauces.

° Influenza; catarrhal fevers; and bronchitis.

## Back and Extremities.

° Acute rheumatism, confined to the large joints, with much pain and swelling.

° Pains in the limbs.

[I would urge a trial of this remedy in rheumatism, when *Colchicum* and *Cimicifuga* seem inefficient.—*Hale*.]

# ATROPINE.

### (*The active principle of Belladonna.*)

OFFICINAL PREPARATIONS.—Triturations, (centesimal) up to the third, then the dilutions.

[No complete provings of *Atropine* have been made. Allen's new Encyclopediæ of Materia Medica contains the most complete pathogenesis yet collected. The symptoms obtained are all like those of *Belladonna.* We do not believe *Atropine* can produce *all* the symptoms of *Belladonna,* because it does not contain all the forces and medicinal constituents of that plant. To the mere chemist, who cannot discern anything left in the plant after the *Atropia* is extracted, this assertion may seem absurd; but the chemist looks at drugs from a point of view widely divergent from the physiological experimenter. There are intangible remedial forces in plants which escape the subtlest analysis of the chemist, and can only be evolved by careful provings. One object of giving this pathogenesis is to give an idea of the scope and sphere of action of this isolated constituent. While we should never think of prescribing *Atropine* in febrile states, acute exanthemata, inflammations, erysipelas, glandular diseases, etc., where we usually use *Belladonna,* we have a high opinion of its value in neuralgia, acute congestions, painful spasmodic affections, especially of the sphincters, nervous jactitations, hyperæsthesiæ, and other affections due to purely functional nervous derangements.—*Hale.*]

PHARMACOLOGY.—The Sulphate of *Atropine* is the best preparation to use in making triturations. The pure alkaloid is too insoluble. An "Atropine," or so called active principle is sold and used by a class of Eclectic physicians, but it is unreliable, and should not be used in homœopathic therapeutics. The pure Atropine is composed of slender fasciculated crystals. The sulphate is a white crystalline powder. The spurious "Atropine" is a powder.

ANALOGUES.—*Belladonna and its analogues.*

### Mind.

* Rambling, incoherent speech, spectral illusions, with frequent fits of wild uncontrollable laughter.

° Furious delirium, especially at night.

Quiet, dreamy delirium, with nervous startings.

Muttering and smiling, with sleepiness.

Delirium, with picking, and other motions of the hands and fingers in the air, as if they were in contact with real objects.

He carries on conversations with imaginary beings.

When conversing, had to stop in the middle of a sentence and inquire what he had been talking about.

Imagines he has epilepsy.

He lost the power of estimating distances; he reached at
objects which were across the room, and stumbled on
objects which he supposed were far off.

### Head.

\* Beating and throbbing of the carotids, with red face, etc.

Fullness of temples and of forehead, with dizziness.

Feeling as if the brain was being pressed out in all directions.

\* *Feeling as if the head was screwed up; walking caused
the most severe sticking pains;* relieved toward 11 A. M.,
and disappeared toward evening.

\* *Fine, drawing, very sensitive stitches across the forehead
and temples,* recurring every four to ten minutes, and
lasting several seconds.

\* *Dull pain in the temples, coming on at intervals of perhaps a quarter of an hour,* and lasting a few minutes.

\* *Very sensitive sticking in the left temporal region on
waking in the morning;* it extended to behind the ear,
and scarcely permitted him to open the left eye; disappeared after moving about in the open air.

\* Neuralgic pains commencing under the left orbit, and run
ning back to the ear.

Vertigo upon turning the head suddenly.

Vertigo, with staggering, and inability to walk.

° Neuralgic hemicrania, of the severest character.

° Symptoms simulating cerebral meningitis.

° Cephalalgia, generally nervous or congestive.

° Headaches of a nervous or neuralgic origin.

### Face and Eyes.

Dark red, livid and puffed face, with burning heat in face.

\* Twitching of the facial muscles, especially around the mouth
and eyelids.

\* Congested eyes and eyelids, with feeling of dryness in eyes.

\* Deep-seated, dull pain in the back part of the eye.

\* Bright flashes before the eyes immediately upon closing then

Intolerance of light (rare.)

*Dimness of vision; can neither read nor thread a needle.*

Pain in the eyes; dull, or sharp and increased at each cardiac
pulsation.

Eyes fixed and glassy; cannot compare objects or estimate their distances.

*Dilated pupils*, to an extent not caused by any other drug.

Can read well for a few moments, when the words run together and become indistinct.

When reading, the words seem to contract and expand with the action of the heart.

*Spasmodic winking.* Eyelids feel heavy and difficult to open.

Double vision; all objects seem elongated.

Dryness of the conjunctiva. (*Apparent* dryness.)

When closing the eyes he sees all kinds of spectres and unpleasant objects. (*See Allen's Encyc. of Mat. Med.*)

The field of vision is covered with colored phantasms.

Everything looks yellow. (*See Santonin.*)

° Neuralgia of the eyes, and orbital regions.

° Used extensively (and sometimes *abused*) by oculists to dilate the pupil in cases of iritis, cataract, etc., and to assist in examinations with the ophthalmoscope.

### Ears.

Hearing morbidly sensitive—at night. (*p.*)

Illusions of the sense of hearing, ringing, roaring, etc. (*p.*)

Dullness of the sense of hearing, deafness. (*p.*)

### Nose.

Redness and heat of the nose.

Great dryness of the mucous membrane of the nose.

### Mouth.

*Intense dryness* of the mouth, tongue, fauces, soft palate, and the lips and throat, followed by a sensation of a viscid, sticky, acid secretion of a peculiar and very sickly, offensive odor.

The mouth becomes foul and clammy, and the tongue covered with a sticky white fur.

Smoking does not excite the secretion of saliva.

Mucous membrane of mouth dark and mottled.

ᵓ Mercurial salivation. (It arrests the profuse secretion.)

### Tongue.

Loss of sensation in the buccal cavity

Tongue dry, with red tip and edges.

Tongue sticky and coated white.

Cannot move the tongue around in the mouth.

Difficulty of protruding the tongue.

Tongue feels thick; cannot articulate distinctly.

Teeth feel " on edge."

° Dry, parched and cracked tongue, in typhus.

° Paralytic symptoms of the tongue.

### Throat.

Dryness of the pharynx, making it *almost impossible to swallow.*

No natural sensation when drinking; the water did not seem to touch the mucous membrane.

Cannot swallow solids without washing them down with liquids.

Mucous membrane of throat feels raw and irritated; it looks darker than usual, and mottled.

Swallowing appeared to give pain.

\* Great difficulty in getting the child to swallow. Each attempt to do so produced paroxysms of suffocation, which appeared to threaten its existence.

### Taste and Appetite.

*Loss of taste;* nothing tastes natural.

Everything tastes *salt.*

*No appetite;* partly owing to the dryness of the mouth and throat, which obliges him to *wash* his food down.

### Gastro-Enteric.

*Nausea,* from the foul, sticky saliva.

Vomiting, profuse, hurrying him out of bed at night.

Easy vomiting of bitter liquid at first, afterwards tasteless.

Eructations, tasting like the yolk of eggs.

° *Gastralgia,* purely neuralgic: (very prompt cures.)

Violent, severe *sticking* pains in the umbilical region, during attacks of vomiting, at night.

Diarrhœa, hurrying him out of bed at midnight, preceded by urgent desire.

Stools copious and watery, coming out with a *gush,* relieving the pain at the umbilical region.

° Spasmodic or neuralgic colic.

° *Constipation*, cured permanently by very minute doses continued for some time. (*Allopathic authority.*)

### Urinary Organs.

The kidneys are active in the elimination of *Atropine* from the minute when it enters the blood until it is entirely removed from the system.

It causes an *excess* of uric acid in the urine.

It causes an increased flow of blood through the kidneys, and thus increases the urea.

The phosphates are increased by its administration.

Profuse and frequent urination. (*p.*)

"It is a most powerful *diuretic.*" (*Harley.*)

Retention of urine; the catheter has to be used daily.

° Nephritic colic, from passage of calculi.

* Violent, irresistible and ineffectual urging to urinate, with agonizing tenesmus. (*Hale.*)

* Paralysis of the bladder — probably the sphincter.

° Dysuria; it relieves the pain in many cases.

° Dropsy from Bright's disease.

° *Chronic albuminuria;* the albumen decreased rapidly.

### Generative Organs.

° Neuralgia of the testes, with extreme sensitiveness to touch.

° Irritable uterus, with neuralgic pains in it, in paroxysms.

° Uterine colic, neuralgic and paroxysmal.

° *Ovarian neuralgia*, acute pains, in paroxysms.

° *Vaginismus*, a spasmodic disorder of the vagina, often an undoubtedly neuralgic disease.

* *Hyperæsthesia* of the vagina and uterine cervix. (*Hale.*)

[In these cases give the 6th + trit., and apply a cerate of 1 gr. to 1 oz., of cocoa butter or lard.]

### Respiratory Organs.

Dryness of the *larynx*, causing a constant inclination to cough.

* The tough mucus in the larynx causes paroxysms of coughing, very severe, occurring every fifteen or twenty minutes, attended with difficult expectoration of thick, tenacious mucus, and followed by burning in the larynx.

° *Whooping-cough*, cured by the 3d centesimal trit.

' Spasmodic cough, in adults, after influenza. (*Hale.*)

Sensation of a glow of heat in the lungs.

* Violent and suffocative constriction of the chest.

° Spasmodic asthma (by hypodermic injection).

### Heart.

Pulse feeble and heart's action almost imperceptible.

Pulse rising from 60 to 140 beats, but no increase in the respirations. (*Harley.*)

Fluttering sensation in the cardiac region. (*Ib.*)

° Nervous palpitation of the heart, with red face and throbbing in the carotids. (*Hale.*)

° Palpitation at night, with debility and distress.

### Extremities.

Trembling of the limbs.

Anæsthesia of the extremities; the sense of touch seems blunted and sometimes almost abolished; numbness and prickling of the hands, extending to the tips of the fingers.

Cannot tell when the hand touches an object.

Continued desire to open and shut the hands.

Jerking of the muscles of the extremities.

While drinking, the arm suddenly contracted, causing him to spill the water.

While walking, the flexor muscle would contract suddenly, throwing him to the ground.

Staggering, tottering gait.

On picking up a pin, it feels as if there were five or six of them.

Spasms of the muscles of the extremities.

Spasmodic contractions of extremities at night.

Coldness of extremities.

### Skin.

[Dr. Sadler, of London, (*Med. Times and Gazette,*) reports an interesting case showing some of the physiological effects of *Atropine*, and the smallness of the dose capable of affecting a child.

He gave a child, three months old, a mixture containing 1-200th of a grain of Sulphate of Atropine. *In a few minutes the child turned a deep red, "like scarlet fever,"* over its face and upper part of its body; the perspiration was checked, and the skin became hot and dry. This continued for five hours. The next morning only half the quantity was given; the same effect was produced, but only lasted for two hours. The third morning only four drops were given (60 drops contained 1-200th of a grain) and this time without any effect. Six drops were given the next morning; the same redness appeared, but this time only lasted for half an hour. The six drops contained 1-800th of a grain. No narcotism was produced, even by the larger dose first given. The paroxysm of whooping-cough, for which it was given was slightly but not decidedly improved.]

*Dark red or mottled efflorescent redness of the skin,* like that in scarlet fever.

Dark red or purple redness of the face.

Scarlet red, hot and dry skin, on the upper half of the body.

*Anæsthesia of the skin:* the sense of touch is lost or perverted.

Thrusting pins into the skin causes no pain.

Water poured over the skin produces no sensation.

Skin *seems* unnaturally smooth, like glass.

Cold, pale and clammy skin.

° Useful in some cases of scarlet fever.

᷎ In cases of retarded or suppressed eruptions, it will cause their re-appearance. (*Hale.*)

### Sleep.

Sleepiness, or drowsiness with inability to sleep.

Deep, heavy, comatose sleep.

Heavy sleep, with muttering, incoherent talking.

He sits in a dull, apathetic or drowsy condition, and frequently gives a prolonged yawn.

Deep sleep, with red, bloated face.

### Fever.

Continual chilliness all over.

*Chills alternating with flashes of heat.*

It stimulates the action of the heart, causing the pulse to rise from 60 to 140, with flashes of heat, red-hot skin, dry mouth and throat, with throbbing all over; a kind of erethistic fever, with general ebulition of blood. (*p.*)

Chilliness, with cold skin, pulse feeble, action of the heart feeble, cold extremities. (*s.*)

Fever, with low muttering, incoherent delirum.

° Useful in some typhoid fevers.

### Generalities.

General anæsthesia of the skin and extremities. (*p.*)

Hyperæsthesia of the whole organism. (*s.*)

° *Tetanus:*

[In a late number of the *British Medical Journal* is a case of Tetanus successfully treated by *Atropia.* On the fourth day of the attack one-sixteenth of a grain was administered every three hours.

Within twenty-four hours the clonic spasm became less severe and of shorter duration, and the tonic rigidly gave way, first in the legs and neck, then in the back, and last of all in abdomen and masseters. On the sixth day of treatment by *Atropia,* rigidity of masseters only remained. He was kept under the influence of *Atropia* for three weeks, and made a good recovery. The patient was "a healthy-looking lad, aged 14, who was seized with lockjaw and severe pain in the cervical and dorsal region, with fever, a few days after jumping from a coal wagon."

The reporter asserts that it cures on the theory of Brown-Sequard, namely: "Reducing congestion of the blood vessels of the spinal cord." It was certainly homœopathic to the condition, for the primary effect of *Atropine* is to cause spinal anæmia, the *secondary,* spinal congestion. For this reason the large dose cured.]

---

# ARSENITE OF COPPER.

### (*Cupric Arsenite. Scheele's Green.*)

PHARMACOLOGY.—This salt may be prepared by boiling three parts of pulverized white arsenic, with eight parts caustic potassa, in sixteen parts of water until the arsenic is deposited in the shape of a powder; pour this liquid into a hot solution composed of eight parts of the sulphate of copper and forty-eight parts of distilled water, stirring the mixture all the time; wash the precipitate well, and dry at a moderate temperature.

It is a bright green insoluble powder.

OFFICINAL PREPARATION.—Triturations to the 6th ×; then dilutions.

ANALOGUES.—*Arsenic, Agaricus, Belladonna, Cuprum, Æthusa, Œnanthe,* etc.

## Mental Sphere.

Confusion of ideas, vertigo, and headache between the temples.

Dullness and fullness of the head.

Intense anguish of mind and body.

A kind of intoxication.

## Head.

Severe headache, with dull pain in the forehead, and soreness of the orbital bones.

Throbbing pain in the right temple.

Headache between the temples; the pain seems to meet in the centre of the forehead, and thence to pass down the nose.

### Eyes.

Persistent boring pain in a small spot above the left superior orbital arch, with soreness when touched.

Dimness of the eyes, with profuse lachrymation.

Dark specks before the eyes; eyes are very sensitive.

Sparks before the eyes.

### Ears.

Boring pain in the right ear.

### Nose.

Soreness of the nose, with watery discharge from the nose.

### Face.

Soreness of the bones of the face.

Œdema of the face.

Paleness of the face.

Violent twitching and jerking of the facial muscles of the left side, between the eye and the corner of the mouth.

### Mouth and Throat.

Heavy white coating of the tongue.

Shooting pains in the upper jaw; the pains are intermittent and throbbing.

Burning sensation in the throat; soreness of the glands of the neck, with stiffness of the neck; moving the head aggravates the pain in the neck.

### Stomach.

Nausea, with headache between the eyes, and metallic taste in the mouth.

* Vomiting and purging, with cramps and collapse.

Vomiting of mucus tinged with bile.

Great sensitiveness of the epigastric region to the least touch.

° Cramps in stomach and bowels, followed by tonsillitis.

° Nausea, with burning pain in the stomach and bowels; palpitation of the heart, with trembling of the limbs; headache, particularly in the forehead; jerking in the limbs.

### Abdomen and Stool.

* Violent colic; frequent vomiting, with purging; cold sweats; intense thirst.

Great distension of the abdomen.

Pains in the abdomen, sharp and cutting.

*Diarrhœa;* slimy stool.

° Asiatic cholera, with cramps in hands and feet.

### Urinary Organs.

Strong-smelling urine.

Dark-red urine; burning pain during and after urination.

### Generative Organs.

*Male.*—White, purulent discharge from the urethra; soreness
of the penis, with pain in the prostate gland; tingling
and burning in the urethra.

Perspiration of the scrotum, which is constantly moist and
damp.

Boils frequently forming on the scrotum.

### Chest.

Dull, stitching pain in left chest, between the sixth and
seventh ribs, with a weak, numb feeling in the left chest,
left side of the back, left shoulder and arm.

Constricted feeling of the chest.

Sudden debility, with dull pain in the heart, and sensation of
oppression around that organ.

Palpitation of the heart, with trembling of the limbs.

° Angina pectoris. (*Hale.*)

### Back.

Lameness of the back.

Severe pain under the scapula; worse when moving or breathing.

### Upper Extremities.

Numb, weak feeling in left shoulder and arm.

Left arm feels numb and powerless, and a similar sensation
soon afterward appeared in the left leg.

### Skin.

Aggravation of a chronic irritation; itching of the arms and
legs.

Pustular tumors(?) on the wrists and ankles.

Eruptions of the skin; œdema of the face; boils on scrotum.

### Sleep.

Persistent sleeplessness.

## Fever.

Chilliness all over the body; creeping sensation produced by the contact of the clothing.

Intense thirst; cold sweats.

Pulse frequent, skin cold, with great depression.

Small, quick, irritated, or else spasmodically contracted, pulse.

### Generalities.

Cerebro-spinal irritation; staggering gait.

° Chorea; syncope; spasms; severe convulsions.

° Epilepsy; death-like syncope.

---

# ARSENIATE OF IRON.
### (*Ferri Arsenias.*)

PHARMACOLOGY.—The arsenite of iron may be substituted for the above if necessary, although I do not consider it as assimilable as the arseniate, for the reason that the former is made with arsen*ic* acid, the latter with arsen*ious* acid. I have, therefore, made the *arseniate* officinal. (*Hale.*)

It may be prepared as follows: To a solution of the sulphate of iron add a solution of the arseniate of potassa (or soda) as long as a white precipitate falls. Wash the precipitated arseniate of iron on a filter, and dry it.

It is white when first formed, but quickly becomes green on exposure to air; is an amorphous powder, without smell or taste, insoluble in water, but readily soluble in muriatic acid.

OFFICINAL PREPARATIONS.—Triturations to the 6th ×.

*(See Therapeutics, Vol. II.)*

---

# ARSENIATE OF QUINIA.
### (*Quinia Arsenias.*)

PHARMACOLOGY.—The arsenite of quinine is used by many practitioners; but as I consider the arseniate the best preparation, I have made it offi. cinal. (*Hale.*)

The *arseniate* may be prepared by placing one and a half drachms of arsenious acid in a glass vessel, with five drachms quinia, and six fluid ounces of distilled water; boil till all is dissolved; filter and allow to crystalize spontaneously. To purify, dissolve these crystals, and then crystalize again.

*The Arsenite of Quinia* is prepared by placing sixteen grains of arsenious acid, eight grains carbonate of potassa, and one fluid ounce distilled water in a glass vessel; boil till all is dissolved, adding water to keep the quan tity of the solution at one fluid ounce. To two and a half drachms of the solution add twenty grains sulphate of quinia, previously dissolved in distilled water by boiling. The arsenite of quinia precipitates in the form of a white, amorphous substance, which must be well washed and dried.

Soluble in alcohol, but not in water.

OFFICINAL PREPARATIONS.—Dilutions with alcohol; triturations.

*(See Therapeutics, Vol. II.)*

---

# BADIAGA.

### *(Fresh-water Sponge.)*

OFFICINAL PREPARATIONS.—Tincture and triturations from the dried sponge.

ANALOGUES.—*Spongia, Silicea, Carbo animalis, Kaolin, Kali bichromicum, Clematis, Sulphur, Iodine, Mercurius, Phytolacca, Baryta jod.*

## Mental Sphere.

In spite of the headache, he is still clear in his mind, and more inclined to mental activity than before.

Upon the slightest emotion or thought, forcible pulsation of the heart

## Head.

Dull, dizzy feeling of the head.

Congestion in the forehead.

Headache from two P. M. till seven in the morning, with slight aching pains in the posterior portion of both eyeballs, and in the temple.

During the day more or less headache, with pain in the eyeballs, worse in the left; more from one o'clock in the afternoon till seven in the evening.

Frontal headache during the forenoon, worse in the temples, and extending into the posterior portion of the left eyeball, aggravated by moving the eye.

Headache, with inflamed eyes.

During the afternoon, heat, pain and congestion in the forehead, worse at seven P. M.

In the temples and eyeballs, pain; to the temples from the eyeballs.

A very severe headache on the top of the head; remains the same in all positions; better at night after sleeping and better in the morning, returning violently after breakfast, lasting several days.

Headache, commencing between one and two P. M., lasting till between six and seven in the evening.

Headache and soreness of the body, aggravated, from seven to ten in the evening.

An excess of dandruff or dry, tetter-like appearance of the scalp, with slight itching.

Scalp sore to the touch, with tetter-like eruption on the forehead and dull, dizzy feeling of the head during the forenoon.

### Eyes.

° Slight intermitting pains in the posterior portion of right eyeball and temple; more during the afternoon.

Pain in the posterior portion of both eyeballs, more in the left one; more between one and seven in the evening.

Inflammation of the eyes, especially the right.

Pain in left eyeball and temple, quite severe, extending to the left side of the head and forehead.

Twitching of the left upper eyelid (from triturating the Badiaga.)

Left eyeball quite sore, even upon closing it tightly.

Scrofulous inflammation of the eyes, with hardening of the meibomian glands.

Bluish-purple margin of the eyelids and blue under the eye.

### Nose.

Itching of the left wing of the nose (while triturating the Badiaga.)

*Profuse coryza, mostly from the left nostril*, worse in the afternoon and P. M.

Discharge of thick, yellowish mucus from left nostril, during the afternoon.

Occasional sneezing, with more profuse coryza, most on the left side, with occasional stoppage of the nose; worse in the afternoon and evening.

Coryza and cough.

### Face.

On forehead tetter-like eruption.

Pale, ashy, or lead color of the face.

Stiffness in the maxillary joints.

### Mouth and Throat.

Mouth hot and dry, with thirst for large quantities at a time

° Throat inflamed and sore, *especially* on *swallowing;* tonsils red and inflamed.

Mouth and tongue feel as if scalded.

Hawked up a viscid, solid lump of bloody mucus, in the morning.

### Stomach and Abdomen.

Severe, lancinating pain in pit of stomach, extending to the vertebræ opposite and to the right scapula, and at times to the right side, resulting in a pleuritic pain.

A lancinating pain, with a bounding movement in the region of the liver.

Bowels costive; hæmorrhoids.

### Urinary Organs.

Sharp pain in the right kidney.

Urine high-colored and reddish.

Severe, sharp lancinating pains in and near the orifice of the urethra.

### Groins.

° Indurated, inguinal glands. (*Hering, Mat. Med.*)

° Syphilitic bubo in the left groin; a longish swelling, as hard as a stone; border rugged, like a scirrhus; at night violent lancinations, as if with red-hot needles. (*Ib.*)

° Buboes originating with consensus or cellular irritation, with shooting pains, if suppuration has not commenced, will disappear in three days completely, if with rest, low diet, cold local application, the tincture of *Badiaga* is given, one drop in a tablespoonful of water, every three or four hours. (*Ib.*)

ᶜ Buboes, with decided fluctuation, are scattered and absorbed from six drops of the tincture, every day in water. (*Ib.*)

### Cough and Chest.

While lying on the right side in bed, and at the moment of becoming unconscious by sleep, severe oppressive suffocating attacks, from suspended respiration, causing a quick effort to prevent suffocation, by changing position.

On full inspiration, pleuritic pain; aggravated pain in side.

Occasional severe paroxysms of spasmodic cough, ejecting viscid mucus from the bronchial tubes, which at times comes flying forcibly out of the mouth, more during the afternoon; caused by a tickling in the larynx.

Cough, with yellowish mucous expectoration; better in the warm room.

A sense of sharp, lancinating pain in the right supra-clavicular region, in or near the sub-clavian artery, lasting several minutes during the evening.

Pain in the upper part of the right chest.

Pleuritic pain in right side, also on the left; increased with stitches on both sides, aggravated on motion or full respiration, with soreness of the whole body, especially the chest.

Severe stitches in the side, especially the right side, from the seventh to the eighth rib; aggravated by the least motion.

### Heart.

Severe vibrating tremulous palpitation of the heart, even while sitting or lying quiet, upon the least elation or other emotion of the mind.

While lying in bed, forcible pulsations of the heart felt and heard, extending from the chest up into the neck, upon the slightest emotion or thought.

Palpitation of the heart, with a fluttering and vibrating upon the slightest emotion.

Occasional spells of severe jerking, fluttering palpitation of the heart upon a sudden elating thought or emotion of the mind, even while sitting or lying.

While lying on the right side, the heart is both heard and felt to pulsate from the chest up to the neck.

Midnight, while in bed, vibrating palpitation of the heart, lasting but a few minutes, after which, while lying on the right side, a sensation as if the lower lobe of the left lung was settling down, or being collapsed—relieved by changing position.

6

## Neck.

A very stiff neck.

Soreness and lameness, with stitches in the nape of the neck, aggravated by bending the head back and forth.

° Glandular swellings on the left side of the face, throat and neck, nearly all of the size of a hen's egg, some hard, some suppurating; they disfigured and enlarged the whole region considerably, since his early youth, now twenty years; in often repeated doses, lessened it more than half the former size. (*Hering's Mat. Med.*)

## Back.

Painful drawing near the spine to the left, downwards from the shoulder blade.

Severe lacerating pains and stitches in the posterior right side below the scapula, aggravated very much by throwing the shoulders back and the chest forward.

Pain in small of the back, hips, and lower limbs.

Pain in the front of the upper part of the right shoulder, afterwards in the left shoulder and arm.

## Limbs.

Palms of the hands hot and dry, dry and husky.

An intermitting pain in the muscles of the lower posterior third of the right leg, with a sore, contracted, clumsy, bruised feeling of the arterior muscles of the lower third of the right leg, which is *aggravated by flexing the foot and going up stairs*, when the toes have a tendency to drop down, as if the foot were asleep.

The anterior muscles of the right leg sore, as if beaten.

Several small hard lumps along the shin bone.

° Lessened hard-cellular swelling of both legs.

Sharp, stinging pain in the posterior portion of the right heel, aggravated by the slightest pressure.

° Bad ulcers on the feet of horses.—(*Popular remedy.*)

° Hurts of the hoofs of horses.           "        "

° Chilblai ıs.                            "        "

A general soreness of the muscles and integuments of the whole body, especially the integuments; aggravated on motion, and especially by the friction of the clothes.

Flesh feels sore, as if it had been beaten, and very sensitive to touch or friction of the clothes.

### Sleep.

Awoke with frightful dreams and severe crampy pains in the metatarsal bones of both feet.

Restless night, could lie only a short time in one position, on account of the soreness of the muscles and whole body.

° At night violent lancinating pains in the limbs.

In the night palpitation, lying on the right side.

Headache better after sleep.

### Fever.

Feverish, hot breath and mouth.

Hot and dry palms of hands.

### Skin.

Itching on scalp.

° Scrofulous diseases, particularly swollen glands.

° Bruised spots from falls or from being beaten.

Flesh and skin sore to the touch.

---

# BALSAMUM PERUVIANUM.

### (*Balsam of Peru.*)

BOTANICAL DESCRIPTION.—The proper botanical name is *Myrospermum peruiferum*. It is the *myroxylon peruiferum* of Linnæus. It is known by the natives of Peru under the name of *Quinquino*, its bark and fruit as Quinquina, by the Mexicans *Hoitziloxitl*, and by the Brazilians *Cabureiba*.

It is a large tree. with a thick, straight, smooth trunk, and a coarse gray, compact, heavy, granulated bark, of a pale straw color, filled with resin which, according to its quantity, changes the color to citron, yellow, red, or dark chestnut.

It is found in low, warm, sunny situations in Peru, especially near the river Maranon; also in other parts of South America, and flowers from July to October.

The balsam met with in the markets is not constant either in quality or appearance, owing probably to its being procured from different species. That used for Homœopathic preparations should be procured from this species. It is prepared by incising the bark and collecting the juice upon rags, which, when saturated are placed in water. Upon boiling, the balsam rises to the surface, and is removed and put into vessels for purification and exportation.

It has a dark reddish-brown color in thin layers, is black in bulk, is of the consistence of ordinary molasses, an agreeable balsamic odor, a hot, acrid, somewhat bitter taste, and a specific gravity of 1.15.

The purity of Balsam of Peru may be ascertained by mixing ten drops of it with twenty drops of concentrated sulphuric acid, in a watch glass, and then diluting with water. If it is pure, a brittle resin is obtained; if not, a soft resin.

OFFICINAL PREPARATIONS.—A tincture may be made by dissolving in nine parts alcohol, and dilutions made as in other cases. Triturations from the balsam with coarse sugar of milk.

ANALOGUES.—*Aurum mur, Copaiva, Cubeba, Chimaphila, Kali hypophos, Iodine, Myosotis, Stannum, Sulphur, Thuja, Uva ursi.*

### Head.
Heat and fullness in the head.

\* Profuse thick discharge from the nose.

° Chronic, muco-purulent nasal catarrh.

° Ozæna—with ulceration.

### Gastro-Intestinal Sphere.
Increase of appetite and digestion.

Heat and oppression of the stomach.

\* Vomiting of food and mucus.

Nausea, with colic and diarrhœa.

\* Catarrhal state of the stomach.

° Chronic mucous diarrhœa.

° Chronic dysentery, with bloody mucus and tenesmus.

° Irritable bowels after typhoid fever.

### Respiratory Organs.
Heat and burning in the larynx.

Irritating short cough, dry.

\* Cough, with copious expectoration of thick yellow, green, and fœtid muco-pus.

° Chronic inflammation of the larynx.

° Laryngeal phthisis—*not* tuberculous.

° Chronic bronchial catarrh—especially of old people.

° Loose, rattling cough, with thick, yellow, or green and fœtid expectoration—*after* pneumonia. (1-10th dil.)

° Suppression of the accustomed expectoration in bronchial affections. (6th dil.)

° Chronic bronchitis with purulent expectoration and hectic fever. (*Hale.*)

' I have seen persons laboring under perfectly formed phthisis, and seriously affected for several years, happily restored by the use of this balsam. (*Hoffman.*)

° Purulent, fœtid expectoration from vomicæ in the lungs. (*Ib.*)

(In affections of the bronchia and lungs, with scanty expectoration and fever, use the 6th dilution. If profuse purulent expectoration, and absence of fever, use the 1-10th dilution.) (*Hale.*)

### Urinary Organs.

Increased secretion of urine.

\* Scanty urine with mucus sediment.

° Chronic catarrh of the bladder.

° Chronic uterine and vaginal leucorrhœa. (?)

### Fever.

General heat, with excited circulation and quickened pulse, but moist skin.

° Hectic fever in suppurations, phthisis, and chronic bronchitis.

### Generalities.

° Debility, with slow, feeble circulation.

° Indolent ulcers. (*the cerate.*)

° Cracks in the nipples, fingers and hands. (*the cerate.*)

---

# BAPTISIA TINCTORIA.

### (*Wild Indigo.*)

BOTANICAL DESCRIPTION.—This plant is indigenous, growing in most parts of the United States, in dry and poor soils, in woods and on hills. It blooms in July and August, having bright yellow *flowers*, in small loose clusters at the ends of the branches. It resembles a shrub, and grows from one to two feet high. The *fruit* is an oblong pod of a bluish black color. It contains indigo, tannin, an acid, and baptisin. When the whole plant or any portion of it is dried, it becomes black and affords a blue dye, inferior to Indigo.

There are thirteen species of the Baptisia in the United States. The most important are the B. *tinctoria*, B. *alba*, (with white flowers,)B. *leucantha*. (with white flowers.) These grow in the Western States on prairies, etc. and probably possess very similar qualities to the B. *tinctoria*, but none have been proven but the last named. As the other species may be mistaken for the one in use in our school, the botanical description of the B. tinctoria is here given from Wood:

"Smooth branching, *leaves* nearly destitute of a stalk, *leaflets* small, roundish, acute at base, very obtuse at apex; stipules bristly, falling off early; *racemes* loose, terminal; *legumes* nearly round. A plant with bluish

green foliage, frequent in dry soils.   *Stem* very bushy, about two and :ne
half feet high.   Leaflets about seven lines by four to six long, emarginate;
*petiole* one to two lines long.   *Flowers* six to twelve or more in each raceme.
*Petals* six lines long, yellow.   Legume (seed vessel) about as long as a pea-
pod, on a long stipule, mostly one-seeded."

OFFICINAL PREPARATION.—Tincture of the fresh bark of the root, with
strong alcohol.

The B. *leucantha* is equally active and trustworthy.  (*Hale.*)

SPHERE OF ACTION.—It exerts a marked action on the blood and vascular system, the nerves of sensation, and on the intestinal lesions common
to typhoid and other low types of fevers.  (*Hale.*)

On the gastric mucous membrane and the great semilunar ganglion of
the sympathetic nervous system. (*Bayes.*)

ANALOGUES.—*Bryonia, Agaricus, Kali chloricum, Nitric acid, Rhus tox.,
Muriatic acid, Arsenicum, Carbolic acid.*

### Mental Sphere.

* Restless, uneasy frightful dreams, gloomy and cast down for
    several days.

Indisposition and want of power to think; unhappy; mind
    seems weak.

° The patient imagines he "cannot get himself together," as
    if the pieces of his body were scattered about.  (*Bell.*)

° Stupefaction and drowsiness in typhoid, a "wild" feeling,
    with the headache.

### Head.

Sharp pains in both temples.

Dull, heavy, pressive headache, very much aggravated by
    motion.

Dull feeling in occiput, with pain and fullness of the vessels.

Vertigo, a confused feeling, or swimming sensation in the head.

* Peculiar feeling of the head, which is never felt except dur-
    ing the presence of fever, excitement of the brain, such
    as precedes delirium.

* Headache which precedes and accompanies typhoid fevers.

Head feels too large, and too heavy, with numb feeling of head
    and face.

*Soreness as if in the brain* in frontal region, with pain, heat,
    and vertigo, worse on stooping.  (*Muriatic acid.*)

Great tightness of the skin of the forehead, it feels as if it
    could be drawn to the back of the head, with pain in right
    eye, and pressive pain in right temple.

Pressive pain in the forehead, as if it would be pressed in, with sharp pain in both temples, very much aggravated by motion.

Severe pain in occiput, with dull, stupid feeling all over the head, with sharp pain over the eyes.

Brain feels numb with stitches, or shocks in various parts of the head.

Head feels heavy, as if he could not sit up, day and night, causing a "*wild*" feeling, aggravated by noise.

Severe frontal headache with severe pressure at the *root* of the nose.

Burning in the top of the head, with soreness of the scalp.

Head feels very heavy with pain in the occiput.

Stiffness and lameness of the cervical muscles.

Frontal headache with fulness and tightness of the whole head.

Heavy pain at the base of the brain, with lameness and stiffness of the cervical muscles.

[The last five symptoms are from a new proving by Dr. Wallace.]

° The peculiar headache preceding and during typhoid and cerebro-spinal fever, also from brain exhaustion.

° Her head feels as though scattered about, and she tosses about the bed to get the pieces together.

### Eyes.

Feeling as if the eyes would be pressed *into* the head, with great confusion of sight; cannot place anything till after looking at it a few seconds.

Vertigo, with sensation of paralysis of the lids, eyes smart and ache.

Bloated feeling of the eyes; eyes unusually glistening; disposition to have the eyes half closed; soreness in front part of the head upon moving the eyes or turning them upward; soreness of the eyeballs, eyes feel swollen, with burning and slight lachrymation; congestion of the vessels of the eye, they look red and inflamed.

Eyes feel sore and lame on moving them.

### Nose.

Thick mucus discharge from the nose.

Severe drawing pains along the nose.

Catarrh, with dull pain at the root of the nose.

### Face.

Burning heat of face; face flushed and hot; external vessels
of face distended and full; flashes of heat over the face,
which feels flushed and very hot; cheeks burn.

### Ears.

Deafness, or dullness of hearing, * during typhoid.

Roaring in the ears, with confusion of the mind.

### Mouth, Tongue, etc.

* Profuse flow of saliva, with small vesicles and ulcers in the
mouth.

Tongue feels as if it had been scraped or burnt.

* Tongue coated yellow along the centre, with flat, bitter taste
in the mouth.

* Tongue feels dry on rubbing it against the roof of the
mouth; smarts and feels as if burned.

Saliva abundant, viscid, with flat or filthy taste.

* Tongue coated white, with red papillæ protuberant, followed
by yellow, brown coating in the centre, the edges red and
shining.

Tongue feels swollen, thick, with numbness.

Teeth and gums feel sore, with bloody oozing from gums.

* *Great dryness of mouth and tongue, in fevers.*

° Chronic mercurial sore mouth, with fœtid breath.

° Stromatis materna, in feeble women, with offensive breath.

° Ulcerations of the mouth and fauces in diphtheria or small-
pox, with fœtor.

(The Baptisia should be used topically as well as internally. *Hale.*)

### Throat.

Sore throat, extending to the *posterior nares;* the throat feels
sore and contracted.

Soreness of the throat, with scraping and burning.

Raw sensation in pharynx, with abundant viscid mucus.

Constrictive feeling in throat, with frequent desire to swallow.

Pricking sensation in upper part of pharynx.

Throat feels swollen and full; tonsils and soft palate injected
with pain in root of tongue when swallowing.

The dryness of the mouth and tongue extends to the throat.

° Angina, with swelling, but with *unusual absence of pain.* (*Dr. Miner.*)

° *Diphtheria,* with fœtid breath, ulcerations of throat, and great prostration.

## Stomach.

Much distress in the stomach; severe pains every few moments in the cardiac region.

Dull pain in the epigastric region, frequently recurring, aggravated by turning over or walking.

Nausea, with eructations, followed by painful vomiting.

Disposition to vomit, without nausea.

\* "Gone," empty feeling in stomach.

° Dyspepsia, following typhus, with great sinking at stomach, frequent fainting, and brown tongue in morning.

Feeling as if there was a hard substance in stomach.

Stitching pain in the cardiac portion of stomach.

Nausea, with want of appetite, and constant desire for *water*

## Abdomen.

Constant pain in right hypochondriac region, with sharp, shooting pains in the bowels.

Severe colicky pains in the umbilical and hypochondriac regions, recurring every few seconds, with rumbling and desire for stool.

Pain in abdomen on pressure, with dull aching pain in the lumbar region on going to bed.

\* Fullness of the abdomen, with borborygmus and diarrhœa.

Pain in the hypogastrium, with soreness of the abdominal muscles as if from a cold, or from severe coughing.

\* Distension of the abdomen, with rumbling, and a feeling as if it would be a relief to vomit.

The small and large intestines filled with bloody mucus. (pathological appearance in a cat.)

° Abdominal typhus, with ulcerations of Peyers glands.

## Liver.

Pain in the right hypochondriac region aggravated by walking; constant dull pain in the region of the gall bladder; the pain extends to the spine.

Soreness in the region of the liver; pain in the liver.

᷄ C.ngestion of the liver during typhoid fever.

## Stools and Rectum.

In large doses Baptisia is a drastic cathartic.

Stools are generally dark, offensive, mucus and bloody

Vomiting and diarrhœa, with dark stools.

Rumbling in the bowels and desire for stool, with soft papescent stool with much mucus. ( *p.*)

Severe constipation and hemorrhoids after the diarrhœa. (*s.*)

* Frequent, small, offensive, and acrid stools.

Dysentery, with offensive, bloody discharges.

° Dysentery after confinement, with violent colicky pains in
the hypogastric region before stool, with great tenesmus;
stools pure blood with a little mucus, occurring every five
minutes.

° Dysentery, with bloody, mucus evacuations, tormina, brown
coat on the tongue, with low fever.

° Autumnal dysentery, with tendency to typhoid fevers.

## Urinary Organs.

Urine dark red and not very copious, with burning during
emission.

Shooting pains in the region of the left kidney

## Genital Organs.

Menses too soon and too profuse.

It is said to produce abortion.

° Fœtid lochia, with much prostration.

° Puerperal fever, with typhoid symptoms.

° Threatened abortion in typhoid fever.

## Respiratory Organs.

Hoarseness even to complete aphonia.

Tickling in the throat, provoking a cough.

Difficult breathing increased.

Increased compass and frequency of the pulsations of the
heart; pulsations seem to fill the chest.

Difficulty of breathing; the lungs feel tight and compressed;
cannot get a full breath.

* Tightness of the chest; feeling of want of power in the
respiratory apparatus, such as is felt during fever.

Constriction and oppression of the chest.

Oppressed respiration; sharp pains in the chest when taking a long breath; throbbing in the heart so as to be distinctly heard.

Awoke with great difficulty of breathing, the lungs feel tight and compressed; could not get a full breath; felt obliged to open the window, to get my face to the fresh air.

° Dyspnœa during the low stages of typhoid.

### Back.

Dull heavy pain in the lumbar region, very much aggravated by walking.

Back and hips are very stiff and ache severely.

Chills up and down the back as if ague were coming on.

Dull heavy aching in the lumbar region on going to bed at night; flashes of heat from the small of the back in all directions.

### Upper Extremities.

Stiffness of the joints as if strained, and twitching in the left deltoid, and latissimus dorsi of left side.

Soreness of muscles of neck; muscular debility; feeling of weariness in the right arm and shoulder.

Hands feel too large, and are tremulous with a thrilling sensation as if going to sleep.

### Lower Extremities.

Dull drawing pains in right groin and testicle; also in the legs and knee joints.

Burning heat of feet; feeling of pulsation.

Dull pain in the sacrum, extending round the hips and down the right leg.

Extremities feel hot, except the feet, which are cold.

Cramp in the calves when walking.

Aching in the limbs; heat and burning in the lower extremities so intense as to prevent sleep most of the night.

### Skin.

A general redness, like Erythema, all over the body.

° A hot, pungent, but moist skin (in typhoid fever).

° Intense heat of the skin, which may be dry or moist.

### Sleep.

*Heavy sleep,* with feverish feeling on waking.

Sleeps well till two A. M., then very restless till morning.

Very restless sleep, with *frightful dreams*.

Dreams of being bound down with a chain across his mouth.

Cannot sleep after midnight.

### Fever.

Feeling of greatly increased compass and frequency of the
   pulsations of the *heart*.

Pulsations of the heart seem to fill the chest.

The pulse (usually seventy) is ninety, full and soft.

Uncomfortable *heat* of the whole surface, especially the face.

\* The feverish heat, at night, compelled him to move to a cool
   part of the bed, and finally to rise and open a window, and
   bathe his face and hands. With these symptoms there
   was a peculiar feeling in the head, which is never felt
   except during the presence of fever—a sort of excitement
   of the brain, which is the preliminary, or rather the
   beginning, of delirium.

Chilly sensations over the back and lower limbs.

\* Burning sensation over the whole body, followed by perspiration, vomiting and diarrhœa of dark stools, debility,
   and slow, round, full pulse.

*Thirst*, and flashes of heat over the face.

General heat after going to bed.

\* Heat and burning in the lower extremities so intense as to
   prevent sleep.

\* Chill all day, with fever at night; rheumatic pains and *soreness all over the body; mouth and tongue very dry.*

\* *Feverishness, with feeling all over as if bruised; the parts
   on which he is lying soon ache, and feel sore and bruised.*

° *Typhoid fever*, in the *premonitory stage* of bilious, gastric,
   or catarrhal origin—or from impure exhalations—it will
   often prevent the *access* of the fever. (*Hughes. Hale.*)

° *Typhoid fever in the first stages;* it will often *arrest* the
   disease, and bring about a rapid convalescence. (*Hale.*)

° *Typhus fever*, with heavy sleep, unconsciousness, delirious
   muttering, etc.

° *Fevers*, with drowsiness; pulse one hundred and twenty, and
   thready; lips parched and cracked; pasty tongue, heavily

coated; gieat thirst; mind wandering; could not give a
direct answer to any question; falls asleep in the middle
of a sentence; delirious at night, and low muttering.
(*Dr. C. C. Smith.*)

*Gastric fevers*, with nausea, vomiting, dry, baked tongue,
rapid pulse, tenderness of the abdomen, diarrhœa. (*J.
Harmer Smith.*)

° *Scarlet fever*, with dark-red eruption; dry, brown tongue,
inclined to be red in the centre; fœtid breath; stupor;
fever; dysenteric stools. (*Hale.*)

° *Catarrhal fever*, or influenza, when the prostration is excessive, and the sore, bruised pains and sensations predominate. (*Hale.*)

° *Bilious fevers; gastric fevers; enteric fevers; septic fevers.*

° Fevers setting in during dysentery, or any intestinal affection, and assuming a low type. (*Hale.*)

° Puerperal fevers, from absorption of purulent matters, or
from infection.

° *Cerebro-spinal*, or "spotted fever." (*Dr. W. S. Searle.*)

### Nervous System.

The hands felt large, and were tremulous, with a peculiar
thrilling sensation through both hands and feet, somewhat like going to sleep — a want of circulation.

Intolerance of pressure on any part of the body—it caused
soreness.

Numb sensations all over the body.

Sensation of paralysis of the eyelids.

Numbness and prickling, followed by temporary paralysis of
the left side of the body.

The left hand and arm entirely numb and powerless.

Prickling numb sensations in the extremities, with burning
and prickling of left side of face and head.

### Generalities.

\* Feels weak and tremulous, as though recovering from a fit of
sickness.

Incapable of making any vigorous mental or physical exertion.

An indescribable sick feeling all over, with great languor.

Stiffness of all the joints, as though strained.

\* *A sensation all over the body as if bruised or beaten.*

Very great prostration of the whole system.

Lying in one position for a few moments, or upon the back, caused the sacral region to become exceedingly painful, as though I had lain on a hard floor all night, and induced the conviction that a short continuance of the same position would cause bedsore; when turning on the other side, the same sensation was produced on the hips. (*Dr. J. S. Douglas.*)

It prevents too rapid metamorphosis of tissues during illnesses, or from too long sustained mental and physical exertions.

---

# BAROSMA CRENATAS.

## (*Buchu.*)

BOTANICAL DESCRIPTION.—It is a slender, smooth, upright, perrenial shrub, between two and three feet in height, with twiggy, somewhat angular branches, of a brownish purple color, growing in various parts of South America.

OFFICINAL PREPARATION—Tincture from the leaves, with dilute alcohol.

ANALOGUES.—*Copaiva, Chimaphila, Erigeron, Terebinthina, Uva ursi.*

[*No proving,* but its importance demands one; it would doubtless cause, secondarily, all the conditions given below. (*Hale.*)]

° *Gastric catarrh,* causing chronic dyspepsia.

° *Intestinal catarrh,* chronic.

° Chronic maladies of the urino-genital organs, characterized by *muco-purulent secretions.*

° *Chronic inflammation* of the pelvis, of the kidneys, and mucous membranes of the bladder. attended with copious discharge of mucus.

° *Irritable bladder,* from vesical catarrh.

° *Irritable* conditions of the *urethra,* as spasmodic stricture.

° *Gleet,* with profuse discharge.

° *Lithiasis,* with increased secretion of lithic acid. (*Pereira.*)

° *Prostatic affections,* with abnormal discharge.

° Incontinence of urine from irritability of neck of bladder.

° Dropsy; idiopathic anasarca.

° *Leucorrhœa,* complicated with vesical diseases.

° Undue secretion from the mucous follicles of the urethra, the vesiculæ seminales or prostate, produced by excessive venery, or self-polution. (*Stille.*)

---

# BROMIDE OF CAMPHOR.
### (*Monobromide of Camphor.*)

[The Monobromide of Camphor consists of one equivalent of camphor united with one of bromine. (C. 10. H. 16 O, Br.) It is a white crystalline salt, having the odor of camphor, and to a slight extent that of bromine. It decomposes readily when exposed to the atmosphere, to a heat of 100. This new medicine, first used by a Belgian Physician, and then by Dr. Hammond, of New York, bids fair to prove a very useful remedy. No experience with its use in homœopathic practice—save my own—has yet come to my knowledge. I give the authority, and the doses used. (*Hale.*)]

OFFICINAL PREPARATION.—*Triturations.*

ANALOGUES.—*Ambergris, Coffea, Cimicifuga,* (?) *Gelseminum,* (?) *Conium,* (?) *Scutellaria, Thea, Valerian.*

### Mind.
Delirium, furious, with red face and threatened spasms. (*p.*)
° Delirium, muttering, incoherent, with sleeplessness. (*s.*)
° Alternate paroxysms of weeping and laughing.

### Head.
* Cerebral congestion, with great nervous erethism. (*p.*)
* Cerebral anæmia, with coldness, torpor and debility. (*s.*)
* Headache from mental excitement or excessive study. (*p.*)
* Headache from anæmia, with sleeplessness. (*s.*)

### Generative Organs.
Debility, coldness and relaxation of the generative organs. (*p.*) (in man.)
Absence of sexual desire or power (*p.*) in both sexes.
* Sexual erethism, spasmodic erections, emissions, etc. (*s.*)
* Hysterical conditions, mania, etc., from irritation of the sexual organs. (*s.*)

### Generalities.
* Epileptiform, hysteric and choreiform spasms. (*p.*)
* Coldness of the body and extremities, with cramps and jactitations.

[In cats and Guinea pigs it causes:
A lessening of the number of the pulsations of the *heart;* and it determines the contractions of the auricular muscles.

Diminishes the number of inspirations.

Lowers the temperature in a regular manner. (*p.*)

Increase of the temperature of the body. (*s.*)

° It calms the cerebro-spinal nervous system and the circulation.

° Tremblings, excitability, insomnia and visual delusions.

° Insomnia with heart disease. (3 grs.)

° Insomnia (in locomotor ataxia) with nightmare. (12 grs.)

° Chorea, not able to walk or lie in bed. (16 grs. palliated.)

° Paralysis agitans. (4 to 15 grs. caused amendment.)

° Chorea in the left arm. (9 grs. daily, cured in five days.)

° Hysterical chorea with vomiting. (9 grs. daily, rapidly cured.)

° Insufficiency of the mitral valve. (Digitaline aggravated; under the Brom. Camph. the heart-beats diminished in frequency and became regular for two weeks after.)

° Nocturnal incontinence of urine. (cured by 6 grs.)

° Paralysis agitans. (much relieved.)

(See Therapeutics, Vol. II.)

---

# BELLIS PERENNIS.

### (*English Daisy.*)

DESCRIPTION.—The only Bellis (Daisy) indigenous to this country—B integrifolia; grows profusely all over the United States; has probably the same properties. The B. perennis is a native of England.

OFFICIAL PREPARATIONS.—Tincture of the plant; infusion.

ANALOGUES.—*Arnica, Hamamelis*, (?) *Rhus.* (?) *Leucanthemum.*

A large boil on the back of my neck, (for the first time in my life,) right side, commencing with a dull aching pain; some difficulty and bruised pain in keeping the head erect; slight nausea, want of appetite, and a little giddiness in the head. Pain in the little finger of the left hand, as of a gathering; at the same time pain in inner side of left forearm, as of a boil developing; afterwards similar pain in right arm.

A boil beginning as a slight pimple, with burning pain in skin, increasing until in six days' time it was very large, of a fiery purple color, and very sore; burning and aching pain in it, accompanied with headache, extending from occiput to sinciput; of a cold, aching character. The brain felt as if contracted, with vertigo. This was followed by other boils. (*From provings by Dr. Thomas, in "Additions to Mat. Med.," London,* 1868.)

° Boils, all over the body. (*Dr. Thomas.*)

° *Bruises,* with extravasated blood. (*Ib.*)

° *Sprains* of ankle and wrist. (*Ib.*)

° *Whitlows.* (*Ib.*) (Dr. Thomas used it in the same manner as Arnica.)

---

# BENZOATE OF AMMONIA.

### (*Ammonia Benzoas.*)

PHARMACOLOGY.—This salt may be made as follows: Take of solution of ammonia three fluid ounces (imperial measure), benzoic acid two ounces (avoirdupois), distilled water four ounces; mix the solution of ammonia and the water, and dissolve in them the benzoic acid; evaporate at a gentle heat, keeping ammonia in a slight excess, and set aside that crystals may form.

It is in minute, white, glistening, extremely thin, four-sided laminæ, having a slight odor of officinal benzoic acid, and a bitter, saline, somewhat balsamic taste, leaving a slight but persistent sense of acrimony on the tongue.

Soluble in water and alcohol, when heated sublimes without residue; but is probably changed into acid benzoate.

OFFICINAL PREPARATIONS.—Triturations; tinctures in distilled water; dilutions to the 3d × with water.

The Benzoate of Potassa is now used more extensively, and may be the best preparation.

ANALOGUES.—*Benzoic acid, Colchicum, Ferr. mur. Lycopodium.* (?)

### Head.

Rheumatic pains about the head and neck.

° Heaviness and stupidity of the head. (in dropsy.)

### Face.

Bloated face, with swollen eyelids.

### Urinary Organs.

\* Very *scanty*, dark-red, bloody-looking urine, with strong ammoniacal odor, and red, thick sediment.

Scanty, dark and smoky-looking urine.

Frequent desire to urinate, with scanty discharge.

The urine is acrid and irritating. (primary effect.)

7

*Profuse* and frequent urination.

Clear, limpid, and abundant urine.

The sediment disappears from the urine.   (secondary.)

˷ Nocturnal incontinence of urine.

\* Scanty, blood-red urine in rheumatic affections.

° Urinary troubles of infants.

° *Dropsy after scarlet fever*, or Bright's diseases.

### Extremities.

° Rheumatic affections of the arms and legs and small joints.

° Dropsical swelling of the legs.

° *Jaundice*, from *suppression* of the biliary secretion (*not* from obstruction of the *ducts*).   (*Harley.*)

*Gout*, when the small joints are red and swollen, or when fluid is deposited in the joint of the great toe; and also in cases when the lithate of soda existed in the joints of the fingers.   (*Seymour.*)

° *Albuminuria;* the albumen in real dropsy diminished under its use.   (*Ib.*)

---

# BERBERINA.

**Pharmacology.**—Berberina is obtained from many plants, notably from Hydrastis, Coptis Columbo, as well as from the Berberis vulgaris, from which plant it takes its name.   It is the *yellow* principle of the roots of all these plants.   The Hydrastia sold as the active principle of golden-seal is principally Berberina.   The true Hydrastia is composed of colorless crystals.   The salts of Berberina, as well as the alkaloid itself, is very sparingly soluble in cold water or alcohol.   The Muriate of Berberina is generally used, although many physicians prefer the Sulphate.   A phosphate is now extensively·used, under the name of Phosphate of Hydrastia. I think the Hypophosphite will be found superior to all others of its salts. The wrongly-named Muria˸e of Hydras*tina*, as well as other salts of Hydras*tina*, are all salts of Berberina.

**Official Preparations.**—Triturations of the alkaloid or its salts.

**Analogues.**—*Aletris, China, (Quinia,) Coptis, Columbo, Berberis, Hydrastis, Helonias, Nux vom., Pte'ea, Ferrum, Gentiana.*

(See Therapeutics of *Hydrastis*, and compare Pathogenesis of Berberis.)

° *Muscular debility*, atony and wasting.

˓ *Myalgia*, and all the pains incident thereto.

° Enlargement of the liver. (and spleen?)

˒ Intermittent fevers; remittent fevers.

° Loss of appetite, with slow and imperfect digestion.
[Useful in all cases where Hydrastis is recommended *except in diseases of mucous membrane.*]

---

# BI-SULPHIDE OF CARBON.

### (*Carburetum Sulphuris.*)

OFFICINAL PREPARATIONS.—Tincture and dilutions.

### Mental Sphere.

Loss of memory, and mental alienation.

Great absence of mind, with difficult comprehension of what is read.

They forgot what they had to do; sought for things which were lying before them; could not find the right words when speaking.

Cheerfulness, with inclination to sing.

Exhilaration bordering on intoxication.

Vehement and irascible.   Dejection of spirits.

### Head.

*Frequent attacks of vertigo* when sitting.

Dullness and vertigo in the forehead.

° Intoxication, to entire loss of consciousness, from drinking whisky.

° Asphyxia, from alcohol and from coal gas.

*Great dullness of the head.*

Pressing headache in the forehead, aggravated by reading and stooping.

Pressing frontal headache, with occasional flying, tearing pains in the temples.

Drawing, tearing pain from the forehead toward the temples; better in the open air than in the room, when at rest.

Frontal headache, more of a tearing nature, which goes toward the temporal bones.

Frequent, transitory, jerking stitches in the forehead; heat in the head and face.

Violent, pulsating pains in the temples (megrim), on awakening in the morning.

Head very painful when brushing the hair, particularly on the verte ..

° Violent pain in the head; headache increasing until it causes confusion of mind; feverish attacks; cold extremities, and spasmodic pulse.

Pain in the head is connected with the discharge of blood with the stool.

### Eyes.

Weakness of the sight; objects seem as if fading away, on account of a mistiness, which spreads out before them.

Pupils enlarged.

Sensation of pressure in the sockets of the eyes.

Jerking stitches in the muscles of the right eye; intermitting and alternating.

Burning in the eyes, with pain in the forehead.

Heaviness of the eyelids, and dimness of the eyes.

A small pustule on the upper eyelid, with itching-burning.

Eye sunken, with strongly marked gray rings.

Quivering of the eyelids.

### Ears.

*Violent stitches and contractive pain in the left ear*, at night.

Pressing, boring pains in the right ear.

Ringing in the ears, lasting several days.

### Nose.

Everything smells like the drug.

Frequent sneezing.

End of the nose burns, and is quite red; eruption on the nose.

### Face.

Face bloated up and red; convulsive jerking of the corners of the mouth.

*In the mornings, after shaving, a red eruption* on the cheeks and nose similar to the eruptions on the noses of hard drinkers, looking like tetter, and lasting till night.

Eruption makes its appearance after drinking a glass of beer.

### Mouth.

Saltish taste of the phlegm hawked up from the fauces.

Constant accumulation of sweetish tasting water in the mouth.

Increased flow of saliva, with increased appetite.

Toothache, with a gradually formed swelling around the painful tooth.

**Drawing,** tearing toothache, from evening until midnight, more endurable in the greatest cold.

Toothache in the molars of lower jaw, right side.

° Toothache brought on by warm food.

° Neuralgic odontalgia.

Sensation of coldness, first on the tongue, then in the mouth, which quickly rises to a stitching burning.

Burning, pungent pain on the tongue, as from peppermint, with peculiar onion or garlic taste.

### Throat.

Immediately after lying down, tickling in the posterior portion of the palate, causing a violent dry cough.

° Rough, scraping pain in the left side of the throat when swallowing.

° Burning and scraping in the whole of the œsophagus, with difficult swallowing.

Severe stitching, contracting pain in the upper part of the œsophagus, as if a piece of bone had lodged there.

° Chronic pharyngitis.

Scraping, scratching feeling, with fine stitches in the throat.

### Appetite—Thirst.

Increased appetite, with a pleasant warmth spreading through the stomach.

Great thirst; beer relished unusually.

After breakfast, headache, pressure in the stomach, diarrhœa.

After dinner, diarrhœa; tickling in urethra; pain in thigh; pain in feet.

After eating, and in the cold, all the symptoms disappear, or are ameliorated.

Aggravation of the symptoms from wine.

### Stomach.

Rising of flatulence, tasting and smelling of the medicine; also disagreeable, putrid-tasting, nauseous fluid.

Acrid, burning eructations.

Heartburn so severe that it causes cough.

Extraordinary amount of loud eructations, and very stinking flatus in the evening; better from belching; inclination to vomit; pain in scrobiculum; pressure of stomach, impeded respiration.

Vomiting of greenish, bilious masses, accompanied with nausea, cold sweat, and dejection of spirits.

Increased amount of saliva in the mouth and stomach, producing nausea; accumulation of water in the mouth; eructations; fullness in the stomach and abdomen; rumbling and cutting in the abdomen, from wind; also cutting, tearing belly-ache; a bubbling in bowels, relieved by copious diarrhœic stools; also producing dullness of the head; attacks of vertigo; pressing frontal headache; surly mood; sleepiness during the day, and sleeplessness at night; confused dreams.

Inclination to vomit on entering a room, or when going out from the room to the open air.

° A single attack; vomiting a small quantity of bitter water.

Fullness of the stomach, with belching, yawning, and inclination to vomit.

Pressing, tearing pain in the chest, stomach and abdomen.

° Pressure in the region of the stomach, and under the sternum, with hepatic depression.

Pressing, stitching pains, of short duration, in the pit of the stomach, beginning at one point and radiating to the cardiac region, like neuralgic colic, followed by loud belching, which gives relief.

Very severe stabbing pains in the stomach.

Burning in the stomach and region of the liver, aggravated by pressure.

Pressure on stomach and abdomen increases nausea.

### Hypochondrium.

Diseased condition of the liver, with swelling of the feet.

Unpleasant, undefined, painful feeling in the region of the left lobe of the liver, coming on in attacks; this pain changes to a pressing (distending), stitching feeling.

Under short ribs, stitches.

### Abdomen.

Pressing, crampy pain in the abdomen; passing much flatus, both up and down.

Pains in the bowels, with twisting, rolling, and rumbling, as if diarrhœa would set in.

<sup>c</sup> Colicky pains, cutting, with diarrhœa.

Griping pains in the bowels, followed by stool; after the stool the pains cease.

On awaking at 4 A. M., cutting in the abdomen, with a moving swelling as if from flatus or incarcerated wind; on taking a deep inspiration, and from pressure, this pain changed into a stitch pain, and settled in the region of the cœcum for about one hour; small passages of wind has no influence on this condition; turning in bed or bending increased the pain or brought it on anew after it had nearly passed off.

<sup>o</sup> Puffiness of the abdomen, with bruised, sore feeling of the abdominal walls.

<sup>c</sup> Fullness and distension of the abdomen.

<sup>c</sup> Flatulent complaints; sour smelling flatus.

Single, fine, jerking stitches, extending from the right side of the umbilical region toward the bladder.

In cœcal region, on taking a deep inspiration or from pressure, a cutting in abdomen changed into a stitching pain, settling in cœcum, often repeating.

<sup>o</sup> Strangulated hernia.

### Stool.

Papescent stool, with urging; during the passage, and particularly afterwards, a feeling of weakness and trembling.

Stool always papescent and small; papescent stool with discharge of blood.

Papescent stools, preceded by the peculiar stitching, distending pains in the abdomen, and followed by griping, stitching pains in the cœcum.

During rumbling in the bowels, violent diarrhœa of sour-smelling stools, with tenesmus.

Awakes at 5½ A. M., with urging to stool; profuse, thin, yellowish evacuations, followed by burning at the anus, as from an acid.

<sup>o</sup> A chronic diarrhœa, which set in every four or six weeks, and lasted for one or two days; yellowish, frothy, sour-

smelling fluid evacuations, with tenesmus and colicky belly-ache, particularly in the umbilical region, in the night.

Difficult, small stools, even when the passage is small and soft, as if from want of power in the rectum.

° Constipation, with belching after eating, with herpes.

No desire for stool for three days, when he had a soft passage, with discharge of bright red blood.

° Griping; urging before; pains before; tenesmus with the stool; with diarrhœa.

Anus and rectum, stitch-like, cramping pain; likewise in the bladder and urethra.

Burning and itching at the anus, with flying stitches in the rectum.

### Urinary Organs.

After drinking a glass of wine, on urinating at midnight, violent, stitch-like, cramping pain in the bladder and neck of bladder, extending through the urethra; at the same time a.similar pain in the anus and rectum.

Burning in the urethra when urinating; slight irritability of the mucous lining of the urethra; urine smells like sulphur; *increase of sulphates and carbonates in the urine.*

Strong urging to urinate.

### Sexual Organs.

Entire want of sexual desire, and of erections; inability to have sexual intercourse (constant); increased sexual desire was observed in only one case.

Complete impotence, with atrophied testicles.

Erection at night, with emission of semen.

Stitching, burning pains in the left seminal cord, up to the abdominal ring.

Jerking, stitching pains in the left testicle and left seminal cord.

Left testicle and epididymis swollen and indurated.

Scrotum and penis shriveled and drawn up during the entire proving.

The previously regular menses appeared three days too soon.

' Labor-pains too weak.

## Larynx.

Hoarseness.

Sensation of contraction of the larynx upon swallowing the drug, producing great irritation to cough, even to strangulation, and expectoration of mucus.

Scratching and scraping feeling in the throat; irritation to cough.

Violent dry cough, from tickling in palate after lying down.

Immediately after lying down, violent, asthmatic, dry cough, brought on by a continued and irritating tickling in the upper part of the pharynx, causing much straining of the chest, and producing pain.

Cough from irritation in larynx, even to strangulation, and expectoration of mucus.

Anxious breathing, with pressure on the sternum; aggravated by the close air of the room and from going up stairs.

Expiration hot; breathing difficult; flying stitches and burning in the chest, quickly passing over, but frequently repeated.

Difficult breathing, with nausea.

## Chest.

Throughout the whole chest, agreeable warmth, ascending from the pit of the stomach.

Congestion of the lungs, which appears to affect the upper lobes most.

Deposit of tubercles in the lungs, some ecchymosis and some infiltration.  (Rabbits.)

Hepatisation of the lower or posterior lower surface of the lungs.  (Rabbits.)

° In the first stage of tuburculosis of the lungs, before any, or yet only slight, fever has set in, flying, burning and stitches in the chest; quickly passing heat of the face; dry cough; difficult breathing when moving.

° *Constrictive, stitching, pressing pains in the chest.*

Jerking, stitching pain, first in the region of the right, and then of the left, lower ribs, quickly coming and going.

Periodical stitches in the left half of the chest, without cough.

Several violent stitches under the centre of the sternum, shooting upwards like a flash of lightning.

### Heart.

° Palpitation of the heart, with anæmic patients in an advanced stage of the disease; nun's murmur in the vessels of the neck; fever symptoms not frequent, and mostly at night. In one case, diminution of the pulse to fifty-two beats in a minute.

### Neck and Back.

Painful stiffness in the neck and throat; rheumatic-like pains. ° Goitre.

Feeling as if a heavy load was hanging on the back (from one scapula to the other), weighing him down so that the head sank forward.

*Continual backache and pain in the loins.*

Violent pains in the back and loins, in the morning when awakening.

### Upper Extremities.

Stitches from the shoulder joint to the elbow, or even to the wrist, especially violent after midnight, and during damp or cold weather.

° Crackling in the right shoulder joint from strong motions of the arms, either forward, backward, or upward.

° Crackling in the right shoulder joint from every motion, connected with more or less severe stitches from the shoulder joint to the elbow, on every change of the weather.

Violent rheumatic pain in the right arm, shoulder and neck.

° Pimples on the right forearm and hands.

Jerking pains in the joints of the hand, coming and going.

° Gout of the hand.

Itching and smarting of the hands, particularly between the fingers, where he discovered small vesicles.

° Vesicular, scurfy herpes on the dorsum of the hand.

Pricking, stitching sensation in the fingers, more or less through the whole day.

### Lower Extremities.

Jerking, stitching pains at different places, particularly on the tuber ischii, and at the insertions of the gracilis and sartorious muscles at the knee.

° Rheumatism of the lower extremities; the slightest motion brings on violent pains, particularly in the hips and knees, with redness and swelling of the feet from a severe cold.

° Dropsical swelling of the feet, arising from diseased condition of the liver.

° Inflammatory sciatica in left thigh, brought on by taking cold, with entire inability to walk.

° Chronic sciatica in right thigh, movements of the limbs impeded.

Tearing pains in the right knee and ankle joint.

° Jerking, flying, stitching pains in the legs.

Violent pains in the ankle joints, as if broken, in the morning in bed; after getting up, the walking, at first, very difficult, but continuing to walk makes it easier.

° Audible crackling of the ankle when walking—ankle was sprained two years ago.

Sudden, violent, stabbing, piercing pain from the metatarsal bones through the toes, while walking.

Tearing pains in the left foot, particularly in the tarsal bones.

Feet, pains; underpart; hollow of the foot; soles of the feet.

Severe painful tenderness and bruised feeling in the soles of the feet; knee to the great toe stitches.

Painful cramp of the limbs; involuntary contractions and stiffness of the limbs; staggering gait, on account of general weakness of the muscles; paralysis; atrophy of the muscles.

° Chronic, rheumatic and arthritic affections without fever.

*Jerking, stitching, tearing, flying pains, returning at regular intervals, for a long time.*

° Rheumatism, either without fever or with slight fever.

° Tearing in the limbs, with herpes of the face.

° Tearing in all the limbs, coming and going, now in one and again in another limb; sour belching, and passage of much sour-smelling flatus; cold feet; stool not increased, but accompanied with tenesmus.

° Rheumatism and gout; after the relief of the acute and inflammatory conditions, to be applied externally, with oil

ot almonds, or, when the sufferings are great, to be taken
internally.

° Gouty swellings when not of too long standing.

### Sleep.

Great sleepiness the whole day, but at night restless sleep.

*Restless sleep*, with continual rolling about in bed; particularly with the head.

Sleeplessness, *disturbed dreams*, starting as from fright, followed during the day by lassitude, want of energy.

Good and long sleep during the night.

### Fever.

Heat of the whole body, with slight headache, followed by
great debility, succeeded by sleep.

Coldness, with succeeding burning pain.

Coldness of the legs, with general warmth of the upper part
of the body.

Cold face; coldness in mouth; cold extremities.

Pulse diminished to 52 beats; pulse, 90–93.

Strong pulse; spasmodic pulse.

### Skin.

° Itch and herpetic diseases.

° Herpes phlyctænodes covering dorsal surface of the hand;
vesicles appearing on a red, inflamed and swollen basis;
partly close together, but mostly separated from each
other. They contain an opaque, yellowish fluid, which is
discharged, and forms thick, yellowish scabs; sometimes
the discharge excoriates the surrounding parts and produces violent itching.

° Impetigo; pimples which form scabs, in the popliteal space
and on the dorsum of the foot and hand.

° A tetter-like eruption on the left cheek, for more than two
years, produced through scratching with the finger nails;
spreads, and is covered with yellowish-brown scabs, dis-
figuring the face; almost unbearable on acount of continued itching.

° Herpes exedens; together with constipation and alternating
of cutting pains in abdomen and flatulency; drawing and
tearing in the limbs, and particularly in the head.

Itching on both thighs, right side of the back to the region of
the kidneys, and on the right forearm, which necessitates
scratching. On inspection, small, colorless pimples are
seen, which, on scratching, are more irritated, and through
the friction they redden, get points, and finally form an
itch-like eruption.

Nodules on scalp, pustule on eyelid, eruption on nose and face.

° Slight burning of the left hand with boiling water; bright
redness without much pain or swelling.

° Wrist joint was scalded with boiling water, several days ago;
wrist much swollen, blisters partially opened.

---

## BROMIDE OF AMMONIUM.

### (*Ammonium Bromidum.*)

PHARMACOLOGY.—This salt may be prepared by dissolving Bromine in
water of Ammonia. The liquid becomes heated, Nitrogen escapes with
effervescence, and the solution assumes a slight yellowish color, in consequence of an excess of Bromine after saturation. After evaporation the
Bromide is obtained in four sided prisms, sometimes crossing each other
at right angles.

A better method than this is by adding to Bromine and water a sufficient
solution of hydrosulphate of Ammonia to discharge the color, filtering to
separate the sulphur, and then evaporating to dryness.

Soluble in 1.5 parts water, and in 13 parts alcohol.

It is incompatible with acids and acid salts.

OFFICINAL PREPARATIONS. — Mother-tincture; (prepared by dissolving
one part in nine parts distilled water). Dilutions in water up to the 3 ×,
afterwards with alcohol.

ANALOGUES. — *Bromides of Potassium, Sodium, Lithium,* ( *Drosera,
Spongia, Secale, Ustilago.* (*?*)

### Head.

\* Sensation as if a band were tied around the head, pressing
the hardest just above the ears.

\* Pain in right side of head, near the eye, as if a nail were
driven in.

° Sharp pain in left side of head.

In cases where there is suspicion of the existence of congestion of the base of the brain, and still more of congestion
of the spinal cord, or its meninges, the Bromide of
Ammonia is preferable to the Bromide of Potassa.
(*Brown Sequard.*)

\* Headache from congestion of the brain.

° Epilepsy, when the predominant symptom is intense congestion of the brain. (*Brown Sequard.*)

° Cerebro-spinal meningitis; in the congestive stage. (*Hale.*)

### Eyes.

° Pain around both eyes, into the head.

° Right eye full of white, stringy mucus.

Looks as if a membrane were growing over the eye, like a
pterygium.

Both eyes very sore and red; lids stuck together in the morning.

Eyeballs unnaturally full, large.

Every evening eyelids droop, and it is painful and difficult to
raise them.

° Strumous opthalmia, conjunctivitis, corneitis, leucoma.

### Nose.

Discharge of stringy mucus from the nose.

° Catarrh of the anterior and posterior nares, of thick, stringy
mucus.

### Mouth and Throat.

White, stringy, tasteless mucus in the mouth.

Accumulation of mucus in the throat.

Fauces, and top of tongue for half its length, feel as if scalded.

Stinging in fauces, inclination to cough, relieved by sneezing.

Tongue very sore, as if burnt; cannot talk or read without
pain.

Throat looks mottled, as if diphtheric deposit were commencing. (*See Brom. Pot.*)

### Larynx and Trachea.

Cough caused by a secretion of mucus in the throat.

Tickling in the throat in the morning, with inclination to
cough.

Irritation of the throat, with inclination to cough.

° Sudden, deep cough, spasmodic, causing a pain in the stomach.

\* Irritation of the organs of respiration and stomach, accompanied with spasmodic cough, and even a distinct whoop,
simulating whooping-cough. (*Okie.*)

° Whooping cough, many cases. (*Drs. Harley, Gibbs.*)

\* Cough deep, spasmodic, and very severe, and at times an
interval of only a few moments, almost continuous for
hours, especially when lying down at night, with a sensation of tickling irritation, with heat and burning. (*Hale.*)

° Cough distressing, hoarse, dry, spasmodic, asthmatic and
exhausting, without expectoration. (*Talbot. Cushing.*)

### Chest.

Tightness across the chest, with pain in the chest; inclination
to take a long, deep breath.

Swallowing anything cold causes a feeling of distress the
whole length of the œsophagus.

Sensation on top of right shoulder as if a heavy load were
upon it.

### Stomach.

Something seems to issue from the stomach, as if it would
stop my breath, causing a faint and disagreeable sensation, and belching of wind, which relieves me.

Sensation as of hot air passing up the throat on the right side,
though the stomach feels cold.

### Back.

Feeling as though something were pressed hard against the
right kidney; relieved by pressure, but leaving a pulling
sensation.

### Uterus.

° In all forms of uterine hemorrhage, whether from lesions of
the uterus itself, from ovarian irritation, excitation, inflammation, or any of the various diseased or deranged
actions peculiar to the ovaries or adjoining parts and
viscera. (*Griffith.*)

° Amenorrhœa, dysmenorrhœa. I have used it with great
alleviation of suffering. (*Griffith.*)

° Premature and profuse menses.

### Superior Extremities.

Great lameness, with sharp pains in back of left leg, midway
from the hip to the knee.

Pains leave the right leg, and are felt in the left in same place.

Pains leave above the knee, and are felt below the knee, then
in the ankle, then in the foot.

## BROMIDE OF. IRON.

### (*Ferri Bromidum.*)

This is obtained by heating gently in thirty parts water, two parts bromine, and one of iron filings.   When the liquid has become greenish, it is filtered and evaporated to dryness in an iron vessel; and the dry mass is again dissolved and evaporated to dryness.

It is a black-red deliquescent salt, very soluble and styptic.

Soluble in water.

OFFICIAL PREPARATIONS.—Tincture; must be made as follows:   Take of Bromide of Iron one part, add three parts of sugar and ten of distilled water.   Dilutions, to the 3d × with distilled water; higher with alcohol.

ANALOGUES.—*Bromide of Potassa, Bromide of Ammonium, Caladium.*
*(See Therapeutics, Vol. II.)*

---

## BROMIDE OF LITHIUM.

### (*Lithium Bromidum.*)

PHARMACOLOGY.—This salt may be made by adding to a solution of iron and bromine in water an excess of the Carbonate of Lithia, filtering to separate the oxide of iron, and concentrating.

It is a very deliquescent salt; is soluble at 32° in .7 its weight of water.

OFFICIAL PREPARATIONS.—Aqueous tincture; ( ℨ i to ℨ ix.)and dilutions to the 3 × with distilled water.

ANALOGUES.—*Bromides of Potassa, Ammonia, and Soda, Chloral hydrate, Belladonna, Conium, Opium.*

° *Threatened apoplexy,* or cerebral congestion, with or without hemorrhage.   A gentleman who had had one attack, and was in consequence hemiplegic, was taken with *vertigo, headache, numbness,* and thickness of speech.   One dose of thirty grains removed the symptoms in less than half an hour!  (Dr. S. W. Mitchell observes that it acts quicker than the other bromides.)

° *Epilepsy.*  When the Bromide of Potassium loses its effect, or disagrees, the Lithium salt arrests the paroxysms.

° Epileptic fit every morning on rising; (cured by ten grains twice a day.)

° Relieved a case in which any prolonged mental exertion flushed the face, caused intense pain between the shoulders, and insomnia.

° It removes obstinate *sleeplessness* more promptly and surely than the other bromides.

## Skin.

It does not cause the *acne,* eruptions, and skin-ulcers of the other bromides.

---

# BROMIDE OF POTASSIUM.

PHARMACOLOGY.—This Salt is prepared by adding a solution of pure carbonate of potassa to a solution of bromide of iron. The iron is pre cipitated and the bromide of potassium remains in solution, from which it is obtained by evaporating. It forms white, pearly, transparent crys tals. They are without smell, and have a sharp saline taste resembling that of common salt, but more pungent. They are unchanged by exposure to the air, and precipitate when heated. It is wholly soluble in water, but sparingly in alcohol.

OFFICINAL PREPARATIONS.—Aqueous tincture, ( ʒ i to ʒ ix,) dilutions to the 3 × in dilute alcohol. Triturations in pure sugar of milk.

ANALOGUES :—*Bromides of Ammonium, Sodium, Lithium; Gelseminum, Conium, Chloral, etc.*

## Mind.

Remarkable slowness of speech, and difficulty of collecting the ideas, and expressing them. (*Turnbull.*)

\* *Profound melancholic delusions.* (*Dr. Wm. A. Hammond.*)

He imagined that he had been specially singled out for Divine vengeance, and he spent the greater part of the evening in loudly deploring his sad fate,—falling suddenly asleep at intervals of a few minutes. (*Ib.*)

He walked the room, groaning and wringing his hands; he thought he had been accused of robbing a friend, and that the officers were in search of him; with unsteady gait; hands and fingers in constant action; face pale and pupils contracted. (*Ib.*)

*Loss of memory.* He forgot how to talk; for instance, when asked what made him take so large a dose (sixty grs.) he was fully two minutes endeavoring to form a reply, and then was obliged to give up the attempt, with the remark "I can't." (*Ib.*)

*Amnesic* aphasia,—there was no difficulty of co-ordinating the movements of the tongue, so as to articulate distinctly any word he was told to pronounce. (*Ib.*)

8

Gloomy ideas relative to his present and future condition, *with* weeping, moaning, and wringing of hands.  (*Ib.*)

She fancied the boarders in the hotel insulted her.  (*Van Beren.*)

Imagined the weekly bills of the landlord were the evidences of a conspiracy got up against her father.  (*Ib.*)

While standing on the guards of the boat she suddenly gave a loud shriek, and declared she had seen her brother fall overboard.  (*Ib.*)

Profound depression of spirits, with melancholy delusions. (*Ib.*)

She is very absent-minded, low-spirited and childish.  (*Hammond.*)

Mental depression, *with* feeling of approaching death and great weakness.  (*Thomas.*)

Feebleness of intelligence.  (*Pletzer.*)

Decided lack of will and mental activity.  (*Brown Sequard.*)

° Removes the delusions during and after delirium tremens.  (*Begbie.*)

° Acute mania, *with* fullness of the blood-vessels of the brain.  (*Ib.*)

° Frightful imaginings at night (in pregnant women during the latter months); they are under the impression that they have committed, or about to commit, some great crime and cruelty, such as murdering their children or husbands.  (*Ringer.*)

° Night terrors of children, (not from indigestion,) with screaming, unconsciousness of what is occurring around them; cannot recognize, nor be comforted by their friends; sometimes followed by *squinting*.  (*Ringer.*)

° Somnambulism in children.  (*Ib.*)

° She is very fretful, crying at trifles, constantly brooding over the loss of a daughter; is almost crazy.  From fretting, loss of rest, and want of nourishment, is seized with nervous dysentery.  Cured by *Bromide of Potassium,* seven grains, every two hours.  (*Caro.*)

° Spasms, from emotional or moral disturbances.  (**Browne.**)

° *Puerperal mania.*  (*Hale.*)

° Delirium tremens,—not so good in the acute attacks of mania as in the "nervousness" which precedes it. (*Begbie.*)

° *Great despondency*—in men and women,—they "feel as if they should go out of their minds." (*Ringer.*)

* Deep depression, with painful delusions, with persistent sleeplessness, and dread of impending destruction of all near to her. (*Begbie, Wesselhœft.*)

*Insanity,* disappearing on suspending the use of the drug. (*Hammond.*)

Delusions that lewd women had got into his mother's house.

He imagined he was pursued by the police. (*Ib.*)

He imagined his life was threatened by members of his family. (*Ib.*)

He believed he had thousands of dollars sewed up in his clothing. (*Ib.*)

He appeared like a drunken man, except that his face was very pale, pulse sixty, skin cool, and pupils contracted. (*Ib.*)

Manner exciting and rambling; his hands constantly busy, either fumbling in his pockets, tying his shoes, picking threads from his clothing, or in searching for the gold which he imagined was concealed in the lining of his coat. (*Ib.*)

His character had undergone a radical change; from having been frank and brave, he had become excessively timid and suspicious of every trifling circumstance. (*Ib.*)

He several times attempted to throw himself from the window, and battered down a door with an axe, in order to escape from some imaginary danger. (*Ib.*)

Her memory was absolutely destroyed; she could not recollect the simplest things, and even forgot her own name and that of her husband, though reminded of both an instant before. (*Ib.*)

Frequently she would burst into tears for no cause whatever, and often from purely imaginary causes. (*Ib.*)

Incoherent, full of delusions, of no fixed character, and

*Remarkably depressed in spirits.* (*Ib.*)

(This was the most prominent symptom.)

She had the erroneous idea that she was deserted by all her

friends, and as a consequence, she passed all her waking moments, which were not many, in *tears.* (*Ib.*)

A fixed delusion that her child was dead; she declared she saw it dead before her; and when it was brought to her, she refused to acknowledge that it was hers, or had any resemblance to the one she imagined was dead. (*Ib.*)

*Most intense melancholy,* attended with fits of uncontrollable weeping, in a man. (*Ib.*)

*Positive delusions* of various kinds.

### Brain.

It lessens the amount of blood circulating within the cranium and produces a shrinking of the brain from this cause. (*Hammond.*)

Heaviness of the head, with confusion of the head. (*Pletzer.*)

In a case of epilepsy, caused by cerebral-anæmia, each dose of 20 grs. *caused* an attack. (*Hammond.*)

Vertigo, both slight and extreme, with dullness of the head. (*Noac.*)

Drooping of the head; difficulty of holding it erect. (*Brown Sequard.*)

° The flushed face, the throbbing of the carotids and temporals, the suffusion of the eyes, the feeling of fullness of the head, all disappear, as if by magic, under its use. (*Hammond.*)

° Violent headache, from concussion of the brain. (*Ib.*)

° Mercurial headache. (*Roberteau.*)

° Convulsions—during acute meningitis, *after* the inflamation has declined, leaving serious damage. (*Ringer, Hale.*)

° *Delirium tremens;* it relieves the delirium (not furious) removes the delusion, and produces sleep. (*Begbie, Hale.*)

° Bad results from overtaxing the brain by intense study; too close attention to business; grief; anxiety. (*Ib.*)

° Calms excitement, removes the giddiness, noises in the ears, and perversions of the external senses from diseases of the brain. (*Ib.*)

Cerebral irritations during cholera infantum; pupils dilated, eyes sunken, eyeballs moving in every direction without taking any notice; feet and hands blue and cold; pulse imperceptible. Fifty cases treated—no deaths. **Dose** one-half grain every hour. (*Dr. Caro.*)

° Head hot, feel as if in a furnace, with coldness and chills, **etc.,** etc. See "Abdomen." (*Caro.*)

° A feeling of "lightness" and exhilaration takes the place of heaviness and depression. (*Simpson.*)

° *Incipient basilar meningitis.* A delicate thin female child aged five years, had complained for several weeks of severe headache, *nearly all the time*, worse at night. She would play a few minutes with other children, then lie her head down on a chair or other support, and cry with the headache. She grew weak, emaciated, dull, heavy-eyed; had no appetite; did not sleep well nights; when sleeping it was disturbed by groans, grinding of the teeth, starting up as if frightened; complains of terrible headache; tongue clean; pulse 90 to 100, quick and wiry; constipation; scanty urine, and too much heat about the head. A careful homœopathist had given Belladonna, Hyociamus, Cina, Bryonia, and other apparently well chosen remedies, without effect. I at first gave Belladonna, 200, then Sulphur, 200th, which mitigated the pain a short time. Agaricus 3d was tried without much effect. Finally *Kali brom.* one-half grain every three hours for a few days,—no perceptible improvement; then one grain every three hours, when decided improvement in all respects set in, and in three weeks she was quite well. As soon as decided improvement occurred the medicine was given at longer intervals. (*Hale.*)

### Eyes.

Sight impaired, weak vision, with greatly contracted pupils.

Diminution of sensibility in the occular conjunctiva, so that the finger may be passed with impunity over the surface of the eyeball without causing winking. (*Turnbull.*)

Weak sight, *with* intoxication and deafness. (*Stille.*)

Dilated pupils, *with* extreme vertigo and confusion of **the** head. (*Hering.*)

Pupils prominent. (**Noac.**)

Pupils dilated, and contract very sluggishly under the influence of a very strong light.  (*Turnbull.*)

Lusterless eyes.  (*Bazire.*)

ᶜ Squinting, after night-terrors of children.  (*Ringer.*)

ᶜ Dilated pupils and sunken eyes (in cholera infantum.)
 (*Caro.*)

ᵒ Eyeballs moving in every direction.  (*Ib.*)

ᵒ Photophobia (as a collyrium, 2 parts to 30 of water.)  (*Cam-
bron and Rosignol.*)

### Ears.

Diminution of hearing.  (*Hammond.*)

ᵒ Ringing in the ears.  (*Begbie.*)

### Nose.

ᵒ Erythematous swelling of the nose.

### Mouth—Tongue—Fauces.

Loss of speech.  *Amnesic* aphasia.  (*Hammond.*)

Much difficulty in talking.  (*Ib.*)

Slight redness of the buccal and pharyngeal mucous membranes.  (*Pletzer.*)

Slight tracheal and bronchial catarrh.  (*Ib.*)

The fauces do not *contract* when touched, tickled, or even cut
with instruments.  (*Ib.*)

ᵒ Tongue pale and cold.  (*Ib.*)

ᵒ Tongue red and dry (in cholera infantum.)  (*Ib.*)

ᵒ Infants are choked every time they attempt to drink *fluids,*
although they can swallow *solids* without difficulty,—no
malformation of the throat.  (*Ringer.*)

ᵒ Hot, dry mouths of teething infants.  (*Caro.*)

### Face.

A papular rash on face and nose, with heat and itching.  (*Mc-
Gregor.*)

Successive crops of small boils in the face, with troublesome
itching.  (*Bazire.*)

Acne-like eruption on the face, neck and shoulders.  (*Brown
Séquard.*)

ᶜ Expressionless face.  (*Bazire.*)

ᶜ Acne, in young persons.  (*Hale.*)

### Jaws and Teeth.

ᵒ Difficult dentition of children.  (*Caro.*)  (*See Brom. Calc.*)

° *Odontitis* in children. "I have never failed to relieve the child by its local application." (*Ib.*)

° After the first rubbing on, the gums, from being turgid, swollen, and red, they assume their natural color, and a certain amount of ease is felt. (*Ib.*)

° The salivary secretion is restored (in teething children), and as if by enchantment, agitation, carpopedal involuntary motion, vomiting, and looseness of the bowels disappear. (*Ib.*)

### Mouth.

Irritation of the mucous membrane of the mouth and fauces, painfulness of the tongue, prominent pupils, rough and burning sensations in the whole buccal cavity as if burnt with caustic. (*Noac.*)

Increased secretion of saliva and mucus. (*Ib.*)

Short-lasting titillation in the fauces. (*Ib.*)

A state of insensibility of the *larynx* and *palate;* the fingers may be carried to the base of the tongue, touch the amygdalæ and posterior nares, and tickle the uvula, without inducing any effort at vomiting or deglutition. (*Huett.*)

° Restoration of the suppressed salivation in teething children. (*Caro.*)

\* Fœtid breath; a peculiar sickening odor. (*Hale.*)

White tongue, involving the *edges* as well as the *dorsum*, and not necessarily furred, with great *languor, sleepiness,* and *anorexia*. (*Ib.*)

### Gastric Symptoms.

Increased appetite. (*Noac.*)

Thirst in the afternoon. (*Ib.*)

Repeated repulsive eructations. (*Ib.*)

Violent nausea and efforts to vomit, with vomiting of a small quantity of mucus, with salt taste in the mouth. (*Ib.*)

° Troublesome pressure at the stomach after dinner. (*Hering.*)

° Loss of appetite. (*Noac.*)

### Liver.

° Enlargement of the liver; under the use of half a grain three times a day, the belly rapidly assumes the natural size. (*Magendie.*)

## Stomach.

Slight catarrh of the stomach.  (*Pletzer.*)

Peculiar pressure in the region of the stomach, succeeded by violent colic.  (*Hering.*)

Weakness of the stomach, for some time.  (*Ib.*)

° Vomiting when the ganglionic system is affected.  (*Begbie.*)

° Vomiting during pregnancy.  (*Cersoy, Hale.*)

° Vomiting in whooping cough.  (*Dr. Bearfoot.*)

° Vomiting of *meconium.*  (*Caro.*)

° Vomiting, with intense thirst.  (*Ib.*)

° *Vomiting of drunkards* after a debauch.  (*Hale.*)

° Chronic morning vomiting of drunkards.  (*Ib.*)

° Vomiting, diarrhœa, cramps, coldness and collapse in cholera infantum.  (*Ib.*)

° Vomiting with diarrhœa of teething children.  (*Caro.*)

° *Cholera infantum*—many cases (160 cases treated); only three deaths.  (*Ib.*)

## Spleen.

° Enlargement of the spleen.

° Small tumor in the region of the spleen.  (*Turnbull.*)

## Abdomen.

° Ascites of hepatic or splenic origin.

° Constipation of years continuance.  (*Hale.*)

Obstinate constipation.  (*Pletzer.*)

Sensation of warmth in the abdomen.  (*Heimerdinger.*)

Flatulence; frequent rumbling.  (*Ib.*)

Frequent soft stools, preceded by colic.  (*Ib.*)

Several papescent and afterward liquid stools.  (*Ib.*)

° Bloody muco-purulent diarrhœa, with intense thirst, vomiting, eyes sunken, pupils dilated, skin corrugated and spotted blue, body cold, tongue red and dry, pulse imperceptible, urine suppressed.  (*Caro.*)

° *Colic* in young children; the walls of the belly are retracted and hard, while the intestines can be seen at one spot contracted into a hard lump, of the size of a small orange, and the contraction can be seen through the abdominal wall to travel from one part of the intestines to another; these attacks are frequent and excruciating;

are unconnected with diarrhœa or constipation, but are often associated with an apthous condition of the mouth. (*Ringer, Hale.*)

° Periodic colic, in infants, occurring about 5 P. M. every evening, with the above symptoms. (*Hale.*)

° Abdomen sunken, almost stuck to the vertebral column, in cholera infantum. (*Caro.*)

° Retention of *meconium*, with vomiting of all food, and obstinate constipation; in a child three days old, cured by 1-50 of a grain every hour. (*Caro.*)

° Painless diarrhœa, fifteen or twenty passages in twenty-four hours, *with* great chilliness, even in a hot room; burning in the chest; abdomen cold internally; pulse one hundred, weak; urine scanty, dribbling a few drops at start. "At every evacuation felt as if my intestines were sinking from me. I was restless and shaky as if from palsy." Dose five grains; after the second dose fell asleep for six hours, perspiring profusely. (*Caro.*)

° Summer complaint, or cholera infantum, is not an inflammatory affection, but arises from an *over excitement of the nervous* and vascular systems, and therefore the b. of p. is a specific. (*Ib.*)

° *Asiatic cholera*, in the first stage, arrests the vomiting, the cramps, and the rice-water discharges; restores the secretion of urine; the warmth and color to the previously cold and livid skin. (Dose twenty grains every hour.) Its use should be suspended when reaction or fever sets in. (*Begbie.*)

° Discharge of a considerable quantity of tar-like substance (decomposed blood), having a fœtid smell; accompanied with tenesmus in animals. (*Noac.*)

° *Spasmodic stricture of the sphincter ani.* (Hom. *World.*)

## Sexual Organs. (Men.)

*Diminution of sexual desire.* (*Huett et al.*)

Absence of sexual desire, *with* impotence. (*Ib.*)

Semen is not secreted. (*Pfeiffer.*)

° *Nocturnal emissions, with amorous dreams and erections.*

° Excessive sexual desires, with constant erections at night.
    (*Hale.*)

° *Chordee*, during gonorrhœa.   (*Ib.*)

° *Satyriasis.*  (*Thiallman.*)

° Sensual and lascivious fancies and dreams.   (*Hale.*)

The anaphrodisiac power of the b. of p. is due to contraction
    of minute afferent vessels of the corpus cavernosus.
    (*Pelvet.*)

### Sexual Organs.  (Women.)

Abolition of all sexual feelings.   (*Hale.*)

Loss of enjoyment during coition.   (*Ib.*)

° *Nymphomania.*  (*Hale, Couch, Hammond, et al.*)

° Excessive sexual desires during the menses.   (*Hale.*)

° Erotomania, a few days after the menses.   (*Ib.*)

° Nymphomania during the puerperal state.   (*Ib.*)

° Voluptuous itching, tingling and irritation in the external
    genital organs.   (*Ib.*)

° Epilepsy from *ovarian* irritation.

° Epileptic attacks at or near the menstrual periods.   (*Lay
    cock.*)

° Enlargement of the uterus ("sub-involution") after parturi-
    tion, with abnormal discharges.   (*Simpson.*)

° Diminished the size and alleviates the pain in fibrous tumors
    of uterus.   (*Ib.*)

° Menstrual ailments.   Before the menses: *headache;* during
    the menses: *epileptic spasms, nymphomania, itching,
    burning and excitement in the vulva, pudenda and
    clitoris; after the menses: headache, insomnia, and heat
    in the genitals.*  (*Hale.*)

° Metrorrhagia from reflex irritation, or of nervous origin. (*Ib.*)

° Menorrhagia at the climacteric period.   (*Garrod.*)

° Sterility from excessive sexual indulgence.   (*Hale.*)

The menses are more scanty.

### Urinary Organs.

In a few cases the urine contained albumen.   (*Pletzer.*)

Pain in the region of the *kidneys*, spreading in the direction
    of the colon ascendens; afterwards copious secretion of
    urine.   (*Noac.*)

Diminution of the sensibility of the urethra. (*Caro.*)

Profuse urination, *with* thirst. (*Hering.*)

Thin, yellowish-white, copious urine. (*Heimerdinger.*)

Pale, thin urine, having a peculiar fœtid smell. (*Noac.*)

Diminished secretion of urine. (*Ib.*)

° Convulsions from Bright's disease.

° Abnormal irritability of the urinary passages. (*Ib.*)

° Nocturnal involuntary emissions of urine. (*Hewson.*)

° Suppression of urine in cholera infantum. (*Caro.*)

° *Diabetes millitus.* (Two cases.) Symptoms: emaciation; paleness; skin cold and dry; pulse rapid and feeble; tongue red and tender; gums spongy and bleeding; thirst excessive; appetite voracious; bowels constipated; *urine* pale, frequent, large quantity, of high density, and loaded with sugar; liver tumid and tender. (Twenty grs. b. of p. three times a day.) All the symptoms disappeared in six weeks; no relapse. (*Begbie.*)

° Neuralgia of the neck of the bladder. (*Pfeiffer.*)

° Spasmodic affections of the neck of the bladder. (*Hale.*)

° [The b. of p. is found in the urine two weeks, even four weeks, after it was taken in an animal.] (*Roberteau.*)

### Larynx.

Loss of sensibility in the larynx.

Hoarseness, extremely painful and disagreeable. (*Hering.*)

Hacking cough, with dullness and confusion of the head. (*Ib.*)

° Hyperæsthesia of the laryngeal nerves. (*Mayhofer.*)

° *Whooping-cough, uncomplicated* by other affections.

° *Laryngismus stridulus,* uncomplicated. (*Mayhofer.*)

° *Diphtheria,* with quick pulse; fever; dry tongue; offensive breath; highly injected and dusky-red fauces; with patches of wash-leather exudation on tonsils or pharynx. (*Snelling, Belcher.*)

° Follicular and catarrhal laryngitis. (*Mayhofer, of Nice.*)

° Membranous croup, with *whitish* exudation. [Kali bich., when yellow.] (*Ib.*)

[A solution of b. of p. dissolves false membranes.] (*Laboulbene.*)

* Whooping-cough—the spasmodic action disappears in about

five days, leaving a simple bronchial catarrh. It removes
the anxiety and the vomiting; improves the appetite, and
increases the strength. (*De Beaufort.*)

° *Nervous cough* during pregnancy, threatening abortion; the
cough was dry, hard and almost incessant. Auscultation
or percussion gave no evidence of disease of the head or
lungs. Opium, Belladonna, etc., were tried for two
months, without benefit. *Bromide of Potassium*, thirty
grains a day, cured in two days. (*Dr. Cerson.*)

° Spasmodic croup, as the chief remedy, almost to the exclusion of other articles. (*Dr. G. T. Elliot, Hale.*)

### Chest.

Slight bronchial catarrh. (*Pletzer.*)

Tightness of breathing. (*Noac.*)

Violent congestion of blood to the respiratory organs, occa-
sioning spitting of blood.

° *Asthma* of a nervous origin. (*Begbie.*)

° Breath hot and hurried, with burning in the chest. (*Caro.*)

° Breathlessness, with nervous headache, and want of sleep.
(*Begbie.*)

° Spasmodic asthma of children. In one case, great dyspnœa,
no sleep, urine suppressed, general œdema, six grains
every two hours; remarkable improvement now set in;
the dyspnœa subsided; the lividity of the face and œdema
disappeared, secretion of urine returned, and sleep was
obtained; cured in seven days. In another case the result
was similar. It did no good in old asthmatics. (*Hebr.*)
*Browne.*)

" The respirations are affected in a secondary manner only." It
appears to be influenced only mechanically, that is to say,
its muscles are paralyzed, like the other muscles, more or
less rapidly; early in frogs, and at the moment of death
in birds and rabbits. (*Demourette and Pelvet.*)

### Lower Extremities.

Debility of lower limbs; step tremulous and uncertain.
(*Stille.*)

Loss of sensibility in lower limbs; pinching and burning
causes no pain. (*Pache.*)

Extremities cold, pulse slow and very weak. (*Turnbull.*)

° Legs and feet cold and blue, and on being touched would leave the white impress of the fingers for more than twenty-five seconds, — in cholera infantum. (*Caro.*)

### Sleep.

*Extreme drowsiness.* Tendency to coma. (*Hammond et al.*)

She slept all night, and would often fall asleep in her chair, and in most uncomfortable positions. (*Ib.*)

He falls suddenly asleep at intervals of a few minutes. (*Ib.*)

A kind of stupor resembling that of the first stages of typhoid fever. (*Bazire.*)

° Deep, profound and quick slumber, (from twenty to thirty grains). (*Hammond.*)

° Obstinate insomnia, in case of mercurial poisoning. (*Roberteau.*)

° Sleeplessness during convalescence from acute diseases. (*Begbie.*)

° Night terrors of children; horrible dreams. (*Ib.*)

° Waking with severe headache, in a child. (*Hale.*)

° Grinding of the teeth during sleep, with moans and cries.

### Skin.

An elevated, dark red eruption made its appearance on the right elbow, from which it diffused itself over the whole body, rapidly becoming pustular. The pustules were very numerous, isolated, distended with pus, and frequently cupped, so as to present a very fair counterfeit of the eruption in discrete variola. They were generally somewhat oval in outline, and varied from two to four lines in their longest diameter. When maturation had taken place there was no apparent base nor areola, and the intervening skin was healthy. If not interfered with desiccation followed, and scabs were formed and thrown off, and leaving the integument beneath reddened but sound. The pustules continued to appear for four or five weeks; the discoloration of the skin, however, remained for as many months. (*Dr. J. C. Merrill.*)

An eruption similar to discrete variola; a dark red elevated eruption, rapidly becoming pustular; pustules very numerous, isolated, distended with pus, often cup shaped.

### Heart and Pulse.

The minute blood-vessels contract immediately in the region of injection, and later throughout the organism, and the contraction is *succeeded by dilation*. (*Pelvet.*)

The *heart* alone survives many hours (in animals); when it stops, its irritability can be again aroused for some instants, to disappear at last totally. But from the commencement of the physiological or toxic action, the *capillary* circulation is diminished, and the pulsations of the heart are retarded. (*Damoeyette and Pelvet.*)

° Pulse imperceptible, with coldness and collapse. (*Caro.*)

° Pulse 100, weak. Pulse 50, small and feeble. (*Ib.*)

° Neuroses of the heart. (*Hale.*)

° It has a sedative effect upon the action of the heart.

### Temperature.

The temperature of the body was reduced one or two degrees centigrade. (*Pletzer.*)

The temperature is sensibly lessened in warm-blooded animals first, and during many hours in the region injected, and afterwards throughout the organism. The phenomena depends upon the diminution of the capillary circulation, at first local, afterwards general.

° Body cold; skin corrugated and mottled. (*Caro.*)

° Shivering with cold, and cold skin, although the child was covered with mustard plasters. (*Ib.*)

### Generalities.

The gait became staggering; false steps became frequent. Weakness of the muscles of the arms—but no vertigo. (*Pletzer.*)

It paralyzes the nerves of the spinal cord. (*Ib.*)

*Intoxication*, with loss of sight and hearing. (*Stille.*)

* Epilepsy from large doses in a case of cerebral anæmia. (*Hammond.*)

*Unsteadiness of gait;* he was frequently taken for a drunken man; was once arrested for supposed drunkenness. (*Hammond.*)

Well marked numbness throughout the body, and very decided diminution of sensibility.

Almost constant twitching of the fingers and a busy occupation of them in matters of no importance.

Unable to stand or walk; face ashy pale; pupils contracted; loss of memory. Great weakness of the extensors of the legs and feet.

Vertigo, fainting and nausea.

Very emaciated, weak, and of a peculiar pallid color. (*Turn-bull.*)

As an agent for lessening reflex excitability, exceeds all other remedies. (*Pletzer.*)

° Neuroses involving the brain and accompanied by convulsions. (*Ib.*)

° Mercurial trembling. (*Roberteau.*)

° *Lead poisoning.* (*Ib.*)

° *Infantile convulsions,* during teetl ing, whooping cough or laryngismus stridulus. *Spasm of the glottis;* it prevents the recurrence of the spasms. (*Ringer, Hale.*)

* *Epilepsy,* chiefly *grand mal;* rarely useful in *petit mal.*

Restless and shaky, as if from palsy. (*Caro.*)

It diminishes the abnormal vascularity of the great nervous centres.

### Temperature.

The temperature of the body was reduced one or two degrees centigrade. (*Pletzer.*)

The temperature is sensibly lessened in warm-blooded animals first, and during many hours in the region injected, and afterwards throughout the organism. The phenomena depends upon the diminution of the capillary circulation, at first local, afterwards general.

° Body cold; skin corrugated and mottled. (*Caro.*)

° Shivering with cold, and cold skin, although the child was covered with mustard plasters. (*Ib.*)

It mitigates those convulsive movements and spasmodic twitchings, which are the results of the rapid conversion of sensory impressions, or of morbid reflex action through the medulla oblongata. (*C. Browne.*)

° *Quotidian ague* after quinine had been given for two weeks without result. " The sweating stage was unusually protracted and exhausting." " A full dose every three hours during a remission, cured." (*Begbie.*)

\* It removes pathological deposits of fatty matter only, while the iodide removes *normal* adipose matter. (*Simpson.*)

It diminishes the *reflex* excitability of the nervous centres. (*Brown Sequard.*) The functions of organic life are not disturbed. (*Huett.*)

° *Epilepsy*—especially occurring at or near the menses. (*Laycock.*)

*Epilepsy* may be arrested by it, but returns when this drug is suspended. (*Ramshill.*)

*Paralysis agitans.* (*Hammond.*)

° Trembling sensation throughout the whole body. (*Hale.*)

° Tetanus; a boy 15 years old, from suppuration of finger nail and exposure to cold by sleeping on the grass. Attacked October 8th. Discharged September 10th. Dose 20 grs. every two hours nearly all the time. A few days took 20 grs. every hour. (*R. Browne.*)

° *Chorea* in a female. The tongue protruded with a jerk; muscles of the face, right arm and legs in constant jactitation, quite violent. Eight grains every three hours; cured in two days. (*Dr. Hume.*)

° *Chorea* in a female, of several weeks. Unable to dress herself or work, and could hardly speak. Face, arm and leg of right side affected. Ten grains every four hours cured her in three days. (*Dr. Hume.*)

\* *Symptoms from an affection of vaso-motor nerves,* namely:

I. Occasional sudden paroxysmal feeling of "numbness," a term employed by some to denote the sensation of "pins and needles;" by others that of "deadness" and "weakness," and by a third group an "indescribable feeling of something wrong."

II. A feeling of "largeness," or "as if the limb were swollen," there being at the time of its occurrence no change in the size of the extremity.

III. The occurrence of "aching," of "uneasiness," or of actual "pain," the latter not very severe.

IV. The feeling of "coldness," and occasionally, the obvious fact of coldness.

F.8

v. The fact of sudden "weakness," sometimes termed a "paralyzed" feeling; the patient being unable to retain the grasp of an object, and hastily putting it down, or allowing it to fall. At such times the muscles do not respond readily to the will; the co-ordination of movement is defective. Such acts as writing or needle-work have to be discontinued, and generally such patients rub the limbs by, as it would seem, an almost instinctive impulse.

vi. The occurrence of sensations allied to cramp, or that of actual cramp, with varying amounts of pain. (*J. Russell Reynolds.*)

[Aconite, Gelseminum, Platinum, Pulsatilla, Lycopodium, Veratrum album, and Calcarea carb. have many of the above symptoms. (*Hale.*)]

" The symptoms due to large doses of the Bromide of Potassium may be stated as follows, in the usual order of their occurrence:

1. Contraction of the pupils. 2. Drowsiness. 3. Weakness of the arms and legs. 4. Depression of mind. 5. Failure of memory. 6. Delusions.

The first three of these are, I think, usual accompaniments of an active dose of the medicine. They simply show a sedative effect due to cerebral anæmia. In adults they never follow a less dose than ten grains. Doses of five grains produce no obvious effects. No permanent difficulty results from very large doses." (*Hammond.*)

Dr. Hammond asserts that to a condition of *cerebral anæmia* most of the obvious phenomena which follow its administration should be ascribed.

---

# CACTUS GRANDIFLORUS.

### (*Night-Blooming Cereus.*)

DESCRIPTION.—Stems cylindrical, rooting and very long, provided with five or six slightly prominent ribs, and furnished with small spines or thorns, disposed in radicated forms. Fruit shaped like an egg, covered with scaly tubercles, fleshy, of an orange or fine reddish color, filled with very small seeds of an acid taste. Flowers have an extremely sweet odor of benzoic acid and vanilla.

9

OFFICINAL PREPARATION.—Tincture of the stems and flowers, equal parts; dilutions.

SPHERE OF ACTION.—Specifically on the heart and blood-vessels.

ANALOGUES.—*Aconite, Agaricus, Belladonna, Crotalus, Gelseminum, Iberis Kalmia, Lachesis, Naja, Lilium, Stramonium, Spigelia, Veratrum viride.*

## Sensorium.

Hypochondria and invincible sadness; unusual melancholy.

Fear of death, extreme and continuous.

Love of solitude.

## Head.

\* Vertigo from sanguineous congestions to the head.

Heavy pain like a weight on the vertex; worse from noise.

\* Face bloated and red, with pulsating pain in the head.

Feeling of emptiness in the head.

Very severe pain in the right side of the head, which is increased by the sound of talking and by a strong light.

\* Pulsating pain in the temples, becoming intolerable at night.

## Eyes.

Loss of sight; there appear circles of red light before the eyes, which dim the sight.

° Dimness of sight; weakness of sight recurring periodically.

## Ears.

Pulsations in the ears day and night.

Noise like the running of a river, continuing all night.

° Hearing diminished from the buzzing in the ears.

° Otitis, from checked perspiration.

° Rheumatic otitis

## Nose.

Dry and unpleasant coryza.

Fluent and very acrid coryza; nostrils sore.

Profuse epistaxis, soon ceasing; from acute congestion.

## Throat.

° Constriction of the throat, preventing swallowing.

Fetid breath in the morning.

## Appetite and Gastric Symptoms.

° Loss of appetite and loss of taste for food, with nausea.

Great appetite, but weak and slow digestion.

Bad digestion; all food causes weight and suffering in stomach.

° Nausea in the morning, and all day long.

### Stomach.

Acrid acid in the stomach, making food taste acid.

Violent burning in the stomach

Great thirst during the fever.

° Continuous pulsation in the stomach, in an old lady at the change of life.

*Heaviness* in the stomach after eating.

### Liver.

° Acute and chronic engorgement of the liver from cardiac diseases.

### Abdomen.

Distressing sensation in the bowels.

Very violent pains in the bowels, with burning sensation.

° Enteritis; also peritonitis.

### Stool and Anus.

Bilious evacuations, with pain in the abdomen.

Morning diarrhœa, watery, preceded by great pain.

Sensation of great weight in the anus, with itching, with or without copious hemorrhage.

° Constipation from hemorrhoidal congestion.

### Urinary Organs.

Constriction of the neck of the bladder.

Great desire to pass water, but cannot.

Frequent desire to urinate, with copious flow, straw color.

Urine passed by drops, with burning.

Urine reddish, turbid.

### Generative Organs.

*Women.*—Painful constriction around the pelvis, which gradually extends upwards to the stomach.

Pain in the uterus and its ligaments, returning every evening.

Pulsating pain in the uterus and ovarian regions, extending to the thighs.

° Very painful menstruation.

Menstruation copious and painless.

Menstruation eight days too soon.

### Larynx, Cough, etc.

Obstinate, sterterous cough, worse at night.

Spasmodic cough, with copious mucous expectoration.

Cough, with thick **yellow** expectoration.

Dry cough from **tickling in** the chest.

° Various kinds of **cough** due to cardiac disorders. (*Hale.*)

### Heart.

* Sensation of an annoying movement from before backward in the cardiac region, worse by day than by night.

* *Sensation of constriction in the heart, as if an iron band prevented its normal movement.*

Dull heavy pains in the region of the heart, increased by external pressure.

Pricking pain in the heart, impeding respiration and the movements of the body.

* *Very acute pain and such painful stitches in the heart* as to cause him to cry out loudly, with obstruction of respiration.

* *Palpitation of the heart, continues day and night, worse when walking, and at night, when lying on the left side.*

° Nervous palpitation of the heart, aggravated by the near approach of the menses.

° *Functional disorder of the heart,* from mental emotions, aggravated at the menstrual period.

° *Angina pectoris.*

° Palpitations, acute and chronic, even in organic diseases of the heart.

° Acute inflammatory affections of the heart, *idiopathic,* and even from rheumatism.

° *Acute carditis,* with blueness of the face; oppression of breathing; dry cough; pricking pain in the heart; cannot lie on left side; *pulse* quick, throbbing, tense and hard.

° *Chronic carditis,* with œdematous and cyanotic face, suffocating respiration, continued dull pain in the heart, dropsical effusion all throughout the body; cannot drink or speak, hands and feet cold, *pulse* intermittent.

° *Hypertrophy with dilatation;* patients pulseless, extremely exhausted, panting and sad, cannot lie down, or speak; has scarcely slept for fifteen days; forgetful, feet œdematous. (Is soon relieved, lies down and sleeps 12 hours.)

’ *Organic diseases of the heart; valvular diseases,* (an invaluable palliative for many distressing symptoms.)

° Heart disease, **with** œdema of *left* hand only, (no other remedy has this symptom.)

° A constant *fluttering* sensation in the stomach, over the location of the cœliac axis, in a spot about the size of a dollar; a burning line extends down from it to the lower ribs on either side; a hot flash shoots downward, frequently, (cured by a few doses.)

° Rheumatic inflammation of the heart, with severe pain in apex of heart, and pain shooting down left arm to the end of the fingers; dyspnœa, pulse feeble, 120, etc.

° Palpitation of the heart from any exertion, with excessive pain all over the left side between the scapulæ and sacral region.

° A whizzing, to and fro sound, or *bruit de soufflet.*

° Endocardial bruit, increased præcordial dullness, excessive impulse of heart's action, and evident enlargement of right ventricle.

° Great irregularity of heart's action—intermittent at times and of varying character—great *frequency* of action alternating with *slowness.* (Enlargement of left ventricle, with great irritation of cardiac nerves.)

° Irregularity of heart's action, from reflex irritation.

° Palpitation, with vertigo, dyspnœa and loss of consciousness.

### Extremities.

Formication and weight in the arms.

Œdema in the hands—worse in the *left.*

° Pain in left arm, down to fingers, (in disease of heart.)

Œdema of the feet and legs, up to the knees.

Restlessness in the legs—cannot keep them still.

### Sleep.

Sleeplessness without apparent cause; or from pulsations at the stomach, or in the ears.

Delirium during sleep.

### Fever.

Chills, with chattering of the teeth; at 10 o'clock A. M., followed by burning heat with shortness of breath.

Burning heat at night, followed by a chill, then perspiration.

° *Intermittent fever, quotidian,* with chill, heat, dyspnœa, headache, stupefaction, great thirst, then perspiration.

# CAFFEINE.

PHARMACOLOGY.—Caffeine may be obtained by treating ground coffee with benzine, which dissolves out the caffeine and fixed oils. Distill the benzine solution to dryness, and boil the residue in water, dissolving the caffeine, which, on filtering and concentrating, is deposited.

Caffeine crystalizes in white, silky, long needles, which are slightly flexible and transparent, and have a specific gravity of 1.23. Taste weak, but bitter and unpleasant. It is fusible, volatile and soluble in water, alcohol or ether. The Citrate of Caffeine may be substituted for the pure alkaloid.

OFFICINAL PREPARATION.—Triturations up to the 3×; afterwards, alcoholic dilutions.

## Head.

* Congestion of blood to the head, with flushed face and nervous excitement.

* Obstinate sleeplessness, especially in children and nervous women.

It increases the reflex excitability and may produce *tetanus*.

[The tetanus is considered by most authors a medullary tetanus, for it is not produced in the leg of a frog if the ischiatic nerves are cut; and it takes place in a limb, the circulation of which has been stopped by a ligature, before the subcutaneous injection of caffeine.

It produces at first an increased frequency of the pulse, but a diminution of its bulk takes place very quickly (one minute after the injection), and sometimes determines the immediate death of the heart.

The increased rapidity of the heart-beats, and the rise of arterial pressure observed, may be attributed to a paralysis, more or less complete, of the nerves proceeding from the ganglia to the muscles of the heart.

*Three* grains did not kill a dog in which artificial respiration was produced. *One fourth* of a grain killed other dogs in the same condition.]

(See "*Coffea;*" and "*Therapeutics,*" Vol. II.)

---

# CALABAR BEAN.

## (*Physostigma Venenosum.*)

BOTANICAL DESCRIPTION.—This is an irregular, kidney-shaped bean, about an inch in length and three-fourths of an inch in breadth; the product of the Physostigma Venenosum, a perennial woody creeper of Calabar, Africa, where the bean has been used by the natives as an ordeal test for criminals, witches, etc., since time immemorial.

It contains an alkaloid known as *physostigmia*, or *eserine*.

OFFICINAL PREPARATION.—Tincture with strong alcohol; dilutions.

ANALOGUES.— *Agaricus, Belladonna, Gelseminum, Solanum, Conium, Curare, Passiflora.*

## Head.

A feeling of buoyancy; desire to move and talk continually.

Dullness of the mind; sluggishness of the brain.

Dizziness, with great fullness of the blood-vessels of the brain.

° Congestion of the brain, with epileptiform attacks.

Constriction of the forehead and eyes, with heaviness of the lids; numbness and dizziness.

Dizziness and sensation of wavering in the brain, when walking, half an hour after tea. (*H. L. Chase.*)

Deep-seated pain in the forehead, with desire to rub it. (*Chase.*)

Dizziness in walking; it requires an effort of the will to keep from staggering.

Severe pressing pain in the forehead, as though something hard was bound tightly on it, accompanied by dizziness when walking.

Difficulty in concentrating the thoughts. (*Chase.*)

Confusion of the head, vertigo with loss of strength in the legs, as if he had been drinking. (*Cullis.*)

He staggers like a drunken man, and goes to bed with his head swimming.

Some headache over the right eye, lasting two days. (*Cullis.*)

Strange vertigo at night; she holds to the bedstead to keep from falling, and makes an effort to shake off that feeling. Her whole frame seems loosened and powerless.

Her thoughts wander and she has difficulty in fixing her attention.

Feeling of constriction around forehead and temples, changing into oppressive pain over the left orbit and extending to the forehead and temples, very troublesome in reading.

Heat and redness of the face.

Dull weight along the vertex, mostly on the left lobe of the brain. (*Wesselhœft.*)

Feeling of constriction around the entire top of the head, as if a tight cap were being pressed down as far as the temples, at the same time severe pressure along the sagittal suture, as if from fulness of the longitudinal sinus and dull aching in each temple. (*Wesselhœft.*)

Dulness; was obliged to make an extra effort in speaking with people. ( *Wesselhœft.*)

Pressing from within outwards in vertex and temples.

During the forepart of the day he has at times a feeling of weakness, though there was uncommon mental activity. (*Cullis.*)

Sudden attack of headache with nausea and bitter rising, followed by dull pain under the sternum, increased by suddenly turning the head, bending forward or throwing the shoulders forward.

Headache with fullness and a sense of faintness, with a numb feeling down the left arm, pulse 50 to 60 with feeble impulses.

## Face and Eyes.

Face hot and red.

Sensation of contraction of eyelids with difficulty of opening them, and a suffusion of tears, when opened wide. (*Chase.*)

Sensation of contraction of the whole left side of the face, with slight numbness; it required an effort to keep the eyelids open.

Eyes unusually free from black spots. (*curative.*)

For three days attacks of partial blindness, on attempting to write he was unable to see a line.

Alternation of dilatation and contraction of the pupil from oscillatory motions of the pupillary muscles, ending in permanent contraction. (*Leven.*)

Nystagmus. (*Leven.*)

Severe pain in the right side of the upper jaw, like toothache.

Sensation of contraction of the alæ nasi and upper lip, with frequent desire to rub them, which relieved for a time. 20 minutes. (*Chase.*)

Severe sharp darting pains in the right malar bone, and in the ramus of the jaw on the right side.

Small boil on the inside of the right nostril, very painful, the pain extending up to the eye and right side of the head. It broke on the fourth day with very little discharge.

It stimulates the *sphincter pupillœ* and the *ciliary* muscles to contraction.

It contracts the pupil even in dilatation the result of injury.

A decided tight feeling, referable pretty accurately to the ciliary region of the left eye (to which the solution was applied), as if something were creeping in it, (in five minutes). Ten minutes after, this continued, with occasional rather sharp pain in the ciliary region. An attempt to read with both eyes instantly increased this pain, and the type was confused, as if by a disturbance of the power of accommodation. Type looked smaller with the right eye than the left. I could see Jaeger 17, at 15 feet, but with a remarkable oscillation in the distinctness; the type came and went, at one instant quite clear, then indistinct, as if the ciliary muscles were undergoing irregular contractions.

*Astigmatism;* the vertical bars of a window were seen clear and sharp at from six to ten feet; the horizontal bars within the same range having their edges slightly hazy, but rendered clear by a concave cylindrical glass of 14 inches focus.

The pupil contracted (to the size of a pin's head) and remains so eighteen hours, then gradually relaxed during four days, resuming gradually its mobility under light whether falling on its own or the opposite retina. With the sudden contraction of the pupil came a sudden twilight gloom, as if an eclipse of the sun, but this gloom soon lessened and gradually disappeared before the pupil dilated.

When applied to the eye of a long-sighted person it restores vision (temporarily).

Short sightedness (in the normal eye).

Pain in the eyeballs, over the eyes, and in the head.

Profuse lachrymation.

° Dimness of vision.

° Paralysis of the circular fibers of the *iris*, and of the ciliary muscles of one eye; the dilated pupil and dimness of sight disappeared.

° *Prolapsus of the iris,* from injuries, even when the whole globe is vascular and irritated, and sight impaired; (under the topical use of the alkaloid, the prolapsus retracted as the pupil contracted).

° Prolapsus of iris, from sloughing of the cornea.

### Stomach.

Tongue feels as if scalded.

Dryness and smarting at the tip of the tongue all day. (*Chase.*)

Numbness, tingling and smarting of the tongue and lips, with a constant desire to moisten them.

Soreness of the bowels, painful when moving about, aggravated by riding.

Soreness of abdomen, the spot is not larger than the palm of the hand.

Sense of distension with soreness of abdomen. (*Chase.*)

Colicky pains low in abdomen, succeeded by a copious loose discharge from the bowels. (*Chase.*)

Small intestines in a state of contraction, showing in places circular constriction, like internal strangulation.

Feeling as if he had bolted a piece of solid food of too large a size; the sensation gradually increases until it is very painful.

Burning heat in the stomach, with much belching of wind.

### Urine and Sexual Organs.

Pain in the back, hips and lower part of the abdomen; thought the menses were about to appear, but this did not take place.

Slight stitches on the left side of the abdomen (female).

Dull pain and downward pressure in the back, accompanied by the appearance of the menses. (*Mrs. P.*)

Menses come on at the usual time without the usual unpleasant premonitory symptoms. (*Mrs. N.*)

### Chest and Heart.

Pulsations through the whole body, particularly at the chest, each beat of the heart distinctly perceptible in the chest and temple. (*Wess lhæft.*)

Heart's action retarded with diminished impulse; rate 56; no abnormal sounds, the radial pulse irregular and weak.

Trembling and convulsive agitation of the heart. (*Leven.*)

Respiratory muscles in oscillatory motion. (*Leven.*)

° Chronic bronchial catarrh, aggravated by talking.

° Cough, with inability to raise the mucus.

Heart's action tumultuous and irregular.

Heart's action feeble and irregular.

In some cases the heart goes on beating long after death (in animals).

The heart contained fluid blood and clots in all the four cavities, indicating death from paralysis of the muscles of the heart (in men).

### Back and Extremities.

Sharp darting pains in the right elbow-joints, extending down the outside of the arm to the two middle fingers.

A numb pain in the knees and ankles, while sitting, with a desire to move frequently.

The limbs feel weary, as after great fatigue, with a constant desire to move.

Severe cramp-like pain in the left popliteal space; walking was very painful.

Heavy pain in the back, under left shoulder, continuing severe for an hour, and then slowly passing away. (*Mrs. S.*)

Sharp twinges in the right instep, and various twinging pains about the body. (*Wesselhœft.*)

Throbbing pains in the forehead; worse on moving. (*Wesselhœft.*)

Sharp darts through the right thumb, at the root of the nail, and several weaker ones through the finger joints of the right hand. (*Mrs. P.*)

Dragging pains over the left hip toward the back.

Slight twinging pains in the lower limbs, with sharp momentary twinges in the ankles.

Drawing rheumatic pains through the left shoulder.

Drawing pains low in the back and abdomen, with bearing down, as if the menses were coming.

Feeling of weakness, as though paralyzed, passes downward from the occiput through the back to the lower extremities; the feeling in the legs like that known as being asleep. (*Chase.*)

Slight exertion causes lameness and weakness of the back.

## Sleep.

After falling asleep wakes repeatedly during the night with terrible thoughts. He fears he is becoming crazy, and that he may get up and do some mischief. He dreams that he is a lion. Awakes at 4 A. M., with soreness, not a pain, in the left side of the abdomen, painful to pressure.

Irresistible desire to sleep. (*Wesselhœft.*)

Soporific sleep, extremely distressing, paleness of the face. (*Ib.*)

Drowsiness in the forenoon, even while riding or working.

Profuse perspiration, partly dispelling the drowsiness.

Great drowsiness after dinner; sleeps good, and sleeps just as well at night as if he had not slept in the afternoon.

In the evening not drowsy as usual, but wakeful.

## Nervous System.

° Chorea in a boy of fourteen; the disease had lasted several months, and resisted Ferrum, Arsenic and Zinc; (cured in nine weeks by eighteen drops a day of the tincture).

° Progressive muscular wasting. (*Reynolds.*)

(It did no service in a case of paralysis agitans.)

° Chorea in a girl of twenty; (a rapid cure) with the tincture

° Chorea, of the right side; the tongue seemed too large.

General paralysis of the insane. (*Crichton-Browne.*)

° Traumatic tetanus, several cases; (cured).

° Epileptiform convulsions.

° Cerebro-spinal meningitis, in the tetanic stage. (*Hale.*)

## General Symptoms.

Increase of secretion, particularly of the perspiratory, salivary and intestinal glands; the discharges that follow are occasionally free, producing severe sweating, insalivation, and catharsis.

The operation of the drug is spinal, not cerebral, acting upon the anterior or motor column, so as to suspend or deaden its energy or reduce the activity of its functions.

The powerless parts are those that receive their nervous supply from the spinal cord and its nerves. The muscles of the extremities and of respiration are most enfeebled; and the paralysis is primarily and always seated in the striped muscles.

There is no failure of volition; the will is strong, but a difficulty lies in the way of carrying out its purpose.

Unable to move, though he makes the attempt.

The mind exhibits no defect.

Suspension of the functions of the motor tract, by which it does not conduct the impulses of the will through the cord to the muscles.

The paralysis is not exclusively owing to poisoned blood, as the lower limbs are first paralyzed, then the upper, then the trunk, then the neck.

A cramp-like condition in organs that are supplied with involuntary muscular fibres.

Pain ceases during rest, but commences again during motion; but by continued motion it is relieved.

Muscular trembling in different degrees; from a mere tremor up to a jerking of the muscles.

The muscles retain their normal contractility unimpaired, and still respond to direct irritation when artificial stimuli are applied.

The paralysis is commonly preceded by twitching or trembling of the muscles; in the lower animals these are often convulsive.

When movements occur, they have sometimes been uncoordinated; again, the palsy has been found to include the unstriped muscles; and furthermore, the functions of the brain may be disturbed. The first is only met with after entire loss of exercising the will. The second is, perhaps, due to extension of the poisonous influence to the sympathetic system.

*Trembling, dizziness, and loss of power in the limbs in half an hour.*

*Fatal syncope,* from paralysis of the heart.

Stupid and giddy; a sense of feebleness over the whole body, rendering progression difficult.

Sharp pains, shifting quickly from one place to another.

When the pain remained in any place for a short time the *spot became disagreeably sore.*

A sensation of heat, accompanied with sweat, extending from

the fourth or fifth cervical vertebræ to the last lumbar. (*Beckwith.*)

° *Dyspepsia*, with great pain *immediately* after eating. (*Beckwith.*)  * Also, Arg. nit. and Dioscorea. (*Hale.*)

Constriction of the intestinal canal (general).

° Constipation of years duration, from atony of the bowels.

---

# CANCHALAGUA.

BOTANICAL DESCRIPTION.—The proper botanical name is not known to me. I give the name as it appeared in the *Philadelphia Journal of Homœopathy.* "A small grass-plant, growing in patches; has a small, red blossom, not unlike the Forget-me-not (*Myosotis*), a round, woody stem and branches, lanciform leaves; indigenous to California." (*Dr. Richter, Philadelphia Journal of Hom., Vol. II.*)

OFFICINAL PREPARATIONS.—Tincture of the whole plant; dilutions.

## Head.

Congested feeling, with pressive pains in the forehead; a sensation of fullness.

Tightness of the scalp; it feels as if drawn together.

## Ears.

Piercing and stitching pains in the ears.

Buzzing and roaring in the ears.

## Eyes.

Burning, first in the left, then in the right.

## Stomach.

Increase of appetite.

Eructations and regurgitations.

Water-brash, with spitting of white mucus, and a **trembling** nervousness.

## Sleep.

Sleeplessness.

## Fever.

° *Fever and ague;* (tertian).

* Soreness all over, especially in the lower **extremities.**

Heat in the whole body.

° Intermittent fever; obstinate. (*Dr. Richter.*)

# CANNABIS INDICA.

### (*Indian Hemp.*)

BOTANICAL DESCRIPTION.—This plant is a native of Persia and the northern part of India. It is an annual, covered with a rough but very fine hair, almost invisible to the naked eye. Stem erect, branched, green, angular. Leaves opposite or alternate. Each leaf consists of five long, narrow, sharp-pointed leaflets, spreading from the extremity of a long lax leaf stalk. Flowers in axillary clusters; in the males drooping, and leafless at the base; in the females erect, and leafy at the base.

There are two species of the Cannabis, or Hemp, recognized in our Materia Medica—the Indica and the Sativa. Their difference, however, is rather in their physiological action than in the botanical characteristics, and these are undoubtedly owing to locality and cultivation.

OFFICINAL PREPARATIONS.—Tincture and dilutions.

ANALOGUES.—*Aconite, Arnica, Belladonna, Berberis, Bryonia, Camphor, Cannabis sat., Cantharides, Clematis, Copaiva, Digitalis, Dulcamara, Hyoscyamus, Lachesis, Lycopodium, Nux vomica, Opium, Petroleum, Pulsatilla, Sepia, Spigelia, Stannum, Stramonium, Terebinthina, Thuja, Uva ursi, Veratrum.*

## Mind.

Moaning and crying.

Great anguish and despair.

Great apprehension of approaching death.

Horror of darkness.

*Incoherent talking.*

Stammering and stuttering.

Exaltation of spirits, with great gaiety and disposition to laugh at the merest trifle.

Full of fun and mischief, and laughs immoderately.

*Exaltation of spirits, with excessive loquacity.*

Uncontrollable laughter, till the face becomes purple, and the back and loins ache.

Laughs indiscriminately at every word said to him.

He begins a sentence, but cannot finish it, because he forgets what he intended to write or speak.

Imagines he is gradually swelling, and that his body is becoming larger and larger.

*Very absent minded.*

Imagines some one calls him.

Inability to recall any thought or event, on account of the number of different thoughts crowding on his brain.

He fancies he hears numberless bells ringing most sweetly.

*Imagines he hears music, shuts his eyes, and is lost for some time in the most delicious thoughts and dreams.*

While listening to the piano he loses consciousness, and is seemingly raised gently through the air to a great height, when the strains of music become perfectly celestial; on regaining consciousness his head is bent forward, his neck is stiff, and there is a loud ringing in his ears.

His mind is filled with ridiculous speculative ideas.

Constantly theorizing.

His head feels very heavy, he loses consciousness, and falls.

*On regaining consciousness, violent shocks pass through his brain.*

In the daytime, dreams, returning periodically, or dreamy attacks.

He could not read, partly on account of dreamy spells, and partly because he had not full power of vision.

*Fixed ideas.*

He forgot his last words and ideas, and spoke in a low tone, with a thick voice, as if tired.

*Every few moments he would lose himself, and then wake up, as it were, to those around him.*

*He was in constant fear that he would become insane.*

Unpleasant shuddering through all the limbs, with a painful feeling of weight in the occiput, and a tetanic intermittent contraction of the muscles of the nape of the neck.

° Hallucinations and illusions following excesses in wine, and venery, and also arising from or during religious excesses, seem to me to demand this drug with the dietetic use of Phosphate of Lime. (*Gray.*)

° It has proved of great service against illusions of a spectral character, not accompanied by terror; such as arise in some forms of nervous fever and in puerperal mania. In this class of hallucinations my dose has not been less than 1-100th of a grain of the extract (*Gunje*) rubbed in sugar. (*Gray.*)

### Head.

Vertigo on rising, with a stunning pain in the back part of his head, and he falls.

Fullness in the forehead, as if it would burst.

Burning pain in both temples.

Heavy insurmountable pressure on the brain, forcing him to stoop.

Severe stitch in the right temple, gradually changing to a pressing pain.

Aching in both temples, most severe in the right.

Throbbing, aching pain in the forehead.

Dull, drawing pain in the forehead, especially over the eyes.

Dull, heavy, throbbing pain through the head, with a sensation like a heavy blow on the back of the head and neck.

Dull, sticking pain in the right temple.

*Frequent involuntary shaking of his head.*

Jerking in the right side of the forehead toward the interior and back part of the head.

Pain in the whole right side of the head.

° In my practice it has proved a wonderful remedy in subacute inflammation of the brain, in delirium tremens, and in a few cases of epilepsy. It has been eminently serviceable in hypochondriac affections of females, especially those somewhat advanced in life. It exercises a peculiar control over this class of maladies, and has sometimes effected speedy cures of cases which were bordering upon actual insanity. Some years since I made a few experiments upon Guinea pigs and rabbits with a tincture of Cannabis indica, and in most instances it caused an injection of the blood vessels of the entire brain; but its chief influence appeared to be exerted upon the tubercular quadrigemina and the parts in immediate vicinity. Indeed, the appearances it produced were very similar to those which have been observed from Opium, Belladonna, Alcohol, and from the ethers.—(*Marcy*.)

° A lady, aged about forty years, had been confined to her bed for seven months, with a morbid sensitiveness and great prostration of the entire nervous system. Her allopathic

physician had treated her with Iron, Cinchona, Opium,
and the other usual remedies of his school, without any
benefit, until she had been in her bed almost constantly
for the period above indicated. At this time she was
placed under my care in the following condition: no apparent organic derangement in any part of her body. The
organs all performed their functions with considerable
regularity, but sluggishly. On attempting to make the
slightest effort, in rising up in bed, or in making any
exertion, she experienced a great sense of prostration, and
a death-like sinking and weakness at the pit of her stomach, and to some extent in her chest. Pulse seventy-six
and regular, but weak. Respiration and temperature of
the skin natural. We put her on Cannabis indica, and
after six days she was able to sit up for fifteen minutes
without any serious inconvenience. The remedy was
persisted in, and her improvement continued until at
the expiration of six weeks she was able to sit up the
entire day; to walk for half an hour at a time, and to
ride out for an hour or two, with benefit. All her un
pleasant symptoms in the chest and stomach have disappeared, and she is now quite well with the exception of
a slight debility. (*Marcy.*)

### Eyes.
*Injection of the vessels of the conjunctiva in both eyes.*
The vessels of the conjunctiva of both eyes are injected in a
    triangular patch extending from the internal canthus to
    the cornea; worse in the right.
Twinkling, trembling, and glimmering before the eyes.
Jerking in the external corners of the eye and eyelids.
*Fixed gaze.*
*While reading the letters run together.*

### Ears.
Noise in the ears like boiling water.
Periodical singing in his ears, that always ceased as soon as
    he came to himself, and renewed itself whenever a dreamy
    spell came on.
Aching in both ears.

*Throbbing and fullness in both ears, and ringing and buzzing in the ears.*

Sensitiveness to noise.

### Face.

*He looks drowsy and stupid.*

Wearied, exhausted appearance.

Coldness of the face, nose, and hands, after dinner.

*Profuse sticky sweat standing out in drops on his forehead.*

### Mouth.

*Dryness of the mouth and lips;* the lips are glued together.

*White, thick, frothy and sticky saliva.*

### Throat.

*The throat is parched, accompanied by intense thirst for cold water.*

### Appetite and Taste.

Increased appetite; every article of food is extremely palatable.

Ravenous hunger, which is not decreased by eating enormously; he ceases eating only from fear of injuring himself.

° Pastry and fat food, which previously he never ate without suffering from rancid risings and headache, are now digested readily.

### Gastric Symptoms.

While eating, his stomach felt swelled and his chest oppressed as if he would suffocate, so that he was forced to loosen his clothes.

### Stomach.

*Pain in or near the cardiac orifice.*

### Stool and Anus.

° Costiveness.

Sensation in the anus as if he was sitting on a ball; as if the anus and a part of the urethra were filled up by a hard round body.

### Urinary Organs.

Aching in both kidneys, keeping him awake at night.

Sharp stitches in both kidneys.

Burning in the kidneys.

Pain in the kidneys when laughing.

*Profuse colorless urine.*

Urinating frequently, but in small quantities.

*Urine dribbles out after the stream ceases.*

He has to force out the last few drops with his hand.

He has to wait some time before the urine flows.

Urging to urinate, but he cannot pass a drop.

Frequent urination, with burning pain in the evening.

*Burning and scalding before, during, and after urination.*

Urging to urinate, with much straining.

The urging continues after urination.

Pain and burning during urination.

*Stinging pain before, during, and after urination.*

Uneasiness, with burning sensation in the penis and urethra,
     accompanied by frequent calls to urinate.

Intense burning at the orifice of the urethra during urination,
     and continuing afterwards.

Sharp pricklings like needles in the urethra, so severe as to
     send a thrill to the cheeks and head.

Feelings in the urethra as if there were a gonorrhœal dis-
     charge.

*On squeezing the glans penis a white glairy mucus oozes out.*

° It has also been useful in debility of the bladder with a para-
     plegic state of the lower limbs, used in alternation with
     Nux vomica of the same strength and continued many
     weeks. (*Gray.*)

### Genital Organs.

*Male*—Itching of the glans penis.

Itching and burning of the scrotum.

*Satyriasis;* violent erections; priapism; chordee.

Excessive venereal appetite, with frequent erections during
     the day.

Erections while riding, walking, and also while sitting still;
     not caused by amorous thoughts.

*Female.*—° Menorrhagia, dysmenorrhœa, and inefficient **or**
     absent labor pains.

° Profuse menstruation and metrorrhagia. (*Hirschel.*)

' Metrorrhagia of parturient women. (*Hirschel.*)

### Larynx and Trachea.

*Rough cough scratching the breast immediately under the sternum.*

### Chest.

Oppression of the chest, with deep, labored breathing.

He feels as if suffocated, and has to be fanned.

*Anguish, accompanied by great oppression; ameliorated in the open air.*

Pressing pain in the heart, with dyspnœa the whole night.

Anguish at the heart.

Painful sticking, as with the prongs of a fork, in the heart.

Pain in the heart, with palpitation when lying on the left side.

Stitches in the heart; accompanied by great oppression; the latter relieved by deep breathing.

It requires great effort to take a deep inspiration.

Palpitation of the heart, awakening him from sleep.

### Back.

*Pain across the shoulders and spine, forcing him to stoop, and preventing him from walking erect.*

### Upper Extremities.

*Agreeable thrilling through the arms and hands.*

The hands feel monstrously large.

Coldness of the right hand, with stiffness and numbness of the right thumb.

### Lower Extremities.

Weariness in both limbs, almost amounting to paralysis; worse in the left.

*Agreeable thrilling in both limbs, from the knees down, with sensation as if a bird's claws were clasping the knees.*

The right limb feels paralyzed when walking.

The right limb suddenly gives way and falls.

He is unable to walk up stairs, on account of an almost entire paralysis of the limbs, with stiffness and tired aching in both knees.

*Entire paralysis of the lower extremities.*

Numb feeling of the sole of the left foot, then of the foot, increasing to a numbness of the whole limb. On attempting to walk he experienced intensely violent pains, as if he trod on a number of spikes, which penetrated the soles of his feet and ran upward through his limbs to his hips, worse in the right limb, and accompanied by drawing pains in both calves; these pains forced him to limp and cry out in agony.

Shooting pains in the joints of the toes of the left foot, worse in the great toe.

Aching and stitching pain in the ball of the left big toe.

Pricking and aching in the joints of the big toe of the left foot.

° One case of complete paraplegia was permanently cured by the Cannabis indica and Nux vomica, some three years since, in my practice. (*Gray.*)

### Fever.

*Pulse below the natural standard, as low as 46.*

General chilliness; loss of animal heat.

° Dr. L. Warner has successfully prescribed the Cannabis in many cases of ship fever (*Typhus petechialis*).

### Sleep.

*Excessive sleepiness;* day sleepiness.

Starting of the limbs while sleeping, which awoke him, when he feared he would have a fit.

Grating and grinding of the teeth while sleeping.

Talking during sleep.

He wakes before midnight, in a state of semi-consciousness; with inability to move; palpitation of the heart, slow, deep, labored and intermittent breathing, and a feeling as if he were dying.

He wakes before midnight overcome with dreadful sensations; imagines he is going to be choked; cries and moans for some time, when all the objects in the room appear double their respective sizes, and he falls asleep again.

Nightmare every night as soon as he falls asleep.

Sound sleep with melancholy dreams.

Dreams of danger and of perils encountered.

Dreams of dead bodies; vexatious dreams; prophetic dreams.

Voluptuous dreams, with erections and profuse seminal emissions.

## Generalities.

*Agreeable thrilling through the body and extremities.*

Great desire to lie down in the daytime.

*Thoroughly exhausted from a short walk.*

He feels so weak he could scarcely speak, and soon fell in a deep sleep.

*Paralysis of the lower extremities and right arm.*

---

# CARBOLIC ACID.

### (*Acidum Carbolicum.*)

PHARMACOLOGY.—This is an acid obtained from coal-tar, by fractional distillation and subsequent purification.

Carbolic acid, in its pure state, is a solid, at ordinary temperatures crystalizing in minute plates of long rhomboidal needles, white or colorless, of a peculiar odor, similar to creosote, and an acrid burning taste. Its specific gravity is 1.065. If colored brown under the influence of light and air, it is impure. It deliquesces on exposure, and ultimately becomes liquid. It is soluble in 20 parts water, its solution, if pure, colorless and remaining so; but if impure, colored brownish by exposure. It is very soluble in alcohol, ether, acetic acid, glycerine, and the volatile and fixed oils. It is neutral to test paper.

OFFICINAL PREPARATION. — (1) Tincture (one grain to ten drops pure alcohol); (2) Triturations of the crystals with coarse sugar of milk.

ANALOGUES.—*Arsenicum, Baptisia, Bromide of Potassium, Bromide of Ammonia, Cimicifuga, Creosote, Lachesis, Mercurius corrosivus, et wd., Phosphorus, Nitric acid, Muriatic acid, Rhus tox., Sulphur, etc.*

[The symptoms here given are mainly taken from Dr. Hoyne's pathogenesis, given in the *Journal of Homœopathic Materia Medica* for May, 1872, to which I have added Dr. Mitchell's symptoms and my own observations. (*Hale.*)]

### Mental Sphere.

*Entire disinclination to study;* what he had accomplished seemed trifling.

Disinclined to work; even correcting proof is fatiguing.

Cross, loses control of temper readily.

Affection bestowed seemed distasteful.

Reading increased all the head symptoms, especially the pressing in the occiput, while the intellect was unusually quiet

Dullness of intellect, which passed away after breakfast.

### Head.

*Forehead—Aching pain in the forehead* (transient).

*Feels as if a band was around the forehead.*

Headache in the forehead of a neuralgic character.

Burning pain in the forehead.

*Dull* (or heavy) *pain running from the forehead to the occiput.*

Feels as if a band was around the forehead.

Felt a dull feeling in the frontal lobe of cerebrum, which increased to a severe headache.

Awoke with a dull, hot, constricted feeling in the head, more especially in the forehead; followed before rising, by an acute piercing pain in the left supra-orbital ridge. This was circumscribed and might have been covered with a silver ten cent piece.

The acute piercing pain lasted only five or ten minutes, and ceased on my rising, leaving the spot where it had been sore to the touch for more than one day.

*Vertex*—burning pain in the top of the head.

Hard headache in the morning confined to the upper half of the head.

Sensation as of fine electric sparks in vertex, changing to a pricking itching, with desire to rub the part and relief from it.

In the vertex a feeling as if the brain was swashing about.

*Temples*—Burning pain in the right temple and top of the head.

Dull aching pain in both temples and back of the head, when leaning forward.

*Occiput*—Dull aching pain in back of head, and right side and temple.

Back of head feels sore.

Constant dull, pressure and pain in the *occiput* and the muscles of the back of the neck, especially just behind the ears. (*Mitchell.*)

*A very great sense of weight on my neck*, with a *tenderness, even to the touch, on the seventh cervical vertebræ.* (A persistent symptom. *Dr. F. N. Mitchell.*)

*Constant vertigo, not* relieved by shutting the eyes; *better* when walking fast in the open air; much worse when sitting down. (*Ib.*)

Constant humming, buzzing sound in the ears, with the head-ache, *without* dullness of hearing. (*Ib.*)

*Sides*—Beating pain in right side of head.

The pains are the most severe on the right side.

Neuralgic pain in left side of head.

*Scalp*—*Itching of scalp*, first on right side, then on left.

Head feels sore when moving it; sore feeling after the head-ache.

The dull, hot, constricted feeling which was severe enough to become an ache at times, (relieved by pressing the head with the hands,) lasted all day long and late in the night.

Confused feeling in the head.

Feel as if I had a cold in the head.

Head seemed to swell and felt hot, even as though it radiated heat as from a hot stove.

Hard headache most of the night.

The headache did not locate anywhere in particular, but was as bad in the forehead as anywhere else.

Headache worse when bending the head forwards.

The headache continued until I went to sleep at night (all day.)

° Periodical sick-headache, generally just before or after the menses.

Headache with nausea; better from drinking a cup of green tea.

Pressure at first relieves the pain for a moment, but if continued increases the headache. However, if the pressure was removed, if only for an instant, and then re-applied, it would bring relief for a moment.

The head pains are the most severe and worse on the right side.

Feels very dizzy from the slightest motion.

A sensation, when stooping, of a coldness in one spot, followed by a clammy sweat on the head.

### Eyes.

Very severe orbital neuralgia, worse *over right eye.*

Burning pain in the eyes, worse in the left.

° Pupils contracted.

Things look as if they were moving backwards and forwards.

Cannot see across the room.

While writing, the letters seem to run together, so that it is
     with difficulty I can read what is written.
Eyes sensitive to light.
A constant dark spot in front of left eye.

### Ears.

Beating pain, with a humming sound in both ears.
Constant humming, buzzing sound in the ears.

### Nose.

Both nostrils plugged up.
Dryness of posterior nares.
When blowing the nose the mucus was bloody—bright red
     blood.
Feeling of expansion in the nasal passages.
*Smell* decidedly *more acute.*
Watery discharge from both nostrils while in the open air;
     ceasing when in doors—returning when entering a cold
     room.
Sensation at left wing of nose as of fine electric sparks; wants
     to rub the part repeatedly.
° Œzena, even malignant, with great fœtor, and ulceration.
     (*Hale.*)

### Face.

Sharp pain about the centre of the cheek, as if bitten by a
     mosquito.
*Face flushed* and burns.
Slight heat of face and forehead, especially the left side.
ᶜ Face blanched and bathed in perspiration.
Drawing pain in the jaw, right side.

### Mouth.

Nasty taste in the mouth.
Swelling and soreness, internal side of left cheek, opposite the
     molars: the cheek is in the way of the teeth when biting.
° Interior of the mouth very white.
ᶜ Slight lividity of the lips and tips of the fingers.
° Tongue dry and chippy.
Aching of teeth of right upper jaw; grinding of the teeth.
ᵒ Toothache from caries, or from a cold.
ᵓ *Thrush* in children and consumptives (a weak wash).

### Throat.

Throat sore; felt slightly hoarse, as if taking cold.

Throat sore only when swallowing, and pressing upon the upper part of the larynx; worse on the right side.

*Soreness worse on the right side.*

Soreness of the throat on empty deglutition.

Sharp stitches in the throat.

The pain in the throat comes on every few moments; the pain is sharp and pricking.

Pricking burning in the throat, as if she had eaten something strong.

Much mucus in pharynx.

Dryness of pharynx and posterior nares.

*Hawking of clear white mucus* while in the open air.

Hawking from pharynx and posterior nares of much white mucus.

° Spasmodic contraction of the œsophagus.

Slight nausea in the throat.

Mucous membrane of the œsophagus dry and shrunken and of a brownish color.

° Ulceration of the throat, tonsils, palate, etc.

### Gastric Symptoms.

*Constant belching* up of large quantities of wind.

Sensation as if the stomach was filled with wind, which ought to come up.

Wind in the stomach very troublesome; better after raising a sort of sweetish-sour liquid.

Nausea in the stomach.

Slight nausea in the throat.

\* *Nausea nearly all the morning.*

After tea the nausea was better, but she was very drowsy.

After tea the nausea returned, and was increased by taking a little sherry wine.

Regurgitation from the stomach which tastes like buttermilk and cabbage.

In the afternoon, after dinner, long continued hiccough

Dull aching, uneasy feeling in the stomach.

Burning pain in the stomach.

° Chronic vomiting of sarcinæ.
° Chronic vomiting of every meal.
° Vomiting in pregnancy.
° Inflammation of the stomach and duodenum.

### Abdomen.

Aching pain in lower part of abdomen.
Burning pain in lower part of abdomen and top of the head.
Rumbling and rolling in the abdomen, with a sense of disten-
sion.
Rumbling in the bowels; a feeling as if diarrhœa would come
on, after walking about.
While sitting, a crampy stitch in left inguinal region.
Abdominal muscles feel sore.
Constant sensation of distension in the abdomen.

### Anus and Stool.

The anus itches and feels as if the skin was rubbed off.
Bowels seem torpid but not costive.
Desire for a stool all day, although I had had a natural move-
ment in the morning.
Two natural stools per day, which is unusual, having generally
but one passage in two days.
° Diarrhœa from bad drainage.
° Cholera infantum, with putrid, rice-water discharges, like
foul eggs.

### Urinary Organs.

Passed an unusual quantity of saccharine urine.
*Urine increased*, and had a strong smell.
Passed urine oftener than usual during the night.
Unusually free flow of urine—normal in color, odor and quan-
tity.
The urine was voided about once in two hours, and was large
in quantity—quality normal.
° Greenish urine, after scarlet fever.

### Genital Organs.

Lascivious dreams, with emissions, followed by weakness and
dejection.
*Male*—Sexual appetite very much decreased.
Awakened by unusual strong sexual excitement.

Itching of scrotum and inside of thighs, relieved by scratching, but it soon returns.

Intense burning itching of the genitals.

*Female*—Menses came on two days later than usual, and were more profuse.

*Menses much more profuse*, and darker color than usual, followed by headache and great nervous irritability for twelve hours.

\* Mucous tubercles on the labia and inside of the thighs, with discharge from the vagina.

ᶜ Puerperal fever, *with* putrid symptoms.

ᶜ Ulceration of the cervix uteri; obstinate. (*Hale*.)

## Larynx.

\* Short hacking cough, with tickling in the throat.

Constant inclination to cough.

Left side of larynx very sore when pressed upon—not true of the right side.

Irritation of the throat, causing a short, dry cough.

Expectoration of a large quantity of thick *whitish mucus.*

ᶜ Catarrhal laryngitis.

ᶜ Large granulations in the throat.

Coughed to clear the bronchi; expectorated a little.

ᶜ Catarrhal croup.

ᶜ *Chronic laryngitis*, threatening phthisis laryngea. (*Hale*.)

## Chest.

Stitches in region of the heart.

Slight uneasy pains in right lung.

Dull aching pain whole left side of chest and abdomen, running around to the shoulder-blades.

While walking out of doors, feeling of expansion (of lightness) in the lungs; also in the nasal passages.

Sensation as of fine electric sparks on the sternal end of right clavicle; later on middle finger of left hand; later on vertex, changing slowly to a pricking itching, with desire to rub the part, and relief from it.

Respiration free and deep; inclination to take a deep breath.

Respiration stertorous, and smelling strongly of the fluid.

### Back.

Aching pain across the small of the back and in the lower limbs.

General soreness; worse in back, abdomen, chest and muscles of neck.

Neck feels lame and stiff, when moving the head.

Drawing in muscles of neck (right side)—think in splenitis capitis.

Soreness of the seventh cervical vertebræ.

While walking rapidly, after dinner, had spasm of the left common carotid artery.

Spasm of the left external carotid artery.

### Upper Extremities.

Drawing pain in the left arm, from the shoulder to the elbow.

Constant tired, heavy feeling in left arm.

Lameness and soreness of right shoulder while walking.

Aching pain in right shoulder when bending forward.

Numbness of the skin of the hands.

Peculiar feeling of stiffness and discomfort (puckering) of the entire hand, which remained until night.

Sensation as of fine electric sparks on middle finger of left hand.

Appearance of a small pimple on middle finger of left hand, which increased in size until it became a sore resembling a carbuncle. The flesh suppurated until a probe could be passed nearly through the finger. (From the direct application of the acid.)

° Lividity of the tips of the fingers.

### Lower Extremities.

Occasional pains in hips and shoulders.

Dull pain in right hip, ankle and left knee, most of the morning.

The pain in the hip has gone to the left shoulder.

Very severe aching pain in right hip joint, felt only while walking, not when sitting still.

Tingling in the left great toe, followed by a feeling as if pressed on.

Sensation, just below the knee on the shin, as if it was touched with a piece of ice.

## Fever.

° Miasmatic fever.

° Typhoid or enteric fever, in the stage of ulceration

° *Scarlatina maligna*, with putrid sore throat, etc.

° Pulse quick, feeble, *intermittent*, small, slow (60 to 100).

*Chilly sensations;* pulse 78.

## Sleep.

*Incessant yawning;* feel languid and sleepy.

Slept heavy; awoke sore all over, especially legs (gluteal muscles), back, chest and arms.

*Wakes often during the night.*

Woke up in the middle of the night and found that he was bathed in perspiration.

Wakes frightened; paralyzed with fear.

Awakened by unusual strong sexual excitement.

Awoke with a dull, hot, constricted feeling in the head.

Passed urine oftener than usual during the night.

Dreams of fire; so vivid was the dream that he was awakened.

*Had a great many dreams,* some amorous, *others I was unable to recall.*

Dreamed that she could not get to sleep on account of thinking about the body I had enbalmed; thought she tossed about and then tried to wake me, to give her some medicine to stop thinking; she thought she could not wake me, and pulled me out of bed; and that I was bathed in perspiration, pale face; thought I was dead. She could not at first be persuaded that she had been asleep. Gave her a dose of *Nux* and she dropped to sleep at once, and slept soundly.

## Skin.

*Itching of the skin of various parts of the body;* scalp, back of neck, left shoulder, left elbow, arms, right forefinger, buttocks, right thigh, outside of thigh, inner side of left knee, shin, calf of leg, ankles, face, nose, right cheek, abdomen, scrotum, genital organs.

Slight *eruption of a vesicular character* all over the body.

Vesicular eruption on the hands and all over the body, which itches excessively; better after rubbing, but leaves a burn ing pain. Neither *Arsenicum, Rhus,* or *Sulphur* had any influence over it. Disappeared after eighteen days without treatment.

\* Pustular eruption.

\* Acne; eczema; impetigo; scabies; psoriasis inveterata.

<sup>c</sup> *Confluent variola,* the pocks began to dry up on the eighth day, tongue clears off, *no secondary fever;* the pocks were dry all over the body on the twelfth day. (*Dr. Middleton, Hahnemannian Monthly, April,* 1872.)

<sup>c</sup>Indolent or irritable ulcers, with unhealthy granulations, and foetid pus, (externally).

° Leprosy; prurigo; pityriasis; lupus; carbuncles.

° Pediculi, and vermin of all kinds on the body.

### General Symptoms.

Complains of being very tired.

Cannot walk straight.

The pains seem to affect the right side first, and afterwards the same parts of the left.

*Itching of various parts of the body.*

*Feels as if he had taken a violent cold.*

General soreness, worse in back, abdomen and chest

Soreness as if I had taken much cold—think I have not.

° Body much swollen a short time before death.

All the muscles prominently used are sore and stiff.

° Cancerous affections.

---

# CARDUUS MARIÆ.

### (*Blessed Thistle.*)

DESCRIPTION.—*Root* perpendicular, strong, simple, with few fibres. *Stalk* from three to six feet high, upright, stem round, ribbed, arachnoid-wooley, branching half way up. *Leaves* longish, heart-shaped at the base, lanceolate sheathing; the very large radical leaves spreading in a circle, narrowing almost to a footstalk, pinnatifid, tipped with spines, the upper ones only serrate, the lower more or less folded or recurved; all naked, smooth, almost shining, green, *marked with broad white stripes along the veins. Flowers* reddish-purple or white. It grows in waste places in Southern Europe; found wild in middle Europe; common in England; scarce in Scotland; seldom, if ever, seen in America, except when cultivated in gardens. It is an annual, blooms from June to September.

PHARMACOLOGY.—The root is bitter, the young leaves sour, the farinaceous seeds tasteless without the hull, bitterish with it, astringent. The *root* and *hull* of the seeds contain the medicinal principle.

OFFICINAL PREPARATION.—(1) Tincture of equal parts of the root and seed with the hull on. (2) Tincture of the hull; dilutions.

[Rademacher's tincture, with which most of the cures reported were made, was prepared as follows: To five pounds of the unbruised seeds add five pounds of highly rectified alcohol and five pounds of water; digest (macerate) with frequent agitation for a week; press and filter. (*Hale.*)]

ANALOGUES.—*Bryonia, Chelidonium, Chionanthus, Nux vomica, Podophyllum, Leptandra, Benzoic acid, etc.*

### Mind.

Depressed, sad, hypochondriacal.

### Head.

\* Dull, heavy in the forehead over the eyes and in the temples
\* Vertigo, with want of clearness of thought.

### Gastric.

Bitter taste, and want of appetite.

Great nausea, pyrosis, eructations, and distension of bowels.

Violent nausea, painful retching, and vomiting of sour green fluid.

Tongue coated white in the middle.

### Stomach.

Feeling of malaise in the epigastric region

Empty eructations after food taken against his inclination.

Pains in the stomach, continuing for two hours, preceded by vomiting.

° Morning vomiting in a pregnant woman; food remains undigested all day.

### Liver.

\* Swelling and painfulness of the liver.

° Tenderness and hardness of the right hypochondria, especially the left hepatic lobe; pressure there caused oppressed breathing and cough; stools brown; urine yellow; respiration asthmatic; expectoration thick and tough, with violent cough.

° Pain in the liver, with œdema of the feet, scanty bright yellow urine, and asthma.

° *Jaundice* (many cases).

° *Gallstones*, with jaundice, pain in stomach, vomiting of bile.

11

etc. (Two cases cured by ½ ℥ tincture in a pint of water; a teaspoonful every two hours. (*Dr. Liedbeck.*)

° *An epidemic* of influenza with *hepatic* symptoms, viz: peculiar brown, gray, dirty complexion of patient, sometimes real jaundiced tint; sensitiveness of left hepatic lobes to pressure; bright, pale yellow, seldom dark green stool; dark brown urine; oppression of the chest; stitches in the side; debility; fever; frontal headache. Nux, Chelidonium, Pulsatilla did no good; only Carduus promptly cured. (*Dr. Reil.*)

° Painful tenderness and swelling of the gall bladder.

° Hepatic affections, with hæmoptysis, asthma and cough.

° Portal congestion and obstruction and its consequences.

° Hypertrophy of left hepatic lobes, with tenderness of the cervical and dorsal vertebræ.

### Abdomen.

Feeling of fullness in the hypochondria, obliging him to draw a long breath.

Inflation of the abdomen, especially on the right side.

Sensibility of the hepatic region to pressure.

Painful sensation of an undefined character in the abdomen, producing deep breathing, increased by violent movement.

Cutting colic in bowels here and there.

Stitches in the abdomen, as well as in the chest.

° Pain in the whole abdomen near the cœcum; cramps; urine normal; complexion smutty, yellowish; sleeplessness; great emaciation; hectic fever.

### Stool.

Stool tardy, knotted, hard, brown. (primary.)

Stool soft, yellowish, thin, loamy, chocolate colored, pappy, and without bilious tinge. (secondary.)

### Urine.

Urine at first normal, then as the bile disappears from the stools, it appears in the urine.

Golden yellow urine, diminished in amount, depositing a sediment; finally scanty and brown.

### Female Sexual Organs.

° Affections of the climacteric period; megrim, metrorrhagia, leucorrhœa, and asthma, with consensual disorder of the liver. (*Reil.*)

### Larynx, and Chest.

° Painful cough at night, obliging him to set up in bed.

° Expectoration of pure blood, or blood and mucus, generally connected with liver troubles.

° Expectoration of tough, clear mucus.

° Influenzas, which appear to cause severe derangements of the liver, even to jaundice.

° Cough of consumptives, and asthmatics.

\* *Stitches in the side*—It relieves, but does not appear to remove the fever and oppression as well as Aconite.

° *Pleurisy*, in the first stage or chronic pleuritic pain.

° *Asthmatic symptoms*, connected with hepatic disorders.

### Fever.

Heat followed by sweat, with full pulse and quotidian aggravations.

---

# CASTANA VESCA.

### (*Chestnut.*)

DESCRIPTION.—The common chestnut tree of the American forests.
OFFICINAL PREPARATIONS. —Tincture of the ripe leaves.

ANALOGUES:—*Bromide Potassium* (?), *Drosera* (?), *Corallium* (?).
(No Provings.)

### Larynx and Cough.

[I have found in all cases that it would, in from five to ten days, relieve the spasms in *pertussis*, and in about two weeks cure it; the little sufferer would whoop no more, but go on to a speedy recovery, to the great delight of myself and friends.—*Dr. Unzicker.*]

[One-half ounce of the leaves in a quart of water; the infusion was drank by the children. The same curative effects would probably follow the use of the lower dilutions.—*Hale.*]

---

# CAULOPHYLLUM THALICTROIDES.

### (*Blue Cohosh, Squaw Root.*)

BOTANICAL DESCRIPTION.—This is a perennial smooth herb with matted, knotty rootstalks, sending up in early spring a simple and naked stem, terminated by a raceme or panicle of yellowish-green flowers supported on pedicels, and a little below, bearing a large compound leaf composed of three ternate leaves, without any common petiole. The whole of the plant is covered with a greenish grey powder when young. Stem smooth, purple when young, one to two and a-half feet high, dividing above into two parts, one of which, a large divided leaf stalk; the other bears a smaller double ternate leaf at the base. Flowers appear in April and May, while the leaf is yet small. Sepals six, with three small bractlets at the base, egg shaped and oblong. Petals six, thick and gland like, somewhat kidney shaped, and a hooded body, with short claws, much smaller than the sepals, one at the base of each. Pistil enlarged on one side, style short. Stigma minute and one sided: ovary bursting soon after flowering (by the presence of the two erect enlarging seeds), and withering away; the spherical seeds remain naked on thin, thick-set seed stalks, looking like berries, the fleshy integument turning blue; albumen of the texture of horns; seeds, one or two about the size of a large pea, erect and globe-shaped, and ripen in the later part of summer, and are said to form an excellent substitute for coffee, when roasted. Fruit, dry, sweet, and insipid. The root, which is the officinal part, is sweetish, bitter, and pungent, and affords a yellowish infusion, and yellow brown tincture. It is yellow inside, brown outside; hard, irregular, knotty, branded with many fibres. Grows all over the United States, in low, moist, rich ground, or on mountains and shady hills, deep woods, or near running streams, or on grounds which have been overflowed with water. An active principle or resinoid is obtained by precipitation from the saturated alcoholic tincture, called Caulophyllin. It is soluble in water, and partly so in alcohol.

OFFICINAL PREPARATIONS.—(1), Tincture from the root, with strong alcohol dilutions; (2), triturations of the pulverized root; (3), triturations of Caulophyllin.

ANALOGUES.—*Pulsatilla, Cimicifuga, Viburnum, Asarum, Ruta, Senecio,* (*Secale,*) *Cannabis ind., Uva-ursi, etc.*

### Head.

Swimming in the head, a sort of vertigo, with dimness of sight.

Sensation of fullness of the head, with pressure behind the eyes, and fullness of the temporal arteries.

Dullness of the head, with contracted feeling of the skin of the forehead.

Sensation as if pins stuck in the forehead, with hard headache.

By spells a very severe pain in the temples, as if both temples would be crushed together.

° Rheumatic and neuralgic headaches; or headaches dependent upon uterine disorder, or spinal irritation.

### Eyes.

Dimness of sight.

Pressure behind the eyes; profuse flow of tears.

### Mouth.

Sensation of dryness and heat in the mouth.

Distress in the fauces that causes frequent inclination to swallow.

Teeth feel sore and elongated

Tongue coated white.

° Aphthæ of the mouth in pregnant and nursing women.

### Stomach.

Heat and fullness in the stomach.

Great thirst.

Distress in stomach and bowels, with drawing in right hypochondrium.

Empty eructations.

Canine hunger, with white-coated tongue.

Frequent gulping up of sour, bitter fluid, with vertigo.

° Spasms in the stomach, cardialgia, spasmodic vomiting, and excessive nausea, attending uterine irritation.

° Dyspepsia, with spasmodic irritation of stomach and bowels.

### Abdomen.

Distension of and rumbling in the abdomen, with tenderness.

Severe colicky pains every few minutes near the umbilicus.

° Spasmodic and flatulent colic.

° Spasmodic action of the muscular tissues of the intestines, from irritation of the motor nerves, or from rheumatism.

### Stool.

Constipation; stool every other day.

Watery stool, great quantity, but no pain.

Soft stool, very white.

### Urinary Organs.

Copious emissions of pale or straw-colored urine.

Every few minutes sharp, stinging pain in glans penis.

### Respiratory Organs.

° Spasmodic affections of the thoracic organs.

### Back.

Dull pain in the lumbar region.

Severe drawing pain in the sterno-cloido mastoid that draws the head to the left side.

### Upper Extremities.

Elbows and wrists ache.

Constant flying pains in the arms and legs.

\* Severe drawing pains in the joints of the arms and legs; also in wrists and fingers.

\* Shutting the hand produces severe cutting pains in the second joints of all the fingers; they are very stiff.

° Inflammatory rheumatism of the joints of the hands.

### Lower Extremities.

Drawing pains in the thighs, knees and legs.

Very sharp pains in left knee joint.

Ankle and toes of left foot are painful.

Knees feel very weak when walking.

All his joints crack frequently when walking and turning.

Pain in feet and toes, worse at night.

### Generative Organs.

\* Sensation as if the uterus was congested, with fullness, heaviness, and tension in hypogastric region.

\* Spasmodic pains in the uterus, and various portions of the hypogastric region.

° Suppression of the menses, with spasms of the uterus.

° Dysmenorrhœa, spasmodic pains in the uterus.

° Menorrhagia, with threatened abortion; from want of good contractions after confinement.

° *False* pains during pregnancy.

° Prevention of premature labor, almost a specific.

° Deficient labor from rigidity of os uteri.

° Suppressed lochia, with uterine cramps.

° Retroversion of the uterus, causing paraplegia.

° Drawing in the groins (uterine ligaments.)

° Labor-like pains, occurring in any uterine disease.

° Abortion, with little or no flooding.

° Gonorrhœa (?)

° *Intermittent* uterine contractions. (Secale causes *continuous.*)

Menses too soon. (three days.)

Relaxation of the os uteri.

Profuse secretion of mucus from the vagina.

Increases the natural pains of labor.

*Male.*—Stinging pains in glans penis.

# CEANOTHUS AMERICANUS.

### (*New Jersey Tea. Red Root*)

BOTANICAL DESCRIPTION.—The Ceanothus is a small shrub, growing from three to four feet high, from a dark red root, which varies widely. During the Revolutionary war, the leaves were used as a substitute for tea. *I have tasted tea made from them; it tastes very much like a poor quality of black tea.*) The leaves are egg-shaped, the broad end at base, with three ribs, toothed edges, downy beneath, very beautiful green in summer, but in the autumn turn a very bright and beautiful red; have a long leaf stalk. The branches are downy. The flowers grow in white clusters. The calyx has five lobes, which are colored, and curved in, the lower part with a thick disk cohering with the ovary, the upper part separating across the fruit. The petals are spreading, hood-shaped, on slender claws, longer than the calyx. The fruit has three lobes, and when ripe splits into three carpels.

OFFICINAL PREPARATIONS.—Tincture of the leaves; dilutions.

ANALOGUES.—(?).

### Mind.

Used as a substitute for *tea;* said to have slightly exhilarating effects.

### Mouth.

Sore mouth after fever. (?)

Aphthæ of nursing children. (?)

### Throat.

Ulcerated sore throat after scarlatina. (?)

### Spleen.

[During the late civil war I used this plant for splenitis, and so well satisfied have I been with the results that for six years I do not remember using anything else for enlarged spleen. I have used it in the worst cases I ever saw, from tender infancy to old age. I have yet to see or hear of its failure in a single case, however inveterate.—*Dr. ——, Atlanta Med. Jour.*]

Enlarged spleen in a child a few weeks old, congenital.

Enlarged spleen after ague, and abuse of quinine.

[The dose was a few drops, or teaspoonful, of the tincture, and the application of the tincture over the spleen.]

[In chronic cases, when the organ is no longer tender, under the use of the tincture, even without the friction, *it soon becomes painful and tender,* then sinks very rapidly to its normal size, and so remains, the patient no longer conscious of its presence.—*Atlanta Medical and Surgical Journal.*]

### Respiratory Organs.

Chronic bronchitis.

### Generative Organs.

Leucorrhœa. Gonorrhœa. Syphilis. (?)

# CEDRON.

*(Simaruba Cedron.)*

DESCRIPTION.—The origin of this drug was for a long time unknown. Even so late as 1870 Hughes wrote: "CEDRON.—It is the fruit of a South American tree, (Simaruba Cedron—supposed to be a kind of cedar,) whose exact description is not yet ascertained."—*Pharmacodynamics*, and edit., p. 203.

He was probably misled by Dr. Casanova's papers in the *Monthly Homœopathic Review*.

Cedron is the *seed* of the fruit; and by consulting Hooker's *London Journal of Botany*, Vol. VI, p. 556, it will be seen that M. Planchon had given a name and botanical station to the so-called "nondescript Cedron," long before Dr. Casanova had penned his paper.

The earliest mention of the Cedron is found in *The History of the Buccaneers, Anno* 1699.

The native Indians first offered the seeds for sale in Carthagena in 1828

Dr. S. A. Jones, who has written up this drug, published in the *American Observer*, said of his work: "When this *resumé* was begun, a more painstaking piece of work was designed. It has long been laid aside; and now that other and more pressing duties are upon us, it is published simply because from no other single source can the practitioner get all that is pathogenetically known of *Simaruba Cedron*. The remedy certainly appears capable to fill a larger sphere than our meagre clinical reports show it to have occupied."

OFFICINAL PREPARATIONS.—Tincture of the seed of the fruit; dilutions

ANALOGUES.—*Arnica, Cimicifuga, Cornus, Cinchona, Quinine, Sepia Sanguinaria, (Nux? Eucalpytus, and perhaps Eupat. perf.)*

## Mind.

Gloomy, depressed spirits; disposition to weep; inquietude and excessive anguish.

Dullness of the senses; torpor of the mental faculties, and uneasiness; dread of friends, (in females particularly.)

## Head.

Head dull and heavy in the morning; distensive headache, increased during the night; temporal arteries enlarged.

Bending of the head backward, with pressure on the occiput and parietal regions, as if these parts were going to burst.

Forehead cold, and as if it were empty, in the morning.

Pressure at the right temple, causing a dull pain in the whole right side of the head; disappears wholly toward noon.

Headache increases in the open air, (toward 9 A. M.)

Pressive pain over the eyes, as if a band were tied round the parts.

Pressure at the top of the head, slight in the daytime, somewhat violent just at the moment when the shivering begins; it never wholly ceased during the whole proving.

Toward 6 P. M. shuddering soon followed by a dull and heavy frontal headache, spreading to both parietal regions.

Pulsating sensation in the temple, and a twisting pain behind the right ear, changing to a dull pain and extending to the temples.

The whole head feels swollen and heavy, most on the right side.

Pressure on the occiput in the morning; in the forenoon, occasional sharp, jerking pains in the occiput; successive sharp pains in the occiput, abdomen and lower limbs. (These pains in the head are dull, except those in the occiput, which are acute.)

At 10 P. M. dull pain in the top of the head, with sharp flying pains in all the joints of the extremities; worse in the feet, particularly the first joint of the great toe.

Awoke late in the morning, after a sound sleep, with dull pain in the vertex, and with dull pain in the whole upper head.

Throbbing in the temples increasing to pain; pain across the forehead, over the eyes, from temple to temple; beating in the temples, increasing to pain and extending over the ears.

Headache, especially in the bottom of the orbits (compelling him to close the eyes), and extending to the occiput.

### Eyes.

Eyes protruding and red, with pressive pain extending to the forehead.

Pupils fixed and dilated; dimness of sight.

Objects appear red at night and yellow in the daytime.

Eyelids injected bright red, and painful when pressed.

Enlargement of the meibomian glands and conjunctiva.

Sensation in the eyes as if one had wept a good deal; itching of the eyes; redness of the eyes, and itching of the inner and outer surfaces of the eyelids.

Conjunctiva inflamed and dry.

Rose early, dizzy; could not see to light a candle, and could not tell when it was lighted.

### Ears.

Singing in the ears as of crickets; buzzing of the ears toward noon; hardness of hearing at night.

° Antidotes the effects of Sulphate of Quinine on the auditory nerves.

### Face.

Flying heat of the face alternated with chills, toward evening, with bloated appearance.

Cheeks red and burning at night, pale and cold in the morning.

Pressing or tearing pain in one or both cheeks, with occasional shoots under the orbits.

Spasmodic twitchings of the *levator palpebræ superioris* during three successive nights.

Toward 6 P. M. constant heat in the face, which looks animated.

Icy coldness of the tip of the nose, even in the midst of febrile reaction, the face being red and burning.

° Prosopalgia, more frequently in women than in men, generally on the right side, recurring in regular paroxysms of indefinite duration, with spasmodic distortion of the muscles corresponding to the affected region (the *zygomatic* process almost always).

ᶜ Chronic intermittent prosopalgia always coming on at 7 or 8 P. M., and lasting from two to four hours.

### Mouth, Tongue, Throat.

Mouth dry, with viscous saliva when talking; lips dry, with desire to moisten them often.

Intolerable prickling itching of the tongue, obliging her to rub it incessantly against the palate.

Slightly yellowish coat on the root of the tongue, with a nasty, sickish, bitter taste of the mouth.

On rising in the morning, gulping up of a bitter wind; tongue coated yellow; bitter taste in the mouth.

Awoke with dull pain in the whole head; tongue coated yellow; sickish taste; sour taste; the saliva becomes sour at night.

After talking, the saliva becomes white and thick like cream.

Taste as of iron in the mouth, causing a profuse flow of saliva; constriction of the throat, which scarcely allows her to swallow the saliva.

ᶜ Mouth and tongue very dry; difficulty of speech; great thirst all the time.

She felt at times as if the tongue was paralyzed, with pricking of the tongue.

(These symptoms *appeared only with* the catamenia, and lasted as long as that discharge; at the termination of which she had a profuse ptyalism and leucorrhœal flow.)

### Appetite—Thirst.

Loss of appetite; appetite is impaired as the proving progresses.

Thirst; desire for cold water at noon and warm during night.

Aversion to cold water during the evening; great thirst and desire for cold water; thirst, and craves only warm drinks.

### Stomach.

Fructations of bitter wind from the stomach before rising in the morning, with dull pain in the temples.

Sensation as of a stone on the stomach; rolling pain in the stomach; sensation of heat and fullness in the stomach.

Distension of the stomach, and disposition to nausea, generally aggravated by rest, but relieved by walking, and by eating.

ᶜ Uncomfortable feeling of the stomach, which obliged him to lie down; great sensitiveness of the præcordial region; pulse small and hard; dryness of the mouth and fauces; depressed spirits and inquietude, relieved by food and drink.

(These symptoms appeared every day from 10 to 11 A. M., lasted from one to two hours, after which there was prostration of body and mind for an hour or two.)

### Abdomen.

Abdomen hard and distended toward evening; flatulence in the morning, with slight colic and discharge of fœtid wind.

Borborygmi in the left side of the abdomen.

Sharp pain alternately in the cœcum, liver, and spleen.

Successive sharp pains in the occiput, abdomen and limbs;

pains only in one place at a time; on getting warm in bed, flying pains in the region of the ascending colon; liver and spleen—kept him awake most of the night.

### Stool.

Constipation; unsuccessful urging to relieve the bowels.

Copious stool, with excessive tenesmus.

Yellowish loose evacuations (three days after taking large doses of Cedron).

Whitish stools, mixed with fragments similar to clotted milk (in other provers, three days after large doses).

Slight colic, followed almost immediately by a copious evacuation of a substance that looked like curdled milk, white, with a slightly yellowish tint (from chewing the nut as an antidote to the bite of a *coral snake*).

° Semi-liquid, whitish fæces, somewhat like starch; white, frothy, and papescent evacuations immediately after meals, accompanied with slight colic and discharge of inodorous wind.

° Involuntary discharge of urine and fæces.

### Urine.

Scanty urine; frequent ineffectual urging to urinate.

Frequent emission of large quantities of pale urine.

Dark urine with sediment; urine of a dark-red color; scanty urine, with deep yellow color.

### Genitals.

Nocturnal erections and intense venereal excitement (many provers.)

Genital excitement at daybreak, with a discharge similar to leucorrhœa, and swollen mammæ with some pain (in two married women.)

A discharge like gonorrhœa, continuing three days and ceasing spontaneously on omitting the drug (in a young man.)

Dreamed all night (I seldom dream) of pleasant social interviews with female acquaintances, and woke with firm erections in the morning.

### Larynx.

Larynx constricted and tender; difficulty of swallowing; difficult respiration with partial loss of voice recurring at intervals.

## Chest.

Oppression of the chest and throbbing of the heart.

Oppressive pain in the chest every now and then, extending to the back, with frequent desire to moan and take a long breath.

Palpitation of the heart and hurried breathing with headache.

Pulse increased from 12 to 15 impulses per minute, in from 20 to 30 minutes after the dose. (This was a constant phenomenon in all the American provers—three women and two men. The doses were from one to three drops of the crude tincture.)

The oppression of the chest and throbbing of the heart occurred in nearly all the provers in whom febrile paroxysms were developed.

## Back.

Pains in the loins and back on rising in the morning.

° Rigidity of the nape of the neck.

° Pain all along the spine.

## Superior Extremities.

Laming and weary pains in the shoulders; passing pains in the elbows and forearms, with a cold sensation extending to the hands toward noon; sharp flying pains in all the joints of the extremities; arthritic flying pains continue, more or less, for more than four weeks, most in the feet and hands, some in the elbows.

Laming passing pains in the joints, especially the right elbow; pain at the elbow and right forearm, as from a shock or blow, lasting one quarter-of-an-hour.

Various unpleasant sensations, such as contusive pains at the elbow, etc., recurring periodically every morning at nine o'clock; hands unusually pale; hands cold; pains (when not febrile concomitants) relieved by friction.

° Numbness of the arms and legs.

° Irregular and uncontrollable movements of the left arm and legs.

## Inferior Extremities.

On getting warm in bed, severe, sharp flying pains in all parts of the system; the pains in the limbs seem to be

in the cartilages of the joints, particularly in the first
joint of the great toe, and streaking *up* the bones; lanc-
ing pains in the joints of the knees; sharp flying pains
in all joints of extremities, worse in the feet, particularly
the great toe joint; smart rheumatic pains in all the
joints of the limbs; sharp, lame pain in the right ankle;
swelling of the feet, with extreme pain in all the joints;
in the morning, pain at the heel as from an abscess, only
when walking, for an hour, after which period it ceases
entirely.   Various unpleasant sensations, such as contusive pains in the elbow, or pains as from an abscess of
the heel, recurred periodically every morning at nine
o'clock; arthritic flying pains continued, more or less, for
more than four weeks, most in the feet and hands, some
in the elbows, more in the hips and knees; but most
troublesome in the first joint of the great toes; pain
relieved by motion and cold before *soreness* of the joints
came on, when they are aggravated by motion and cold,
worse at night.

### Sleep.

A general feeling of fatigue after awaking, if the sleep has
exceeded more than six hours, and a general weakness of
body and mind.

No sleep, with a flow of confused ideas until five in the morning; all night very restless, frequently waking fatigued
from lying in one position.   Dreamed of quarreling with
a dead sister and other dead friends, cried about it and
awoke with a nightmare, and sensation of a stone on the
stomach.

### Fever.

Feverish paroxysms every day in some provers, every other
day in others, toward eight P. M., preceded by depressed
spirits, dullness of the senses and pressing headache at
noon; cramps, then contracting and tearing pains in the
upper and lower extremities, with a cold sensation in the
hands and feet; mouth dry, great thirst and desire for
cold water; chills and shivering; sometimes very strong
shuddering of the whole body; palpitation of the heart

and hurried respiration; pulse weak and oppressed. These symptoms lasted from one to two hours, varied much in intensity, and were followed by a sensation of dry heat, and then of profuse perspiration, full and quick pulse with animated red face; cold and pale in the apyrexia; thirst and desire for warm drinks.

At three o'clock p. m., shuddering all over the body, with malaise and desire to lie down; the shuddering is renewed by motion; hands, feet, and nose are cold; flying heat in the face several times; lastly, toward six o'clock in the morning, constant heat in the face, which looks animated, with smarting in the eyes, especially when closing them; lips dry, with desire to moisten them often; headache, especially in the bottom of the orbits, compelling him to close the eyes, and extending to the occiput.

While this congestion of the head lasts, the shuddering continues all the time; the hands, feet, and nose remain cold; urine of a dark-red color.

Toward six o'clock in the evening (immediately after dinner) cold all over; shuddering in the back, icy coldness in the feet; the hands are burning; sensation in the eyes as if one had wept a good deal.

In the evening toward $6\frac{1}{2}$, half-an-hour after dinner, shuddering in the back and legs; unusual paleness of the hands; red face; heaviness of the head, stretching toward seven in the evening; general coldness all evening; increase of the headache in the open air (toward nine o'clock); pressive pain over the eyes as of a band of iron tied round the parts; no thirst during the shuddering; dry heat at night.

At $6\frac{1}{2}$ p. m., feverish paroxysms with itching in the eyes, which is only stopped for a moment by rubbing; laming and weary pains in the shoulders; profuse emission of watery urine. Toward 5:30 p. m., prickings in the tongue; itching of the eyes; half-an-hour later shiverings, with heat of the face, hands pale, feet and tip of the nose cold.

Toward six p. m., shuddering, soon followed by a dull and heavy frontal headache spreading to both parietal regions, with redness of the eyes, itching of the internal and ex-

ternal surfaces of the eyelids; icy coldness of the hands
*and tip of the nose*, even in the midst of the febrile reaction (the pulse is 80), the rest of the face is red and
burning; lastly, dimness of sight, dilatation of the pupils;
objects look red; mouth dry, with thick, viscous saliva;
constriction of the throat, which scarcely allows her to
swallow the saliva; anxiety, restlessness, general malaise.

The medicine being taken by the healthy prover, was followed
by—

1st.   A certain state of mental excitement, and augmentation
of vital energy; florid face, and a sensation of heat
throughout the body; full and strong pulse; more or
less perspiration and no thirst.

This group lasted from twenty to forty minutes in some, and
disappeared after that time to return no more, without
any other abnormal manifestation in their health; whilst
in others, the symptoms were prolonged for one to two
hours, and were followed by—

2nd.   Depressed spirits; dullness of the senses, and torpor of
the mental faculties; general debility, languor and faint-
ings in some. When these symptoms are followed by
those of the first group, the phenomena of both sets are
often repeated, and at certain intervals of time; but
neither of the two occur periodically, unless when they
are together. Nor are they absolutely concomitant to
pyrexia; for the paroxysms generally take place without
them, as in the natural disease. It is for this reason that
such phenomena were disconnected from category of the
physical group; but whenever pyrexia occurs, or follows
that condition, the symptoms, after weakness of the mind
and body, are as follow:—

3rd.   Great thirst; yawning; cramps and painful feelings of
contraction in the lower extremities; cold sensation in
hands and feet; chills and shivering of the whole body;
palpitation of the heart; pulse weak and oppressed; hurried respiration; chattering of the teeth and shaking of
the whole body; scanty and highly-colored urine; slight
nausea in some, with yellow color of the skin and face in

others; great debility; dilated pupils and confused sight. These symptoms lasted from one to two hours, and varied much in their intensity; after which—

4TH. Dry heat follows, with full and quick pulse; animated face; profuse perspiration; longing for cold in some, and for warm drinks in others; and discharge of pale urine in large quantities. These symptoms lasted from two to three hours, and were generally followed by a desire to sleep. The provers felt as if they were contused; sound sleep in some, and somewhat agitated in others during the night.

The apyrexia generally lasted from fifteen to seventeen hours, after which and *in about the same time as the previous day*, the paroxysms were repeated as per group third, and continued almost quotidian.

*The chief characteristic of this remedy is a* PERIODICITY *which is often clock-like in its regularity.*

---

# CERASUS VIRGINIANA.

### (*Choke Cherry.*)

BOTANICAL DESCRIPTION.—This is a small tree or shrub, from **five to** twenty feet high, growing in woods and hedges. Leaves smooth, oval, or egg-shaped, the broad extremity at base, sharp pointed, thin, not shining, with edge serrate, the teeth being oval-shaped and sharp, veins bearded on each side toward the base; the leaf-stalk with two glands. The flowers are in short, loose and spreading branches; petals circular and white, appearing in May; outer bark greyish; inner bark green; leaves two or three inches long. The fruit is abundant, of a dark red color, very astringent to the taste, but not disagreeable.

OFFICINAL PREPARATION.—(1) Tincture of the inner bark; and dilutions to 3 × dilute alcohol: above, strong alcohol.

ANALOGUES.—*Digitalis, Laurocerasus, Lycopus, Collinsonia, Hydrocyanic acid, Amygdala, Ammonia, etc.*

## Head.

Heavy, dull feeling in the head.

## Stomach.

* Dyspepsia, with tendency to *acidification* of food.
° Slow digestion, with pyrosis.
° Loss of appetite, with weak, intermittent pulse.

12

### Generative Organs.

° Debility from spermatorrhœa.

### Chest.

° Cough from functional or disease of the heart.
° Irregular and intermittent action of the heart, *with deficient impulse.*
° Hypertrophy, with dilatation.
° Pulse quick, weak and irregular.
° Debility after fever or any exhausting disease, especially in heart affections.
° Whooping cough.   ° Phthisis pulmonalis (palliative).

### Fever.

° Hectic fevers.   ° Intermittent fevers. (?)

### Skin.

° Ulcers.   ° Scrofula.

---

# CHELIDONIUM MAJUS.

### (*Great Celandine.*)

DESCRIPTION.—Root cylindrical, reddish-brown, with many fibres; stem upright, hairy, branched, one to three feet high. Leaves soft, pinnate, netted, bright green above, glaucous beneath, with large trifid terminal lobes; tip oval, sinnate, or crenate; petioles winged, hairy. Flowers of four petals, yellow, in four-to-nine-flowered axillary cymes, each flower with a peduncle and bract; petals nearly round; calyx of two convex, green, deciduous, nearly smooth sepals; stamens twenty; divergent, equal. Fruit a siliquose, many.seeded, knotty capsule, with two carpels.

Seeds shining, blackish-brown, with little pits. Duration, perennial.

There are, besides, but two species known as yet—one of which grows in Japan (Ch. Japanicum, Thumberg), and one in North America (Ch. diphyllum, Mich.)

In the whole of Europe no other plant grows which, when injured, gives out golden-yellow milk; and from this peculiarity, no plant is so well known to every village child. The milk of the root has a redder tinge than elsewhere.

This fluid is contained in special canals which reticulate over the leaves and open into main vessels along the ribs. Schultz first made known the movement of the juice, called by him Cyclosis.

If a recently gathered tender leaf be placed under a good microscope, one can see the reticulated canals colored by the yellow juice, and plainly distinguish the slow movement of the fluid, whilst crowds of globules pass through the petioles

If a leaf be torn across, the yellow juice issues in drops out of the larger veins on both sides of the ribs.

On the skin the juice makes yellow spots, which on drying turn brownish-black, and also colors the dried root black.

The smell of the recent plant is disagreeable; the taste sharp and bitterish, especially of the root.

On drying, it almost entirely loses the smell.

The milk, when dry, tastes more bitter than sharp.

After chewing the plant, the taste remains for several hours, and gives a sensation of heat in the mouth, throat, and stomach. Eight pounds of the fresh plant lose one pound eight ounces by drying in the shade.

OFFICINAL PREPARATION.—Tincture of the whole plant; dilutions.

ANALOGUES.—*Agaricus, Æsculus, Bryonia, China, Carduus, Dioscorea, Lycopodium, Leptandra, Mercurius, Nux vomica, Podophyllum, Phosphorus, Sulphur, Sanguinaria, Myrica.*

## Mental Sphere.

Depression of spirits; extraordinary dejection.

Incapacity for thought.

Cross, quarrelsome disposition. (*p.*)

Great calmness of spirits and cheerfulness. (*s.*)

° Restlessness and uneasy conscience, as if she had committed a great crime and could find rest nowhere.

° She thinks she must die.

° Thinking becomes difficult to her, and she easily forgets what she wants to do or has done.

## Head.

* Tearing in left side of the occiput, over the ear and toward the front.

* *Repeated attacks of violent throbbing pains from nape to occiput.*

* *Frontal headache* and itching of the skin.

Shooting in the forehead under the skin.

Aching pains in both temples.

Tensive, heavy feeling in the top of the head extending to the occipital protuberance, and the head feels as if surrounded by a band; inwardly a pressing heaviness.

* Great weight in the occiput, and drawing in the nape from above downwards.

Giddiness, with weight in the upper part of the head.

On moving the head the neck is stiff on both sides, and painful on taking a deep breath.

Feeling of undulation and weight of the whole head.

Shooting in the frontal bone over the left eye; thereafter on left side of the occiput.

Violent throbbing in the temporal arteries with headache; aching pain in right temple, then in right parietal bone, lastly close over the right eye.

° Throbbing headache.

° Twitching here and there in the head.

Congestion of blood to the head.

° Feeling of a cord about the forehead and temples, close over the eyebrows, as if the head were compressed.

° Pain in the head, increased by fresh air, cough, blowing the nose, and stooping.

Twitching here and there in the head.

° Vertigo on sitting up in bed.

Vertigo, with shivering over the upper part of the body.

Vertigo on closing the eyes, as if everything were turning in a circle.

° Vertigo, with tendency to fall forwards.

*Great pain in the head*, passing from within outwards, *especially toward the forehead, all day.*

Pressive, tearing pain between the eyebrows and over the right eye, tending to close the eyes.

° *Neuralgic pain over the right eyebrow*, periodically, every morning.

*Violent throbbing in the temples, with great anxiety.*

Periodical stupefying pains in the crown and left temple, so that her ideas are lost.

° *Violent drawing pain from the crown to the nape*, so that she is forced to draw up her shoulders, close her eyes, and tread lightly.

° Splitting pressure, and painful throbbing, in the occiput, worse on lying down.

Sensation of cold mounting up from the nape to the occiput.

When she wants to sit up in bed she has to raise her head with her hand, because the occiput seems to be fastened to the pillow and broken off from the rest of the skull.

Creeping on the whole of the hairy scalp, and also on individual spots, passing off more or less when scratched.

Scalp on the crown painful; hot to the touch.

° Great falling off of the hair on the occiput when combed.

*Pain in the roots of the hair when combed*, as if there was ulceration beneath.

° Pressive headache, and heat in the head with the pains.

° Pressure as if from a band around the forehead and temples

° Weight in forehead, as if it were falling outwards.

° Pressing pain in left parietal region.

° Drawing pain in the occiput, with feeling as if the head were drawn backwards.

### Eyes.

\* Lids of both eyes are closed with dry mucus in the morning.

\* Tearing, pressure and shooting in right eye, soon afterwards in left.

Pressure in the orbits.

Shooting in left eyelid; ° burning in lower eyelids.

\* Tearing pain in the left eye and close above it.

° Photophobia, with pain in forehead.

° Violent pressive pain in left eye, in the middle of the ball, as if it was so large that the upper lid could not be let down over it.

\* On moving the eye, pain in the eyeballs and feeling of sand in the eyes.

Increase of the pain by lamplight, relief on closing the eyes.

Pricking between the eyebrows toward the right eye.

Stupefying pressure in the right orbit, as it were from without inwards.

\* Pressure and pain in the upper part of the eyeballs, as if they were squeezed in, *more in the left than the right eye.*

Sudden jerk in the left eye, in the middle of the ball, as if it was so large that the upper lid could not be let down over it.

Continual pricking and burning, as if from a grain of sand, in the inner canthus of the left eye.

Redness and swelling of the lower tarsal edges.

Twitching and burning in the eyelids.

<sup>c</sup> In the morning the lids are swollen and agglutinated.
*Flickering and dazzling and brilliant specks before the eyes.*
She sees blackish-gray specks before the eyes.
When reading or writing the letters run into each other.
Blackness before the eyes, with a sensation of faintness.
Yellow, jaundiced color of the eyes.

### Ears.

*Ringing, buzzing and rushing in the ears.*
Burning in the left ear, while the right is cold.
Shooting in the ears.
Tearing in the meatus auditorius and temporal bone.
Frequent tearings from right ear into right teeth.
*Hoarse roaring in the ears like a distant storm of wind.*
A tearing pain behind the right ear, downwards.

### Nose.

° Dryness and itching in left nostril.
Fluent coryza, with frequent sneezing.
On blowing the nose in the morning, thick blood appeared
 among the mucus. (Was subject to epistaxis.)
Prolonged pressing pain from the root of the nose to the nasal
 bone.
Itching and burning in the tip of the nose.
Tearing in the nostrils, most severe in the left.
° Feeling of soreness in the nostrils.

### Face.

* Sunken countenance, with grayish-yellow face.
* Complexion strikingly yellow, as if from jaundice.
* *Redness of the left cheek*, passing gradually from bright red
 to dark red.
A small, defined, burning, dark red, circular, somewhat ele
 vated spot on the left cheek.
Feeling of great cold in the face; cheeks pale and feeling cold.
Glowing heat in the face, with dark, obscure red complexion.
Vesicles on the lip and *alæ nasi*, forming scabs.
Burning, as if from nettles, here and there on the face.
Isolated stitches in the face, worse in the evening in bed;
 warmth aggravates, cold water relieves, the pain.

° Pains in the teeth, lasting several weeks, chiefly in the whole of the left cheek, especially at night.

Toothache every night (for eight days).

Drawing pain in the molars of the right side.

Sudden jerk in the teeth, as if torn out.

Violent pains in the molars of the left side, which extend to the left ear and draw into the left eye, with swelling and redness of the left side of the face, whereupon an abscess formed on the hard palate (after rubbing the tincture into the eyelids).

° Jerking pain in right zygoma, as if torn to pieces.

### Mouth.

Dry, chapped, and scabby lips.

Vesicle full of serum, as clear as water, on the mucous membrane of the lower lip.

Bleeding of the gums.

Dryness, so that the tongue almost clave to the palate.

Abscess on the left side of the hard palate, near the furthest molar, of the size of a bean (after rubbing the tincture on the eyelids).

Tongue in the morning covered with gray, shaggy, thick coat, which can be partly rubbed off.

Pricking on the end of the tongue; stitch in end of the tongue, left side.

*Collection of water in the mouth*, with nausea and giddiness.

° Dryness in the mouth and lips, with thirst.

° Redness and swelling of the uvula and tonsils.

### Appetite and Taste.

° Bitter taste, whilst food and drink taste naturally.

Bitter in the mouth and burning in the stomach.

Loss of appetite, especially in the evenings (for six days).

Increased appetite, such as occurs in bilious affections.

* Great thirst, with dryness in the mouth and throat.

Much thirst for milk, (it previously produced flatus).

Longing for wine, which relieves the abdominal pain.

Whilst taking the medicine, inclination for warm drinks; after the proving, continual thirst for cold water.

Great dislike to cheese, boiled food, especially flesh, and cold drinks.

### Fauces and Œsophagus.

Slight irritation in the œsophagus, imperceptible when swallowing.

Slight shooting in the tonsils on empty swallowing.

Contractive spasm in the gullet, forcing him to swallow.

Scraping and pricking in the throat; roughness.

Smoking causes burning pain and acidity from the cardia up into the throat.

Heat and burning from the mouth down to the stomach.

A feeling as if some foreign body was mounting up in the throat, obliging him to swallow, and then going down again.

Hawking up of lumps of mucus.

° Feeling of dryness in the throat, with difficulty of swallowing.

### Gastric Symptoms.

Bitter eructations, and bitter taste in the mouth.

*Great nausea*, with increased temperature of the body.

Nausea, with inclination to vomit; (from the external application).

° Nausea and retching during a fit of anxiety.

° Vomiting of tough mucus after severe nausea.

° Eructation, with heartburn.

### Stomach.

\* Pressure and oppression of the stomach, drawing up toward the chest.

Pinching, pressing pain in and below the scrobiculus cordis, increased by the touch.

Stomach pain for one hour, with eructation of wind, relieved by lying on the left side with the legs drawn up.

Spasmodic pain in scrobiculus cordis, toward the right.

° Violent pain in the scrobiculus cordis, as if the stomach was constricted.

° Digging pain in the epigastric region.

Feeling of heat in the stomach, with pressure and pricking.

Stitches in the pit of the stomach.

Cutting in the stomach, increased by pressure.

Peculiar feeling of gnawing and clawing in the stomach, which passes off after eating. (*See Arnica and Lachesis.*)
' Pressure on the stomach, with eructation of wind.
' Pressure in the pit of the stomach, with oppression of the chest and difficult breathing.
° Distension of the stomach.

### Hypochondria and Liver.

Stitches in the liver.

Dull throbbing and pressing pain in the region of the liver.

\* Pressing pain in the region of the liver, on the edge of the ribs; the pressure of the clothes increases the pain.

\* Pain in the region of the liver, which extends quickly downwards across the navel into the intestines.

° Spasmodic pain in the region of the liver.

° *Congestion of the liver*, also chronic disease of the liver.

° *Jaundice*, even the most obstinate functional kinds; also when caused by obstruction of the gall ducts from calculi, or biliary concretions. (*Hale.*)

° *Biliary calculi;* specific in many cases. (*Hale.*)

### Abdomen.

Spasmodic contraction of the navel, with transient nausea.

Constricted feeling over the navel, as if the abdomen was tied round with a string.

\* Violent pressing, periodically returning, and also continued spasmodic pain in the umbilical region.

\* Painful distension.

\* Pinching about the umbilical region as if stool were coming on.

Pain over the left hip, as if there was something thick and bulging there.

Spasmodic drawing pains in the inguinal regions, with pressure on the bladder.

Tensive, spasmodic pain on each side, extending from above down and inwardly, followed by a discharge of turbid lemon-colored urine.

Labor-like pain, drawing from the lumbar vertebræ over the hips toward the hypogastrium.

° Abdomen distended and hard, without pain on being touched.

When coughing, the whole abdomen is painfully contracted.

Cutting in the intestines, as if from knives.

° Accumulation of flatus, with a full, bloated feeling in the abdomen.

Burning in the bowels.

Cold feeling and pressure in the abdomen, especially below the umbilical region, with cold of the whole body.

Pinching, extending toward the chest and back, relieved by passing flatus.

Constant pinching and commotion here and there in the intestines.

Feeling as if the intestines were torn out of the abdomen.

Sensation of turning and moving about the navel, as if an animal was wriggling through the bowels.

Rumbling, with diarrhœa following.

### Stool and Anus.

Stool very hard and difficult, with pains in the anus in consequence.

Costiveness; stool like sheep-dung for two days.

Repeated thin fluid stools daily, from four to eight days duration.

° Mucous diarrhœa; ° painless diarrhœa.

Brown watery stools.

ᶜ At night, once, severe watery, whitish diarrhœa, with nausea after severe chill in the evening.

* Small, thin, bright yellow stools (characteristic of its primary action).

Soft, greenish stool, with cutting pain in rectum and higher up.

Pressure in the rectum, with urging to stool.

Periodic straining and pressure on the rectum, as if before stool, without result.

Sensation as if the rectum was forced out, with spasmodic constriction of the anus, lasting all day.

Cutting pains in the anus and rectum during a hard stool.

Burning and cutting in the rectum, with alternation of itching in the anus; vertigo; fainting sensation and failure of appetite.

Painful nodule on the margin of the anus.

Crawling, pricking, and itching in the rectum, and on the perineum.

° Soft bright yellow stool, with straining and moderate pain in the anus afterwards.

° White, clay-colored stool, destitute of bile. (*Hale.*)

### Urinary Organs.

Pressing pain in the left renal region.

Stitch in the left kidney on deep inspiration.

\* Pain in region of both kidneys, which are very sensitive to pressure, even the bands of the underclothing give pain there.

In the morning on rising, violent stitches in renal region, making her cry out and then fall down.

She cannot lie on her back owing to pain in the renal region, and must also often change from side to side. Gets most relief by lying on her face.

Spasmodic pain in right kidney, with sweat on forehead and hands.

Spasmodic pain close above the os pubis, with frequent urging to pass urine.

Burning in the urethra when passing urine.

Shooting and cutting in the urethra on passing urine, and on moving the body.

° Shooting pains in the region of the bladder.

Frequent call to pass *urine; pale,* watery.

Call to make water every quarter-hour, passing some five times within one and one-half hours.

Had to make water ten to twelve times a day, and two or three times a night, and a great deal each time.

° Urine reddish and turbid immediately after being passed.

° Napkins reddish-brown from the urine; after drying still more darkly colored.

° Urine dark brown, turbid, forming bubbles on the edge like brown beer.

Urine has an excess of uric acid salts.

° Urine turbid as soon as passed, lemon yellow after previous pains in the inguinal region. In four hours a grayish yellow, mucus, cloudy sediment, without the urine being cleared.   The inner surface of the utensil is covered with reddish crystals of uric acid as far as the urine reaches. The urine is turbid from an excess of acid uric salts, is deficient in chlorides, contains crystals of hippuric acid, mucous epithelium, and compact urinary cylinders.

° Urine bright red, *with a sharp acid smell.*

Urine with a strong ammoniacal smell.

### Generative Organs.

*Male.*—Pressure and forcing toward the root of the penis.

Shooting and creeping on the glans.

Frequent erections even in the day time.

Pressure and tensive pain in the testicles downwards, with pressive pain in the occiput.

Drawing and stitching pain in the testicles.

Redness, heat and swelling of the scrotum.   On the following day, on both sides there is here and there a raising of the epidermis from yellowish serum in flat vesicles the size of a pin's head, and from that to a small lentil, painful to the touch.   In the evening the vesicles burst and the red and swollen skin, stripped of the epidermis, discharges a little fluid.   On the morning of the third day the scrotum is covered with dry, thin, cracked, red scales.

*Female.*—Daily for 14 days constant burning in the vagina at precisely the same hour, forenoon and afternoon.

Menstruation set in two days earlier than usual, but more copious.

Menstruation four days too early, and rather in excess, after vertigo, staggering, pricking, itching pains in the head and limbs.

Menses very copious the ninth day, going on increasing for three days; about four days too late, with pains, lasting seven days.

A mucus discharge from the vagina for some days, coloring the linen yellow.

Menstruation passing gradually into leucorrhœa (suffered from this previously.)

### Larynx and Trachea.

Sensation as if the larynx were pressed from without on the

œsophagus, whereby swallowing, not breathing, is rendered difficult.

Severe shooting in the larynx, with a constrictive sensation.

Choking sensation in the throat, aggravated by breathing.

Pressure, with sense of constriction in the trachea, mounting from the sternum towards the larynx.

° Sense of constriction in the trachea, with deadly anguish, and a wish for eructation without success (at night on awaking.)

Rapidly following stitches in the larynx toward the outside and inside of the throat.

Scraping in the larynx, exciting a cough.

Frequent hoarseness, with dry cough.

Heat mounting from the chest to the throat, quite into the larynx.

Congestion of blood toward the larynx, with dull throbbing there.

Sensation of dust in the trachea, and throat, and behind the sternum, which could not be removed by cough.

### Cough.

\* Infrequent, slight fits of coughing, with spasms of the glottis on expectoration.

\* Dry, hollow cough; violent spasmodic cough.

Cough, with severe tickling in the larynx in the evening.

° Whooping-cough. (Specific in certain epidemics.)

° Short cough, with short breathing.

° Frequent fits of short cough, with stitches in right side and difficulty of breathing.

° Much exhausting cough, especially in the morning, with much expectoration deep out of the lungs.

Strong fit of coughing, without expectoration.

Dry cough, lumps of phlegm being sometimes thrown out.

° Pain in the larynx when coughing, with pains in chest and sacrum.

° Shooting pain in the throat and region of the larynx.

### Chest.

\* Tightness of the chest, with oppression.

Shortness and difficulty of breathing, with tightness and anxiety of the chest.

Difficulty of breathing, with shooting in the left thoracic region backwards.

* He can only breathe short, and with difficulty and anxiety,
as if he must choke.

° Respiration impeded in the evening in bed.

° Short breathing and oppression, as if the breast were constricted and the breath could not pass.

Her clothes cause tightness of the chest, so that she has to
loosen them.

Longing for fresh air to breathe more easily.

He cannot at each breath inspire as much air as he wishes,
therefore expires quickly in order to be able to inspire
again soon.

° Difficult respiration, with short fits of coughing, preceded by
pain first in the right then in the left side of the thorax.

She must breathe quick and short in order to make somewhat
tolerable the pains in the chest and back.

She cannot take a deep breath for violent stitches in the right
side.

° Anxiety in the chest and oppression.

Congestion in the apices of the lungs, with dull throbbing in
them.

* At each breath pain inside the chest, with short dry cough,
which increases the pains and returns after short pauses.
(Pulse 90.)

On stooping low, pain deep in the chest, especially toward
the bodies of the vertebræ, so that the stooping could not
be continued; also after walking fast, blowing the nose,
and sneezing; at the same time more externally along the
spinous processes.

Inward burning between the chest and shoulder-blades, with
internal heat and want of breath.

On deep inspiration, painful tension around the inside of the
base of thorax.

Stitch in the chest, with interruption of the breathing.

Stitches in the right side behind the ribs.

Stitches in the lower part of the left lobe of the lungs.

*In the left lobe soreness like a wound*, aggravated by *deep breathing*, coughing and sneezing.

High up behind the sternum a spot which smarts like a wound.

Spasmodic pressure behind the sternum, in the middle, on a surface about two inches in diameter, on awaking in the night.

High up behind the sternum a feeling of dust, not to be removed by coughing.

Tensive pain in the whole thorax.

Constrictive pressure under each arm, as if the chest was tight-laced.

Drawing pressure from the right shoulder-blade, through the chest towards sternum.

On inspiration fine stitches like needles in the chest, passing from the left to the right side.

The seventh and eighth rib of each side are painful to the touch, and on drawing the breath, as if they were wounded, worse on the right side; a cold sensation steals from the spine to those ribs on the way to the sternum, worse on the right side.

Pains and jerking in the left clavicle.

*Oppressive pain under the left clavicle up the neck.*

*Shooting in the right side, close under the mammary gland.*

Tensive pain from the left pectoral muscle up toward the neck.

*Lancinating pains* in pectoral muscles.

° Violent pains in the sternum at each respiration.

° *Shooting*, jerking pain a little to the right from the lower part of the sternum right through toward the back, aggravated by breathing. By laying the trunk forwards the pain is worse in the chest; by laying it backwards, worse in the back.

° She must sit upright, and dare not move; otherwise the pains in the chest are intolerable.

Deep, pressive pain on the right side without cough, which does not allow deep inspiration.

Pain as if from a deep seated abscess.

Pain in the lower part of the wall of the chest on the right,

quite to the right side, for the breadth of a hand, **aggra**
vated by each inspiration.

° Sudden, violent pain of the right side in the region of the
seventh and eighth ribs, increased by respiration and
movement for two hours, preceded and followed by burning headache.

Drawing pains from lower part of the sternum toward the
right, quite round to the spine, with *sore pain* there, so
that even the touch of the clothes increases the pain.

Repeated stitches, lasting some minutes, compelling short
breathing; on attempting deeper breathing, intolerable
stitches.

Stitches in right side for two hours, with chill, heat, and red
cheeks.

° Violent stitches in the under part of throat, right side, aggra·
vated by breathing, movement, and cough.

° Violent stitches for three hours, in right side, obliging her to
inspire slowly and carefully, and also to speak softly;
sometimes not to move or speak at all.

Tearing pressure in left axilla and thence toward the nipple.

Pain in left side as if bruised, *aggravated by movement.*

Awaking with stitches, confined chest, and anxiety; she cannot
take a deep inspiration for the stitches.

### Heart.

Stitches in the cardiac region on coughing.

Oppressive pressure in cardiac region.

Stitches in the region of the heart through the left side of the
chest, so that she has to breathe short and quick.

Lancinating pains in the heart; and stitches under the heart.

Palpitation toward evening, after sitting down somewhat tired;
and in the evening directly after lying down.

° Violent stitches in the cardiac region, followed by strong
palpitations, with anxiety and agitation all day.

° Sudden great anxiety, with palpitation. (The beating of the
heart is not accelerated nor irregular, but so strong that
the clothes are lifted by the movement communicated to
the thoracic parietes, and she hears it so plain that she
fancies others must hear it too.)

### Neck.

* Drawing pain, tearing and stiffness in the muscles of the nape.

Weight in the nape of the neck and occiput.

Sensation of constriction in the muscles of the nape, as if the head were drawn back.

° Sensation as if the neck was broken.

Cracking and creaking in the cervical vertebra on moving the neck.

Pains in the first cervical vertebra for seven hours, increased by moving the head and by pressure.

Feeling as if the vertebra in the nape were torn out of their place.

### Back.

* Drawing pains in the muscles of the back, with stitches and stiffness.

* Drawing pain between the shoulder-blades down to the sacrum.

* Burning in the back.

Shudder running down the back.

Tensive and pressive pain in the whole of the back, extending around toward the chest.

° Pain in the back, as if after excessive muscular straining.

° Wound-like pain in the lower dorsal vertebra, the five lowest ribs on the right, and the lumbar vertebra, aggravated by pressure and movement.

Violent pain at every breath, around the lower angles of the shoulder-blades.

*Tearing pressure on the lower lumbar vertebra* forward toward the haunch bones, *as if the vertebra were broken asunder,* only on bending forward and when he bends back; perceptible for many days even when walking.

*Wound-like pain in the lowest lumbar vertebræ, as if it were dislocated or smashed.*

### Upper Extremities.

* Pinching, spasmodic pain on the inner edge of the right shoulder-blade, which hinders him from moving the arm.

* Stitches under right shoulder blade.

13

\* *Violent pains on the lower angle of the left blade;* from thence violent stitches right through the chest forwards.

The hands hot up to the middle of the forearm, and swollen, with distension of the superficial veins.

° Paralysis and weight of the arms, as if weights were hung upon them.

Drawing pain from the right shoulder down to the wrist, with cold and stiffness of the arm.

° Paralytic pains in the left shoulder and the whole arm.

Drawing pain from the left shoulder to the fourth finger.

In the evening in bed, violent pains in the right shoulder, with a feeling on moving the arm as if it was smashed; the arm is cold and stiff.

° Pain in left shoulder, as if broken or dislocated, with cold feeling in the upper arm.

° Pain in the right shoulder.

Tearing in the muscles of the right upper arm.

° Pain in the deltoid and biceps on moving the arm, all day.

Rheumatic pains from left shoulder to the elbow.

Paralytic drawing in the wrist joints.

Distension of the superficial veins of both hands.

Tearing, shooting pain in right metacarpals, much increased by pressure.

Burning in the ball and scalpel joint of the right thumb.

Tips of the fingers cold.

Stitch in the second and third joint of the right forefinger.

Fine tearing in the tips of the fingers.

Itching in the fingers (constant symptom).

### Lower Extremeties.

° Lancinating pains.

° Bruised pain from the thighs to the calves, worse on walking and when touched.

From the hip bone to the toes of the right foot paralytic drawing pain, continuing the same whether walking, lying, or sitting, disappearing suddenly.

Legs feel as if bruised.

Tensive pains and sense of swelling in the thighs, for the breadth of two hands, midway between the hip and knee.

° Shooting in the right hip.

Pain as if from a blow in the middle of the right thigh.

Burning, itching, and shooting pain in left hip joint.

Pain like dislocation in the left hip, preventing walking.

° Pain in right hip when on rising from a seat.

Giving way of the knees when standing and walking.

Weight and stiffness, and jerking and trembling in the knee joints.

Boring, drawing pain in the right knee.

° Pain in right knee, aggravated by movement.

Violent pain in the left knee.

° Feeling of stiffness in left knee joint, with burning.

She cannot extend the left leg without violent pains in the knee.

° In walking she is obliged to advance the left leg at full stretch, and can only extend it slowly for pain like a wound in the knee joint, when it is once bent.

Feeling of icy coldness in the legs, especially the calves and sides.

The right foot up to the knee actually cold while the other is warm.

*Great weight in the legs.*

Shooting, boring sensation in the bones of the left leg.

Drawing pains in the calves, aggravated by pressure.

Some burning, painful spots, with stitches in the middle above the tendo-Achilles; the pain is increased by scratching.

° Painful pressure on the outside of the ankle.

° Ankle joints painful, especially the right; worse when walking.

° Pressive pain in right ankle joint when sitting.

° Pain in left ankle joint, especially when walking.

Feet first cold then burning hot.

° Feet as if dead, and cold.

Tensive, burning pain in the bones of the right foot, on the joints of the toes.

Continued dryness of the feet, which usually perspire.

Stitches in the right heel; violent pain, hindering walking.

Cramp in the sole of the right foot, which near the toes was bent under; the cramp ceased on compression with the hand.

Burning; itching in soles of the feet.

Shooting in the right great toe.

Pain as if from a blow in the toes in bed.

° Weight in the legs, as if she could not step out, and as if she had to drag a great burden.

° Œdematous swelling about the malleoli.

### Skin.

On the upper part of the right cheek many red, elevated pimples, raised in the centre and feeling pointed.

° Elevated exanthema on the face.

Red, inflamed, elevated spot, with a pimple in the middle; in the centre of the forehead itching and pricking, which disappeared again in a few hours.

Large pustules on the forehead.

The whole face, except the forehead, is covered on awaking in the morning with bright red, lentil sized, round spots, with pointed pimples in the centre.

Vesicles on the lip and also nose forming scabs.

Papular exanthema on a red base on the upper lip and right cheek.

° Red, round, burning spots on the forearm.

Pimples like pocks on the back of the right nates, with red areola.

Eruption of the face like miliary rash and measles.

Reticulated, red, itching, coroding spots, with swelling on the back of the hand.

* *Skin yellow all over, as in jaundice.*

° All the skin feels cool in spite of a very warm room.

### Fever.

Chilliness and shuddering all over toward evening.

Cold all over, especially in the hands and feet.

° Chill, with cold feet, in the morning on awaking.

Chill, internal and external, with weight in the occiput, and drawing in the nape.

° *Heat.*— Heat without thirst, after lying down in the evening.

° Glowing heat in the head, with sharply defined, darkish redness of the cheeks; pulsation in the arteries; full pulse (at 90); faintness; difficulty of speech; nausea; short breath; and cold feet.

Much dry heat all over, especially in the face, with full pulse, and thirst.

Increased temperature all over, especially in the hollow of the hands, from whence the heat seems to proceed.

° Rigor in the evening, with chattering teeth and rigor; thereafter great heat, especially all over the head.

° Perspiration at night on awaking, especially in the palms of the hands.

° When lying in bed at night, a rigor comes over him, lasting nearly an hour, with external warmth all over, yet with goose skin; then follows perspiration for the whole night.

° Heat inside and out, with warm perspiration on the face.

Pulse 62, full and hard.

Pulse 50; after previous palpitation of the heart, with withered looking, pale face.

### Sleep.

\* Sleepy condition; she falls asleep as she sits; lethargy in the daytime in jaundice and hepatic congestion.

Sleepiness, with yawning, and stretching, and languor.

When awakened she falls asleep again directly.

° From 10 till midnight, phantasies in a half-waking state, without meaning or connection, and images of death and soldiering.

° Restless sleep, full of dreams.

" She cannot get to sleep for a long time, then sleeps well.

° Frequently in the evening, in bed, restlessness and excitement till toward midnight, preventing sleep.

° Sleep prevented by a sensation of numbness and coldness in lower extremities.

On awaking he cannot remember what he has dreamed.

Dream of a journey, remembering most minute particulars.

Dreams of corpses and burials.

### Generalities.

\* Periodical neuralgia of the facial nerves.

* After food, **very great** distaste for work, and laziness with sleepiness.
° Great distaste for mental occupation.
° Prostration, exhaustion, and languor, with weakness in walking.
° Weariness and exhaustion of all the limbs, as after a long walk.
° Feeling ill, as if from influenza.
° Loss of consciousness.
° Drawing pains through the whole body.
° Wandering pains in the joints of the extremities, especially left side.
° On awaking, slight twitching in the muscles here and there.
° Twitching in arms and legs.
° Great emaciation, with total loss of appetite.
Sudden restlessness of all the limbs, compelling her to move; she cannot stand still, and on trying to do so steps with her feet.
Anxiety, vertigo, and heat of the head drive her into the fresh air; she feels better.
Long-continued fainting, with cold extremities.

---

# CHELONE GLABRA.

## (*Balmony.*)

DESCRIPTION.—A smooth perennial, with upright, branching stem, and large, white, rose-color, or purple flower. (It is called *Turtle-head* and *Snake-head*, because of the appearance of the corolla, resembling in shape the head of a reptile.) The flowers are sessile, in spikes or clusters; leaves lanceolate, on very short stalks. It grows in wet places; blooming from July to September. All its parts are very bitter.

OFFICINAL PREPARATIONS.—Tinctures; of the whole plant; dilutions.

ANALOGUES.—*Hydrastis, China, Myrica, Chelidonium, etc.*

### Stomach.
Increase of appetite, with powerful digestion.
° Dyspeptic ailments, with hepatic disorder.

### Liver.
° Jaundice, with loss of appetite and disgust for **food**.

**Stool.**

᪲ Constipation from hepatic torpor.

° Expulsion of lumbrici.

**Fever.**

᪲ Specific in cases of quinine cachexia. (*Drs. Ball and Price.*)

ᵓ Intermittent fever after abuse of quinine. (*Ib.*)

---

# CHIMAPHILA UMBELLATA.

*(Prince's Pine.)*

DESCRIPTION.—A small, evergreen plant, with a perennial, creeping root, which gives rise to several simple, erect, or drooping stems, from four to eight inches high, woody at their base. *The leaves* are wedge-shaped, leathery, serrate, smooth, a shining green on the upper surface, paler beneath, or irregularly white. *Flowers* in a terminal corymb, on nodding penduncles; they are white, tinged with red, and exhale an agreeable odor. The *C. maculata* is a variety only, with spotted leaves, or veined with greenish-white. It may be used for our tinctures, as it possesses identical properties.

OFFICINAL PREPARATIONS.—Tincture of the root and leaves; dilutions.

ANALOGUES.—*Cubeba*, (?) *Copaiva, Buchu, Galium, Pareira, Uva ursi, Cannabis sativa.*

*(No Proving.)*

**Urinary Organs.**

* Scanty urine, containing large quantity of muco-purulent sediment.

° Dropsy, from disease of the kidneys.

° Albuminuria, occurring during Bright's Disease.

° Increased amount of urine, with diminution of the lithates.

° Chronic catarrh of the bladder.

° Disease of the prostate, with waste of prostatic fluid.

° Hæmaturia, from chronic gonorrhœa.

° Dysuria in plethoric, hysterical women; scanty, frequent urination, and pressing, scalding, smarting pain; high-colored urine, depositing a copious mucus sediment.

ᵓ Urine thick, ropy, of brick color, and copious bloody sediment, with hectic fever and night sweats.

**Stool.**

Constipation, when connected with renal or cystic disease.

° Enlargement of mesenteric glands.

### Generative Organs.

\* Excessive itching and painful irritation of the urethra, from the end of the penis to the neck of the bladder.

\* Sensation of swelling in the perineum, as if on sitting down a ball was pressing against it.

᙮ Atrophy of the mammæ.

° Tumors of the mammæ.

° Scirrhous tumor of the mammæ. (?)

### Fever.

\* Flushing of the cheeks and general heat, with accelerated pulse.

° Hectic fever, from chronic renal disease.

### Skin.

° Glandular enlargements, especially of the lymphatics.

° In scrofula it seems to rank with some of the anti-psorics.

---

# CIMICIFUGA RACEMOSA.
### (Black Cohosh.)

BOTANICAL DESCRIPTION.—This indigenous plant is very stately in appearance, and is found growing abundantly in shady and rocky woods, on rich grounds, from Maine to Michigan, and southward to Florida. The Cimicifuga is the Macrotys racemosa, or Botrophys serpentaria of Rafinesque; the Actea Racemosa of Linnæus. It is also known by the common names of squaw root, black snake root, rattle weed, etc.

The stem is simple, smooth, from four to eight feet high. The leaves are fine, alternate, the lower one nearly radical, divided several times, the upper one two-pointed. The leaflets oblong, egg-shaped, with the stem opposite, incised and from three to seven-toothed. The flowers are one styled, white, fœtid, in long slender racemes; sepals four or five, falling off early; petals white, four to six, and small; stamens slender, white, about one hundred to each flower, giving to the raceme the appearance of a long slender plume; one pistil with a broad stigma. The fruit is a capsule, ovoid and dry, having only one cell, containing numerous flat, smooth seeds, which are loosely packed, horizontally, in two rows. In the late autumn and winter any motion of the plant causes a rattling of the seeds, so much resembling the alarm of the rattlesnake as to cause the hunter to start involuntarily; hence its name of rattle weed, given by the country people. The root consists of a thick, irregularly bent, contracted body, from one-third to an inch in diameter, often several inches in length, furnished with many slender radicles, and rendered extremely rough and jagged in its appearance by the remains of the stems of succes sive years. The color is extremely dark brown, almost black; internally yellowish white. The odor is feeble but disagreeable; taste bitter, some what astringent, leaving a slight sense of acrimony. It yields its virtues partially to boiling water, and wholly to alcohol. The taste of the tincture reminds one strongly of laudanum.

The root is the officinal portion, and should be gathered early in autumn. An *active principle*, named at the time it was discovered, *Macrotin*, is very extensively used by all schools, under the supposition that it contains all the virtues of Cimicifuga. Some of the following symptoms were caused by Macrotin, but it cannot represent all the pathogenesis, nor cure all the symptoms caused by this plant. It stands in about the same relation to Cimicifuga, as Atropine to Belladonna.

The *Macrotin* is a brown, dry, very bitter powder, and nearly ten times stronger than the tincture, by weight. It should now be called *Cimicifugin*.

OFFICINAL PREPARATIONS.—Tincture, with strong alcohol, of the fresh root; triturations of the dried root. Macrotin (Cimicifugin); triturations.

ANALOGUES.—*Caulophyllum, Colchicum, Digitalis, Stillingia, Glonoine, etc.*

### Mental Sphere.

Miserable, dejected feeling; mind dull and heavy.

Delirium, with nausea, retching, dilated pupils

Vertigo; impaired vision; dizziness.

She feels grieved, troubled, with sighing.

\* *Great melancholy, with sleeplessness (primary,*.

Exhilaration, with pleasant thoughts (*secondary*).

\* She is often startled by the illusion of a mouse running from under her chair.

\* Delirium tremens, with nausea, retching, dilated pupils, tremor of the limbs, incessant talking, and changing from one subject to another, sleeplessness, imagines strange objects about the bed, as rats, sheep, etc., with quick, full pulse, and peculiar wild look out of the eyes.

\* Apprehensiveness and sleeplessness in pregnant women.

\* *Mental disorder:*—" Sensation as if a heavy black cloud had settled all over her and enveloped her head, so that all was darkness and confusion, while at the same time it weighed like lead upon her heart." (Cured by 1×.) (*Hale.*) She was suspicious of everything; would not take medicine if she knew it; indifference, taciturn, takes no interest in household matters; frequent sighs and ejaculations. (Cured by *Cimicifuga* 200th.) (*Dunham.*)

### Head.

\* *Pain over the eyes,* and in the eyes, extending along the base of the brain to the occiput.

\* Severe pain over the *left* or *right* eye, extending to the eye and base of the brain, with dejection of spirits.

Sensation as if the temples were compressed.

Head feels as if pounded full of something.

\* Dullness and heaviness in the head, as if he had been on a "spree."

Brain feels too large for the cranium; a pressing from *within*, *outward*.

Excruciating pain in the forehead, extending to the temples, on waking at 2 A. M., with coldness of the forehead.

° Severe remittent headache of long standing, occurring every day at same hour.

Moving the head, or turning the eyes, caused a sensation as if the cranium was opening and shutting.

Acute pain through the head during the day.

Dull boring pain in the forehead, over left superciliary ridge, at 10 A. M.

\* Severe pain in forehead, extending to the temple and vertex, with fullness, heat and throbbing; when going up stairs sensation as if the top of the head would fly off.

° Pain in the head relieved in the open air.

° Excruciating pain in the forehead, with coldness of forehead; pain in the eyeballs.

° Nervous, rheumatic and menstrual headaches.

° Headache, with severe pain in the eyeballs, extending into the forehead, and increased by the slightest movement of the head or eyeballs.

° Dull pain in occipital regions, with shooting pains down back of the neck.

° Cerebro-spinal meningitis. (*See Therapeutics, Vol. II.*)

### Eyes.

\* Aching of the eyes, which feel heavy, lasting for days.

\*Eyeballs exceedingly painful; with increased secretion of tears.

Stinging in the eyelids, with inflammation.

Eyes feel as if swollen; black specks before the eyes.

\* Congestion of the eyes during the headache.

° Intense and persistent pains in the eyeballs.

Ocular hyper-æsthesia

* Severe pain in the centre of the *eyeballs*, worse in the morning, lasting all day, aggravated by going up stairs.
* Sensation of *enlargement* of the eyeballs; they feel as if they would be pressed out of the head.
* Pain, as if situated between the eyeball and the orbital plate of the frontal bone.

Heat and swelling of the *eyelids*, with stinging pain.
*Dilated pupils, with black specks before the eyes.*
* Neuralgia of the eyeballs, without much congestion.
° Catarrhal and rheumatic ophthalmia.

The myopia was aggravated by large doses.
° Amaurosis; amblyopia; double vision.

### Jaws.

Very severe pains in teeth and jaws, worse in under jaw and its articulations.
Pain in right superior maxillary bone and teeth.
° Rheumatic and neuralgic toothache.

### Nose.

Stinging sensation in the nose in the evening.
° Frequent sneezing and fluent coryza during the day.
° Catarrhal condition of the mucous membrane.
Very profuse greenish and slightly sanguineous coryza.
Stuffed condition of the nostrils.

### Face.

Severe pain in left jaw.
Heat on one side of the face, with lassitude all over.
° Pains in the head and face are constant.
° Catarrhal-rheumatic prosopalgia.

### Mouth and Throat.

Offensive breath.
Dryness and soreness of the lips, with swelling of the back part of the tongue.
Accumulation of thick mucus upon the teeth.
° Swollen condition of mucous membrane in rheumatism.
Dryness of the pharynx, in a small spot, with inclination to swallow.

Soreness of the throat when swallowing, and on pressure, with stiff neck.

Inflammation of the uvula and palate, worse on the left side; with copious coryza.

° Hoarseness, roughness and scraping in the throat.

° Dry cough, from irritation and tickling at the lower part of the larynx.

° Rheumatic sore throat.

### Stomach.

\* Eructations, with nausea and·vomiting, with headache.

° Acute, darting pain in the stomach.

Slight pain in the epigastrium, extending to the left hypo-chondrium.

\* Faintness and emptiness in the epigastrium, almost constant; (a very characteristic symptom.)

Sensation of internal tremor in the epigastrium.

### Abdomen.

Flatulence, causing sensation of fullness in the abdomen.

Acute cutting pains in the umbilical region.

Severe pains in the bowels, with weight and pains in the lumbar region.

Dull griping, twisting at the umbilicus, more toward the left.

Periodic colic, with inclination to bend forward, relieved after stool.

° Rheumatism of the muscular structures of the abdomen.

° Neuralgia of the abdominal plexuses.

° Puerperal peritonitis, with suppressed lochia, delirium, etc.

° Abdominal myalgia, after confinement.

### Stool.

Disposition to diarrhœa, with large papescent stool.

Constipation; fæces hard and dry.

Scanty diarrhœa with tenesmus.

° Non-inflammatory colics and diarrhœas of children.

### Urine.

Frequent urination, with increased flow.

° Retention for eighteen hours, followed by profuse urine.

Profuse flow of pale, watery urine. (*primary.*)

Urine scanty and high colored. (*secondary.*)

° It increases the excretion of the *solids* of the urine in rheumatism.

### Generative Organs.

(*Female.*)  * A sensation of weight and bearing down in the uterine region, with a feeling of heaviness and torpor in the lower extremities.

* The menses appear eight days before the time.

* Troublesome labor-like pains during pregnancy.

* Abortion in the early months of pregnancy.

Premature labor, with serious hemorrhage.

Prickling sensations in both mammæ.

Leucorrhœa, with bearing down pains.

° Vaginal and cervical leucorrhœa, without ulceration.

° Amenorrhœa, with excessive pain in the head, back and limbs; with dark circles around the eyelids.

° Retarded menstruation, with pressive, heavy headache, etc.

° Suppression from a cold; febrile symptoms; rheumatic pains in the limbs; uterine cramps.

° Congestive dysmenorrhœa, and of rheumatic origin.

° Uterine ailments of a neuralgic type.

° Dysmenorrhœa, with aching in the limbs, severe pain in the back, down the thighs, with heavy, pressing down, labor-like pains, cramps, tenderness of the hypogastric region.

° Menorrhagia; profuse flow, of a passive character, dark coagulated, with the characteristic pains.

° Uterine inertia during and after labor.

* Spasmodic, painful and intensely powerful but intermitting contractions.

° Suppression of the lochia, with severe uterine pain and threatened peritonitis.

° Threatened abortion, and habitual abortion.

° Prolapsus uteri, from deficient innervation.

° Ovaritis.  ° Irritable uterus.

° Post-partem hæmorrhage.

° Spasms of the broad ligaments.

° Sterility, from various causes.

° Puerperal melancholy and mania, with sleeplessness.

*Male.*—Pain and tenderness of the testicles.

### Larynx.

Constant inclination to cough, from tickling sensation in the larynx.

Hoarseness; short dry cough; fluent coryza.

° Troublesome hacking cough.

° Catarrhal cough of children, especially at night.

### Chest.

Acute pain in right chest, extending from top to bottom, about two inches to the right of the sternum, aggravated by inspirations.

Lancinating pain along the cartilages of the false ribs, left side, aggravated by inspiration.

Transient and fugitive pains all through the chest, with cardiac palpitations.

° Aching, wearing pains in under left mammæ.

° Neuralgic pains through the chest.

Stitches in the region of the heart, and pain in left side of the chest.

\* Pleurodynia, rheumatic or myalgic.

\* Pleurisy, sub-acute (after Aconite and Bryonia).

° Chronic cough, dependent on nervous debility.

° Pains in the left side so common to females.

° A *sore, aching* pain in left side, below the nipple, relieved by a long inspiration. (in a man.)

### Heart.

Pain in the region of the heart, with palpitations, and stitches flying through various parts of the thorax.

Pain and anxiety in the heart, with pain in left shoulder; the arm feels bound to the side.

Transient but severe cardiac palpitations.

Pulse weak, irregular, eighty per minute.

° Paroxysms, several times a day (in a woman at the change of life), of intense pain in the region of the heart; great anxiety; livid or purple color of the face; cold perspiration on the hands; numbness of the whole body, especially the arms; the heart's action seems suspended by spasms; she cannot speak or move; she feels as if suffocating; head forcibly retracted, and unconsciousness.

° Palpitation of the heart; numbness of the arms; (pain down the left arm into the hand, and great exhaustion).

° Intense anxiety and pain about the heart, with pain in the shoulder, extending down the left arm.

° Rheumatic affections of the heart.

° Pericarditis, sub-acute, during rheumatism.

° Cardiac myalgia (with pain, irregular action, etc.)

° Functional disorder, from mental depression.

° Angina pectoris.

° Palliation in some organic heart affections, hypertrophy, etc.

### Back.

* Stiffness of large muscles of the neck.

Drawing and pulsating pain in lumbar region.

* Dull, heavy aching in the small of the back, relieved by rest, increased by motion.

Stitches in the back, aggravated by motion or respiration.

* Cramping in the muscles of neck on moving the head.

* Rheumatic pains in the muscles of the neck and back.

Trembling and weakness in the back—sacrum.

In the morning, on bending the neck forward, a severe, drawing, tensive pain at the points of the spinous processes of the three upper dorsal vertebræ.

Dull pain in region of lower dorsal and upper lumbar vertebræ.

Weight and pain in lumbar and sacral regions, sometimes extending all around the body, somewhat below the crest of ileum.

Feeling of stiffness and constriction in muscles of the back.

° *Lumbago*—one of the most useful remedies.

° A painful affection known as "crick in the back."

° *Spinal myalgia*, falsely called spinal irritation, with pain, soreness, tenderness along the spinal column; a disease seated in the ligaments and muscles of the vertebral column, and generally of a rheumatic origin, or due to weakness of the muscular fibres.

### Superior Extremities.

Dull pain in right arm, deep in the muscles, from the shoulder to the wrist.

Itching and redness of **dorsal** surface of the hands.

\* Neuralgic pains in all the extremities.

Pains which are cramping, with lameness and numbness.

° Muscular rheumatism of the extremities.

### Lower Extremities.

Twitching of fingers and toes.

Dull, aching, burning pain in the great toe, extending up the limb.

° Sciatica, with numb, crampy, and laming pains.

° Rheumatic-neuralgic pains.

ᶜ Articular rheumatism; also muscular, especially in the large muscles.

### Skin.

Prickling, itching, and heat of the whole surface.

Eruptions of white pustules over the face and neck, sometimes large, red, papular.

Papular eruption on back of hands and wrists.

° Varioloid — useful in some cases.

### Sleep.

\* Sleeplessness, from nervous irritation.

° Sleeplessness of children during teething.

° Sleeplessness, with melancholy mood.

### Fever.

° Rheumatic fever of an acute character.

° Typhoid fever in some cases.

° Night sweats without organic disease.

### Generalities.

*Nervous system.*—\* *Chorea*, from suppressed menses.

° *Chorea*, from undue exposure to cold.

° *Chorea*, from rheumatic irritation of motor nerves, or anterior column of spinal cord.

° *Chorea*, from deranged menstrual functions; always worse at the menstrual periods.

° *Chorea;* the whole body in constant motion, with loss of speech, and mental depression.

° Spasmodic jactitation of limbs, or single muscles.

° Cerebro-spinal irritation, when the motor side is excited and there exists atony of the muscular system.

It causes first great irritability of the nervous system, and secondarily, great exhaustion of that system.

Nervous exhaustion after the least excitement.

Great sensitiveness to cold air; it seemed to penetrate the system.

Continual restlessness in afternoon; desire to move about, not knowing what to do, or where to go.

General weak, ill, trembling, sinking feeling.

*Tremors;* so weak and trembling as not to be able to walk or study.

General lame and bruised feeling, as if sore all over.

It affects the left side most.

Severe *aching* in joints and back, as if attacked with variola

---

# CHIONANTHUS VIRGINICA.
### (*Fringe Tree.*)

DESCRIPTION.—This is a singular looking shrub or low tree, from ten to thirty feet high, growing from Pennsylvania to Georgia, on river banks and sandy plains. It presents clusters of snow-white flowers in May and June. (It is called the "Virginian Snow-Flower Tree," "Snow-drop Tree," etc.) The small fruit is a *drupe*, berry-like, with a "bloom" on it, containing a striated nut.

The leaves are often a foot long and nearly half as broad. There are three *varieties*, but all have the same properties.

OFFICINAL PREPARATION.—Tincture of the bark with strong alcohol; dilutions.

ANALOGUES.—*Chelidonium, Chelone, Carduus, China.* (?)
### (*No Provings.*)

° Hypertrophy of the liver. (*Dr. Goss.*)

° Chronic *hepatic disorders, jaundice, etc.*

° The bark of the root, bruised, is sometimes used for healing wounds. (*Browne, " Trees of America.*")

### (*See Vol. II. " Therapeutics.*")

---

# CISTUS CANADENSIS.
### (*Rock-Rose.*)

DESCRIPTION.—Sometimes called Frost-plant, because the roots throw off small icicles, with all the colors of the rainbow, which can be seen on frosty mornings—even when other plants show little dew-drops. It is a

14

perennial herb, with simple, ascending, downy *stem*, about a foot high. *Flowers* large and bright yellow, in terminal corymbs; they open in the sunshine, and cast their petals the next day. It grows on sandy plains and rocky places, preferring limestone ground.

OFFICINAL PREPARATIONS.—Tincture of the whole plant in strong alcohol.

ANALOGUES.—*Ampelopsis, Belladonna, Calcarea, Corydalis, Graphites, Hepar sulphur, Kali bichromicum, Paris quadrifolia, Phytolacca, Stillingia, Lachesis, Lobelia cerulea.*

[All the following symptoms are marked by Hering as (°)curative.]

## Mind.

All mental excitement greatly increases the sufferings.

Bad effects from vexation.

After supper, until bedtime, cheerfulness.

Mental agitation increases the cough.

Every mental excitement is followed by stitches in the throat, producing a cough.

## Head.

Head drawn to one side by swellings on the neck.

## Eyes.

Scrofulous inflammation of the eyes of long standing.

## Ears.

Discharge from the ears.

Tetters on and around the ears, extending into the external meatus.

## Nose.

Evenings and mornings frequent and violent sneezing.

Painful tip of nose, which at first grew worse and then was cured.

## Face.

Flushes of heat in the face.

Caries of the lower jaw.

## Teeth.

Very scorbutic gums, swollen, separating from the teeth, bleeding easily, putrid, disgusting.

## Tongue.

Dryness of the tongue and roof of the mouth.

## Throat.

Impure breath from disease of the throat.

Inhaling cold air causes pain in the throat.

Inhaling the slightest cold air causes a sore throat, which he
has not when inhaling in the warm room.

A feeling of softness in the throat.

Rawness, extending from the chest into the throat.

A feeling as if sand were in the throat.

The patient is constantly obliged to swallow saliva to relieve
an unbearable dryness, especially during the night.

Continuous feeling of dryness and heat in the throat.

Dryness of throat from 12 o'clock noon, until 1 to 3 A. M., at
night, then better until the next noon.

A small dry spot in the gullet for one year, then general dryness of throat—better after eating, worse after sleeping—
as if tearing asunder, the patient must get up and drink
water.

The inside of the throat looks glassy; on the back of throat
there appear strips of tough mucus.

Periodical itching in the throat.

Tickling and soreness in the throat.

In the morning sore pain in the throat and dryness of the
tongue.

Tearing pain in the throat when coughing.

Stitches in the throat, causing cough when mentally agitated.

Fauces inflamed and dry, without feeling dry; tough, gum-
like, thick, tasteless phlegm brought up by hawking,
mostly in the morning.

Hawking of mucus, constantly.

Expectoration of bitter mucus.

After discharging phlegm from the throat he feels generally
much relieved.

° Ought to be specific in catarrh of the larynx, trachæa, and
posterior nares. (*Hale.*)

### Stomach.

Drinking water relieves the dryness in the throat.

After eating the dryness of the throat is relieved.

### Abdomen and Stool.

All night till daybreak thin hot stool squirting out, of a gray-
yellow color: three more before noon.

° Chronic dysentery. (*Dr. Comstock, of St. Louis.*)

° *Chronic diarrhœa*—a very successful remedy in many cases
The wind is not incarcerated as often as before.

### Chest.

Feeling as if the windpipe had not space enough.

Pain in the windpipe; itching and scratching in the larynx.

Feeling as of rawness, extending from the upper part of the
    chest into the throat.

Cough from stitches in the throat.

Cough, with a very painful tearing in the throat.

Cough, and her neck thinly studded with tumors.

He bled at the lungs, and his scrofulous symptoms had re-
    turned.

In the evening, after lying down, and at night in bed, once
    a week or oftener, attacks of a kind of asthma; he draws
    his breath with such a loud wheezing that it wakens
    others sleeping in the same room.

He has the feeling as if the windpipe had not space enough.

Pressure on the chest.

### Neck.

Scrofulous swelling and suppuration of the glands of the
    throat.

Mrs. C., of delicate constitution, when nineteen years of age,
    was afflicted with a cough, and her neck was thickly
    studded with tumors; using the Rock-rose she was re-
    stored, and has not been afflicted with any such symptoms
    since. (*Dr. D. A. Tyler.*)

### Back.

Scrofulous ulcers on the back.

### Lower Limbs.

A lad seven years old had the "white-swelling" of the hip for
    three years. The bone was dislocated upward and out-
    ward; there was a large opening on the hip, leading to
    the bone, into which I could thrust my finger. I counted
    three ulcers. He had been under several physicians who
    had given him up. After using a decoction of the Rock-
    rose, in two days his night sweats ceased; thirty-nine
    days after he was entirely well. (*Dr. J. H. Thompson.*)

### Sleep.

In the night swallowing of saliva on account of dryness.

Must get up in the night on account of dryness in the throat.

The dryness in the throat worse after sleeping.

On awaking pain under the hypochondria.

Night sweats attending suppurations.

### Skin.

Tetter on the ears and hands.

Lupus on the face.

For scrofula a popular medicine in domestic practice.

Mr. C., from a child was afflicted with the scrofula, and had also grandular swellings on the neck; at the age of sixteen he was much worse, had eight abscesses on the neck, three ulcers on the shoulder and three on the hips; at forty years of age he had his head drawn on one side, and was unable to labor. After using the Rock-rose for four weeks, the ulcers broke, discharged and healed; the tumor lessened in size, his head resumed its natural position, and he went regularly to work. Later his scrofulous symptoms returned again, and he also bled at the lungs, for which he used it again with the same beneficial results. (*Professor Ives.*)

Hard swelling around all her syphilitic mercurial ulcers on the lower limbs.

Furunculi, commencing with small blisters. (boils.)

### Conditions.

From noon until midnight the dryness of throat is worse; all the symptoms are worse in the morning.

Belladonna, Carbo veg. and Phosphorus acted favorably, between repeated doses of Cistus.

---

# COCA.

### (*Erythroxylon coca.*)

[A plant used by the natives of Peru, for the purpose of stimulation, and to enable them to perform arduous labor. These symptoms are collated mainly from Hering's pathogenesis.—*Hale.*]

PHARMACOLOGY.—This is a shrub growing wild, in South America, and largely cultivated in Bolivia, for the sake of its leaves, which are much used in that country for chewing. The plant which is propagated from the seed in nurseries, begins to yield in eighteen months, and continues productive for half a century. The leaves, on being picked, are dried in the sun, and then packed in bags. They are known in South America by the name of Coca. They were in general use among the natives of Peru, at the time of the conquest, and have continued to be much employed to the present time.

The leaves resemble in size and shape those of tea; being oval-oblong, pointed, two inches or more in length, by somewhat over an inch in their greatest breadth, and furnished with short delicate footstalks; but they are not, like the tea leaves, dentate, and are distinguished from most other leaves by a slightly curved line on each side of the mid-rib, running from the base to the apex. When well dried, they resemble, in odor, tea, and a peculiar taste, which, in decoction, becomes bitter and astringent. It has been found so impossible to import the leaves to this country without injury to their medicinal properties, that the tincture ought to be prepared from them as soon as gathered.

OFFICINAL PREPARATIONS.—Tincture with strong alcohol, from fresh leaves, dilutions.

ANALOGUES.—*Coffea, Thea, Scutellaria, Ignatia, Paullinia, Cannabis indica, Cypripedium, Phosphoric acid, etc.*

### Mental Sphere.

\* Slow in finding the words to express himself at times.

\* Brain feels so muddled that he cannot read understandingly.

° Mind much clearer; spirits much better.

A peculiar sensation of isolation from the outer world.

On any one speaking to him, it seems as if the person were at a great distance.

Their excited imaginations conjure up the most wonderful visions; at one time consisting of indescribably beautiful and delightful forms; at another, however, of the most horrid figures.

Inclination to work, with sleeplessness all night; disinclination.

An irresistible inclination to feats of strength.

Shy; they flee the society of their fellow-men; seek concealment in gloomy woods or lonely dwellings.

Instinctive desire to make no motions at all.

° Always relieves him from unusual fatigue; producing perfect calmness of mind and body, and is never followed by any depression.

A kind of numbness, with a feeling of security, with retention of clear self-consciousness, and the instinctive desire to make no motion, not even to move a single finger, for an entire day.

During the evening, after the first dose at six o'clock, his hearing became painfully acute; he felt something like expectation; brain excited; and a rather painful pressure on the sides of the head.

° Mental depression.

Great anxiety, palpitation, humming in the ears the whole day, and sparks before the eyes.

° Peevish temper; hypochondria.

Nausea and vertiginous feeling, incapaciting for carrying on literary labors.

° Loss of energy.

### Head.

Giddiness and dizziness; involuntarily stopping quickly when walking; the head inclined forward, with giddiness and fear of walking.

Giddiness, though slight, on going out in the open air early in the morning; objects appearing to turn before the eyes, for an hour's time.

Great dullness in the head, like the effects of a debauch.

Fullness of forehead; dull feeling over the whole brow; slight shooting pains in right temple; sensation of tension over forehead, as if an india rubber band were stretched over it.

Violent headache immediately over the eyes, with low ringing in the ears.

Dull frontal headache, which vanished with the setting of the sun, followed by a state of mental exhilaration.

A pressing headache on the right side of the occiput as well as of the right side of the forehead, with giddiness and chill after dinner, disappearing toward evening.

Headache in the afternoon, with chilliness.

Rather violent *headache*, with sensation of dryness in the throat.

° Migraine; a one-sided headache.

### Eyes.

Great intolerance of light, with remarkable dilatation of pupils.

Black spots flying lightly before the eyes several times while reading.

White spots before the eyes, so that on reading the book seems moulded white. (Chloral has "everything looks white.")

Flickering before the eyes; the letters seem to run together on the paper; it seemed as if he were writing with two pens; fiery specks float before the eyes. A sensation comes on as if some one were knocking about the eyes, with loud ringing in the ears; two hours later he can write without double vision or swimming.

Dullness of the head, with flying of fiery points from above downwards, and swimming together of the letters.

White spots and glittering serpentine lines before the eyes, with great uneasiness on going out after dinner, for an hour.

The eyes become very sensitive, reading cannot be endured long; some are troubled with slight headache, while others suffer from nausea and various disorders of the digestive apparatus, which may be compared with seasickness.

Disposition on the part of the upper lids to fall, without being sleepy.

After using for a number of days, on himself and others, there broke out a circumscribed erythema—on one an exanthema resembling herpes—around the eyelids.

### Ears.

Acute hearing, and excited brain.

Loud ringing and buzzing in the ears.

Difficulty of hearing; it seems as if the sounds came from a great distance.

### Nose.

Running of clear water from nose, and occasional sneezing, without having properly a coryza as he usually has it.

### Face.

Burning, redness of cheeks, first left then right; white spot in the centre of latter.

Small boils on the face.

Quivering, trembling lips; pale lips and gums, with green, blunt teeth.

Ugly, blackish border around the angles of the mouth.

On the lips a nettle rash; scabs; bleeding.

### Mouth.

Toothache in a hollow tooth, at noon till evening, violent.

\* Prevents caries of teeth.

\* No taste in the morning.

\* Much furred tongue.

Dryness of mouth on waking.

### Throat.

Irritability of the pharynx, so that the stomach would not retain food.

\* A distinct feeling of swelling of the uvula; difficulty of swallowing.

Swelling of the uvula without any particular redness, lasting from five o'clock in the afternoon and through the whole evening.

Feeling as if some mucus were at back of pharynx; not removed by coughing or hawking.

Early in the morning, after a very comfortable sleep, a sensation of dryness in the throat, very disagreeable on swallowing, as if swollen.

### Appetite.

Not hungry at noon, as usual, nevertheless ate a good deal, and with appetite.

Quickly satiated, notwithstanding great hunger and good appetite at noon.

Wants food at an earlier hour in the forenoon, notwithstanding a distension of the abdomen, as if from overloaded stomach.

Digestion goes on with great activity.

An intense gnawing, hungry sensation at the pit of the stomach. (*Abies.*)

Morbid hunger, even to swallow animal excrements; (chronic symptom of chewers.)

Very little need of food, even with hard labor; incredible fatigues are endured with unusual vigor on the most meagre diet.

Always felt a sense of great satiety after taking the infusion in the morning, and did not feel a desire for his next meal until after the time at which he usually took it.

Prevents getting hungry; feels no hunger.

Retards approach of hunger, when taken as tea.

Enables the body to feed upon itself, without the hunger pains and weakness usually accompanying prolonged abstinence from ordinary food.

Drinking the decoction at three or four o'clock P. M., it has invariably and totally deprived him of all appetite for dinner, and of his rest at night; under these circumstances he always passed the night in reading or writing; he feels no fatigue or hunger on the following morning.

° Want of appetite (a remedy of doubtful value). (*Hale.*)

### Stomach.

At noon, a peculiar feeling of emptiness in the stomach and abdomen; when walking, a painful contractive sensation in the stomach, and close to the latter, on the left side, a pain similar to the so-called stitches in the spleen.

Debility of the digestive organs; at first it seems to be slight uneasiness; soon reaches a frightful intensity.

° Catarrh of the stomach; a cup of Coca after dinner.

° After taking for five days twenty drops of the tincture, once or twice a day, his digestion became extraordinarily good, and continued so.

When walking, a pain about region of cardiac end of stomach, gradually increasing; would have amounted to a cutting pain; after standing it went off, returning in a week.

° Gastralgia, similar to that caused by coffee.

### Abdomen.

* Violent belly ache, with rumbling, as if from flatulence; tympanitic distension of the abdomen, diminished by a frequent discharge of inodorous flatus.

° Spasmodic colic; given in the hospitals in Bolivia; had no effect in Valparaiso.

° Pituitous disease of the abdominal organs.

* Tympanitic distension of abdomen, diminished by frequent discharges of inodorous flatus.

° Hypochondriac pressure and tension after meals.

## Stool.

The dangerous obstructions which would result from the diet of the Indians—roasted maize and roasted barley, pounded into meal, and swallowed dry without anything—are prevented by the well-known purgative action of the Coca.

Stool easier than usual in the morning, and thinner; for three minutes after a feeling of want of further evacuation, without any; the soft stool of a normal color.

Teaspoonful musty diarrhœa, four stools during the early afternoon, without pain; stools different from his habitual looseness; stopped taking Coca, and had natural stools.

Ineffectual urging to stool; constipation, with abdominal distension.

## Urine.

° Absence of the usual incontinentia urinæ nocturna.

Rose at night to urinate, as he had to do constantly a long time ago, but not lately, and it ceased after the proving.

Urine had an unbroken film over its surface, iridescent in certain lights, with an appearance like fissures in it, mapping it out, and a flocculent, pale sediment floating at the bottom, seen through the film.

## Generative Organs.

*Women.*—Menses delayed for two days, came on about noon; got very profuse during the night, with some pain in the lower part of the abdomen; not in a steady flow as usual, but in gushes, awakening from sound sleep; after drinking the infusion morning and evening for a whole week.

## Larynx.

Hoarse voice on waking at night.

Hoarseness, with tickling in the upper part of the trachea, and some cough.

° Feels much stronger in voice; can sing much louder and clearer.

° In phthisis laryngea, when from irritability of the pharynx, the stomach would not retain food.

After a strong infusion he could, during the whole day, climb the heights, and follow the swift-footed wild animals, without experiencing any greater difficulty of breathing than in similar rapid movements on the coast.

Great ease in ascending high mountains, and running amongst them, without any difficulty of breathing.

° Mitigates the difficulty of breathing, hæmoptysis, and sleepiness, incident to traveling among the hills, four thousand feet above the sea level.

° A strong tea prevents the usual breathlessness in climbing hills.

° Shortness of breathing, especially on making an ascent; in the forenoon, a tickling cough would cause a tingling.

° Expectoration of small lumps, like boiled starch, which he has had for some time, immediately after rising in the morning.

° Hawking up of small transparent lumps of mucus, chiefly in the morning.

° Asthma; (a useful palliative.) (*Hale.*)

° Oppression of breathing during nocturnal hours.

### Chest.

Rather painful weight on the chest, with constant necessity to imbibe deeply, when sitting in the evening; sensation as if the lungs were too much distended; difficulty of breathing, even in bed; palpitation, with a weakness of the whole body, though not disagreeable, as if from great exertion.

° Emphysema; (a palliative, like Chloral.)

### Heart.

After an infusion of the leaves, pulse becomes much accelerated, the beats of the heart being nearly quadrupled.

Great anxiety, and strong palpitation; he broke out in a copious sweat in the evening, nine o'clock, while in bed.

° Disease of the heart, functional, from over exertion.

### Sleep.

° Inclination to sleep, but can find no rest.

### Skin.

Dry, papular eruption on back of the hand, of three years' standing, not cured by Kali. chrom., Sulph. ac., Fluor. ac., etc., soon ceased to spread, gradually got paler, and has in some spots, where it was worse, disappeared.

° Protection from cutaneous diseases. (?)

### Generalities.

Numbness of hands and feet.

° Suffered frequently from rheumatism, came on from the slightest cold; now not from the first of October till first of November, even not with very unfavorable weather.

During manual labor Coca has very little influence.

Ease in breathing, and feeling of freshness and vigor of the whole body, with great pleasure 'in walking quickly and far, notwithstanding the great heat and great power of the sun, in the forenoon.

Great bodily vigor, and endurance of great fatigue, notwithstanding extremely little nourishment and no sleep.

* Can nowhere find rest; nervousness and nightly restlessness of children during dentition.

° Erethism in the sensitive sphere; ° hysterical complaints.

° Debility during convalescence from typhus.

° Fainting fits from nervous weakness.

The Stramonium patient likes company, the Coca patient solitude; the Stramonium patient light, the Coca patient darkness.

---

# COCCUS CACTI.

## (*Cochineal.*)

PHARMACOLOGY.—This insect is found wild in Mexico and Central America, inhabiting different species of Cactus, and allied genera of plants. It is also cultivated to some extent in Texas and New Mexico. The female insect is the one used in commerce, and the one we use in medicine. They are collected and killed either by immersing in boiling water or over the heat of a fire.

Cochineal has a faint, heavy odor, and a bitter, slightly acidulous taste. When powdered, it is of a purplish carmine color, tinging the saliva intensely red. It is composed of animal matter, and a peculiar coloring matter, or principle, called by most authorities, Cochinilin. This is a brilliant purplish red, very dry powder, unalterable in dry air, soluble in water and alcohol, insoluble in ether, and is without nitrogen.

OFFICIAL PREPARATION.—Triturations of the *insect;* tincture with strong alcohol.

ANALOGUES.— (1) *Bromide of Ammonia, Drosera, Corallium, Ipecac, Hyoscyamus.* (2)

I have only given the symptoms relating to cough, larynx, kidneys, and bladder, because they are the most characteristic of the drug. The complete symtomatology can be found in the third volume of Allen's Encyclopedia. It was first published in Medcalte's New Homœopathic Provings, 1863.

## Cough.

Paroxysm of short cough, with expectoration of globular mucus.

Paroxysm of coughing produced by a tickling in the larynx and throat.

Paroxysm of cough for half-an-hour, and expectoration of a great quantity of mucus.

Cough which wakens him at six A. M., having remissions of a minute; it is at first clear, dry, and barking; subsequently some thick mucus is detached, and the effort of doing this causes desire to vomit, accompanied by an excoriated feeling of the throat, and a pressive headache.

The paroxysm of cough is renewed by the heat of the bed.

He can scarcely speak for coughing, in a warm room.

Very violent cough, which, notwithstanding the expectoration of mucus, is constantly excited by a tickling in region of bifarcation of the trachæa, the attacks go on increasing.

Dry cough in the morning, which lasts several minutes, and finally produces vomiting of mucus.

The cough annoys him all day, and at three P. M., an hour after dinner, is so violent as to vomit him.

The cough is so violent as to cause vomiting, and the expectoration of a great quantity of thick, viscous and albuminous mucus.

Violent cough, without expectoration, which lasts a long time in the morning.

A little greenish yellow mucus, tasting like liquorice, is detached by the cough.

° Cough of drunkards. ° Whooping cough.

## Kidneys.

Pressive pain in the renal region, extending by degrees to the bladder and its sphincter, accompanied by vesical tenesmus and frequent emissions of deep colored urine.

Pain in the kidneys, with increased secretion of urine.

Lancinating and boring pain in the region of the kidneys, in the evening in bed.

Sudden, acute, prolonged lancinations, extending from the left renal region along the ureters into the bladder.

Attacks of *nephritic colic*, but seldom and not violent—with very copious urine, and dull pain in the urethra.

He jumps about, bends himself, and rubs his hypogastrium in order to relieve the *spasmodic pains in the kidneys.*

Excessively violent pain in the renal region seizes him suddenly when sitting quietly in the afternoon; it radiates from the two sides of the kidneys, and differs from the pressive and drawing pain previously felt there, by its spasmodic character and extension, and can only be compared to the pain experienced in the testicles in consequence of a bruise.

Pressing pain through the ureters into the bladder; relieved by discharge of flatus.

At five A. M., wakened by a drawing pain in right kidney, extending along the ureters into the bladder, at the same time a single lancinating thrust, and continual pressure in the urethra and navicular region.

Bruised pain in the sacro-lumbar region and in groins (on waking.)

° Hæmorrhage from the kidneys.

### Bladder.

Alternations of cramps, coldness and heat in the bladder.

Pain in the bladder during the night, with fruitless desire to urinate.

Excoriated, sore pain in the bladder.

Sensation of fullness and tension in the bladder, without desire to urinate.

She is obliged to urinate very often after dinner, which, together with a pressure analagous to that which is experienced at the period (of the menses), makes her think her bladder is diseased.

Feeling of fullness and pressure in the bladder extending towards the urethra, with constant desire to urinate and frequent discharge of normally colored and slightly acid urine.

Attack of pressure, tenesmus, and cutting pain in the bladder, during which the face becomes red.

The pressure and pain in the bladder continue even after the evacuation of urine.

Strong tenesmus of the neck of the bladder *after* urination with tension.

Very violent twisting pain in the neck of the bladder, lasting a quarter-of an-hour, and not ameliorated by the dis charge of urine or flatus.

The sensitiveness of the epigastrium extends throughout the abdomen; lancinating, drawing and pressive pains especially appear in the groins and vesical region, which obliges her to keep her bed.

Lancinations, as if from needles, extend from the bladder through the urethra, toward the glans.

### Urethra.

*Burning* in the urethra *when* urinating, and continuing *after*.

The burning in urethra and titillation in meatus cease after the discharge of clear straw colored urine; the sensation returns, however, several times in the day before urinating.

The burning in the urethra and swelling of the vulva continue fifteen days.

Very violent *lancinating* thrusts in the anterior portion of the urethra and glans, a long time after having urinated when in bed at night; they force him to groan and cry out, and last a minute-and-a-half.

Burning pain in urethra, with sensation as if a little stone were sliding along the urethra.

Sensation in anterior portion of urethra *before* urinating, as if pricked with a blunted needle.

Very *violent lancinations*, along the urethra, toward the glans, lasting several minutes, after urinating (urine dark color.)

The meatus is so contracted and constricted that the urine flows very slowly, and as the vulva is excoriated the burning is very violent, and lasts an hour.

Violent *pruritus* and *itching* at the orifice of the **urethra,** obliging them to rub it constantly.

### Urine.

Very *frequent, copious* discharges (with more powerful stream) of *pale, watery* urine, both by *day* and *night* (primary effect.)

Frequent, scanty discharges of urine, but it is difficult, slow in coming, and takes place with *straining* and vesical tenesmus (secondary.)

Urine first normal in color; it then becomes citron-yellow, then brown, and finally red.

The urine becomes cloudy, and finally jumentous (namely, like that of a horse.)

The *odor* of the urine is sometimes *alkaline*, often *ammoniacal*, also *cadaverous* (the latter when it is dark colored and cloudy.)

The urine seems to be *thicker*, like oil.

Very *acrid* irritating urine.

The urine contains mucus in the form of filaments, clouds and flocks and sediments, and the sediment is entangled with much mucus.

Lateritous sediment; also a reddish sediment of the color of brick-dust, which adheres to the vessel.

[Purulent or bloody urine did not appear in the provings; but we do not know whether any chemical or microscopic tests were applied.]

(See Therapeutics, Vol. II.)

---

# CODEINE.

[An alkaloid of Opium. Provings by Dr. Marcy and others.]

DESCRIPTION.—This substance was discovered in 1832, by Robiquet, in the muriate of morphia, prepared according to the process of Gregory. It exists in opium, combined with meconic acid, and is extracted along with morphia in the preparation of the muriate of morphia. When this solution of the mixed muriates is treated with ammonia, the morphia is precipitated, and the Codeine, remaining in solution, may be obtained by evaporation and crystalization. It may be purified by dissolving in hot ether, which, by spontaneous evaporation, leaves the Codeine in colorless crystals, which are octohedral. It is soluble in water, which takes up at

15

60° 1.26 per cent; insoluble in alkaline solutions. **Gives an alkaline re**action to test paper, and combines with acids to form salts.

ANALOGUES.—*Opium and its analogues.*

## Mental Sphere.

Great mental exhilaration. (*p.*)

Depression of spirits, with dull headache. (*s.*)

Inability to apply the mind.

## Head.

Heat in the head.

Dull headache soon after getting up in the morning, worse on the left side, and lasting about two hours.

Pulsating pain in the right temple, in the afternoon.

Dizziness on blowing the nose.

* Morning headaches, of a dull character, coming on after rising and lasting until noon.

° Headaches from fatigue and excessive mental excitement.

## Face.

Itching and heat of the face and head, extending over the whole body.

## Eyes.

* Involuntary twitching of the left eyelid, sometimes relieved by rubbing. (*Marcy.*)

Burning sensation in the eyes, worse in the left.

* Involuntary twitching of both eyelids, whenever he attempted to read or write (cured by the 5th.) (*Marcy.*)

## Nose.

Entire loss of smell.

## Mouth and Throat.

Lips dry and parched.

Tickling sensation in the throat in the afternoon and evening.

## Larynx and Chest.

Sharp pain in the right lung on inspiration.

Severe pain in the chest and shoulder on motion.

Fullness and oppression of the chest, with stitching pains in the left lung on breathing.

Tickling in the larynx, which causes a cough.

Drawing pain around the heart, which beats loud and full.

Painful pulsations of the heart on attempting to study or write.

° Short and irritating cough, worse during the night.

° Troublesome cough, with copious mucus, and sometimes purulent expectoration. (*Marcy.*)

° Night cough of phthisical patients. (*Marcy.*)

Irregular action of the heart from derangement of the ganglionic system. (*Marcy.*)

Violent pulsations of the heart and carotids.

### Gastric Symptoms.

\* Nausea and vomiting.

\* Acute pains in the stomach, with empty eructations.

Great thirst, with a particular desire for bitter substances.

° Tenderness in the stomach, with violent pulsations of the heart and carotids.

° Gastric and abdominal neuralgia.

° Violent spasmodic pain at the pit of the stomach.

### Abdomen.

Extreme tenderness of lower part of the abdomen.

Dull pains throughout the entire abdomen.

### Stool.

Constipation, tenderness of the bowels, especially the transverse and descending colon.

### Urinary Organs.

Increase of urine, it being lighter in color.

Semi-paralysis of the bladder.

### Sexual Organs. (Men.)

Sexual excitement during the night.

Lascivious thoughts, causing frequent erections day and night

### Back.

Sharp pains extending from the stomach and chest through to the back, between the shoulders, worse on right side.

Convulsive movements of the muscles of the back of the neck.

Acute pains in the region of the kidneys.

### Neck.

Convulsions in the muscles of the neck.

Neuralgic pains from the occiput to the back of the neck.

Painful pulsations in the left side of the neck.

### Superior Extremities.

Involuntary twitching of the muscles of the arm.

On moving the arm a severe pain in the deltoid muscles.

Numbness of the hands and arms.

Pulsating pain in the left upper arm.

### Inferior Extremities.

Sensation and power of motion impaired.

Involuntary twitching of the lower limbs.

Sudden pain in knee joint, rendering walking impossible for a few minutes.

° Neuralgic pains in the thighs and legs, and sub-acute rheumatic pains in the knee and ankle joints.

° Paralytic affections of lower extremities, with extreme restlessness.

---

# CHLORAL HYDRATE.

### (*Hydrate of Chloral.*)

PHARMACOLOGY.—Chloral itself is not used in medicine. It is an oily substance—a liquid. At ordinary temperatures it gives off pungent fumes. It is manufactured by the action of Chlorine on alcohol. United with water, this oily liquid is converted into a hydrate.

Chloral Hydrate is a volatile, crystaline solid, of a hot, burning taste; insoluble in cold chloroform, but very soluble in water, ether, and alcohol It occurs generally as transparent, colorless tablets, but sometimes acicular, or even in rhomboidal crystals. The compound of alcohol and chloral—*chloral alcoholate*—which resembles closely the hydrate, can be distinguished at once by its solubility in cold chloroform.

If an alkali be added to a solution of Chloral Hydrate, it breaks up into foresnic acid and chloroform, which, when water has been the solvent, at once separates in the form of oily drops.

OFFICINAL PREPARATIONS.—Tincture with strong alcohol; dilutions. (Watery solutions; usually 20 gr. to ℨ i.)

ANALOGUES.—*Ether, Chloroform, Bromides, Conium, Gelseminum, etc.*

[When given to cause sleep or allay suffering, in material doses, it is best prescribed in Syrup of Tolu, 10 grs. to the dram. It should be administered largely diluted. 20 grs. is the average soporific dose for an adult.]

### Mental Sphere.

Great excitement and intoxication, without sleep.

Restlessness, with delirium and parched, dry skin.

*Insanity.*—The following results have been gained by giving to insane persons a daily average quantity from twenty to thirty grains:

When patients are destructive and violent, the Chloral acts as an excellent hypnotic by night, and soothing agent by day.

Free from destructive habits, and gain in weight and strength.

Action of the bowels and bladder improves.

Appetite of the paralytic patients increased.

Those suffering from abnormal sensations are benefitted.

Cuts short the hallucinations in those predisposed.

Desire to maim and hurt themselves passes away.

Patients who suffer incessantly from hearing voices, some benefitted.

Melancholia has been benefitted.

That the greater the disorganization of the brain and the cord (as judged by the symptoms), the sooner does the system come under Chloral action.

Very easily irritated at trifles.

° Puerperal mania, it causes sleep when all other remedies fail.

Wandering of the mind; incoherent talking.

° Delirium tremens, when the brain is congested.

### Head.

Congestion of the brain, with some mental excitement. (*p.*)

Cerebral congestion (fatal.) (*Hammond.*)

Pain which is excruciating in the occiput.

*Great heaviness of the head;* he cannot lift it.

Head feels as if compressed in a vice.

ᵛ Cerebro-spinal congestion, in several cases. (*Hale.*)

### Eyes.

Aching heaviness in the eyes.

The eyelids feel so heavy that he can hardly lift them. (*Gels.*)

* Intense itching of the inner canthi and edges of lids.

* Red, injected, and blood-shot eyes.

* Puffy swelling of the lids.

* *Burning in the eye and eyelids.*

Watery eyes, especially when looking at anything

Eyeballs feel *too large.*

Congestion of the retina. (*p.*)
Contraction of the vessels of the retina. (*s.*)

### Sight.

Blindness, or great dimness of vision.
Disturbances of the power of accommodation. (*Crabbe.*)
Great hyperæsthesia of the retina.
He cannot see small objects, such as printed letters, but a few
moments, when they gradually fade away.
If one eye only is used until objects fade, the other sees objects
plainly for awhile. (*Gelseminum.*)
Everything looks white (*Coca*); color-blindness.
Dark spots before the eyes, as in amaurosis.
Gorgeous visions of arches, tapestry, of various vivid colors,
pass before the eyes when shut, or open in the dark.
All colors are unusually bright.
Vibrations apparently in the eyes and head when lying down
Great sensitiveness to *light* and noise.

### Mouth and Tongue.

Apparent swelling of the tongue, with sensations of stiffness,
vibrating, quivering, etc.
Fears of suffocating from swelling of the tongue.
A choking sensation at the root of the tongue.
A black streak down the centre of the tongue.
Foam at the mouth; a kind of salivation.

### Face.

° Neuralgia of the inferior dental branch of the fifth nerve.
(*Ringer.*)
° Neuralgia of the temporal region. (*Ib.*)
Congested and livid face.

### Teeth and Jaws.

° Neuralgia from decayed teeth, (a grain or two in the cavity
stops the pain quickly.) (*Hale.*)
° *Odontalgia traumatica*, from pressure of the filling; the pain
unbearable; worse when lying down. (Cured by ten grains.
See *New England Medical Gazette, March* 1872.) (*Hale.*)

### Stomach.

Retching, lasting an hour, during a surgical operation.
Does not usually disturb the stomach.

Sudden and violent vomiting.

### Stool.

° Diarrhœa, worse at night. during dentition; **excessive** nervous excitement.

Does not usually cause abdominal symptoms.

[In the very severe colic of children, when the pain **threatens to cause** spasms, 3 to 5 grs. will give prompt relief. (*Hale.*)]

### Urine.

° Nocturnal incontinence of urine — in children.

### Generative Organs.

(*Male.*) Loss of sexual power, with absence of desire and erections.

Impotence.

° Chordee, during gonorrhœa, very severe.

(*Female.*)  ° It quickly mitigates the pain of *labor*, of *dysmenorrhœa* and *uterine spasms*, but should not be given when there is a tendency to hæmorrhage, **as it** increases that tendency, even to the production of purpura. (*Hale.*)

### Heart and Circulation.

＊ Great dyspnœa, a sense of suffocation, oppression at the base of the chest (in front), and urgent thirst.

[The following case of poisoning from fifty grains illustrates its action on the circulatory system: *Cold extremities, an excessively rapid, weak, irregular and intermittent pulse; jactitation of the limbs; an intolerable sense of sinking and oppression at the pit of the stomach; gasping breathing, aud confusion of thought.* I observed at this time and for three-quarters of an hour subsequently that the *radial, temporal, and tibial pulses* were all of the character I now describe—*frequent, weak, irregular in both force and rythm, and frequently intermittent, but that the heart was acting regularly,* although with *increased frequency and diminished force.* Stimulants, with white of egg were administered freely, warmth was applied to the extremities, sinapisms placed on the cardiac region, fresh air was introduced plentifully into the room, and at the end of an hour from my first seeing the patient, the pulse had become much steadier, though still very frequent and very weak. The syncopal feeling had diminished; the feet were warm, and there was a tendency to sleep. This state of comparative freedom from urgently dangerous symptoms lasted for longer than an hour, when, without any apparent cause, they returned with increased severity. The patient now seemed in the greatest danger. *The superficial pulses were almost imperceptible,* and when they could be detected, presented the character I have described. Still the heart was regular in its beat, although feeble, and intensely rapid in its pulsations. *The mind wandered much, there was utter prostration of muscular strength, the limbs being extended, the head low, and the aspect was at times that of impending dissolution.* There was great depression, *a sense of suffocation, oppression at the base of the chest* (in front), *and urgent thirst.* The treatment previously adopted was again pursued vigorously, and at the end of an hour and a half relief was obtained and sleep followed. The next morning I found the pulse quite regular, and of its normal frequency. The points of interest that occurred to me were: 1st, the dose; 2d, the time between its administration (one hour) and the appearance of symptoms; 3d, the recurrence of symptoms after their temporary cessation; 4th, the curious effect on the muscles, which was obviously not due to effect on the heart; 5th, the relief by food and stimulants. I found that the albumen of two eggs was followed by a calming effect, and a tendency to sleep.]

### Skin.

*Purpura hæmorrhagica,* as the following cases show:

[M. A., female, aged 69, who had been an inmate of this asylum* for many years, and who was subject to periodical attacks of mania, occurring every six months, and ushered in by convulsions and coma, entered upon one of her wonted paroxysms on the 1st of March, 1870, and was ordered twenty grains of Chloral Hydrate three times a day. This produced sleep and cutaneous anæsthesia, and on the 4th of March, a very unexpected result in the form of a bright red blush, erythematous in aspect but permanent under pressure, over the chest and shoulders. This blush on March 6th had pervaded the whole trunk and limbs, and had become mottled with livid patches and deep red spots. The lips and buccal mucous membrane had contemporaneously become red and raw-looking, the gums spongy, and the tongue blistered and ulcerated in several parts. The breath was fœtid, the pulse 120, feeble and compressible, and the general condition that of great debility, with delirious excitement. On March 9th no material change had taken place, except that the ulcerations in the mouth had become more extensive and distressing; but on the 11th the petechial eruption showed signs of vanishing over the thorax and abdomen, where it had never been so severe as on the arms and legs, and where intervals of yellowish and white skin were now visible. The arms were of a red color, speckled with shreds of white, dead epidermis partially separated from the adjacent cutis, and the lips were covered with sordes and dried blood. On March 15th a sort of general desquamation had set in, the cutis being raised in thick round patches, like blisters from which the scrum had been absorbed, the skin beneath being of a dull purple color, and in some places yellow. After this a large bed-sore formed over the sacrum, and some superficial cracks and fissures presented themselves in the neighborhood of the joints. Convalescence was, however, steadily maintained, and the patient was soon restored to her usual health.]

[L. T., female, aged 46, laboring under heart disease, left hemiplegia,

* West Riding Asylum. Cases reported by Dr. Crichton Browne. Monthly Homœopathic Review, June 1871.

and dementia, with excitement, who was ordered, as a calmative, on February 24th, 1870, fifteen grains of *Chloral* thrice daily, and who seemed to derive benefit from the prescription until March 15th, when numerous reddish purple blotches were observed around the left elbow, which, on the following day, had enlarged and united with others of a similar kind which had come out on the shoulders and forearm. On March 17th several livid marks had broken out on the face, while the left arm had become swollen and indurated, and showed upon its red surface a mass of minute points or stigmata, of a much deeper red, and not disappearing under pressure. On the next day dull purple spots and discolorations—some small, round and circumscribed, others large and regular in shape—were seen on the legs, abdomen and back; being restricted in the latter situation to a band two inches in breadth along each side of the vertebral column. Along with these petechiæ there was great prostration of strength, a tendency to somnolence, weakness and irritability of the pulse, a raw state of the lips, which were entirely denuded of epithelium, and a fissured and thickly-coated tongue. On the 19th of March the spots and discolorations had spread in every direction, and had lost their vividness of hue, having assumed a deep purple tinge. Symptoms of pulmonary congestion also appeared. Strength gradually ebbed; and, after several slight attacks of syncope, death took place on the 22d of March. At the autopsy, thirty-one hours after death, the body was found covered with livid vibices and ecchymoses of various shapes and sizes, largest upon the limbs, smallest upon the abdomen. The ankles and feet were of a diffused purple color, and there was much sugillation of dependent parts. Rigor mortis was present. The outer layer of pericardium was adherent to the heart, which weighed seventeen ounces, had thin walls, dilated cavities filled with discolorized clots, and valves incompetent and enormously thickened and puckered. There was a sort of cartilaginous deposit on the outside of the right auricle. The right lung was congested and œdematous; the liver was fatty; the capsules of the kidney were thickened and adherent, with wasting of the cortical substance. In the head a large arachnoid cyst was found coexistent with the right hemisphere, which was flattened beneath it. It presented a reddish-green appearance, and contained several ounces of a bilio-sanguineous looking fluid. The whole brain weighed forty ounces; the right half weighed eighteen ounces, the left half twenty-one and one-half ounces. There were the rusty-brown traces of an old clot in the right corpus striatum.]

[*Note.*—Whether Chloral will prove a curative agent in this dreadful disease, must be shown by experience. The blood-disorganization may not be a *dynamic* effect of the drug, but due to its presence in the blood, and acting chemically. *Hale.*]

In several cases, and even several times in the same person, Chloral caused all the eruption and symptoms of an attack of scarlatina. (*British Journal of Homœopathy, April*, 1872.)

### Sleep.

Quiet sleep, apparently natural.

Comatose condition lasting for days, ending in fatal cerebral congestion.

Restless; screaming, noisy in sleep.

\* Night terrors, especially in teething children.

Somnolence, during which he is conscious of all his actions, such as coughing, spitting, etc.

[20 grs. usually causes quiet sleep for six hours, 40 grs. for 12 hours.]

### Nervous System.

° *Traumatic tetanus* (many cases).

° Puerperal convulsions in the last stages of labor. (*Dr. F. A. Lord.*)

° Chorea (many severe cases).

° *Infantile tetanus;* (two grs. at time of each spasm).

° Puerperal convulsions, arrested by 20 grs. (*Dr. F. A. Lord, U. S. Med. & Surg. Jour., May,* 1872.)

° *Tetanus,* from various causes, and trismus.

° Neuralgic and rheumatic pains.

### Pathological Effects.

Ocular and palpebral mucous membrane is injected.

Vascularity of the ears without increase of heat.

Pulseless, with contracted pupils; temperature 91–2.

Experiments on rabbits, they exhale the odor of Chloral through their nostrils, a fact which would lead one to think that it was not decomposed in the blood.

Congestion of the abdominal viscera; mesenteric vessels are turgid, all the mucous membranes are injected, particularly that of the trachea, if examined during the experimentation.

The brain, cerebellum, and their membranes show an intense vascularity.

The duration of its action is in proportion with the feebleness of the patient.

In two cases of delirium tremens, quiet sleep was induced.

In a patient suffering from bronchitis with asthma, the Chloral gave relief.

Deep and prolonged narcotism can be produced by the Chloral.

During a portion of the period of narcotism there may be complete anæsthesia, with absence of reflex action; a condition, in short, in which every kind of operation fails to call forth consciousness.

In fatal cases the functions are destroyed in the following order: *a*, the cerebral; *b*, the voluntary muscles; *c*, the respiratory; *d*, the heart.

The Chloral prevents in some small degree the coagulability of the blood, and in large quantities stops the process of coagulation altogether. In large quantities it also destroys the blood corpuscles, and produces general destruction of blood. But to produce deep insensibility, the dose administered need not be so large as to produce serious derangement of blood.

Hydrate of Chloral should be taken, to secure safe and satisfactory effects, on a neutral condition of the stomach.

If the stomach be acid, the Chloral is not taken into the circulation, and acts imperfectly.

If the stomach be alkaline, the Chloral is absorbed too rapidly.

An acid stomach should be neutralized before the Chloral is given.

---

## CROTON-CHLORAL.

### (*Croton-chloral Hydrate.*)

PHARMACOLOGY.—Croton-chloral Hydrate is formed by the action of chlorine gas upon aldehyde. It crystalizes in small glittering tablets, and is soluble, with difficulty, in water. Although its name would seem to signify it, Croton-chloral has no relation with croton oil. Chemically, it is a chlorated aldehyde of crotonic acid. When subjected to the influence of an alkali, there is first formed allyl-chloroform, a trichlorated body, which is rapidly decomposed into a bi-chlorated substance called bi-chlorallylene.

OFFICINAL PREPARATIONS.—Solution ʒ i to ʒ ix; dilutions.

It destroys the sensibility of the cranial nerves, affecting only the brain and nerves of the head; while chloral hydrate affects the whole nervous system.

(See Therapeutics, Vol. II.)

# CLEMATIS VIRGINIANA.

*(Virgin's Bower.)*

BOTANICAL DESCRIPTION.—The Clematis Virginiana is a native of the United States, growing by river banks, in hedges and thickets, from Canada to Georgia and the Mississippi. It flowers in July and August. We use the bark, leaves, and blossoms. The leaves and blossoms should be gathered when mature, and used immediately.

It is a perennial, climbing plant, with a stem from eight to fifteen feet or more in length, supporting itself on shrubs, fences, and brush-work, by means of its long footstalks. The leaves are deep green, three fold; leaflets, egg shaped or heart shaped, sharp pointed, in lobes, dentated edges, and from two to three inches in length, by one to two in breadth; flowers in clusters, irregularly branched, often having the stamens on one plant, and the pistils on another; the clusters, in the junction of the leaf, footstalk and stem; sepals four, white, spreading oblong and obtuse; stamens from twenty-eight to thirty-six; fruit furnished with long plume-like tails, appearing in large downy-like tufts; seeds compressed.

OFFICINAL PREPARATIONS.—Tincture of fresh leaves, bark, and flowers, with strong alcohol; dilutions.

ANALOGUES.—*Pulsatilla nig. and Nutt, Scutellaria, Ranunculus, Rhus, Aconite, Lilium tig., Coffea, Cimicifuga, Bromides, Clematis erecta.*

*(See Therapeutics, Vol. II.)*

---

# COLLINSONIA CANADENSIS.

*(Stone Root.)*

BOTANICAL DESCRIPTION.—The stem is simple, smooth, round, straight, from one to three feet high. Leaves with broadly toothed edges, pointed, having long footstalks, and only two or three pairs, heart shaped at base, broadly egg shaped, sharp pointed, a smooth surface, and small veins. Flowers opposite, on long footstalks, with short, oval shaped floral leaves, forming terminal, leafless, irregularly branched clusters. Corolla two-thirds of an inch long, yellow (exhaling an odor like lemon), tube-shaped at base, spreading above in two lips, the upper lip being very short and notched, the lower lobed on the sides, and fringed around. Stamens, two, long and protruding; anther oval, style protruding; seeds often aborting, only one ripening; root, perennial, knotty, depressed, very hard, with many slender fibres. It is called Ox-balm, Knot-root, etc.

This plant is indigenous, and found in rich moist woods, from Michigan to New England, and southward. It is, I believe, the only species of the genus in the Northern States. It flowers in July and September, and should be gathered while in bloom.

OFFICINAL PREPARATIONS.— Tincture with strong alcohol, from the whole plant, or fresh root; dilutions.

ANALOGUES.—*Æsculus, Arnica, Aloes, Dioscorea, Digitalis, Hamamelis, Ignatia, Lycopodium, Lycopus, Nux vomica, Podophyllum, Sulphur, Sanguinaira.*

## Head.

Dull frontal headache, with lassitude and desire to sleep.

* Headache from suppressed hæmorrhoids.

Slight fullness in the head; throbbing in the head.

## Mouth.

*Tongue* coated yellow along the centre or base, with *bitter* taste in the mouth.

## Stomach.

Vomiting, with pain and heat in the stomach.

* Cramp-like pains in the stomach, with nausea.

° Indigestion associated with constipation and hemorrhoids.

° *Flatulence and spasms of the stomach.*

° Congestion of the pelvic viscera.

° Severe colicky pains in the hypogastrium.

Constant sensation of heaviness in stomach.

Sick feeling at the pit of the stomach.

## Abdomen.

Sharp, cutting pains in hypogastric region.

Severe colicky pain in the hypogastrium, with desire for stool; nausea and faintness.

* Very severe pain in the hypogastrium every few minutes, compelling him to sit down.

° Colic, with flatulence and nausea, in cases where Nux and Colocynthis failed. (*Dr. Palmer.*)

## Stool and Anus.

* Constipation, chronic, with much flatulence, and with hæmorrhoids.

Heat and itching of the anus.

Loose, papescent stool.

* Diarrhœa, mucousdischarges, or watery, with cramp-like or spasmodic pains in the bowels, with vomiting.

° Hæmorrhoidal dysentery.

° Hæmorrhoids, bleeding, with alternate constipation and diarrhœa.

Stools preceded and followed by severe pains in the hypogastric region.

Copious stools of yellow, bilious matter, mucus, bile, blood, and with tenesmus.

\* Light-colored, lumpy stool, with distress in the anus.

° Chronic diarrhœa after confinement; stools of mucus and black fœcal matter, with colic and tenesmus. (*Burt.*)

° *Hæmorrhoids*, obstinate and *chronic*, always attended by constipation; bleeding or not. (*Drs. Fowler, Holcombe, Barnes, Franklin, and many others.*)

° Chronic diseases of the rectum.

° Congestions of the pelvic viscera, with piles.

° Diseases of the rectum, associated with disease of the uterus.

### Urine.

Urine increased in quantity.

° Chronic cystitis and nephritis.

° Catarrh of the bladder, especially with piles.

° Dropsy from cardiac irritability.

### Generative Organs.

*Female.*—Amenorrhœa, from congestion of the uterus and pelvic viscera.

° Dysmenorrhœa complicated with piles and constipation.

° Prolapsus, with pruritus, dysmenorrhœa, and most obstinate constipation.

° Uterine diseases dependent upon diseases of rectum and bowels.

° Pruritus in a pregnant woman; violent itching of the genitals, parts badly swollen, dark red and protruding; she cannot lie down. (*Dr. Cushing.*)

*Male.*—Gleet (?)

° Varicocele, with extreme constipation. (*Fowler.*)

° Spermatorrhœa kept up by piles and constipation. (*Hale.*)

### Respiratory Organs.

° Pulmonary hæmorrhage, with a short, hacking cough; he spat very tough and dark coagula, enveloped in viscid mucus; with uneasiness in the chest, but no pain, but with bleeding from the rectum the first day. (*Dr. Liebold.*)

° Hard, shaking cough, with bloody expectoration.

° Cough and dyspnœa, in connection with cardiac difficulties.

° Chest pains, alternating with hæmorrhoids.

### Heart.

° *Irritation of the cardiac nerves; cardiac hyperœsthesia.*

A functional disorder of the heart, with rapid, regular or irregular beating of the heart; pulse 130 to 140 per minute; the slightest motion or excitement aggravates the symptoms; periodical spells of faintness and oppression; attacks of syncope, with fullness of the chest and difficult breathing; and attacks of dyspnœa, with great weakness. (*Dr. Fenner.*)

(If these symptoms occur in persons subject to hæmorrhoids, or after suppressed hæmorrhoidal flux, the Collinsonia would be specially indicated.—*Hale.*]

° In cardiac disorders it seems to act by increasing the heart's tonicity; or after the heart is relieved, old hæmorrhoids appear, or suppressed menses return. (*Hale.*)

° Valvular diseases after rheumatic endocarditis. (*Paine.*)

° Palpitation of the heart in patients subject to hæmorrhoids, dyspepsia and flatulence. (*Hale.*)

° Disease of the mitral valve, the murmur diminished, and the patient greatly improved under its use. (*Dr. Shepherd.*)

### Generalities.

° Used by the country people as a vulnerary, much as the Germans use Arnica, for bruises, wounds, sprains, etc.

° Dropsy, probably from heart disease, or feebleness of the circulation.

---

## COMOCLADIA DENTATA.

### (*Guao.*)

BOTANICAL DESCRIPTION.—A tree growing in St. Domingo and Cuba. The stem erect, not much branched. Leaves divided, shiny and green above, with a round foot-stalk six inches in length. Six to ten leaflets on each side, with an odd one, which are oblong, sharp-pointed, toothed, furry and somewhat downy at the back. Juice milky, glutinous, becoming black by exposure to air, staining the linen or skin the same color, and cannot be washed off. It is supposed by the natives of Cuba to be death to sleep beneath this tree, especially for persons of a sanguine or fat habit of body.

OFFICINAL PREPARATION.—Tincture with strong alcohol, of the leaves or bark; dilutions.

ANALOGUES.—*Anacardium, Rhus tox., Rhus rad., and Rhus ven., etc.*

### Head.

Feeling of heaviness in the head—aggravated by holding the head down.

Shooting pains through the left temple.

On arising from bed everything looks dark; pains, relieved by motion and in the open air.

### Face.

° Left side of face swollen; the left ear also all cracked and desquamating a substance like powdered starch. Cured in five weeks. (*Navarro.*)

### Eyes.

Aching soreness in the eyeballs, which feel heavy.

*Inflammation of the eyes;* sees from right eye a red ring around the light of the lamp; closing the eye, the ring disappears.

Eyeballs seem too large.

Pains in the eyes increased by being near warm room, with profuse lachrymation.

Severe pains through the eyeballs, extending to occiput.

Painful, pressing out sensation in the head, as if something was pressing on top of the eyeballs.

### Nose.

Intolerable itching of the nose.

### Mouth, Teeth and Jaws.

Aching pains in the teeth.

Sensation as if the tooth was drawing out of its socket.

Sensation as if all the molar teeth on the right side were loose.

Pains in the teeth, relieved by pressure.

Inflammation of the gums of the lower jaw.

Tongue coated dirty yellow.

Lower lips blistered and swollen.

When the toothache stops the head feels large.

### Larynx.

Spasmodic dry cough at night, with tickling in the throat, and constant dull pain under the left nipple.

Tittilating cough; hacking cough in the daytime

### Abdomen.

A pale red flush, as if an eruption would make its appearance across the abdomen.

Acute, sore pains extending across the abdomen above the umbilicus, affecting the breathing.

### Genital Organs.

Continued tingling, itching of the scrotum during the night.

Intense itching on the lower part of the penis, also on inner side of the prepuce.

### Chest.

Acute, sharp pains in left mammary gland, about one inch above the nipple, and leaves a burning sensation; it goes to right side and down right arm.

Oppression of breath, on account of sharp pains in left side.

° A sloughing ulcer on the right breast of a lady of thirty eight. (Cured in six weeks.) (*Dr. Navarro.*)

Constant pain across the chest.

Rheumatic or pleurodynic pains in chest.

### Back.

Rheumatic pains and stitches in the back; the stitches leave a burning.

### Superior Extremities.

Frequent rheumatic pains in the hands, arms and legs.

Vesicular eruption on the arms and hands.

### Lower Extremities.

Severe pains in both knees; pressing down to the feet on the inside of the legs.

Pains, relieved by movement.

* Vesicular eruption on the legs; changing to pustules, and sometimes to deep, unhealthy ulcers.

° An indolent ulcer on lower third of right leg, near the external malleolus—of irregular shape and hard edges; the ulcer was deep, and discharged a sanious and fœtid pus; it had lasted six years. (Cured in four weeks by *Comocladia 30th.*) (*Dr. Navarro.*)

° Inflammation of left leg and foot, with violent fever; the swelling increased enormously, when the pain subsided; the skin became white and covered with shiny scales; cracked and discharged a sanious fluid. (Cured by *Comocladia 6th.*) (*Navarro.*)

16

### Skin.

Violent itching, redness and erysipelatous swelling of the face, hands, and other parts of the body, followed by yellow vesication and desquamation of the cuticle.

Painful burning on face and arms; face enormously swollen

Rash resembling scarlet fever.

° Erysipelas, herpes, zona, etc.

Inflammation of the skin, followed by deep, hard-edged ulcers, discharging a thick, purulent, greenish-yellow matter, having a very fœtid smell; the parts looking like raw meat; the skin covered by small shiny scales.

---

# CORNUS FLORIDA.

### (*Dogwood, Boxwood.*)

BOTANICAL DESCRIPTION.—This is a handsome little tree, usually from fifteen to twenty feet high: common throughout all our forests; conspicuous in spring-time by its festoons of large white blossoms, and equally so during the autumn for its clusters of scarlet berries.

In this genus of Cornaceæ there are about twenty species, of which America has, north of Mexico, eleven. The flowering Dogwood is the most beautiful and showy plant of its genus. It is too well known to need description.

OFFICINAL PREPARATIONS.—Tincture with strong alcohol from the fresh bark; dilutions.

ANALOGUES.—*China,* (?) *Nux vomica.* (?)

### Head.

Sensation of fullness and pains in the head, with gastric derangement.

Severe headache, with quick pulse and violent pains in the bowels.

Cerebral fullness, with constant tendency to sleep.

### Stomach.

Nausea, vomiting, pain in the stomach, with headache.

° Acid pyrosis; painful and slow digestion.

### Abdomen and Stool.

Violent pain in the bowels, with purging.

### Fever.

Increased temperature of the body, hot sweat, fullness in the head.

° Intermittent fever; the paroxysm preceded for days by sleepiness; sluggish flow of ideas; headache of a dull, heavy character; nausea, vomiting, loss of appetite; sometimes bilious or watery diarrhœa; chill, with cold, clammy skin; nausea and vomiting; and violent pain in the bowels; fever, with violent headache; hot but moist skin; stupor; cerebral fullness; pulse quick and hard; confusion of intellect, etc.

## CORNUS CIRCINATA.

(*Round-leaved Dogwood, Green Osier.*)

BOTANICAL DESCRIPTION.—A shrub found all over the Northern States, from six to ten feet high, growing on the hillsides, near water courses. *Leaves* longer than in any other species, round-oval, abruptly pointed, wooly and white beneath, about as broad as long, wavy on the edges, opposite on the branches. *Stem* grayish, upright, with opposite, cylindrical, green, spotted, or warty branches. *Flowers* white, small, in flat or depressed bunches, without any leaves or bracts. *Fruit* light-blue, round, hollowed at the base, soft, crowned with the remains of the styles. The *bark*, when fresh, is bright green; when dried, in quills of a whitish or ash color; its taste is bitter, astringent and aromatic.

OFFICINAL PREPARATIONS.—Tincture with strong alcohol, from the fresh bark; dilutions.

ANALOGUES.—*China, Hydrastis, Eupatorium perfoliatum, Nux vomica, etc.*

### Mental Sphere.

Drowsiness, with indifference.

Mind confused, with inability to concentrate it upon any subject.

° Feeling of indolence, and loss of energy.

Great depression of spirits, and petulance.

Indifference with respect to subjects which usually interest.

### Head.

° Dull, heavy pain in the whole head, with drowsiness.

Headache, increased by walking, stooping, or shaking the head.

° Sense of fullness in head, relieved by a copious stool.

Congestion of blood to the head and face.

Deep-seated, pulsating pains in the occipital and parietal regions.

° Shooting pains through the whole brain.

° Bilious cephalalgia.

### Eyes.

Aching pains through the eyeballs.

Yellowish tinge of the conjunctivæ; hollowness of the eyes.

Sense of weight around the eyes.

Eyes dull aud heavy.

### Nose.

Itching of the nasal mucous membrane.

Coryza early in the morning.

Severe prickling sensation in the bony part of the nose.

### Mouth and Throat.

Tongue coated with a thin, yellowish fur.

Bitter taste in the mouth.

Smarting in the mouth and throat.

White fur on the tongue, with desire for cold drinks.

° Apthous stomatitis of children; stomatitis materna.

° Apthous ulceration of the mouth in children.

### Stomach.

* Nausea, with bitter taste, and aversion to all kinds of food, and desire for sour drinks.

Burning sensation in the stomach.

° Heavy pulsations in the stomach, with nausea and impaired appetite.

Nausea, with great debility and eructations.

Sensation of faintness in stomach and bowels.

Fullness and oppression in the stomach, with bad taste and dry mouth.

Smarting and burning in the mouth, throat and stomach, with desire for stool.

### Abdomen and Stool.

Griping pains in the abdomen, with rumbling of wind.

Pressing down pain in the rectum and stool, smarting at the anus; tenesmus, with griping in the umbilical region.

Urging to stool, with fullness and uneasiness of the bowels.

Abdominal pains, more acute during stool.

Constant working in the bowels.

Distension of the bowels with wind, relieved by a copious, dark and bilious stool.

Urging to stool, but little passed, the discharge consisting of a few slimy lumps, with pressing and smarting at the anus.

° Stool thin and scanty, with burning at the rectum.

° Stool thin, scanty, and slimy, with griping in the umbilical region.

* Copious thin and bilious discharge, with tenesmus and burning.

° Dark green, thin, and very offensive stools, with copious emission of offensive flatus.

° Copious, dark stool of the natural consistence.

Hard, dry, and scanty stool, with pressing in the rectum.

° Dysentery, with ulceration of mucous membrane of the rectum.

° Bilious derangements.

* Diarrhœa, with excessive debility and nervous excitability.

### Urine.

Urine scanty and red, or pale; sensation of fullness in the region of the bladder.

Frequent inclination to pass water.

### Generative Organs.

Increased sexual desire during the evening and night, with diminished power.

### Chest.

Stitches in the chest and back.

A fine scarlet rash upon the chest, with itching.

Sore, bruised feeling in the chest and back.

Shooting pains from the centre of thorax to the lower part of the abdomen.

Choking sensation in the upper part of the thorax.

### Back.

Dull pain in small of the back, with drowsiness and lassitude.

Sore pain in the lumbar region, worse on bending forward or to either side.

### Upper Extremities.

Burning and itching sensation in the hands and arms.

Coldness of the hands, following a loose stool.

### Lower Extremities.

Weakness and weary feeling in the legs.

Itching on the legs and thighs; burning sensation in the feet

Coldness of feet, following a loose stool.

## Skin.

Itching of the scalp, legs and feet, increased by scratching or rubbing.

Paroxysms of itching of the skin of the back, legs and feet, mostly at night.

Fine scarlet rash on the breast, attended with itching.

Skin covered with a copious, clammy perspiration.

Itching around the genital organs.

## Fever.

Flushes of heat, followed by perspiration.

Chilly sensation, succeeded by transient flushes of heat.

Congestion of the head and face.

Flushes of heat and coldness in alternation, followed by cold perspiration.

Bilious remittents, and the characteristic gastric and intestinal symptoms present.

## Sleep.

Very great drowsiness, and disposition to perspire.

Great disposition to sleep, with entire loss of mental and physical energy.

Stupid and sleepy feeling, with nausea, etc.

Sleepy and weak during the day, with dull pains in the head, back and limbs.

---

# CORYDALIS FORMOSA.

### (*Turkey Corn.*)

BOTANICAL DESCRIPTION.—This beautiful little plant is indigenous, found westward and southward of New York, to North Carolina, growing in rich soil on hills and mountains, among rocks and old decayed timber, flowering very early in the spring. It is also known as Wild Turkey Pea, Staggerweed, and Choice Dyelytra. It is a perennial plant, from six to ten inches high, having a tuberous root. *Leaves* radical, rising from ten to fifteen inches high; somewhat three fold, with the incisions quite variable. The *flower stem* is radical, naked, rising from eight to twelve inches high, with from four to eight bunches of flowers, each bunch consisting of from six to ten reddish purple, nodding flowers. The *inflorescence* compound, having at the end of the branches a small tuft of hair. *Corolla* from eight to ten lines long, broad at the base; the *spines* very short, obtuse and incurved; the flower leaves purple, and at the base of the pedicles; the *style* extended; the *stigma* two horned at the apex; *sepals* two, falling off at a stated time; the *capsule*, pod-shaped and many-seeded.

OFFICINAL PREPARATIONS.—Tincture with strong alcohol, from the fresh root; dilutions; triturations of the dried root.

ANALOGUES.—*Chimaphila, Iodide of Potassium, Mercurius corrosivus, Stillingia, Aurum; Phytolacca.*

### Head.

° Syphilitic nodes on the skull.

° Syphilitic and scrofulous eruptions on the scalp.

### Mouth and Throat.

° Syphilitic ulceration of the fauces.

° Chronic ulceration of the mouth and fauces.

### Stomach.

\* A peculiar derangement of the stomach, attended with profuse morbid secretion of mucus; tongue always coated,
with fetor of the breath; loss of appetite and indiges
tion; (acute and chronic catarrh of the stomach).

### Generative Organs.

° *Syphilis, primary and secondary.*

° Syphilitic nodes, with nocturnal pains.

---

# COSMOLINE.

PHARMACOLOGY.—Is manufactured by subjecting crude Petroleum to distillation for the purpose of expelling the light hydro-carbons. The residue is purified without the use of chemicals, and deodorized by animal charcoal.

Cosmoline does not evaporate below 400°; has no affinity of oxygen, and never becomes rancid. It probably consists essentially of Paraffin and some of the heavy coal oils.

OFFICINAL PREPARATIONS.—Triturations; dilutions. (Cerates.)

ANALOGUES.—*Urtica urens, Dulcamara, Petroleum, Calendula, Carbolic acid, Rhus.*

[Cosmoline is purified and concentrated Petroleum, the substance which remains after all ethers, coloring matter, impurities, etc., have been re_ moved. To obtain it, crude Petroleum is distilled and refined, *without the use of acids or alkalies*, until only a pure, dense, neutral, concentrated, oleaginous body, *having an absolute non-affinity for oxygen or moisture*, remains.]

[The following results were obtained from provings of the 3d × tritura. tion, and its effects on the workmen engaged in its manufacture.—*Dr. Malcom MacFarlan, of Philadelphia, Penn.*]

In all cases, speaking generally, the appetite failed. There was a feeling of uneasiness and distress about the epigastrium; eructations, mouth filled with sour water, and bowels disposed to be loose. Several of the persons had diarrhœa (watery and offensive) on the second or third day; great indifference and weariness; urination was free (profuse) and frequent. (*Provers.*)

Loss of appetite, with a feeling of disgust at the sight of food, especially fat meats; a distressed feeling about the epigastrium; *extreme weariness and prostration,*—at times a congestive headache. They are unrefreshed by sleep, feeling tired and stiff on awakening. In some instances they have had a severe diarrhœa, watery and offensive, without pain. They have a constant desire for vegetable acids and fresh fruits. (*Workmen.*)

The skin symptoms in all the cases were alike,—great apparent dryness of the skin and itchiness everywhere, with a constant disposition to scratch one's self. In two cases the skin became dry and scurfy, in irregular patches or blotches, which were very itchy. The skin, on being scratched slightly, would raise in welts or blotches.

In regard to the curative effects of it, I may say that I have cut short two cases herpes zoster, of a very violent character. The eruption disappeared in both cases within ten days.

At the Clinic of the Hahnemann College, and before the class, Cosmoline has been used with wonderfully curative effect in the different varieties of eczema. As far as I know, it is the most reliable remedy we have in that obstinate disease,—Petroleum, highly potentized, acting in a similar manner.

The local application of Cosmoline removes the stinging, burning, and itching of eczema.

It has proved valuable as a topical application, not only in skin diseases, but for burns, scalds, blisters, cuts, bruises, sprains, and acute inflammation; also for hæmorrhoids.

(See Therapeutics, Vol. II.)

# COTYLEDON UMBILICUS.

### (*Navelwort.*)

[A pathogenesis and provings were published in the *British Journal of Homœopathy*. I find nothing concerning the domestic or pharmacological uses of the plant, except an assertion by Culpepper that it was useful in erysipelas, inflammations, etc. Is seems to affect the mental sphere, like *Ignatia*, causing alternate states of exaltation and depression. On the nerves and muscular system—a decided action. This species is a common weed in the west of England, growing on the sides and in the crevices of damp rocks and walls. We have none of this *genus* in the United States. See pathogenesis in Allen's Encyclopedia of Materia Medica.]

OFFICINAL PREPARATIONS.—Tincture of the plant; dilutions.

ANALOGUES.—*Ambergris, Asafœtida, Aconite, Gelseminum, Hyosciamus, Hepatica, Ignatia, Phosphorus,* etc.

(*See Therapeutics, Vol. II.*)

---

# CUNDURANGU.

### (*Condor-plant.*)

[This medicine is prepared from the bark of a climbing plant or shrub found in Ecuador, South America. A decoction of the bark is advised.]

OFFICINAL PREPARATIONS.—Tincture of the bark; dilutions.

ANALOGUES.—*Arsenicum, Baptisia, Conium, Lapis alb., Pæonia, Silica.*(?)

\* A cachectic state of the system, such as obtains in patients in surgical wards of hospitals — and in which ordinary wounds and ulcers tend to take on a bad appearance, fester, etc.

\* Indolent ulcers, with hard callous edges, discharging a fœtid, sanious smell.

° Old, indolent ulcers, appearing cancerous.

(*See Therapeutics, Vol. II.*)

---

# CYANIDE OF POTASSIUM.

### (*Potasii Cyanidum.*)

PHARMACOLOGY.—This salt is prepared, according to the U. S. pharmacopœia, by heating together the ferrocyanide of Potassium and the Carbonate of Potassium. It occurs in white, amorphous, opaque masses, having the odor of Prussic acid and a taste of similar character, but somewhat alkaline.

It is deliquescent, and readily soluble in water. When the Nitrate of Silver is added to its solution, there falls a precipitate of the Cyanide of Silver, which is wholly soluble in ammonia.

OFFICINAL PREPARATIONS.—Mother Tincture; one grain to ten grains of distilled water; dilutions to the 3d × with water, higher with strong alcohol.

ANALOGUES.—*Acidum hydrocyanicum, Amygdala amara, Prunus, Laurocerasus, Digitalis.*

[A most violent poison, very similar in action to Hydrocyanic acid. Three grains are sufficient to destroy life.]

### Sensorium.

*Sudden* loss of consciousness.

### Head.

Severe, sudden pain in the head.

Vertigo, and sensation of weight in the head.

Great pain in *back part* of the head.

° Torturing neuralgic headache in orbital and supra-maxillary region; the pains recurring daily at the same hour, with much flushing of that side of the face.

° Agonizing attacks of neuralgic pains between the temporal region and ciliary arch and maxilla, with screams and apparent loss of sensibility, as if struck with apoplexy; pulse, eighty-four; face flushed.

° Severe neuralgic pains in temporal region and left upper jaw, daily at 4 A. M., increasing till 10 A. M., and ceasing at 4 P. M.; in the interval anorexia, fever, headache, etc.

° In headaches depending on dyspepsia, imperfect menstruation, known as "sick-headache," the *external* application of a solution, not stronger than two or four grains to one ounce of water, applied on compresses, will give prompt relief. (*Trousseau.*)

### Face, Eyes and Ears.

*Face* flushed, with neuralgic headache.

*Eyes* fixed, pupils dilated; dim vision.

*Ears*, rushing sound in the ears.

### Gastric.

Sense of constriction in the throat.

Intense *burning* in the stomach.

*Nausea*, with sense of choking when trying to swallow fluids, followed by copious vomiting.

A feeling as if the bowels were about to act.

### Chest.

He cannot take a deep inspiration, but has no definite pain.

Respiration slow and difficult.

Abdominal respiration (in animals).

° Troublesome cough, preventing sleep at night, with dullness on percussion; respiration feeble, mixed with crepitant and bronchial rales.

### Heart.

It paralyses the heart in tetanic spasm; general convulsive action of the whole body ten minutes after the heart ceased to beat.

### Trunk and Extremities.

Spasmodic tetanic stiffness of trunk and limbs, with shuddering of the limbs.

Skin about the joints fissured, with oozing of blood; the inflammation extending to the nail and its root.

Ulceration of the soft parts of the hands down to the bone, with great pain.

### Generalities.

She fell as if struck by lightning, and died in forty minutes; (from twelve grains).

General convulsions; eyes fixed and limbs contracted.

° Acute articular rheumatism.

---

# CYANURET OF MERCURY.

### (*Hydrargyri Cyanuretum.*)

PHARMACOLOGY.—This salt is prepared by dissolving in sixteen parts of water, in a glass flask, two parts of crystallized Ferro-cyanuret of Potassium, and then adding three parts of dry per-sulphate of mercury. Boil for half an hour in a sand bath, filter, and evaporate to dryness, stirring constantly. Powder the dried mass, digest it with eight times its weight of 80° alcohol, for some hours, filter while hot, wash the residue on the filter, with hot alcohol, and set aside to crystallize. Collect the crystals, evaporate the molten liquor to dryness, and preserve the whole in a well closed bottle, excluded from the light.

It is formed in white, more or less transparent, four-sided prisms and pyramids, which are odorless, but have a pungent, nauseous, metallic taste. Heated in a close glass tube the crystals fly in pieces, and decompose. Water at 60° F. dissolves 1-11 part of its weight of the salt; at 212° F. 2-5 its weight; 80° alcohol dissolves 1-22 its weight, and when boiling 1-5 its weight.

OFFICIAL PREPARATIONS.—(1) Mother tincture —with 80% alcohol, 1 part to 20, by weight; dilutions. (2) Triturations.

ANALOGUES:—*Arum triphyllum, Causticum, Hepar sulph., Kali bichromi cum, Kali causticum, Mercurius iodat., Phytolacca, Muriatic acid, Lachesis, etc.*

[In the treatment of malignant diphtheria the 6th dilution has been used. Owing to the intensely poisonous nature of the drug, this is as low as should be used, especially for children. (*Hale.*)]

### Mental Sphere.

Cerebral excitation, with sleeplessness at night.

Loss of consciousness; syncope and general debility.

### Head.

Headache, with vertigo, and burning in the ears.

### Face.

Face pale and wan; bluish cast.

Copious epistaxis.

Blue face and lips.

### Eyes.

Eyes are sunken.

Pupils contracted.

### Mouth and Throat.

Tongue pale with yellowish streak on the base; swollen, red on its borders.

\* Throat looks rough; pharynx red and injected.

Gums swollen and covered with a white adherent layer, under which was found a violet border.

\* A white opaline layer formed on the columns of the velum palati and the tonsils; on the inside of the right cheek was a round ulcer with a grayish base, the borders as if cut out and surrounded by great redness.

\* Pseudo-membranous inflammation of the throat.

\* Lips, tongue and inside of the cheeks dotted by ulceration, covered by a grayish-white coating.

Mucous membrane of the throat was very red.

Inflammation over the whole buccal cavity.

Salivation, a thin, foetid, excoriating discharge.

Great difficulty of swallowing.

° Pseudo-membranous croup; (considered a specific in the most malignant cases by many physicians).

° *Diphtheria maligna*, with phagadenic ulceration.

### Stomach.

Nausea, vomiting, and frequent diarrhœic stools, with icy coldness of the body.

Drinks are immediately returned.

Burning sensation in the stomach.

Increased thirst, with violent irritation of the throat.

Vomiting of green mucus.

Violent retchings.

Hiccough constant for twenty-four hours.

### Abdomen.

Abdomen slightly painful.

Violent abdominal pains, increasing with every stool.

Colic, followed by hard stool, then a soft one.

### Stool and Anus.

Fluid stools, tinged with blood.

Diarrhœic stools, smelling badly; green and glairy.

Very copious diarrhœa, which is persistent, with moist and icy-cold skin.

Frequent inclination to stool, preceded and accompanied by tenesmus; stools scanty and mixed with blood.

Great inclination to go to stool (with incessant vomiting), followed by liquid stool.

Dark-colored stool.

On making the effort at stool passes pure black blood.

A fœtid liquid oozes from the rectum, having the characteristic smell of gangrene, and forming on the linen large black spots.

Pains in the rectum when sitting down, also around the anus, which is swollen.

Hæmorrhoidal tumors around the anus, and knobby swelling of the mucous membrane.

Diphtheritic, grayish layer around the anus, similar to that on the cheeks.

° Malignant or putrid dysentery.

### Urinary Organs.

Retention of urine during five days.

Suppression of urine.

Urine yellow, amber-colored; painful.

Urine clear, but scanty.

Urine scanty and dark.

Numerous whole cylinders, or broken down, with fine detritus; no blood globules; a quantity of albumen.

Urine contained in the bladder is extremely albuminous.

° Bright's disease.

### Generative Organs.

(*Male.*)   Penis is of a dark color, is in a state of semi-erection. Scrotum is of a dark color.

### Heart.

Pulse small, depressed, 76.

Pulse stronger and more frequent, 90.

Pulse weak, 130, with cold extremities and cyanosed face.

Pulse 102, irregular in the morning (noticed only at one time).

Beating of the heart is violent and rough.

Severe contractions of the heart, repelling the hand.

### Lower Extremities.

Severe pain in the left calf; the veins form two strings which unite in the neighborhood of the ankles; the least touch is extremely painful; leg much swollen (varices).

### Generalities.

General debility, syncope, icy-coldness of the body.

Extreme prostration, frequent vomiting, hiccough.

Great sensation of chilliness.

Extremities agitated by light convulsive motion.

---

## CYPRIPEDIUM PUBESCENS.

### (*Lady's Slipper.*)

DESCRIPTION.—*Root* fibrous and branching; *stems* single, a foot or more high, bearing three or four broad, ovate, rather downy, ribbed leaves, clasping the stem at the base, and one or two large flowers.   These consist of two lanceolate, brown-purple sepals, and a pair of somewhat narrow, wavy petals crossing each other at right angles; from the midst of them projects a great yellow pouch or bag, resembling a moccasin, a shoe, or a slipper, as the imagination wills.

OFFICINAL   PREPARATIONS. — (1) Tincture of the root;  dilutions. (2) Cypripedin; triturations; (Tincture of the whole plant when in bloom, for future provings?)

ANALOGUES.—*Ambergris, Coca, Paullinia, Coffea, Thea, Scutellaria, Zinc, Valerian, Bromides.   (Rhus?)*

## Mind and Brain.

Exhilarates the mind and nervous system. (*primary.*)

A sense of quiet, or mental lassitude. (*secondary.*)

Talkative, and more disposed to work. (*p.*)

A sense of weight and oppression on the mind. (*s.*)

*Profound indifference to everything,* even to his studies duties, and the common courtesies of life.

Inability to study, think, or listen to lectures.

Feeling of intense soreness and irritation of the eyes every evening about *five* o'clock.

Slight disposition to drowsiness. (*s.*)

Slight heaviness, and fullness in the brain, with sleeplessness. (*p.*)

Irritable; fretful; angry at trifles; hysterical. (*p.*)

° Disorders of the gray-nerve matter from mental over-exertion, or reflex nervous excitement. (*Paine.*)

° Delirium tremens, mild attacks. (*Hale.*)

° Mental despondency—in spermatorrhœa. (*Ib.*)

## Sleep.

\* Sleeplessness, with desire to talk, or with constant crowding of pleasant ideas. (*Ib.*)

\* Sleeplessness, with restlessness of the body; twitching of the limbs. (*Ib.*)

## Generalities.

° Hysterical complaints.

° Chorea, and reflex epilepsy.

° Functional irritation of the brain, especially in very young children, from teething, or intestinal irritation.

° Incipient cerebral disorder, when the child is sleepless, and laughs and plays in the night.

° Jactitation and trembling in typhoid fevers.

## Skin.

It has not been known heretofore that *Cypripedium* had any specific action on the skin, but a communication from Prof. H. H. Babcock, a scientific botanist of Chicago, would seem to show that its effects are often mistaken for *Rhus* poisoning. It seems strange, however, that it has not been observed before, especially in school children in the country, who gather the flowers of the Lady's Slipper daily, during the season of flowering. I have attended Prof. Babcock several times for attacks of what was supposed to be *Rhus* poisoning. The symptoms were identical with those of *Rhus*. He says, in his letter to *The Pharmacist:*—" Working botanists have so often been poisoned by *Rhus toxicodendron* that many of them have come to regard it as their special bane. In the five seasons commencing with 1868, I was particularly careful not to touch this poisonous plant, not to pluck a specimen growing in its immediate vicinity, nor to receive from the hands of another person a freshly-gathered plant, for fear it might have come in contact with *Rhus*. In spite of these precautions, in the latter part of May or first of June in each year, I was poisoned so severely as to be confined to my room for several days. In June, 1872, after gathering many specimens of *Cypripedium spectabile*, I observed that my hands were stained with the purplish secretion of the glandular hairs with which its stem and leaves are densely clothed, and shortly after experienced a peculiar irritation about my eyes. The next day my whole face presented the appearance of a severe case of *Rhus* poisoning. On reviewing my notes of the previous years, I found that in each season the poisoning had appeared on the day after I had collected *Cypripedium spectabile* or *C. pubescens*. In 1873 and 1874, I collected more extensively than ever before, but suspecting that my previous sufferings had been caused by these two species of *Cypripedium* rather than the *Rhus*, took no unusual pains to avoid the latter, but refrained from touching either of the former with the bare hand. The result was what I had expected, for I escaped entirely the poisoning that I had begun to regard as inevitable, and am now convinced that upon myself, at least, *Cypripedium spectabile* and *C. pubescens* are capable of producing effects similar to those caused by *Rhus toxicodendron*. Is it not possible that others, also, have wrongly attributed to *Rhus* the annoyance caused by

F.16

these plants hitherto considered inoffensive? A decisive answer, either affirmative or negative, must depend upon the results of future experiment. Who will undertake it?"

In a proving by Dr. Vanderberg, he observed that "every evening, about five o'clock, the eyes became sore," *i. e.*, were affected by sensations of itching, burning, and *sore* feeling, but without any apparent redness or swelling. This symptom may be corroborative of the above, for if the proving had been continued, the itching, burning, etc., might have extended to the face and body. Perhaps if the proving had been made from a tincture of *the whole plant*, cutaneous symptoms would have appeared.

---

# DATURA ARBOREA.

## (*Bougmancia Candida.*)

DESCRIPTION.—A native of Peru, growing along the Pacific coast in California, cultivated in gardens and conservatories. Leaves large, their sides unequal. Flowers; corolla funnel shaped, long tubed and bent downward; color, snow-white, with a yellow tint by the fundus, of very sweet odor. Dr. Poulson, of Council Bluffs, Iowa, communicates the following pathogenetic symptoms.

OFFICINAL PREPARATIONS.—Tincture of the leaves and flowers; dilutions.

ANALOGUES.—*Agaricus, Æthusa, Belladonna, Hyoscyamus, Cannabis indica, Stramoniam, etc.*

### Mind.

*Toxicological effect* much slower than *D. Stramonium,* but dynamically very intense and lasting.

The odor of the flowers in a room causes considerable psychological aberration.

Causes such deep impression upon the mental sphere and faculty of concentrating ideas that I was sensibly affected a long time. (*Dr. Camaun.*)

A very strange feeling of pleasant ease and comfort, as if I scarcely touched the earth with my feet, and had to gather my ideas from afar, as if they were floating in the clouds.

A longing for beauty and fine scenery.

17

The brain seems floating in thousands of problems and grand
ideas, without being able to concentrate itself, or get to
any point and carry out any system of thought.

It acts mostly as a pure dynamic and semi-spiritual agent
upon the sensations, without perceptible pain. (*Poulson.*)

He experienced a slight *vertigo*, and found himself involved
in a most beautiful atmosphere, bright and calm as the
sunlight at noon. (*Camaun.*)

A confusion of ideas across the cerebrum. (*Ib.*)

° Recommended by Dr. Camaun as a remedy in some forms of
emotional or functional *insanity*, or when the patient is
happy and contented and imagines himself or herself to
be some extraordinary emperor, prince, etc. (*Poulson.*)

**Head.**

A drawing, nervous irritation, from the cerebrum back to the
cerebellum, and a spinal irritation, or depletion of nervous circulation in the medulla oblongata. (*Ib.*)

A contraction of the front cerebrum of a convulsive nature,
sometimes as if a string was tied close around the head
from sinus frontalis to os occipitis. (*Ib.*)

The cramps of both hemispheres (cerebro-frontalis) made me
careful in experimenting more. (*Ib.*)

A feeling as if my forehead was expanded, and my ideas were
floating outside my brain. (*Ib.*)

A sharp, constrictive sensation across the spine in the region
pars dorsalis, extending upward to the pars cervicalis,
into ventriculus quartus, or the lower region of the cerebellum, with irritation of nervous accessories. (*Ib.*)

[Dr. Poulson's estimate of the power of this remedy is, perhaps, over-
rated; his theory of its action rather vague. It would have been better if
he had couched his language in less transcendental terms.

---

# DIOSCOREA VILLOSA

### (*Wild Yam Root—Colic Root.*)

DESCRIPTION—This is a plant with slender twining stem, herbaceous,
rising from large, matted, knotty rootstalks. It climbs bushes, old fences,
etc. The *stem* is smooth, rarely villous, green or greenish brown, dying
every fall. *Leaves*, mostly alternate; sometimes nearly opposite or in fours;
more or less downy underneath, heart shaped, conspicuously pointed, nine

to eleven ribbed. *Flowers*, pale greenish yellow, very small, the sterile in drooping panicles; the fertile in simple, drooping racemes. *Fruit*, a membranaceous, three-angled, or winged pod. *Seeds*, one or two in each cell, a minute embryo in hard albumen. It grows in thickets, from New England to Wisconsin, and very common in all the Southern States. It flowers in July. The roots should be procured in September in the North, later in the South.

OFFICINAL PREPARATIONS.—Tincture of the fresh root; dilutions; Triturations of the pulverized root, and of Dioscorin; Infusion.

ANALOGUES.—*Æsculus, Aloes, Bryonia, Chamomilla, Colocynth, Collinsonia, Hyoscyamus, Nux Vomica, Senna, Podophyllum.*

## Moral Symptoms.

**Nervous**, easily troubled; or nerves uncommonly steady.

**Feel cross**, desire to be alone; company is disagreeable; **conversation** is troublesome.

**Feel tired**; still keeps walking around the room.

**Great depression** of spirits.

## Head.

Dull, stupefying pain in both temples.

Dull, dizzy, confused feeling in head, worse during stool.

Dull pain deep in centre of the head.

Severe dull pain in back of neck, extending to head and shoulders; worse on left side.

Dizzy, severe deep-seated pain in left occipital region.

Sharp, deep-seated pain behind right ear.

Dull, stupefying pain in both temples, as if from pressure; relieved at once by pressure, but when the pressure is removed, the pain is sharper and worse than before.

A pressing pain from front to back of head, as if he would become unconscious.

Pain in front of head and temples, as if the top of the head were lifted·up.

Severe pain in both temples and front of head; head feels cold.

Head feels heavy, with pain between the eyes and near the top of both ears.

Faintness is increased by sitting up in bed; numbness increased by lying down.

Head feels as if a band was tied around it.

Dizzy, inclined to go to the right when walking.

Head after breakfast, feels tight as if squeezed.

Pulling pain in front of both ears as precedes vomiting.

Sharp pain in both temples, not changed by walking, riding, or shaking the head.

Sharp pain in left temple, with nausea and chills, beginning on back, worse over left scapula.

Pulling pain in occiput, causing a stupid sensation; feel confused; call things by wrong names.

Belching large quantities of wind, with a sensation as if both temples were in a vise.

Frequent dull, then stabbing, pain in left temple; feel dull and stupid.

Head feels strange; inclined to fall backwards.

Constant, dull, frontal headache, more in the top of the forehead.

° Vertigo and giddiness, with heat in the head; with sharp cutting pains in right side of the forehead, extending to the ears; a remittent pain, aggravated by pressure; fullness in the head, speedily followed by some spasmodic pain in the abdomen. (*Cushing.*)

### Eyes.

Itching of both eyes; smarting of both eyes, right one worse.

Internal angle of eyes worse than external.

Eyes feel as if some large, smooth substance was in them.

Eyes feel as if dust or lashes or sticks were in them.

Discharge of hot water from the eyes.

Sharp pain in left eye; sharp pain in ball of right eye.

Both eyes weak, sore, and smart badly.

Eyelids stiff; hard pain just below angle of right eye.

Sharp pain in right eye, extending to occipital region.

Sore on under lid of right eye, like a stye.

Both lids of right eye sore, but do not look sore.

Eyes smart badly in the evening; smarting of internal angle of both eyes.

Eyes smart so badly that it seems as if hot air came out of them, and passed down over the cheeks.

Water runs from the right eye, and smarts so bad that he has to keep it closed most of the time.

Eyes gummed up in the morning.

In open air eyes so full of tears he cannot see plainly.
Wants to keep the eyes closed.

### Ears.
Hard pain behind left ear; hard pain in front of both ears.
Itching of right internal ear, worse than in left.
Loud ringing and buzzing in ears.
Small balls of wax drop out of the right ear almost every day.
Both ears suddenly feel stopped up, and internally sore to the touch.

### Nose.
Irritation of nasal passages, with sneezing.
Discharge of water from left nostril, with smarting of fauces.
Sore place on nose quite painful, but no redness nor swelling.
Discharge of bright red blood from left nostril, followed by one dark clot, then spitting of blood.
Both sides of nose sore and swollen; inside of nostrils sore.
Constant bad smell in nose, as from bilious fever or bilious dysentery.
Dryness of nose, with bad smell.
Any offensive smell remains a long time in the nose.
Nose inclined to be stopped up.

### Face.
° Little pimples with black heads disappear during the proving.
Sharp pain in left cheek or lower portion of temporal region.
Drawing pain at angle of jaw, left side.
Hard aching pain in left side of face, extending to the neck.
Neuralgic pain in the temples.

### Mouth and Jaws.
Sweetish taste in the mouth.
Mouth bitter and sticky in the morning.
Tongue dry and stiff in the morning, worse on the sides.
Mouth dry and sore in the morning.
Tongue coated in the morning.
Tongue coated heavily brown, and sore on sides.
Tip of tongue sore when eating.
Tongue sore on sides near back molar teeth, making talking difficult.
Pain in front teeth, and burning of the mouth and fauces.

Gums on inside of front upper teeth swollen.

Soreness of gums extending to the roof of the mouth.

Corners of mouth sore; sore pain at angle of jaw, left side.

Saliva runs out of his mouth when asleep.

Pain in upper front teeth; pain in lower front teeth.

Spasmodic closing of the jaws, biting the tongue, when neither eating or talking.

Mouth dry, but no thirst.

Tongue feels as if it was burnt on the sides.

Sharp aching pain in right upper molar tooth (which had been filled for years), as if he touched a bare nerve.

### Throat.

Irritation, roughness, burning and smarting of fauces.

Posterior fauces smart and burn, and feel as if the skin was off.

Burning of left tonsil and left side of throat.

Itching and pulling pain in left tonsil.

Stinging in right tonsil; both tonsils slightly congested.

Throat sore with hoarseness; throat seems sore, but is not.

Pain on back and right side of throat, causing a choking sensation.

Pain in both parotid glands, extending to the throat.

Irritation of left side of throat, extending to ear and larynx.

Irritation of larynx, with inclination to cough.

Constant desire to swallow, but it causes nausea.

Hard, aching pain in left parotid gland.

Difficult swallowing.

Constriction of glottis, as if he were choking, or something was tied around the throat.

Dryness of the fauces, with frequent inclination to swallow

### Taste and Appetite.

Bitter, sweet, bloody, flat, clammy taste, with disgust for food.

### Stomach.

Uneasy feeling at stomach.

Sharp pain in stomach, relieved by eating.

* Sharp pain in epigastrium, extending to left hypochondrium, lasting one hour.

Hard pain and soreness at epigastrium.

Very sharp pain in epigastrium, causing me to bend over.

Sharp pain in epigastrium, relieved by standing erect, aggravated by stooping.'

\* Sharp, cramping **pain at pit** of stomach, followed by raising, belching, and **gulping** enormous quantities of tasteless wind for fifteen minutes, then hiccough, and discharge of flatulence from the bowels; hiccough, with simultaneous, involuntary discharge of flatulence from the bowels, with shuddering, after a light supper.

° Constant, dull, weary pain in cardiac region of the stomach, extending to left side and dorsal region.

Sharp, cutting pain in stomach, extending to umbilicus.

Bad, distressed feeling in stomach all day, at times so sharp he had to walk around the room to get his breath.

During the day very often a dreadful, cutting, cramping, sinking sensation at epigastrium and upper portion of bowels, relieved by standing erect or by pressure.

Sharp, cramping pain across the epigastrium, preventing motion.

Sharp pain in left hypochondrium, and in the liver.

Soreness and pain at epigastrium.

Aching pain at epigastrium and left hypochondrium.

Hard, sharp pain in region of gall bladder; aching **pain at** left hypochondrium, and faint feeling at stomach.

Belching of large quantities of wind, relieving the **distress at** stomach for a minute.

Sour stomach, belching of sour water, and belching sour wind, with shuddering.

Distress at stomach, **had to unfasten** his clothes, which were quite loose.

Could taste food ten **hours after eating**, with nausea.

\* Distressing pain at **epigastrium**, relieved by raising sour, bitter wind, with **shuddering**.

Belching large quantities of wind, with a sensation as if both temples were in a vise.

Belching of wind and bitter mouth; worse on sides and back part of tongue.

Inclined to raise wind, but cannot.

Dull pain in stomach and right hypochondrium.

Heavy feeling at stomach, as of undigested food.

Stomach feels faint and distressed after eating a little

Stomach burns and smarts and is sore, after eating.

Belching of wind and bad taste in the mouth.

Belching of wind, with pain in left knee.

Trembling, with faint feeling at stomach.

Belching of wind slightly sour, accompanied with shuddering.

Distress and faint feeling at epigastrium, partially relieved by raising wind.

Aching pain in left hypochondrium.

Sensation as of a stone in the stomach; twisting pain in stomach.

Vomiting (from very large doses).

° Dull, heavy, wearing pain in *stomach*, worse after eating, relieved by copious eructation of air.

Severe, cutting, tearing pains in region of stomach and gall bladder, sometimes spasmodic.

Burning distress in stomach, with sharp pricking pains in it, and faintness.

° Stomach painful on pressure, with faintness.

° Pyrosis in pregnant women.

° Gastralgia; cramps in the stomach.

### Abdomen.

Dull pain in region of *liver*, aggravated by inhalation, relieved by exhalation.

Heavy, distressed feeling in region of *gall bladder* when lying on the right side.

Pain in bowels, as if a diarrhœa would come on.

Griping, and sharp pain in umbilical region.

Griping pain in hypogastric region, as if a diarrhœa would come on, relieved by passing flatulence.

Twisting sensation in region of liver; also squeezing pain.

Sharp pain in liver, extending to nipple.

Wringing, twisting pain at hypogastrium.

Frequent, cutting, cramping in epigastrium, extending to the umbilicus, with a faint, distressing sensation, as if a diarrhœa would come on.

Bowels feel sore on stooping.

Dreadfully troubled with **incarcerated** flatulence.

Distress in bowels, with **raising bitter** wind.

Immediately after lying **down a hard** pain in left hypochondrium, aggravated by **lying on the** right side, not changed by lying on the left.

Dull pain in left hypochondrium when lying on left side.

Dull pain in liver when lying on right side.

Digging pain in left hypochondrium.

Pain in left inguinal region and inguinal glands in the evening; left inguinal glands swollen and painful.

Aching pain in left hypochondrium, with a faint feeling at stomach, with chills in the back.

Constant dull pain in epigastric and umbilical region, with frequent colic-like pains of a cutting, tearing character.

Sharp, cutting pains around the umbilicus, aggravated by walking.

Severe cutting colic pains awaking him at night.

Uneasy feeling in umbilical region with eructations.

Rumbling in the bowels, with bloating and soreness on pressure.

Abdominal pains which intermit, aggravated by lying down.

* Spasmodic, very sharp pains in umbilical and right iliac regions, not modified by pressure, although pressure caused a rumbling.

Severe, griping abdominal pain, followed by diarrhœa.

Continued pain in abdomen, as if the point of a finger was placed upon the naval and pressed upward and backward, followed by soreness on pressure.

Severe spasmodic pains in abdomen, preceded by fullness in the head, and attended by burning sensation in abdomen in the intermission of the pains.

* Intense, cutting, twisting, agonizing pains in the abdomen, commencing in the umbilical region, radiating all over the abdomen, relieved or not by pressure, attended with distension, soreness and sensitiveness of the abdomen; vomiting, cramps, etc.

° *Bilious colic; flatulent colic; spasmodic colic.*

* Spasmodic pains in the abdomen, with severe tenesmus in dysentery.
* Violent, cutting, lancinating pain in the bowels, eliciting shrieks.
* Intense agonizing pains, day and night, occurring in paroxysms.
* Constant pains, worse in paroxysms, **of a violent** *twisting* character, with constipation, thirst, and **sensitiveness** of the right side of the abdomen.
* The pains are steady and *twisting*, aggravated in lying down, and in the morning; pressure does not usually relieve.
° Severe cramping pains beginning just below the umbilicus, extending into the back, thence flying to the fingers and toes, where the pain was intense (in a pregnant woman).
° A crampy, spasmodic pain, commencing near the crest of the ilium (right side) extending into the lumbar region, and hypogastrium; gradually increasing for days; ending in an attack of vomiting or headache; aggravated by physical or mental labor, and by lying on the affected side; relieved by lying on the back and left side; always leaving suddenly.
° Hyperæsthesia of the abdominal nerves; **neuralgia of the** bowels.
° Flatulent colic, occuring every night.

**Stool.**

Dark, costive stool.
Diarrhœa, with white slimy stools; **light colored**, jelly-like stools.
* Loose stools, with much straining.
* Painful diarrhœa, with much straining; **diarrhœa early in the** morning, driving one out of bed in a hurry.
Discharge of large quantity of very offensive flatulence.
Very offensive stools; flatulence has copper odor.
Sharp darting, hard aching, and pinching pain in **rectum.**
Occasional pulling, twisting pain in rectum.
Itching of rectum and moisture around the anus.
During the morning several stools; each one has **more strain-**ing than the preceding one, and is more slimy.

Discharge of flatulence, with great desire for stool.

Great desire for stool, driving him out of bed early in the morning.

Small, light colored stools, with much straining, and pain in the bowels; desire for stool, with a faint burning pain in rectum.

Stools passed with much force, followed by straining.

Frequent stools, each one more slimy and more straining, with less pain before and more pain after stool.

Stools like the white of an egg, but lumpy, with unavoidable straining and burning in rectum, and a sensation as if the fæces were hot.

During the stool, faintness; came near complete syncope.

Hurried, almost irresistible desire for stool while eating.

Sudden, great desire for stool at 8 P. M., two evenings in succession, with small stools and much flatulence.

Involuntary, unconscious discharge of slimy mucus from the anus.

Darting pain from old, hæmorrhoidal tumor to the liver.

Old hæmorrhoidal tumor quite sore.

° Hæmorrhoidal tumor of nearly four years' standing entirely disappeared during the proving, and has not returned.

Hæmorrhoidal tumor larger, and more soreness on moving than for a long time.

Black, hard, dry, lumpy stool, last part of it soft, white and mushy.

Dark, black stool, followed by prolapsus of the anus.

Four hæmorrhoidal tumors protrude, as large as cherries; three are of the color of the normal mucous membrane, the other is of a livid dark blue color.

Obstinate constipation, followed by bilious diarrhœa.

Very profuse, deep yellow, thin stools, followed by a very weak, faint feeling, and without relieving the pain in the bowels; this continued for two days, in the morning, and was followed by constipation; the hæmorrhoidal tumors were prolapsed all the time, with pain and distress.

° *Cholera morbus; cholera infantum; dysentery; diarrhœa.*

• **All the abnormal alvine discharges are attended by the c**haracteristic *twisting, writhing,* severe pain around and extending from the region of the umbilicus.

° Very severe tenesmus, with the colic and dysentery.

### Urinary Organs.

No morbid sensations observed by any prover.

No change in the quality or quantity of the urine.

° Spasmodic stricture of the urethra, with cutting, severe, remittent colic pains around the umbilicus.

### Hepatic Region.

Sharp, cutting pains in the hepatic region; also in the region of the gall bladder.

Dull, heavy, aching pains in the right lobe of the liver.

Stools first yellow (bilious), afterwards too light colored.

° Supposed to be useful in neuralgia and spasmodic affections of the liver and gall ducts; said to facilitate the passage of gall stones, and relieve the pain.

### Genitals (Male.)

Strong smelling perspiration of the genitals.

Constant excitement of the genital organs, with frequent erections day and night.

Erections all night, with amorous dreams.

Emissions of semen during sleep.

Genitals cold, relaxed, and almost insensible; no erections for many days.

Sexual desire greatly diminished, or entirely absent.

Pain in the lumbar and both inguinal regions, extending to the testicles.

In afternoon, pain in left inguinal region, extending to the testicles and penis.

Nocturnal emissions, with erections and amorous dreams. (*Cushing:* Several cases cured with the 2nd and 7th dilutions.)

° Nocturnal emissions, without erections, sensation, or dreams, but with great weakness of the knees, depression of spirits. (Several cases cured by Dr. Pease with the 2nd decimal trituration of Dioscorein.)

° *Nocturnal Emissions Treated by Dr. Cushing.*—Mr. L., aged 35, above medium size, dark eyes, black hair and beard, married, father of three children. When twenty years of age, commenced having nocturnal emissions of semen. Was troubled badly; was under treatment some two or three years, with no relief. By advice of physicians was married, but no change of symptoms. Now, after 15 years, is as follows: During 15 years, thinks he has been once three weeks without an emission. A very few times has been two weeks, usually not over four days at the longest, considerable of the time every other night, at times every night for some time. At times he feels so badly in the morning that he sits up nearly all night to avoid it. Rich or spare diet, excessive labor or rest, make no difference. Has had all kinds of treatment, the last from a traveling physician, to whom he paid fifty dollars a few months since to have the urethra cauterized the whole length, but it gave him no relief. He feels dull and bad; backbone and knees weak.

September 12.—Gave *Dioscorea* 20th decimal, dose every night.

September 19.—Has had no emissions; *Dioscorea* 20th every other night.

October 3.—Has had two emissions; *Dioscorea* 15th every night.

October 10.—No emissions; *Dioscorea* 15th every night.

October 22.—No emissions; *Dioscorea* 20th every other night.

November 5.—Has had two emissions; *Dioscorea* 20th every night.

November 18.—No emissions; *Dioscorea* 20th every third night.

December 5.—No emissions; *Dioscorea* 20th, to take an occasional dose at night. He feels well; back is not lame, and considered cured.

*Female.*—Dysmenorrhœa; uterine colic; after pains; false pains during pregnancy.

### Chest.

Very sharp pain in right lung at the right of the nipple, arresting breathing; relieved by pressure.

Sharp pain in lower portion of right lung, commencing in back side and darting through to the front.

Aching pain in right lung; sharp pain in left lung at the side of the nipple.

Sharp cutting pain in region of heart, arresting breathing and motion.

Pain through from back to front of both lungs.

Very sharp, cutting 'pain from left axilla to nipple, and down on side and deep into the lung.

Sharp pain in region of right nipple, with difficult respiration.

Dull pain through right scapula and lung.

Sharp pain in region of heart; had to stop when walking on the street.

Sudden, sharp, cramping pain in right lung just below the nipple, arresting motion and breathing for a few seconds.

Sharp pricking pain and distress in region of heart.

Burning pain behind top of sternum.

Violent attack of cough from tickling low down in throat; can with difficulty get his breath, with frothy expectoration, seeming to come from the head.

Profuse frothy expectoration seeming to come from posterior fauces.

° Cough, with pain at epigastrium; dull pain in both temples, brownish yellow tongue, and weak knees. (*Cushing.*)

° Pains through the sides of the chest, with headache in the temples. (*Cushing.*)

### Back and Neck.

Chills on back, commencing over left scapula.

Dull pain in back of neck, extending to head and shoulders.

Violent itching over right scapula every evening, with no eruption.

Very sharp, sudden pain in back, left side, at tenth rib.

Dull, lame pain in lumbar region, extending to legs.

Sharp pain in lumbar region, extending to the testicles.

Sharp pain in sacral region, hindering walking or movement.

Sharp, deep pain in lower portion of left scapula, followed by sharp pain through centre of right lung.

Sharp pain in lumbar region that pulled him over back and sidewise, so sharp that it made him groan out loud.

Itching over both hips, extending down the legs, aggravated by getting cold.

Back in region of liver so lame it is almost impossible to turn in bed; relieved by motion.

Soreness of sacral region.

* Hyperæsthesia of the spinal cord (?). (*Paine*.)

* Reflex irritation of the spinal cord. (*Hale*.)

Dull pain on top of left shoulder, extending to neck and head.

### Superior Extremities.

Numbness of left hand and forearm, as if asleep; worse at little finger.

Hard, aching pain in lower third of left forearm, extending to little finger.

Dull, grinding pain in middle of left forearm; quite severe, which returned at intervals during the evening.

Arms and hands numb.

Frequent, sharp, jerking pains in left shoulder.

Frequent, sharp pains in right shoulder.

Hard, pulling pain all day on top of left shoulder, extending to neck and head.

Pain in left lung, extending to back and down inside of left arm.

Pain and soreness in right axilla.

Pain and soreness in left axilla, extending down the arm, aggravated by walking.

Pain in both shoulders; left elbow lame and stiff.

Grinding pain in elbow joints.

Aching pain in elbow, alternating with pain in knees, same kind.

Left thumb, between first and second joints, quite painful for two days, but no swelling, soreness, nor redness.

Pain in right forearm, and hard pain in right wrist.

Frequent, severe, but not very sharp pains between the third and fourth metacarpal bones of left hand.

Hard, aching pain in left forefinger and right hand.

Severe itching of palm of right hand.

Nails on toes and fingers very brittle.

° Severe pains, with cramp in the flexor tendons of the fingers and toes in a pregnant woman, alternating with false labor pains. (*Hale.*)

### Inferior Extremities.

Dull, drawing pain from hip to knee in right leg.

Pain in back side of right leg as if gluteal muscles were too short.

Cramping pain in back side of legs; dull pain whole length of right leg on back side, worse at buttock and heel.

Sharp pain in right hip joint, also dull pain.

A sharp pain went from left hip to head like an electric shock while lying down.

Dull pain in both hips.

Pain in front side of right hip down to the **knee**

Pain in left thigh.

Sudden, stinging itching over right hip.

Dull, cramping pain in back side of both **legs, worse above** the knees.

Dull, tearing pain in right hip, hindering walking.

Left leg feels numb and heavy, and goes to sleep easily.

Right hip lame, as if the gluteal muscles were too short, aggravated by walking.

Cramping pain all day in back side of right thigh, as if the muscles were too short.

Dull pain in right groin, extending down inside of leg, **caus-**ing lameness.

Pain in left popliteal space, hindering walking.

Sharp pain in right popliteal space.

Pain in left popliteal space, then right knee, then right popliteal space.

Both knees very weak, lame and painful, aggravated by walk-ing; continued walking cured it.

Pain in right knee at head of tibia, relieved by motion.

Pain in right knee and ankle; pain in right leg, back side, near the knee.

Hard pain at head of right tibia, extending into the knee joint.

Pain in left knee, as if out of joint, and could not be moved, but relieved by motions.

Sharp, tearing pain in left knee, which is weak and painful.

Right knee very lame and stiff; knees weak and trembling.

Right tibia seemed sore, with pain extending to left side of knee at edge of patella, producing lameness; then the pain moved to lower portion of fibula, same leg.

Both knees lame, as if they could not be moved.

Pain alternates from one knee to the other; right leg from knee to foot feels weak.

Cramping and grinding pain in both knees.

Right tibia quite sore and painful when walking, but not to the touch; is better by contact.

Pain in bones of legs, and is chilly.

When walking, severe cramping pain at head of left fibula, making walking painful.

Dull pain in both sides of right leg below the knee.

Sharp pain in left tibia, near the ankle, that made him limp; then pain at right tibia; then right hand.

Frequent hard, dull pain in left tendo achilles.

Violent itching on front side of left ankle when walking.

Violent itching of right ankle, extending above the joint, while walking.

Sharp pain in right tendo achilles.

Hard pain at middle of right tibia.

Hard, sharp pain in left ankle.

Feet and legs to knees feel numb and strange.

Sharp pain in left tendo achilles that makes him hold his breath.

Sensation as of a bee sting on outside of left ankle.

Burning, aching pain in right little toe.

Very sharp, severe pain in right little toe, relieved by pressure

Corns on second toe of each foot very painful and sore.

Jumping, darting pain in old corns on second toe of each foot; they become very painful and sore.

Sharp pain underneath right great toe, as if a pin were driven in.

Sharp pain in bottom of feet and toes.

Constant dull pain in ankles, feet and toes.

Toes are very stiff, especially in the morning.

18

° Great weakness of the knees (in several diseases). (*Cushing.*)
° Pain and soreness in fourth toe of right foot. (*Ib.*)

### Sleep.

Falls asleep late at night; restless, cannot sleep.
Went to sleep in his room in the afternoon, very uncommon; awoke with bitter mouth and pain in bowels.
Roused suddenly from sleep with slow but hard beating of the heart.
Sleep full of lascivious dreams, with emissions of semen.
Roused from sleep early in the morning by great desire for stool.

### Fever.

Feels as if he had a cold; chilly, bones and back ache.
Chilly, yet perspires easily.
Several severe chills during the evening.
Chilly, then perspiration, no fever, no thirst.
Pain in bones of legs, and is chilly.

### Characteristics.

Pains all relieved by motion; symptoms worse about eight A. M. and ten P. M.; pain in stomach and bowels, relieved by standing erect; chilly in a warm room; frequent sharp pains darting from one part of the body to another; sudden stinging in various parts of the body.

### General Symptoms.

Faintness; came near syncope.
Itching of various parts of the body and limbs.
Sudden stinging in various parts like a bee sting.
Violent itching over right scapula (every evening), and over various parts of the body, without eruption.
Headache, worse in temples.
Cramping, cutting pains in stomach and bowels.
Sharp darting pains in lungs, worse in region of heart.
Restless sleep, with bitter, sticky mouth in the morning.
Back lame, with soreness in inguinal regions, and pain in hips; knees weak, lame and painful.
Sexual desire increased (*p.*), or nearly all gone. (*s.*)

### Special Indications.

Pain in either temple, worse in right; also in back or front of head; one or both eyes sore.

Mouth dry, bitter or sore, worse in the morning.

Sharp pain in either lung, worse in region of the nipple, arresting motion or breathing.

Pain in the stomach, either sharp, dull, cramping or twisting, worse by stooping, relieved by standing erect.

Severe pain in either hypochondrium, either sharp, dull, cramping or twisting.

Bowels sore and distressed; sharp, cutting, cramping pain in bowels.

Back in dorsal or lumbar region lame; aggravated by stooping.

Sexual desire increased, or greatly diminished.

Genitals cold and relaxed.

Emissions of semen during sleep, or no erections for many days.

Knees quite lame, weak or painful.

Cramping pain in legs, whole length.

Rheumatic symptoms, worse at night and early in the morning.

At first the pains are aggravated by motion, afterwards motion relieves.

Morning diarrhœa.

---

# DORYPHORA DECEM-LINEATA.

## (*Colorado Potato Bug.*)

DESCRIPTION.—This insect belongs to the same family as the squash bug, the black potato bug, and the Cantharides—all possess the power of blistering the skin if bruised upon it. The Colorado potato bug has its original home in the Rocky Mountains, where it fed on a species of Solanum indigenous to that locality. It got a taste of the S. tuberosum, the common potato, and rapidly traveled east, until it has reached the Atlantic.

OFFICINAL PREPARATIONS.—Tincture or trituration of the whole bug.

ANALOGUES.—*Agaricus, Apis, Belladonna, Æthusa, Crotalus, Lachesis, Stramonium.*

### Mental.

Delirium, with red, bloated face, protruded eyes, and pulse one hundred and twenty-four.

Irritable temper.

Delirious; talking and muttering about business matters.

### Head.

Congestion of blood to the head.

Meningitis. (?)

Congested brain (post mortem).

### Face and Eyes.

Face bloated, giving the prover the appearance of a confirmed drunkard.

Bloated face, mottled, with red, staring eyes, and high fever, with delirium, vomiting and stupor.

Inflammation of the eyes.

Eyes red, congested, and protruded.

Pupils dilated.

Sight much impaired; a sensation of dimness and blackness before the eyes.

Erysipelas of the head and face.

### Mouth, Throat and Œsophagus.

Burning in the throat down the œsophagus, with pain in the stomach.

Dark brown coating on the tongue.

### Gastric Symptoms.

Vomiting of dark, grumous and acrid matters.

*Vomiting* attending the stupor and delirium.

Vomiting of dirty brown fluid, and diarrhœa.

Pain in the stomach.

No appetite, but great thirst; craving for sour things.

### Abdomen and Stool.

Pain in the bowels, chiefly in hypogastric region.

Discharges of bloody and slimy matters, with intense pain in the *rectum*.

Loud rumbling in abdomen, with stupor.

Violent pain in bowels, in right side, passing downward to the rectum.

Continued bloody, slimy diarrhœa.

The pain in bowels increased by eating or drinking.

° Dysentery, with intense pain in rectum.

### Urinary Organs.

*Retention* of urine from morning till night.

Difficult urination.

Voided a large quantity of urine of a dark red color, dirty sediment, and much pain.

\* *Dysuria*, with burning, stinging pain.
° Gleet and gonorrhœa.

### Extremities.

Swelling of the whole arm, very painful; the abraded spot on the wrist developed into a deep ulcer, angry, red, with sticking, stinging pains through the arms; the ulcer assumed a malignant character, eating until it exposed the bones of the wrist (from the local effects, through an abraded surface).

Great trembling in the extremities.

Could not guide his pen when endeavoring to write.

Trembling in *right* arm and leg as if from a galvanic (induced) current.

Swelling of the feet, with burning and stinging, and sensation as if full of pins.

Icy coldness of the hands and feet.

### Generalities.

*Great weariness*, increased by *talking*.

Fatigued by the slightest exercise.

Fainting sensation when walking.

Sensation as if he would fall at every step, with dimness of sight.

*Enormous swelling of the whole body*, with the mental and cerebral symptoms above named.

The general swelling of the whole body was elastic, would not "pit."

Pain all over the body, especially in the region of the *spleen*.

Nervous restlessness; twitching and spasms.

Great, general prostration, ending in collapse.

### Fever.

Violent fever, with cerebral congestion, vomiting, and delirium; pulse 120 to 140.

Fever; skin alternately cold and clammy then hot and burning.

Violent fever from 8 A. M. to 2 P. M.

Fever of typhoid character.

Pulse very weak, with coldness and collapse.

### Sleep.

Great sleeplessness till 12 at night, then restless sleep, with terrifying dreams.

Comatose slumber; while sleeping has wild dreams, and screams as if in great distress.

Stupor, with muttering and loud rumbling in the bowels.

All the symptoms worse after *smoking.*

The blood will not coagulate; the blood globules are disorganized as after serpent poisoning.

---

## EPIGÆA REPENS.
### (*Trailing Arbutus.*)

DESCRIPTION.—This plant belongs to the Heath family. It is common to New England. A prostrate or trailing plant, bristly with rusty hairs, with evergreen and reticulate, rounded and heart-shaped alternate leaves, on slender petioles, with rose-colored flowers, in small axillary clusters. It grows in sandy woods, sometimes in rocky soil, especially in the shade of pines. The flowers appear in early spring, even under light snow, and exhale a rich, spicy fragrance.

OFFICINAL PREPARATIONS.—Tincture of the root and leaves.

ANALOGUES.—*Uva Ursi, Eupatorium purp.,* etc.

No provings.

Burning in neck of bladder when urinating.

Tenesmus of the bladder; after urinating.

Increased flow of pale, limpid urine.

° Urine with bloody sediment.

° Urine containing mucus and pus.

* Discharge of small brown particles resembling **fine sand.**

° *Dysuria,* from various causes.

---

## ERECHTHITES HIERACIFOLIUS.
### (*Fire Weed.*)

DESCRIPTION.—This common plant is found in moist woods, and is very common in recent clearings, where the ground has been burned over—whence its popular name. It grows from one to five feet high, has a hairy, grooved stem; a coarse looking annual, of rank smell; alternate simple leaves, lanceolate, acute, cut, toothed, sessile; flowers *white,* in a large head. It was once called a senecio. It blooms from July to September.

OFFICINAL PREPARATIONS.—Tincture of the plant; dilutions. The *oil,* and dilutions from it.

ANALOGUES.—*Asarum, Cubeba, Copaiva, Erigeron, Millefolium, Sabina, Trillium, Terebinthina.*

### Head.

Vertigo, everything goes up, down and sidewise.

Dull frontal headache.

Headache, with throbbing in the temporal arteries, with flashes of heat running across the back from one shoulder to the other; the sensation of heat suddenly gives way to cold-ness, which darts across the face and back in a similar manner, accompanied with nausea.

### Nose.

* Epistaxis of bright red blood.

### Mouth.

* Bleeding from the gums and looseness of the teeth.

### Stomach.

Eructations, with burning in the stomach, cramps in the bowels.

Uneasiness of the stomach as if nausea was about to set in.

Vomiting, with burning in stomach, afterwards empty retching.

Feeling in the stomach as if it would be dissolved; after drinking cold water.

Nausea, with giddiness and headache.

Extravagant appetite.

Vomiting of bloody mucus; ° even pure blood.

° Eructations and heartburn after eating warm bread or coffee.

### Abdomen and Stool.

Cramps in the region of umbilicus, recurring every 15 minutes.

Constipation, followed by copious diarrhœa.

Copious diarrhœa of yellow fœcal matter, of a mushy consist-ence, preceded by griping in the morning, followed by two or three days' constipation.

° Hæmorrhage from the bowels (in typhus).

° Excessive hæmorrhage from hemorrhoidal veins.

° Dysenteric discharges of almost pure blood.

Small mucous stools, streaked with blood, with tenesmus.

### Generative Organs.

(*Female.*) * Profuse menorrhagia and metrorrhagia of bright red blood.

° Premature and profuse menses.

(*Male.*) Stimulation of the genital organs, with erection and dreams of nudity and shame.

Erection, with dreams and emissions toward morning.

\* Slight burning pains in meatus urinarius, with profuse urination.

\* Swelling of the right testicle, with painful, continuous aching, tenderness to the touch.

### Urinary Organs.

\* Urine very scanty, painful, scalding and bloody; blood oozed from the urethra after urinating.

\* Urine dark, scanty, and mixed with blood.

\* Hemorrhage from the kidneys and bladder.

Urine contained a large amount of mucus floating about in minute particles.

Specific gravity 10.24; acid reaction; 40 ounces per day.

The urine, after standing, has a milky appearance.

Urine decreased from 42 ounces to 33 ounces.

### Bronchia.

Cough, with muco-purulent expectoration (almost bloody).

### Back and Extremities.

Aching in the small of the back.

Pains in the lower extremities.

### Generalities.

\* Active arterial hæmorrhages, with general excitement of the circulation.

---

# ERIGERON CANADENSE.

### (*Flea Bane.*)

BOTANICAL DESCRIPTION.—*Stem* erect, wand-like, five inches to five feet high, branching, hairy and furrowed. *Leaves* very narrow, with rough edges; those from the root cut-lobed. *Flowers* white, very numerous, small, of mean appearance, irregularly racemous upon the branches, and constituting a large oblong panicle. The *disk* of the flowers *yellow*. This is an annual plant, common all over the world, seldom seen in woods or on mountains, but grows in fields, commons, dry meadows and glades in great profusion, and is deemed by farmers one of the most troublesome weeds. It flowers in June to October. [This genus comprises eight species, three of which are considered to possess similar medicinal qualities, namely: E. canadense, E. philadelphicum, E. annuum. It is quite probable that the plant as found in the shops, and most of the oil in market, is prepared from the three, and perhaps other kinds, mixed indiscriminately. The E. canadense is the largest species, but has fewer rays (forty to fifty), and are white. The two other species are from two to four feet high, rays 100 to 200, and reddish-purple or flesh colored. The E. annuum is a biennial, and the E. philadelphicum a perennial herb.]

MEDICAL HISTORY.—The plant has been used since anterior to the settlement of this country. It is still called by its aboriginal name of "Cocosh." The Indians used it as a vulnerary, much as Arnica is used in homœopathic practice. It has a host of common names. Fleabane is the true English name. Colt's-tail, Mare's-tail, Daisy, Frost-weed, Field-weed, Skevish, etc., are names in common use with the country people, and apply to all the species of the plant. These plants have a peculiar smell, most unfolded by rubbing them, and is not disagreeable. Their taste is astringent, acrimonious, and bitter. The two species having the strongest taste and odor are the E. philadelphicum and E. annuum.

On analysis they are found to contain Tannin, Extractive, Gallic-acid, Amarin, and an Essential Oil. The oil is very peculiar, as fluid as water, of a pale yellow color, a peculiar smell, somewhat like lemon, but stronger, and a very acrid taste. Medical authors do not agree as to which plant shall be decreed officinal. Rafinesque mentions the E. philadelphicum, and botanic writers follow him. Wood and Stille name the E. canadense. Homœopathists settled upon the latter more by accident, perhaps, as that species was first mentioned.

OFFICINAL PREPARATIONS.—Tincture of the plant; triturations or dilutions from the oil.

ANALOGUES.—*Cantharis, Cubebs, Copaiva, Balsamum Peruvianum, Erechthites, Terebinthina, Sabina.*

### Mental Sphere.

Lowness of spirits, with a feeling of great languor.

### Head.

Dull frontal headache on awaking in the morning.

Dull headache, with ringing in the right ear.

Headache, with pain in forehead and right eye; *with* pain in the large joints.

### Eyes.

Smarting of the eyes all day.

Redness, swelling, inflammation, with profuse muco-purulent discharges from the eyes.

° Ecchymoses upon the eyeballs or around the eye, from a blow.

### Nose.

Increased secretion of mucus in the nostrils all the forenoon.

° Epistaxis of bright red blood.

### Mouth.

° Bleeding from the gums; profuse bleeding from the cavity of a tooth.

### Throat.

Dryness of the pharynx; roughness, with a sensation as if
  something had lodged in the upper part of the œsophagus.
Sore throat all night, with frequent inclination to swallow.
° Inflammation and ulceration of the throat.
° Tonsillitis (applied externally) or used as a gargle.

### Stomach.

Nausea, with frequent eructations.
Sharp cutting pains in the region of the stomach every few
  minutes.
Violent retching and vomiting, with burning sensation of long
  duration in the stomach.
° Hæmatemesis, from ulceration, and rupture of blood-vessels

### Abdomen.

Rheumatic (?) pains in the abdomen.
Sharp pains in the umbilicus.
Frequent, dull pains in the bowels.
Sudden, severe pains in the hypogastrium, followed by mushy
  stool.
° Flatulent colic.
° Tympanitis in typhoid fever or dysentery.

### Stool.

Hard, lumpy stool; mushy stools.
Sudden pains in the hypogastrium, followed by papescent
  stools.
Natural stool, followed by severe neuralgic pain in the anus,
  with tenesmus.
Catharsis, with burning sensation throughout the alimentary
  canal.
Thin papescent stool, with burning in the bowels and rectum.
Undigested stools.
Inflammation of the mucous coats of the colon and rectum.
° Diarrhœa and dysentery, bloody and mucus.
° Scybala, with dysentery.
° Hemorrhage from the bowels or from hæmorrhoids.

### Liver.

Dull pairs in both hypochondriæ.
Aching distress in the hypochondriæ.

## Urinary Organs.

Sharp, stinging pains in the region of the left kidney.

Pain in right lumbar region, passing down to the right testicle.

Urine dark color, afterwards pale, double quantity.

Inclination to urinate about every hour, with aching distress in bladder.

° *Dysuria* in teething children; frequent desire and crying when urinating; urine very profuse and of very strong odor; the external parts much inflamed and swollen. (*Dr. Ring.*)

° Vesical irritation from catarrh of the bladder.

Complete suppression of the urine, with pain in the region of the kidneys (primary).

Urging to urinate, with emissions of only a few burning drops at a time (primary).

Copious discharges of pale urine (secondary).

## Generative Organs.

*Female.*—° *Uterine hemorrhage*, with violent irritation of the rectum and bladder. (*Male.*)

° Hemorrhage from the uterus and bladder.

° Abortion, with profuse hemorrhage, diarrhœa and dysuria.

Premature and profuse menses. (*primary.*)

Scanty menses. (*secondary.*)

° Post-partem hemorrhage.

° Dysmenorrhœa, with menorrhagia.

° Profuse lochial discharges.

° Menorrhagia, with spasmodic pains.

° Chronic uterine leucorrhœa.

*Male.*—° Gonorrhœa and gleet.

## Bronchia, Lungs, etc.

Chronic bronchial affections.

° Incipient stages of phthisis, with bloody expectoration.

## Back.

Severe, drawing pains in the right lumbar region.

Dull, aching distress in the whole dorsal region.

## Superior Extremities.

Rheumatic pains in the right thumb all the evening.

Great aching distress in the elbows and wrists during rainy weather.

### Lower Extremities.

Severe, drawing pains in the left ankle joint, aggravated by walking.

Dull pains in the knees.

### Generalities.

Symptoms all aggravated during rainy weather.

The *lower dorsal* region is the location of greatest suffering.

### Skin.

Slightly elevated, sharply defined vesicles on the skin.

---

# EUCALYPTUS GLOBULUS.
### (*Fever Tree—Australian Gum Tree.*)

The Eucalyptus globulus belongs to the natural order of Myrtaceæ, the same as the Clove (*Caryophyllus aromaticus*), the Cajeput (*Melaleuca minor*), and the Pimento (*Eugenia pimenta*).

There are over a hundred species in this genus, of which this is one of the noblest.

It often grows to a size simply gigantic, sometimes being two hundred feet high and fifteen feet in diameter.

The wood is very dense and hard.

The leaves are green, growing on a short stem, are quite thick and leathery, with a well marked nervule through the centre, shaped like a spear, and curved something like a scythe-blade.

They grow in two distinct forms from opposite sides of the stem or branch, and consequently two leaves cannot be superimposed, unless taken from the same side of the stalk.

It is a native of the Australian and Tasmanian forests, but is quite easily acclimated in nearly all parts of the temperate zone. There seems to be a remarkable freedom from malarious diseases in any localities where these trees are grown. I would suggest that their cultivation on some of the malarious districts of our country would not only be practical, but would do more toward preventing intermittents than all our skill in the use of remedies can accomplish.

The chemical analysis made by Cloez of the leaves shows a small quantity of resin and a large quantity of essential oil and tannin.

An essence called Eucalyptol has been obtained from these leaves; its chemical formula is $C_{20} H_{20} O_2$, being almost exactly of the same composition of Camphor—boils at between 170° and 175°—its density is 0.905.

No immediate crystalized substance has yet been found. Eucalyptol has a peculiar agreeable odor resembling camphor, lavender and walnut, and is fragrant.

The taste is aromatic, but bitter and somewhat acrid, and excites the salivary glands.

PHARMACEUTICAL.—The tincture is made by breaking dried leaves finely, and to one ounce add two ounces of distilled water and eight ounces of alcohol, allow it to stand seven days, filter and run up the first and second dilutions with dilute alcohol, above the second with alcohol.

OFFICINAL PREPARATIONS.—Tincture; dilutions.

ANALOGUES.—*Arsenicum, Baptisia, China, Cedron, Carbolic acid, Sodæ Sulphite, Cornus, Copaiva, Cubebæ.*

## Mind.

General mental excitement.

A desire to be constantly moving about.

A general mental exhilaration.

## Sensorium.

Sensation of intoxication (as from a room recently painted with turpentine, or full of the perfume of flowers).

Vertigo.

## Head.

\* Nervous headaches, and other pains of the head, which are not exactly periodic.

Congestive headache, in plethoric subjects, followed by *real fever.*

Dull, heavy, frontal headache, with *fullness* of the head.

Dull, heavy feeling of the head.

° Headache in anæmic persons—it relieves the pain and causes *sleep.*

## Eyes.

Hot, burning, smarting sensation (as from a cold.)

Lids feel heavy.

° Catarrhal and gonorrhœal ophthalmia.

## Face.

Flushed face, with congested appearance.

## Nose.

Stuffed up sensation in the nose.

Tightness across the bridge of the nose, as if epistaxis would set in.

Thin, watery coryza.

° Chronic catarrh of the nasal passages, even when purulent and fœtid (cured by inhalations of Eucalyptus.)

## Mouth and Throat.

⁛ Burning sensation, extending to pharynx and œsophagus, with *thirst.*

\* Excessive secretion of saliva.

Throat feels full; sore on swallowing.

Expectoration of a white, thick, frothy mucus.

Sensation as of phlegm in the throat all the time.

On examination of the throat I found it relaxed and **pale.**

### Stomach.

Strong-smelling eructations.

Eructations tasting of eucalyptus for hours after taking the drug.

Slow digestion; eructations and bloating.

Hot, burning sensation in the stomach.

Improves the appetite.

Sensation of having eaten or drank too much.

A strange sinking, faint sensation at stomach.

Tenderness and burning sensation in the region of the stomach and bowels, with great heat in the rectum, which was followed by tenesmus, with discharge of mucus and great prostration. Violent purgation and hæmorrhage from the bowels ensued.

Burning sensation in the epigastric and umbilical regions, together with tormenting thirst, faintness, vertigo, dimness of sight; a sense of fullness in the head, with dull frontal headache, a tightness across the bridge of the nose, as if profuse epistaxis would set in.

### Abdomen.

Feeling of weight in epigastrium.

Uncomfortable pressure and fullness in the umbilical region.

Slight aching pains in upper part of bowels, then extending all through the bowels.

Sensation in bowels as if he would have a diarrhœa.

### Spleen.

(Dr. Master experimented on animals, and found that it produced, like quinine, contraction of the spleen, which, under its use, becomes more resistant and hard, its surface granulated, and the whole organ diminished in size.)

### Stool.

\* **Dysentery,** with heat in the rectum, tenesmus, discharge of mucus, great prostration; hæmorrhage from the bowels.

Violent purgation, with hæmorrhage from the bowels.

Constipation of short duration.

* Thin, watery diarrhœa, preceded by sharp, aching pains in lower part of bowels.

(The prover, some weeks after getting this symptom, having the same kind of a diarrhœa, took Eucalyptus, and with the best of results.)

° Typhoid diarrhœa and dysentery.

° Chronic diarrhœa, mucous and bloody.

### Urine.

° Incontinence of urine.

° Diuresis, nocturnal and diurnal.

° Vesical catarrh.

° Suppressed urine.

A sensation as if the bladder had lost its expulsive force.

### Generative Organs.

° Ulcer around the orifice of the female urethra.

° Recent cases of syphilitic chancres.

° Gonorrhœa syphilitica.

° Leucorrhœa, of acrid, fœtid mucus.

° Spasmodic stricture of the urethra.

### Chest.

° Bronchitis, in old and feeble persons.

Respiratory movements quickened.

° *Cardiac asthma;* allays the terrible dyspnœa of this affection.

° Strong beating of the abdominal aorta synchronous with the beating of the heart.

° *Aneurisms involving pressure on the vagus and its branches* —No remedy is so efficacious in allaying pain, relieving dyspnœa, calming irritation, and producing sleep in patients suffering from the above conditions. (*Dr. McLean.*)

### Lower Extremities.

Dr. Pignedupritier, of the French Hospital, reports a case of arteritis of the leg, succeeded by gangrene, so high up as to prevent amputation. A large ulcer supervened, the odor from which was horrible. After trying all the disinfectants he knew of, he, as a last resort, applied a decoction of eucalyptus, and says that, without exaggeration, the bad odor was all gone in five minutes.

In both upper and lower extremities, pricking sensations were
first noticed and followed by painful aching in both arms
and legs, together with a sense of fullness in the veins,
and a stiff, weary sensation, as if too lazy to move.

### Skin.

° Ulcers from a varix, of a year's duration.

° Fistulous ulcers, discharging ichorous matter, of a fœtid odor.

° Suppurating wounds; prevents gangrene.

*Eruptions* on the skin, of a herpetic character; glandular en
largements; and foul, indolent ulcers.

A lad thirteen years of age, who appeared to be suffering from
rheumatic fever. The usual remedies were of no service.
On more closely examining the boy's condition, I found
many nodular swellings over the metacarpal and metatarsal joints. He could neither walk nor carry anything
without great pain. Noticing a similarity of the symptoms the Eucalyptus produced on himself, he accused
the patient with having eaten the leaves of the tree,
and on pressing him he found that he had eaten largely of
the gum, and had chewed many leaves. Dr. F. believes
that his symptoms were entirely due to the leaves and
product of the Eucalyptus.

### Generalities.

Rheumatic pains, jerking, tearing, stitching—worse at night—
followed by swellings in different parts of the body; one
below the nipple, a little to the right side; about the size
of a filbert, the seat of stitching and darting pains.

### Fever.

[Infusions, or water containing infusoria, cryptogamic organisms, and
bacteria, are purified by the addition of Eucalyptus.]

° *Remittent fevers; agues.*

° Tuberculous hectic fevers, with profuse sweats.

*Intermittent fever;* quotidian tertian and double tertian.

° *Intermittent fever when quinia fails.*

° *Quinine cachexias.*

° Typhoid fevers, etc.

"Malarious fevers do not exist in localities where this tree grows."

"Travelers who drink of the water in which this tree grows, or in
which the leaves have fallen, are not unpleasantly affected by it."

(*See Therapeutics, Vol. II.*)

# DIGITALINE.

*(The alkaloid of Digitalis.)*

DESCRIPTION. — Digitaline (not the spurious substance called by this name, manufactured by various firms throughout the country, which are generally inert, or less powerful than the dried leaves) is the *crystallized* active principle of Digitalis. It occurs in short and delicate needle-shaped crystals, and possesses an intense and persistent bitter taste; slightly soluble in water—soluble in 12 parts of cold and 6 of boiling alcohol of 90°, less soluble in absolute alcohol; nearly insoluble in ether, very soluble in chloroform.

*Amorphous Digitaline* is a whitish or yellowish powder, odorless, but of a very bitter taste, nearly insoluble in ether and water, readily soluble in alcohol. Crude Digitalis is said to contain 10 or 12 per cent. of crystallizable Digitaline, which is said to be somewhat more powerful than the Amorphous Digitaline.

OFFICIAL PREPARATIONS.—Triturations of either of the above substances (always on the centessimal scale), up to the 3d; afterwards, dilutions with strong alcohol.

ANALOGUES.—*Amygdala amara, Prunus, Cerasus, Hydrocyanic acid, Lycopus, Squilla, Collinsonia, Iberis, etc.*

*(See Therapeutics, Vol. II.)*

---

# EQUISETUM HYEMALE.

*(Scouring Rush.)*

DESCRIPTION.—This rush is sometimes called Horsetail. It is common to the northern and western parts of the United States, growing in wet grounds or river banks: maturing in June and July. The plant abounds in Silex, which it absorbs from the soil. The whole plant is medicinal.

OFFICIAL PREPARATIONS.—Tincture of the fresh plant; infusion.

ANALOGUES.—*Cannabis, Galium, Epigea, etc.*

*(No Provings.)*

° *Dysuria of women;* symptoms, extreme and frequent urging to urinate, with severe pain, especially *immediately after* the urine is voided. (*Dr. J. S. Marsden.*)

° Painful urination, with albuminous urine. (*Ib.*)

° Dysuria after confinement and during pregnancy. (*Ib.*)

[Dr. M. says it is one of the most reliable remedies he has tried, in such cases as the above. He uses it in infusion, pouring hot water on the stalks. A tablespoonful every two or three hours.]

Diuretic and astringent. (*King.*)

° An infusion has been found useful in dropsy, suppression

19

of urine, gravel, hæmaturia, and hepatic affections; also gonorrhœa and gleet.  (*Ib.*)

° The *ashes* of this rush are very valuable in dyspepsia, connected with obstinate acidity of the stomach.  (*Ib.*)

---

# ERGOTINE.

### (*An active principle of Secale cornutum.*)

PHARMACOLOGY.—There are several substances known as Ergotine, viz.: the "Ergotine of Wiggers," and "Winkler's Ergotine," to which may be added the most recent and, probably, the best, "Squibb's Ergotine." They are all *extracts*, not alkaloids.  To be active in its powers, and fully represent the Secale, it must be a compound extract, containing the so-called *Secaline* and *Ecboline*.  It is found in Ustilago.

They are all dark-brown, semi-fluid, or soft-solid substances, having the characteristic odor of the Ergot of Rye, viz.: an odor of herring-brine, or propylamine.  Soluble in water, or dilute alcohol.  Squibb's Ergotine (or Extract), is the most trustworthy preparation.

OFFICINAL PREPARATIONS.—(1) Triturations with pure sugar of milk (for internal administration); (2) Solution, 5 grs. in two drams of water (for hypodermic injection); (3) Dilutions, with dilute alcohol to the 3× afterwards with strong alcohol.

(*See Therapeutics, Vol. II.*)

---

# ERYNGIUM AQUATICUM.

### (*Button Snake Root.*)

DESCRIPTION.—This singular looking plant reminds one of an Endogen. The *leaves* are one or two feet long by half-an-inch to an inch wide, broadly linear, parallel-veined, taper pointed, grass-like, ciliate, with remote, soft spines.  The *flowers* are disposed in a globular head, often over an inch in diameter.  It grows in damp places, *not in water*, and is common on prairies.  The *root* is dark brown, very knotty, rhizoma wrinkled horizontally, fibres of the same color, growing downward.  Internally, it is yellowish-white, with an odor somewhat resembling *Iris v.*, and a sweetish, aromatic taste, like *Aralia rac.*, succeeded by a bitterness and a pungency affecting the fauces.  Dr. Tully says the taste resembles that of *Senega*.

OFFICINAL PREPARATIONS.—(1) Tincture of root; dilutions; (2) Triturations of the dried root.

ANALOGUES.—*Asclepias tuberosa, Copaiva, Gelseminum, Hepar Sulphur, Kali bichromicum, Lachesis, Senega, Spongia, Senecio, Sepia.*

### Mental Sphere.

Unable to concentrate his thoughts.

Depressed in spirits.

## Head.

Vertigo, after dinner.

Dull, heavy pains in the temporal bones.

Dull, dragging pain in the occiput.

Shooting pains in the coronary region.

Frontal headache of a dull, aching character.

Expanding sensation in frontal region, over the eyes, with dimness of sight.

Pain in the occiput, extending into the eyes, and into the neck, and down between the shoulders.

Scalp sore on pressure, and pains on combing the hair.

## Eyes.

Irritated by strong light, producing a smarting, burning sensation.

Eyes congested, with heavy aching, and dull expression.

Severe pains over left eye, of a tearing, burning character.

° Violent ophthalmia in a scrofulous patient.

## Ears.

Burning, tearing pain, as if they were being torn from the head.

## Mouth and Throat.

Tongue and fauces very dry, with insipid taste, thick, tenacious, yellowish-colored mucus in the morning.

Smarting, burning pain; raw, smarting pain on left side.

Sensation as if a lump was in the throat.

Can not bear the clothing close around the throat.

° Chronic laryngitis.

## Stomach.

Slight nausea, with drawing, cramping pains.

Hot, burning pains extending up the œsophagus.

Heavy, dragging pain, with a feeling of emptiness.

Nausea and retching, with inclination to stool.

° Spitting up of bright arterial blood, mixed with black clots, with burning in the epigastrium, after a blow on the stomach. (*Dr. Cushing.*)

## Abdomen.

Severe pain in the left groin, passing down into the left testicle.

Severe colic-like pains in small intestines.

Sharp, piercing pains in the bowels, in the morning, with
  bloated sensation and heaviness in abdomen, and soreness on pressure.
° Hæmorrhoids and prolapsus ani.

### Stool.

Dark leaden color, dry and very hard.
Tenesmus at stool, with a sensation of cutting.
° Mucous diarrhœa of children.

### Urine.

Frequent desire to urinate, after evacuation of the bladder,
  with continued dripping for a few moments after urin-
  ating.
Urine decreased in quantity and darker at night.
Urine deposits a white flocculent matter, s. g. 1016.
° Dropsy, of an asthenic character.

### Generative Organs.

Stinging, burning sensation in the urethra, behind the glans-
  penis, during urination.
Severe pain in left testicle, worse on exercise.
° Gonorrhœa, with painful erections.   ° Gleet.
° Emissions at night, with erections, with great lassitude and
  depression.
Depression of the virile force.
° Leucorrhœa.

### Larynx.

Smarting in larynx and bronchii; slight dyspnœa.
Respirations rather shorter than normal.
° Cough, with sensation of constriction in the throat.
° Laryngeal irritations; short, hacking cough.

### Neck.

Rheumatic pains in the posterior portions.

### Back and Shoulders.

Dull, dragging pains in the lumbar region.
Rheumatic pains in the left shoulder.

# ERYNGIUM MARITIMUM.
### (Sea Holly.)

DESCRIPTION.—This species is a native of Europe, and England. It grows in the sands on the sea shore. A fragmentary proving, by E. B. Ivatts, of Dublin, was published in the "American Observer," 1874, and in the "Homœopathic World," 1875.

OFFICINAL PREPARATIONS.—Tincture of the root.

ANALOGUES.—(Same as of E. Aquaticum.)

### (See " Therapeutics.")

---

# EUONYMUS ATROPURPUREUS.
### (Wahoo.)

DESCRIPTION.—A small shrub or bush, known by several other names, as Indian Arrow-wood, Burning-bush, Spindle-tree, etc., with smooth branches, rising from five to ten feet high. The E. Americanus is a smaller shrub, with smooth, four-angled branches. The name Wahoo is applied to both. They grow all over the United States, in woods and thickets and river bottoms, and flower in June. The flowers of the former are dark purple, enclosed in a crimson, five-angled pod; the latter has yellow and pink flowers, in a dark red pod, rough, warty and depressed.

Both are very beautiful objects in autumn.

OFFICINAL PREPARATIONS. —Tincture of the bark.

ANALOGUES.—China. (?)   Epat. perf. (?)

### Brain.

A sick, weakening sensation all through the nervous system.

She seemed so drawn up from the floor that it seemed difficult to place her foot down when walking, with sufficient firmness to stand.

A tipping-over sensation when sitting and walking.

A dull, heavy pain through the front upper portion of the head.

An enlarged, blurred feeling in the head.

### Stomach and Bowels.

A deathly sickness at the stomach, with perspiration and heat in the face, in alternation with chills on the back, and back part of the arms; (vinegar removed these symptoms).

A drastic cathartic, its operation being attended with death-like nausea, excessive tormina, prostration, and cold sweats.

The evacuations are profuse, violent, and accompanied with much flatus.

° Cholera morbus, and cholera infantum. (?)

° Diarrhœa, with severe colic. (?)

### Fever.

° Intermittent fevers. (?)   A favorite domestic remedy.

---

# EUPATORIUM AROMATICUM.

### (*White Snake Root.*)

DESCRIPTION.—A perennial plant, with rough, slightly pubescent *stem*, about two feet high. It has white, *aromatic* flowers, in small corymbs. The *root* is the officinal portion. It has a pleasant aromatic odor and a bitterish taste. It gives up its medicinal virtues to alcohol and boiling water. It should be gathered in September.

OFFICINAL PREPARATIONS.—Tincture of the fresh root; dilutions.

ANALOGUES.—(?)

° Restlessness and morbid watchfulness.

° Calms the irritability of the nervous system.

° Debility and irritability of the nervous system.

° Relieves tremors, jactitations, chorea, and hysteria.

° Apthous stomatitis in females and children.   (*Hill.*)

° Burning at the stomach in females a few weeks before confinement.

° Nursing sore mouth, with great nervousness.

° Nervous cough.

---

# EUPATORIUM PERFOLIATUM.

### (*Boneset.*)

DESCRIPTION.—The *Thoroughwort* is an indigenous perennial herb, with a horizontal, crooked root. The *stems* are round, stout, hairy, and from one to five feet high. The *leaves* are opposite, connate-perfoliate, each pair resembling a single leaf *centrally perforated by the stem*, and placed at right angles to it. *Flowers* numerous, *white*, in dense terminal corymbs. This well-known plant grows in low grounds, on the borders of swamps, wet prairies, flowering in August and September. It has a feeble, peculiar odor, and a herbaceous, very bitter taste.

OFFICINAL PREPARATIONS.—Tincture of the flowers and leaves of the plant; dilutions with stong alcohol.

ANALOGUES.—*Arnica, Baptisia, Bryonia, Cimicifuga, Chamomilla, Gelseminum, Ipecacuanha, Mercurius, Nux vomica, Podophyllum, Triosteum.*

### Head.

\* Headache, with a sensation of soreness internally, better in the house, aggravated when first going into the open air; relieved by conversation.

Pain extending from the forehead to the occiput.

Throbbing headache; beating pain in forehead and occiput, better after rising.

Darting pains through the temples, with sensation of blood rushing across the head.

Distress on the top and in the back part of the head.

Shooting pains from left to right side of the head.

° Headache, with nausea, every other morning when first awaking, continuing all day; loss of appetite during that day, but good appetite during the intervening day.

° Pain in the occiput after lying, with sensation of great weight in that part, requiring the hands to lift it. (*See Chelid.*)

### Eyes.

* Soreness of the eyeballs, with intolerance of light.

Redness of the margin of the lids, with profuse secretion.

Increased lachrymation.

### Face.

Sickly, sallow countenance; flushed face; redness of the cheeks.

### Mouth.

Increased appetite; causes hunger (*primary*).

Loss of appetite, with disgust for food (*secondary*)

Paleness of the mucous membrane of the mouth.

Tongue coated yellow, or a white-coated tongue.

Sores in the corners of the mouth.

Insipid taste in the mouth; want of appetite; distaste for food.

Nocturnal thirst for something cold.

° The hunger which attends or precedes ague.

### Stomach.

* Belching of tasteless wind, with a feeling of obstruction at the pit of the stomach.

Sensation of something in the stomach that ought to come up.

General shuddering proceeding from the stomach.

Beating in the epigastrium at night.

Sensation of fullness at stomach.

° Nausea, and vomiting of food.

*/Vomiting of mucus and bile, with trembling and pain in the stomach, and weakness even to fainting.

Distressing disposition to, and attempts at, vomiting.

### Liver.

* Soreness around the waist—tight clothing is oppressive.
* Soreness and fullness in the region of the liver.

### Stool.

* Purging stools, with smarting and heat in the anus.

Frequent watery stools, or *bilious* stools.

Tenesmus, with small discharge of loose stool.

Morning diarrhœa (*primary*); constipation (*secondary*).

### Urinary Organs.

Urine scanty and high colored.

Dark brown, scanty urine, depositing whitish, clay-like sediment, voided only once in twenty-four hours.

<sup>c</sup> Dark urine in bilious disorders.

° Watery urine during intermittents.

° Herpes on the scrotum and thighs, even to the anus.

### Catarrhal Symptoms.

* Flowing coryza; sneezing; hoarseness.
* Hacking cough in the evening.
* Cough, with soreness and heat in the bronchia.
<sup>c</sup> Cough aggravated in the evening.
° Hectic cough from suppressed intermittent fever.
° Violent cough, with soreness in the chest.
<sup>c</sup> Epidemic influenza.
° Cough, with flushed face and tearful eyes; he has to support the chest with his hands.

### Chest.

Difficulty of breathing, with anxious countenance, perspiration and sleeplessness.

Painful irritation of the pulmonary organs, with heat in chest.

Aching pain under the left breast, and inability to lie on the left side.

Grating sensation in the chest at every deep inspiration.

° Asthma and bronchitis, when the dyspnœa is great, obliging the patient to lie with head and shoulders high.

### Back.

Weakness in the small of the back.

Pain in the back as from a bruise.

Pain in the back and lower extremities.

Deep-seated pains in the loins, with soreness from motion.

### Upper Extremities.

Soreness and aching *soreness* in the arms and wrists.

Stiffness of the fingers, with obtuseness of the sense of touch

Heat in the palms of the hands.

### Lower Extremities.

Pain, with extreme sensitiveness in left gluteal muscles.

° Stiffness and general soreness of the lower extremities when rising to walk.

Calves of the legs feel as though they had been beaten.

Pains in all the joints of the lower extremities.

Lameness in the right hip and lower extremity.

ᶜ Soreness and aching of the lower limbs when rising **to walk.**

° Rheumatic pains on the inside of the left knee.

° Dropsical swelling of feet and ankles.

° Gouty inflammation of left knee and right elbow.

### Fever.

\* Chilliness through the night and in the morning, with nausea from the least motion; aching pain and soreness, as if from having been beaten in the calves of the legs, small of the back, and in the arms, above and below the elbows; nausea as the chills go off; aching in the bones of the extremities, with soreness of the flesh; chilliness, with excessive trembling and nausea; chilliness in the morning, heat through the rest of the day, but no perspiration; the patient feels worse in the morning of one day, and in the afternoon of the next day.

° Ague and fever, with nocturnal sweat with chilliness from motion or removal of the covering.

° *Belching and vomiting of bile, and trembling in the back during fever.*

° Thirst several hours before the chill.

° The shiverings were severer than the cold would warrant.

° *Intermittent fever,* when the paroxysm commences in the

morning, with thirst several hours before the chill, which
thirst continues during the chill and heat, and vomiting
at the conclusion of the chill; fever attended with great
painfulness, weakness and soreness all over; little or no
perspiration after the heat. (*Williamson, Neidhard,
Gray and Hale.*)

° *Cerebro-spinal meningitis*, with intense soreness and aching
all over, vomiting, pain in back of head and neck, etc.
(*Pratt, Small, etc.*)

° *Remittent fever*, bilious and malarial, with severe gastric
and intestinal irritation.

### Generalities.

Great soreness and painfulness of the whole body and extremities, as if he had been bruised or beaten.

---

# EUPATORIUM PURPUREUM.
### (*Queen of the Meadow.*)

DESCRIPTION.—This plant is known, also, by the name of *Gravel-root*,
Trumpet-weed, etc. It has a perennial, horrizontal, woody root, with many
long, dark brown fibres, which send up one or more solid, glabrous, green,
sometimes purplish stems, five or six feet in height, with a purple band at
the joints, about an inch apart. *Leaves* three to six in a whorl, about six
inches apart; ovate, oblong, or lanceolate. *Flowers* all tubular, purple, varying to whitish, and consist of numerous florets included in an eight-leaved
calyx; heads in lax, very dense and compound corymbs, cylindrical, five
to ten flowers. It grows in wet places, flowering from August to September.

The root is the officinal part; as found in the shops, it consists of a
blackish, woody caudex, from which proceeds numerous long fibres, from
one to three lines in diameter; externally they are covered with a dark
brown, longitudinally furrowed bark, beneath which the interval portion
is white, or whitish-yellow, according to its age, the last color being the
oldest. It has a smell somewhat resembling old hay, and a slightly bitter,
aromatic, and faintly astringent, but not unpleasant taste, and yields its
properties to water, by decoction, or to spirits.

OFFICINAL PREPARATIONS.—Tincture of the fresh root; dilutions, with
dilute alcohol; infusions. Triturations of the Oleo-resin.

ANALOGUES.—*Apocynum cannabinum, Asclepias syriaca, Cannabis sativa,
Chimaphila, Galium, Uva ursi, Senecio.*

### Mind.

The mind is possessed by various delusions.

Talkative; exclamations; feels extremely depressed.

Hysterical mood, weeping, sighing, and a feeling like homesickness, with fluttering of the heart up into the throat.

Illusions of sight, and hearing, with vertigo.

### Head.

*Sensation as if falling toward the left side, with dizziness.*

Lightness of the head; dizzy, as though flying round and
round.

Sensation as if her head were moving in all directions.

Vertigo, as if flying round and round.

Hard, thumping pain in the occipital bones.

Soreness, tenderness, and itching of the scalp.

### Eyes.

Copious flow of tears, filling the eyes with tears, making con
stant wiping necessary.

Eyes fastened, with an earnest look, upon some object.

Wild staring look of the eyes, with wakefulness.

She cannot see as far as usual.

### Ears.

Ears feel as if they were full; crackling in the ears.

Crackling sound in the ears when swallowing.

### Nose.

Abundant discharge of a thin, watery fluid, making the nose
sore and irritable.

### Face.

Congestion to the face, with burning heat, dry and hot to the
touch.

Shining appearance of the face.

### Mouth and Throat.

Increased action of all the glands of the mouth.

Pricking and sticking in the end of the tongue.

Gums red and hot.

*Choking fullness* of the throat; soreness of the throat.

*Smarting and burning in the posterior part of the throat.*

Sensation of *fullness in the throat,* with feeling of homesickness.

She feels like crying.

### Stomach.

Eructations almost constant from wind in the stomach.

Crampy pains in pit of stomach, with weak, sick feeling.
Great nausea, swelling and fullness, mostly on the left side.

### Abdomen.

Fullness and pain in the bowels.
Rumbling, rolling, twisting pain in the bowels.
Pain and soreness, worse on the left side.
Bowels are hard; tympanitic.
Tense cutting pain just above the left ovary.

### Stool.

Feeling as though the bowels must be moved immediately; unable to do so.
Pressure and heaviness upon the rectum.
Pain and suffering as from diarrhœa, although the passages were natural.

### Urinary Organs.

*Deep, dull pain in the kidneys; also cutting pain.*
Strong desire to pass water ten minutes after having urinated.
*Greatly increased quantity of urine,* with large discharges every half hour, but the bladder fills up soon, with cutting, aching pain in bladder.
\* *Smarting and burning very intense in the bladder and urethra.*
Sensation as if she had been a long time without urinating.
° *Diabetes insipidus* and perhaps *mellitus.*
The stream of urine is smaller than natural.
<sup>c</sup> *Dropsy,* when due to renal disorder (low dil. or infusion.)
° *Dysuria,* with *profuse* and watery urine (high dilutions.)
° Strangury from uterine displacement, or during pregnancy.
° Mucus sediment in urine in excess, indicating inflammation.
° Inflammation of the mucous membrane of urinary passages.
° Suppression of urine in infants.
° Chronic inflammation of the bladder.  (*Dr. Dresser.*)
° Renal and vesical calculi.

### Generative Organs.

*Female.*—Inflammation of meatus urinarius.
The external genitals feel as though wet, although they are *not.*
Leucorrhœa quite profuse.

\* Threatened abortions.

° Sterility, from atony of the ovaries.

° Amenorrhœa, dysmenorrhœa (*atonic.*)

° Habitual abortion at the third or fourth month.

A quick, jerking motion in region of left ovary.

Tense, cutting pain in region of left ovary.

° It is a genuine tonic to the female organs of generation.

° Inefficient labor pains.

*Male.*—° *Impotency*, from exhaustion or abuse of the generative functions.

### Chest.

*Palpitation of the heart;* fluttering of the heart up into the throat.

Strong desire to inflate the lungs, of which she was not cognizant.

Pulse 80 to 100, full and bounding.

### Back and Neck.

Neuralgic-like pains from below upwards, mostly on the left side of the back and hip.

Sore pain directly within the spine, its whole extent, from below upwards.

Dull, aching pain in the sacrum, running upward into the kidneys.

Stiff, wry neck, with lame, weak feeling in nape of the neck.

Cutting pain in the neck, running from left shoulder to occiput.

### Upper and Lower Extremities.

Tired, weak, uneasiness in the limbs, with numbness and gnawing pain.

A constant sensation as if her boot-heels were crowding through her boots upward.

Rheumatic pain, changing from place to place, always from below.

Gnawing in the hip bone; legs feel weak, tired, left leg worse.

All symptoms worse on the left side of the body.

### Sleep.

Sleeplessness, with wild, staring eyes.

### Fever.

Intermittent fevers, with chills in the back and aching.

° *Intermittent fever;* miasmatic; paroxysms at various times of the day; *chills beginning in the small of the back,* spreading up and down the trunk and extremities; lips and nails blue; *violent shaking with comparative little coldness;* fever, with nausea and vomiting, followed by moisture, not amounting to sweat, principally about the head and forehead; any attempt to change position, ever so little, during the sweat, a chilliness would pass through the body. (*Van Tagen, Martin, Howard, Gardiner.*)

[This remedy seems specific in ague with the above symptoms; but they have a remarkable resemblance,to those of Eupat. *perf.* (*Hale.*)]

° *Hectic fever,* with night sweats; pulse feeble but regular.

### Generalities.

Faint, dizzy feeling pervading the whole body.

All the symptoms are worse on left side of the body.

*A feeling as if falling to the left;* (compare Anac., Aur., Bell., Dros., Euphorb., Mez., Natr., Nux mosch., Spig., Spong., Zinc.) (*Hering.*)

---

# EUPHORBIA COROLLATA.

### (*Spurge—Wandering Milk Weed.*)

BOTANICAL DESCRIPTION.—A tall, slender, erect plant, one to two feet high, with a large, perennial, branching, yellowish root, which sends up several *stems* from two to five feet in height, round, and generally simple and smooth. The *flowers* are disposed upon a large terminal umbel. The root, when full grown, is sometimes an inch in thickness and two feet in length. It is without unpleasant taste, producing only a sense of heat a short time after it has been taken. The medicinal virtues are said to reside in the cortical portion, which is thick, and constitutes two-thirds of the whole root. They are taken out by water and alcohol, and remain in the extract formed by the evaporation of the decoction of the tincture. This species is one of over thirty of the genus Euphorbiaceæ, indigenous to this country, to which belongs the European species E. officinalis, proved and used by Hahnemann. The E. corollata is found all over the United States, growing chiefly in a dry, barren, and sandy soil, seldom growing in woods or on the borders of streams. Its flowers appear in July and August. The central head is two or three weeks earliest.

OFFICINAL PREPARATIONS.—Tincture of the root; dilutions.

ANALOGUES.—*Croton tiglium, Euphorbia officinalis, Elaterium, Jalappa, Lobelia, Helleborus niger, Veratrum album.*

### Head.

Vertigo, swimming in the head, with faintness.

Excessive vertigo, with ringing in the ears.

Death-like sensation, with anxiety of mind.

### Stomach and Abdomen, Etc.

Burning in the mouth and on the tongue, with nausea.

\* Sudden nausea, followed by sudden and forcible vomiting and diarrhœa of rice-water fluid, with sinking, anxious feeling at the stomach.

\* Profuse colliquative discharges from the bowels, with painful spasms of the intestines.

Cold sweat on the body and extremities with the diarrhœa.

ᶜ Spasms of the legs and feet, with vomiting and diarrhœa.

° Sea sickness; vomiting of pregnancy.

° Acute enteritis and gastritis.

° Chronic diarrhœa from malaria.

\* Diarrhœa which is very obstinate.

° Dysenteric diarrhœa.

ᶜ Cholera morbus.

---

## EUPHORBIA HYPERICIFOLIA.

*(Milk-Parsley.)*

DESCRIPTION.— This *species* possesses widely different properties, although belonging to the same genus. The juice is not irritating, but astringent, of a sweetish taste. It is an annual, smooth branched, leaning with small, white, numerous flowers, disposed in terminal or axillary corymbs. It grows in moist, rich soil. The leaves, which exude a milky juice, should be gathered in July.

OFFICINAL PREPARATIONS.—Tincture of the fresh leaves (infusion.)

ANALOGUES.—( ?)

*(See Therapeutics, Vol. II.)*

---

## FORMICA.

*(Formic Acid—The Poison of Ants.)*

PHARMACOLOGY.—Dr. Constantine Herring, in N. A. J. of H., Vol. XX, pp. 12, says: "The name *Formica* was used by Linnæus as a generic name for a large number of species, all of which appear to common people to be ants." Later entomologists had to separate the species and arrange them under different names, as different genera.

The genus to which the old name, Formica, was left by *Latrielle*, is the one from which we have report of cures, and from which we made our provings. Ants belonging to the genus Formica, as Latrielle has it, when attacked, defend themselves by biting with their mandibulæ, or jaws, and bending, at the same time, their abdomen downward and forward, they eject from the anus a sharp, sour fluid towards the place which they tried to wound with their pincers.

This fluid reddens Litmus paper, and contains the *Fomyl acid*, (Formica or Formic acid,) $C H_2 O_2$.

OFFICIAL PREPARATIONS.—Triturations of the insect; tincture; dilutions.

ANALOGUES.—*Apis, Rhus, Urtica, Croton*, etc.

### Mental Sphere.

Indisposed, forgetful, morose, fearful and apprehensive.

Exhilarated condition after the pain in the vertex had abated

Giddy on attempting to rise.

Dull, sleepy feeling, with heaviness of the eyelids, and inability to study.

### Head.

Dullness and pressure on both sides between temples and ears.

Severe pain in the vertex, like a stitch from a dull instrument.

Headache in the posterior upper and inner part of the head, increased by drinking coffee, and aggravated during washing with cold water.

When waking in the morning headache, with vomiting, stitches in the chest.

### Eyes.

Spasmodic twitching of upper lid of right eye.

### Face.

Entire left side of the face and cheek feels as if paralyzed.

### Nose.

Sneezing and fluent coryza.

### Ears.

Stitches in the left ear (frequent), followed by a small abscess in the external portion of the meatus auditorius.

Pressive pain in both ears (with heat).

Pains in the eyes mornings when awaking, better on washing.

### Stomach.

*Constant pressure at the cardiac end of the stomach, and a burning pain there.*

*Nausea, with headache, and vomiting of yellowish, bitter mucus.*

Burning pain in the stomach, with oppression and weight.

### Abdomen and Stool.

In the morning difficult passages of small quantities of flatus; *afterwards diarrhœa-like urging in the rectum.*

*Diarrhœa, with tenesmus; pain in bowels before stool.*

Dull pain in the region of the spleen.

*Severe pain in the bowels, with shuddering chilliness.*

*Sensation of constriction in the anus.*

Pressure in the rectum, worse in the evening and in bed.

Loose diarrhœic stool, which left a desire for another stool.

Painful desire in the anus and rectum for stool, which, how ever, will not pass.

° Constipation, with sensation of constriction of sphincter ani.

### Generative Organs.

*Male.*—Itching on the scrotum; during coition insufficient erection; jerking pain in the left half of the penis.

Long lasting erections in the morning in bed on returning from urination.

*Female.*—Menses scanty and pale, with bearing down in the back.

Menses appear eight days too soon.

### Chest.

*Violent prickling, pressing stitches in region of left nipple; later on the left side of the back, but more violent; still later, the same sensation on other parts of the body.*

*Violent penetrating itching at the right nipple.*

Palpitation of the heart; fluttering of the heart.

### Upper Extremities.

*Severe pain above the right elbow.*

*Itching in the armpits in the morning.*

*Violent itching on the left shoulder-blade.*

Rheumatic pain in the right elbow joint, and along the course of the ulna.

Violent pain in left side of the nape of the neck, extending down the left arm.

Pain leaves the left arm and goes to the right.

20

**Neck** is very stiff and painful, worse from motion.
**Burning** stitches in the finger ends.

### Lower Extremeties.

**Pains** in the hips (bruised) at night in bed.
**Pains** in the knee joints (rheumatic) increased by walking.
**Lancinating** pain in the left knee joint.
**General** weakness of the whole muscular system.
**Severe** pain across the sacrum and dorsum of each ham, worse on motion.
**Sensation** as if the muscles were strained and being torn from attachment.
**Cramp** in both feet, especially in the soles near the toes.

### Generalities.

**Dr.** Hering (*Hahnemannian Monthly, Jan.*, 1871), gives the following indications for the use of *Formica:*

" *Affections of the spinal cord, paralysis*, spasms.

" *Rheumatism* appearing suddenly, mostly in the joints, with the character of restlessness; the patients desire motion, *although it makes pain more acute.*

" **Pressure** relieves the pains.

" **Sweat** without amelioration.

" *Eye disease*, especially the so-called rheumatic inflammations of the eyes, with their sequelæ; but still more in difficulties of hearing and many diseases of the ear.

" **Lack** of milk in nursing women.

" **Seminal** emissions.

" **The** predominant time of day is from 2 to 4 A. M.

" **The** burning pains are removed by washing in cold water.

" **Consequences** of cold and wet, cold bath, or damp weather.

" **It** often helped when *Chamomilla* only ameliorated, and when *Belladonna* did not agree. *Formica*, therefore, like *Apis*, belongs to the class of acids with ethereal oils, to which the aromatics are complementary. *Formica* seems to be as great an enemy to the narcotics as *Apis* is to the acids (*Rhus*).

# FERROCYANURET OF POTASSIUM.

### (Kali-ferrocyanuretum.)

PHARMACOLOGY.—This salt may be obtained by boiling purified Prussian blue in a solution of Potassa until the blue color disappears, filtering the liquor, evaporating, and crystalizing several times to render it pure. It occurs in broken or entire crystals of large size, whose form is usually a rectangular prism, truncated on the ends and edges. The crystals are large, of a honey-yellow color, transparent. Sp. gr. 1.832. Have at first a sweet-ish-bitter, but afterward a saline taste, permanent in the air; soluble in four parts cold water and two of boiling; insoluble in alcohol, which precipitates them from their aqueous solution in brilliant yellow flakes.

OFFICINAL PREPARATIONS.—Aqueous solution ℥i to ℥ix; dilutions with water.

ANALOGUES.—(Kali. Carb., Ferrum, Digitalis, Lycopus, Collinsonia, Hydrocyanic acid and its salts.)

° Fatty heart, with weak, irregular pulse.
° Fatty degeneration of the heart.
° Hypertrophy, with dilatation.
° Functional disorders of heart, with anæmia.
° Chlorosis, with cardiac debility.

(See Therapeutics, Vol. II.)

---

# FAGOPYRUM ESCULENTUM.

### (Buckwheat.)

BOTANICAL DESCRIPTION.—This plant belongs to the order of Polygonacœæ, or the Buckwheat family, is a native of Asia, and introduced into this country from Europe. It is an annual, cultivated, flowering from June to September.

There is also a wild variety found growing in fields and old pastures, (which it might be worth while to prove,) in the form of a vine.

Emil Wolf, of Wurtemberg, gives us the following analysis: The straw contains 6.15 per cent. of ash and 160. per cent. of water. The dry grain contains 9.2 per cent. ash and 141. per cent. water.

Percentage of Potash, in the straw 46.6, in the grain 23.1; of soda, in the straw 2.2, in the grain 6.2; of magnesia, in the straw 3.6, in the grain 13.4; of lime, in the straw 18.4, in the grain 3.3; of phosphoric acid, in the straw 11.9, in the grain 48.0; of sulphuric acid, in the straw 5.3, in the grain 2.01; of silicia, in the straw 5.5; in the grain .0; of chlorine, in the straw 7.7, in the grain 1.7.

The Fagopyrum contains a crystalizable coloring principle, which is identical with ruteine or rutic acid, discovered in the common rue.

OFFICINAL PREPARATIONS.—Tincture from the whole plant, and seed at maturity, with strong alcohol; dilutions.

ANALOGUES.—*Arsenicum* (?), *Calc. carb.* (?), *Graphites* (?), *Sulphur* (?), *Silicia* (?), *Rumex* (?), *Stillingia* (?), *Juglans* (?).

(These symptoms are selected from the voluminous provings presented to the American Institute in 1873, by Dr. D. Hitchcock, of Norwalk, Conn.)

## Mind.

Very cross and irritable; feeling as of a weight on the mind.

Spirits exhilarated; feels happy.

Inability to study, or to remember what is heard or read, even for a few minutes.

Great depression of spirits in evening. (Never felt before that I did not care to live.)

No desire to speak, or be spoken to.

## Head.

Vertigo, and confused feeling in the head.

Slight vertigo, with nausea.

Vertigo and fullness of the head when rising; better by remaining quiet.

Dull headache in evening, pressing outward, especially in occiput, relieved by pressure, gentle motion, or cool air.

Bursting pressure in temples and forehead, with a feeling as if eyes were pressed out.

Pulsation and pressure in head, slightly relieved by bending head backwards.

Whole head feels composed, as if living in a dream.

Great pressure; occasional sharp, darting pains, more through right side.

A severe, continued pain in head and eyes, came on after an early walk; great heat of head, with red face; slight relief from a cool, wet compress; on its removal the forehead is covered with a measle-like rash.

Congestive headache in afternoon.

Headache and slight vertigo on waking, with tired, dull feeling.

Pressive headache, starting at times with shooting pains from back of eyes to back of neck.

Wavy feeling in head.

A sharp, cutting pain, from over left eye, backward and inward.

Dull pain in left temple, from left eye to occiput, and down left side of neck.

Heat of head and pain in forehead, changing to vertex, and from thence to root of nose.

Severe pressing pain from forehead to eyeballs and root of nose.

Bruised, sore feeling of left temple.

Tensive feeling in upper part of head, followed by a wavy sensation.

Sharp stitching pain in occiput, right side.

Sharp darting pain in left occipital region, radiating to left side, very marked.

Itching of scalp, especially in occiput.

### Eyes.

Objects appear indistinct; eyes feel blurred, have a glassy look.

Things appear obscure and wavy.

The eyes feel sensitive upon closing them tightly; a roughened feeling when moving the lids, especially left.

External canthi sore, with constant burning irritation and itching.

Pain in eyeballs and temples, shooting and darting.

Itching of edges of lids, burning and redness with swelling, but never agglutinated.

Pain in eyes sharp and continued, extending to right ear.

Drooping of right eyelid.

Meibomian glands inflamed.

Itching and smarting of eyes; they feel inflamed and hot.

Muscles of eyes feel sore on moving them.

Eyeballs sore, as if pressed out, and still held back by cords, tender to touch.

Eyes hot, burning and glassy.

Granular lids. (?)

Sensation as of sand in eyes.

Dull, oppressive pain in left eye.

Eyes swollen, hot and watery; secretion bland, and not excessive.

### Ears.

Ears itch internally and externally, and sounds seem muffled.

Burning heat and itching of both auricles.

Momentary buzzing and ringing in ears.

Left meatus externus sore and sensitive to touch.

Dull pain, extending from left ear to throat when swallowing.

Sharp pains, extending from right ear downwards and backwards.

### Nose.

Nose swollen, excoriated and sore within, itching and burning, worse from contact.

Soreness of nose; it fills with loose dry crusts; blood flows slightly when they are removed.

*Fluent coryza;* nose is alternately clear and stuffed up, with catarrhal headache.

Aching pains in nose when in cool air.

Schneiderian membrane parched and dry; it itches and burns, with an intermittent watery flow, followed by dry crusts.

Septum nasi cracked and sore, with a gnawing, stinging pain; ulcer in right nostril.

### Face.

Neuralgic pain in left side of face; a sore, bruised feeling when closing the teeth or moving the jaws.

Face pale and then flushed, with dark circles under eyes.

* A red eruption, with swollen base, with heat, itching and burning.

### Mouth.

Lips dry; they crack and peel, and are sore.

Vesicles on lips and in mouth, with burning.

Deep crack in corner of mouth, dry and sore.

Dryness of mouth and pharynx; lips are black and **dry.**

A very sensitive pimple on chin.

Soreness and swelling of gums; they bleed easily.

Dull pain in teeth, left side, worse from cold water.

Sour, bad taste; bitter taste.

Eructations of ingesta.

Tongue very red all the time, also the mouth and fauces.

Tongue fissured deeply on the edges.

Copious flow of saliva, with yawning and eructations of **air.**

Mouth dry, with tough mucus in throat.

Uvula elongated, with granular appearance of soft palate.

Very offensive breath, with bad taste.

Swollen sensation in roof of mouth.

Rough, sore feeling in roof of mouth and pharynx, with sticking pain in par tid glands.

### Throat.

Throat is sore; feels raw and as if bruised, worse when swallowing.

Aching pain in fauces and pharynx, extending downwards.

Soreness about right tonsil; afterwards expelled a hard, offensive, cheesy mass, the size of a pea.

Dry soreness in throat and pharynx, with desire to swallow.

Smarting on under surface of soft palate when swallowing.

Frequent desire to swallow, with a painful raw sensation of palate.

Sore stiffness and swelling of fauces.

Tonsils swollen and red.

Constriction and darting pain in soft palate.

A small swelling in the trachea, sore and hard.

Submaxillary and parotid glands swollen and painful.

### Stomach.

Faint nausea and loss of appetite, with heat in stomach and throat.

Excessive thirst every evening.

Constant nausea, almost to vomiting, and a sore feeling in stomach, relieved by eructations.

Eructations of scalding, acid, watery substance come up so hot as to nearly strangle one.

Eructations with offensive odor and taste.

Constant acidity of stomach and heartburn.

Belching of wind, with griping.

Heat and a heavy uneasiness in stomach.

Stomach feels as if bruised and hurt, with depression and a gnawing sensation.

Sensation as of something moving in stomach, with a sore, distressed feeling.

### Abdomen.

Aching pains in abdomen, with distension coming on after stool.

Abdomen tympanitic and tender to touch, with suffocative sensation about heart.

Severe aching pain in abdomen early in morning, driving him to stool.

Severe paroxysms of pain, with tenesmus, nausea, and hot flashes and perspiration.

Pain and great soreness in region of liver, with pains around heart.

Sharp sticking pains through liver.

Dull throbbing pain in ascending colon, extending through to small of back.

Sharp pain through hypogastrium, extending into left inguinal region.

Severe griping, cutting pains in hypogastric region, awaking her from sleep, relieved by flexing limbs and by pressure.

Sore, bruised feeling in hypogastrium when she moves.

When seeing an operation, nausea became excessive, extending into bowels, with griping, cutting pains and diarrhœa.

Rumbling and fullness, with flatulence.

### Stool and Anus.

Thin, watery stool, forcibly expelled, preceded and followed by tenesmus.

Stool with severe pain in rectum, extending down into the thighs and legs.

Burning in rectum after a hard, dark brown stool.

Soft, light brown stool, with much flatus; followed by a chill in back.

Frequent desire for stool, which was of oily consistence, and fetid like spoiled eggs.

Great urgency to go to stool, early in A. M.

Feeling as of ascarides in rectum and anus.

### Urinary Organs.

Profuse flow of urine of a light color, acid.

Difficulty in voiding last few drops.

Cutting pain in the urethra, like a knife.

Soon after urinating slight pain in bowels.

### Sexual Organs.

* Profuse sweating of genitals, of an offensive odor.

Pain like a bruise from left testicle upwards.

Menses two days earlier than usual, and not so profuse, but the usual pruritus somewhat ameliorated.

Slight leucorrhœa with pruritus; stains the linen yellow.

Menses two days ahead of usual time, with the usual pains much intensified; unable to keep quiet while pain lasted.

Flow lasts usual time, but not so profuse, less pruritus than usual.

Less mammary tenderness than usual.

Severe bruised pain in right ovary when walking.

(The leucorrhœa and pruritus were aggravated, but other symptoms were ameliorated.)

### Chest.

Desire to take a deep inspiration, which does not satisfy.

Touching neck under right ear occasions a cough with a smarting sensation in ear and throat.

Sharp pain below left clavicle.

Dull, aching, or bruised feeling in chest and around the heart, aggravated by bending over or walking.

Sharp stitches, like the prick of a knife, in right breast when breathing.

Dull, sticking pains in left chest.

Sharp stitches, darting quickly in left chest and under the arm, unaffected by respiration.

Soreness in left chest.

### Heart.

Sharp stitches shooting in cardiac region, with a sense of heat over body; worse when bending forward.

Sharp pain near heart, extending down from shoulder and down arm.

Dull pain around heart and through chest during colic, with depression of spirits.

Sharp stitch through the heart.

"Gnawing pains around the heart, quite severe, with stitches; relieved upon belching wind." (??)

Severe frequent pains seem to pass through heart, and pulse became irregular, on arising in the morning.

Awoke from sleep with a stinging pain through the heart.

Sharp pains around heart during an attack of uterine colic.

Slight constrictive feeling around heart.

[Nearly all the above symptoms seem to be largely due to colic and indigestion, as they were generally relieved by eructations of wind. The erratic pulse of one prover is also mainly due to the same cause, assisted by a lively imagination.]

The pulse seemed to vary greatly; sometimes accelerating rapidly until it would lose a beat; again it begins stronger and soon becomes weaker.

Weak, irregular pulse; constantly changing in quality; each beat seems to be drawn out, holding almost to the next beat.

Pulse ran very fast for ten or twenty beats, and then suddenly changed and gave two or three full, long beats.

Pulse very irregular; not at all alike during the first and last half minute.

Jerking pulse.

The beats run together (after a walk), can count them with difficulty; occasionally a few full, distinct beats.

### Back and Neck.

Neck feels tired and weak, as if unable to support the head.

Pain in back of neck, extending forwards.

Eruption and itching on whole length of the back.

Pains in lumbar region, or small of back.

Stitching pain in right side, in region of kidneys.

Tensive pain under left scapula; better when drawing back the shoulders.

Chills along the back.

### Upper Extremities.

Tearing pains in left axilla, extending into muscles of chest and arm.

Severe pains in left elbow and shoulder, and sharp stitches in region of heart.

Numbness in right shoulder and arm.

A sore, bruised feeling over spine of right scapula, when moving arm.

Sharp pain in superior angle of left scapula.

Rheumatic pains in shoulders, worse when quietly sitting, or in bed.

Disagreeable odor in axillæ.

When writing, the cold table causes severe pains in hands and arms.

Twitching of tendons—of the wrist.

Occasional pains along the course of the radial artery.

Gnawing, stinging pains from ends of fingers, running up the arms.

Hands burn, are hot and uneasy.

Heat and sweat of hands.

One hand hot and the other cold.

A burning, stinging pain in fingers, both internally and laterally, following course of arteries. (The prover believes it is in the coats of the arteries.)

The slight pressure from taking the pulse causes pain up the arm and through the hand frequently.

Throbbing of arteries upon back of hands.

Trembling and unsteadiness of hands.

### Lower Extremities.

Pain extending from hips up to small of back and down to the feet.

Feeling in the right thigh as if the limb would drop off, tired and heavy.

A diffuse pain from knee downwards.

Sharp pain in right knee.

Aching, bruised sensation in right popliteal space when walking.

Numbness and stiffness of legs.

Dull, aching pain in both legs.

Pain on inner side of thigh.

Pain in left heel.

Heel blistered and suppurating, very sensitive to touch, and on walking.

In little toe, a feeling as if a fine cord was cutting it through at the root of the nail.

Numb, prickling pains in feet and toes.

Cold sweaty feet.

### Generalities.

When sitting still, numbness and stinging pains occur along the course of such arteries as seem to be compressed; worse when cold.

Great languor and weariness.

A sore, bruised feeling in whole body.

Lassitude, yawning and stretching.

Sensation as if rubbed all over with rough flannel.

### Skin.

Persistent itching of various parts of the body, especially of left arm and alæ nasi; worse from scratching.

Papillæ sore and itch; worse from touch.

A peculiar feeling over various parts of the body.

Red blotches upon the face and body, very sore; they itch and burn, but do not suppurate.

Itching of knees and elbows, also upon the scalp and face at the roots of whiskers.

Red, itching eruption on back, limbs and body generally; resembling flea bites; also forehead and face.

Excessive burning and itching of the limbs, after retiring.

Severe itching of pubis, as if from pediculi.

Tickling, crawling feeling in various parts of the body.

The eruption nearly heals, then breaks out afresh.

Swelling in back of neck, nearly the size of a hen's egg; another on the left shoulder; they resemble blind boils, and disappear without suppuration.

° Before taking it, he had an itching after retiring, which has since disappeared.

### Fever.

Coldness all over, especially hands and feet.

Chills along the back.

Feels hot and then cold alternately.

Feverish heat of head, with cold hands and feet; after rising.

Intense heat through the body; especially the head, neck and hands, with itching and restlessness.

Perspiration on hands from 3 p. m. until late in evening.

After going to bed, very hot and restless, and soon a light moisture over body.

Aggravation of fever at 4 p. m.; heat with moist hands; back of neck and face burn; pressing out in head; carotids throb, pulse 93; no sense of chill; tongue and fauces scarlet; itching all over; hands burn, although they feel moist and cool to another.

### Sleep and Dreams.

Drops to sleep while sitting up; a headache comes on when retiring, which is unusual.

Awoke at 5 A. M., and could not get to sleep again; bed feels hard.

Extreme lassitude, sleepiness and yawning; could hardly keep awake at 4 P. M.

Sleep disturbed by dreams; am in trouble all night.

Dreams that everything goes wrong.

### Conditions.

All symptoms ameliorated by motion in open air, by eating, and by coffee.

Aggravation in the afternoon and evening; from 3 to 5 P. M., by mental labor; by going up stairs; and the heart symptoms by riding in the cars.

---

Buckwheat bran, when fed to horses will relieve them of worms. When fed to cows, they become poor, and give an inferior quality of milk.

---

# GALIUM APARINE.

### (*Cleavers.*)

BOTANICAL DESCRIPTION.—Galium aparine is decreed by medical writers to be the officinal plant of this genus. Rafinesque says: "Many other species are probably medicinal, but we only use the Galium aparine and G. verum, common in woods, trailing, rough, with white, lateral flowers and rough seeds." This description, however, will only apply to the former species, as the latter has yellow flowers and smooth seeds. The two species above mentioned are the only ones which have eight leaves in a whorl. Gray thinks it " doubtful if the G. aparine is truly indigenous in our district." And the G. verum was certainly brought here from Europe. Only six species of Galium are mentioned by Gray as indigenous to the United States. Rafinesque, however, says we have " twenty or more species in North America." He thinks the G. aparine and G. verum common to Europe and America.

HISTORY, USES, ETC.—This plant is common to Europe and America, growing in cultivated grounds, moist thickets, and along banks of rivers, and flowering from June till September. Its roots consist of a few hair-like fibres, of a reddish color. In the green state some of these plants have an unpleasant odor, others rather the contrary; all are inodorous when dried. They have an acidulous, astringent and bitter taste. They have not been thoroughly analyzed, but chloric acid, galli-tannic acid, citric acid, starch, etc., have been detected in the G. aparine and G. verum. The former contains the most citric, while the latter holds the most galli-tannic acid. According to King, all the species of this genus possess similar medicinal virtues. This seems to be the opinion of Scudder, Beach, and other Eclectic writers. Such generalizations, however, will not be accepted by the Homœopathic school of medicine. In order to meet the requirements of a scientific materia medica, each species of any genus of plants should be studied by itself.

OFFICINAL PREPARATIONS.—Tincture; infusion of the plant.

ANALOGUES.—*Cannabis, Chimaphila, Eupatorium purpureum,* **Althœa** *officinalis, Uva ursi, Triticum.*

### Mouth and Tongue.

° Aphthæ, with urinary disorders, in children.

° Cancerous tumor on the tongue.

### Urinary Organs.

Increases the flow of urine and removes its acridity.

° Scalding and burning during micturition in fevers.

* Dysuria and suppression of urine in young children.

° Strangury of women, from idiopathic or reflex irritation of the urinary apparatus.

° Dysuria, with frequent ineffectual urging and scanty discharge.

° Gravel and the various attendant sufferings.

### Generalities.

Its use causes so much "constant chilliness" that patients complain of it.

It is said to be contra-indicated in atonic or torpid urinary disorders.

° Scurvy; aphthæ, and inveterate cutaneous affections.

° Hard nodulated tumor of the tongue, of a cancerous nature. (See case detailed in New Remedies, second edition.)

It favors the production of healthy granulations on the ulcerated surface of cancers.

# GALLIC ACID
### *(The astringent principle of Nut. Gall.)*

DESCRIPTION.—It is said that Gallic acid differs from Tannic acid only in the latter containing more water. Gallic acid forms white, satiny, needle-like crystals, odorless, of a sweetish, acid, styptic taste. It dissolves in one hundred parts temperate water; much more readily in hot water and alcohol. Exposed to the atmosphere it absorbs oxygen, decomposes, and becomes dark colored.

OFFICINAL PREPARATION.—Triturations.

ANALOGUES.—*Geranium, Rhatany, Kino, Tannin, Plumbum, etc.*

[The symptoms marked " K," are from provings by Dr. D. S. Kimball, in *Observer*, Vol. IX.]

### Eyes.
\* Photophobia, and burning itching of the eyelids.

### Throat.
\* Roughness, and great secretion of phlegm in the throat. (*K.*)

° Mucus in the posterior harp fauces, and throat, especially on washing, in morning. (*K.*)

At night, dryness in the mouth and throat, and bad taste.

### Chest.
In the morning, aching in the right side of the chest and shoulders, and muscles of the neck.

### Abdomen.
Flatulency and pain in the bowels, at night. (*K.*)

Sensation of contraction in the anus, with large, bulky stool. (*K.*)

\**After* stool, a smarting, aching, faint, sick, hungry and gnawing sensation in the *bowels*, extending to the stomach, with *nausea*, with an astringent sensation there.(*K.*)

° Irritable condition of hæmorrhoids, after stool. (*K.*)

° Swelling, smarting and soreness in the hæmorrhoidal tumors. (*K.*).

Uneasy distension of the bladder, with greatly increased flow of pale, tasteless, limpid urine. (*K.*)

° Hæmorrhage from the kidneys. (*Hale.*)

Frequent itching of the skin in various places. (*K.*)

### *(See Therapeutics.)*

# GELSEMINUM SEMPERVIRENS.*

### (*Yellow Jessamine.*)

BOTANICAL DESCRIPTION.—This plant is likewise known by the name of *Field Jessamine* and *Woodbine;* it is the *Bignonia Sempervirens* of Linnæus, and the *Gelseminum nitidum* of Michaux and Purch. It is named the Gelsemi*um* nitidans by some authors. It has a twisting, smooth, glabrous *stem*, with opposite, perennial, lanceolate, entire *leaves*, which are dark above, pale beneath, and which stand on short petioles; the *flowers* are yellow, having an agreeable but rather narcotic odor, and stand on axillary peduncles; the *calyx* is very small, with five sepals; the *corolla* is funnel-form, with a spreading border, and five lobes, nearly equal; *stamens*, five; *pistils*, two; *capsules*, two-celled, compressed, flat, two-partible; *seeds* flat, and attached to the margins of the valves. The berries are black.

This is one of the most beautiful climbing plants of our Southern States, ascending lofty trees, and forming festoons from one tree to another, and in its flowering season, in the early spring, scenting the atmosphere with its delicious odor. On account of its gorgeous yellow flowers, and the rich perfume which they impart, as well as the deep shade it affords, it is extensively cultivated in the gardens of the South, as an ornamental vine. It grows in the North as an exotic. It begins to blossom about the first of March, and its blossoming season lasts until the end of May. The root is several feet in length, with scattered fibres, and varies from two to three lines in diameter, to nearly two inches. The internal part of the root is woody, and of a light yellowish color, the external part or bark, in which the medicinal virtues are said principally to reside, is of a light snuff color, and from half a line to three lines in thickness.

A vine, the root of which is sometimes gathered for the Gelseminum, resembles it very much in appearance, though it is of a lighter color, and the outer bark is covered with white specks or marks somewhat similar to those on young cherry or peach limbs, and the lower part of old vines becomes rough and have small tendrils that fasten upon the bark of trees, and which are never seen on the Gelseminum. The bark of the vine is also more brittle, and the leaves are always on long footstalks which are opposite, at the end of which are two opposite leaves, almost exactly resembling the Aristolochia Serpentaria. The root is almost white, very tough, straight, and about the same length of the medicinal root, and has a slightly bitter, disagreeable, nauseous taste. I never saw any of the flowers, though they are said to resemble the others in shape, but are *snowy white*, with a slight unpleasant odor. The plant is called the *White Poison Vine* and *White Jessamine.*

I am thus particular in giving a correct description of this plant, in order that there shall be no mistake about the matter. Homœopathic pharmaceutists above all others, should be scrupulously careful to prepare

---

* The correct botanical name of this plant is probably *Gelsemium nitidans*, but I have retained the name by which it was first known to the profession. (*Hale.*)

the medicines we use in their utmost purity. The Gelseminum, more than any other vegetable remedy, demands the most careful preparation. It is not known to me whether the leaves possess any medicinal qualities; but I should suppose from analogy that they possess as much comparative power as the leaves of Aconite or Veratrum viride. The tincture made from the flowers is comparatively inert.

OFFICINAL PREPARATIONS.—Tincture of the fresh bark of the root; dilutions.

ANALOGUES.—*Aconite, Agaricus, Belladonna, Conium, Cimicifuga, Hyos-cyamus, Chloral, Iberis, Lachnanthes, Opium, Rhus, Stramonium, Solanum.*

### Mental Sphere.

\* Dullness of all the mental faculties (*primary*).

\* Anxiety; incoherency of thought, aversion to study.

Melancholy and desponding mood.

\* Excessive irritability of body and mind (*secondary*).

° Nervous excitement of hysterical patients.

° Stupid, comatose conditions attending typhoid fever.

° Hysterical conditions in plethoric subjects.

### Head.

Pain in the head, over the eyes, and across the forehead.

Excruciating headache, accompanied by slight nausea; pain slightly mitigated by shaking the head.

Pain most frequently in the forehead and temples.

° Band-like pain surrounds the head, with shooting pains in each jaw.

Pain in the head constant, dull, stupefying and pressive.

Head feels light and large, with vertigo.

° Dull, dragging headache, mainly in the occiput, mastoid, and upper cervical region, extending to the shoulders; relieved when sitting by reclining head and shoulders on a high pillow.

° Congestion of the brain in children during dentition.

° Nervous headaches, from emotional excitement, etc.

° Hemicrania, with dimness of sight and double vision.

*Giddiness, a constant symptom.*

° Headache, extending from the occiput to the os frontis.

° In the morning on rising a dull pain in the head and a slight tendency to throbbing in right side of head.

° A settled, dull, dragging *headache*, mainly in the *occiput,* *mastoid,* and *upper cervical region,* extending to the

21

*shoulders*, relieved when sitting by reclining the head and
shoulders on a high pillow.

° Headache, coming on suddenly, with dimness of sight or
double vision, with dizziness followed by great heaviness
of the head, semi-stupor, dull, heavy expression of the
face, great vascular reaction, full pulse, etc.

Cramp-like pains of drawing or tearing character, aggravated
by study or exertion, following fever and ague.

° Headache (neuralgic) after cerebro-spinal meningitis; "a
terrible neuralgia, commencing in the upper portion of
the spinal cord, proceeding thence gradually through the
upper portion of the cerebrum, and terminating in a
bursting pain in the forehead and eyeballs, with *aggravation* about 10 A. M., *worse* when lying down, with nausea,
vomiting, cold sweat on forehead, and cold feet; vertigo
and obscuration of sight on stooping; *a sensation as of a
band drawn tightly around the head above the ears, and
soreness in scalp and brain;* the vertebræ prominens and
cervical vertebræ sensitive to pressure. (Cured by *Gelseminum* 200*th*, three times a day.) " (*Dr. C. C. Smith.*)

° A relapse of the same patient, with the additional symptoms,
viz.: lameness and stiffness of neck; on waking at night
*retraction of head backward*, relieved by bending head
*forward;* frequent urging to urinate, with partial loss of
power in the sphincter vesicæ; heat in palm of hands and
itching all over the body, preventing sleep; after scratching, a raw sore, surrounded with blisters, would appear.
(These symptoms were also cured by *Gelseminum* 200.)

ᵓ Periodical hemicrania (over one eye).

**Eyes.**

* Great heaviness of the lids; difficulty of opening or keeping
them open.
* Fullness and congestion of the lids.
* Diplopia when inclining the head toward the shoulder.
* Misty or glimmering appearance before the eyes.
* Distant objects seemed indistinct as I rode or walked.
* Dilatation of the pupils; amaurosis; diplopia; blindness;
dimness of sight.

Sense of sight tardy in following the movements of objects.

* Pain in both eyes, particularly the left, with dimness of sight.

ᶜ Inflammation, with great flow of tears at intervals.

Total blindness, with violent dizziness.

° Asthenopia; amaurosis.

Disturbance of the power of accommodation, similar to *Calabar*, *Chloral*, and analagous drugs.

### Ears.

* Rushing and roaring in the ears.

* Sudden and temporary loss of hearing.

Digging in the right ear; also, stitches.

° Neuralgic otalgia, especially when periodical.

° Earache from a cold; (internally, also a drop or two on cotton put in the ear).

### Nose.

* Watery discharge from the nose, with sneezing in morning.

* Tingling in the nose; bloody, mucus discharge.

° Colds in the head, with fluent coryza from the nose, hoarseness, cough, soreness of the throat and chest.

° Epistaxis, with suppressed menses.

° Acute coryza, with dull headache and fever.

° *Hay-fever*, with morning sneezing.

### Face.

* Erythema of the face and neck.

* Sensation of stiffness in the muscles of the jaws.

° Facial neuralgia, with or without contractions and twitchings of the muscles.

° Orbital neuralgia, periodic, every day at the same hour.

Papulous eruptions of the face.

° Trismus.

### Mouth and Throat.

* Stiffness of the jaws; difficulty of opening the mouth.

° Pains of a shooting character in the jaws.

Dryness of the mouth; thickly coated tongue.

* Tongue red, raw, and painful.

* Partial paralysis of the glottis and tongue.

Irritation and soreness of the fauces.

* Paralytic dysphagia.

\* Painful sensation of something having lodged in œsophagus.

° Spasmodic sensation and cramp-like pains in œsophagus.

° Œsophagitis (catarrhal), a *not* rare affection. (*Hale.*)

° Tonsillitis, from acute catarrh.

° Spasmodic affections of the throat.

° Spasmodic croup (catarrhal), with high fever.

Thirst during the sweat, clammy, feverish taste.

Great hunger; eructation; nausea.

Yellowish-white coating of the tongue, with fœtid breath.

### Stomach.

\* Feeling of emptiness and weakness in the stomach and bowels.

Distension, with pain and nausea.

Rumbling and dull pain in the epigastrium, relieved by expulsion of flatus.

° Sensation of weight in the stomach, with dull pain.

### Abdomen and Stool.

Rumbling and roaring in the abdomen, with emissions of flatus above and below.

Periodical pains in the abdomen, with yellow diarrhœa in the evening.

Bowels loose, but great difficulty in discharging anything.

Severe griping in the lower abdomen; no relief till discharge of large, deeply bilious discharges.

° Slow stool, leaving a sensation of more remaining to be passed, and of abdominal repletion.

° Spasmodic and flatulent colic.

° Acute enteritis (catarrhal), during cold, damp, or hot, damp weather.

° Neuralgia of the intestines, periodic, malarial.

° *Diarrhœa, from exciting emotions;* sometimes involuntary.

° Diarrhœa of soldiers from mental and moral excitement.

° Dysentery (epidemic), malarial or catarrhal.

° Paralysis of the sphincter ani, with involuntary diarrhœa, the result of nervous excitement.

### Liver.

Bilious diarrhœa, of the color of green tea (*primary*).

Jaundice, with prostration, clay-colored stool, etc. (*secondary*).

Deficient secretion of bile (*secondary*).

° Passive congestion of the liver, with dimness of sight, vertigo, and fullness of the head.

### Urinary Organs.

Urine much increased in quantity.

\* Frequent urging, with scanty emission, and tenesmus of the bladder.

\* Enuresis, from paralysis of the sphincter, in children at night.

° Spasm of the bladder, with alternate dysuria and enuresis.

\* Profuse urination, with relief of the headache.

° Constant, involuntary discharge of urine every fifteen minutes.

° Paralytic conditions of the sphincter muscles of the bladder.

° Acute catarrhal conditions of the bladder and uterus.

### Generative Organs.

*Female.*—\* *Dysmenorrhœa of a neuralgic or spasmodic character.*

\* Cramps in the abdomen and legs during pregnancy.

° Convulsions during pregnancy, with complete unconsciousness.

° Convulsions (apoplectiform) during labor.

° False pains before parturition.

° Rigid os uteri during confinement.

° Menorrhagia (?) (from lack of contractility).

° Inefficient labor-pains from uterine inertia.

Sensation of heaviness in the uterine region, with increased leucorrhœal discharge.

*Male.*—\* Involuntary emission of semen without an erection.

° Seminal weakness from irritability of the seminal vesicles.

" Spermatorrhœa from relaxation and debility.

° *Gonorrhœa*, in the acute stage; great pain, inflammation, and scanty discharge; (one of the best remedies.) (*Hale.*)

° Suppressed gonorrhœa, with fever, rheumatism, orchitis, etc.; (it will restore the discharge very soon, with abatement of all the other symptoms). (*Ib.*)

\* Sweat of the scrotum, warm. (*Hoyne.*)

### Larynx and Trachea.

Paroxysms of hoarseness, with dryness of the throat.

Cough from tickling and dry roughness of the fauces.

° Soreness in the chest when coughing.

° Acute catarrhal bronchitis.

° Severe cough; pain in the chest; tenderness in the epigastrium, with vomiting in the paroxysms.

° Spasmodic croup, (laryngismus stridulus).

° Periodic *aphonia;* loss of voice only during the menses; (cured with the third dil.) (*Meyhoffer, Diseases of Organs of Respiration, Vol. I.*)

### Chest.

\* Constrictive pain around the lower part of the chest.

Paroxysmal pain in the upper part of right lung, when taking a long breath.

° Periodical pains in the pectoral muscles.

Heavy and labored respirations; expirations sudden and forcible.

° Forming stage in pneumonia.  (*Veratrum v.*)

° Convulsive, spasmodic cough.

° Slow breathing and slow pulse.

### Heart.

\* Stitching sensation in the region of the heart.

\* *Feeling as if the heart would stop beating if she did not move about.*

\* Pulse frequent, soft, weak, almost imperceptible.

Fluttering pulse; pulse full, 120; pulse slow and full, or slow and soft.

Sensation as though the blood had ceased to circulate; pulse reduced from 112 to 56 in twelve hours.

Heart's action slow and feeble; the beats of the heart cannot be felt.

The action of the heart and arteries much depressed, with cold hands and feet; chills and pains in the head.

A sensible motion of the heart as though it had attempted its beat, which it failed fully to accomplish, and the pulse then each time intermitted, worse when lying down in bed, especially when lying on the left side.  (*Wells.*)

° Excessive action of the heart from plethora, congestion, neuralgic or rheumatic irritation, or hysterical palpitation.

## Back and Neck.

Dull, aching pain in back, extending up to the occiput. .

*Pains in the neck, like those of cerebro-spinal congestion.*

° Chilliness and chills running up the back.

° Myalgia of the cervical muscles.

° Congestion of the spinal cord and cerebellum.

## Upper Extremities.

* Severe pain in both extremities, deep-seated in the muscles.

Severe aching pain in left elbow.

° Rheumatic pains in extremities.

Arms become powerless; loss of voluntary motion.

Coldness of the wrists and hands.

## Lower Extremities.

* Deep-seated, aching pains in bones and joints of extremities.

* Paroxysmal pain in the lower extremities.

Pains in left foot and ankle, with spasmodic contraction of
the toes.

Crampy pains in the lower limbs, worse on motion.

Excessive drawing and contracting pains in gastroc nemius
muscle of the left leg.

Coldness of the extremities, especially the feet, often severe.

Rheumatic pain in the right knee, and left side of the neck.

Paralytic symptoms throughout the entire muscular system.

## Skin.

* Papulous eruption, resembling measles.

Pimples on the forehead and neck.

° *Measles* (one of the best remedies, especially for the catarrhal
symptoms).

° Erysipelas, not vesicular or phlegmonous, but a milder
variety, with erythema or papular eruption.

## Sleep.

* Disposition to sleep, a sort of *stupor*.

Drowsiness and long, sound sleep.

Unusually sound morning sleep, with difficult, weary waking.

Languor and drowsiness when trying to study.

° Stupor attending the fevers of children.

° Sleeplessness during dentition.

° Sleeplessness from nervous irritation.

### Fever.

\* Marked decrease in the frequency of the pulse.

\* Chilliness, especially along the back, followed by heat.

\* Febrile chilliness, cold extremities, heat of the head and face.

\* As soon as the reaction takes place after the chill, the pulse rises as much above the normal standard as it was depressed below it.

° Simple fever, without functional disturbance.

° Flushed, crimson face during the fever.

° Remittent fever (infantile or malarial).

° Irritative fever, from abscesses, internal inflammation, etc.

° Intermittents (post typhoids).

° Fevers characterized by severe chill, little shaking, followed by fever.

° *Fever without thirst; wants to lie still and rest; tonsils inflamed, right side.*

° Typhoid fever in the first stages.

° Scarlet fever, with stupor, and flushed, red face.

° Suppressed intermittents, with general prostration, aching and soreness in the body; "dumb-ague."

° Intermittent fever; malarial, generally *quotidian.*

° Rheumatic fever (especially in muscular rheumatism).

° Intermittent fever (tertian type); pain in the head and pains over the body, when he has no chill; tongue not much coated.

° Intermittent fever (tertian type); fever five hours, very hot, with delirium, jerking of the limbs, violent headache; aching in one leg.

° Intermittent fever (tertian type); no chill; fever at 10 A. M.; great pain in the back and thighs.

° Intermittent fever; chills from fifteen minutes to two hours long, followed by heat, often with sleep one to twelve hours long, and perspiration for some time.

° Fever coming on every evening after supper, which gradually increased, and went off before morning, the patient continuing asleep.

° Typhoid fever in a child of five years; nervous movements, every night, like spasms; oscillation of the eyeballs.

° In scarlet fever it determines the eruption to the surface, controls the pulse, calms the nervous erethism, and lessens the cerebral congestion.

° In the forming and inflammatory stage of measles, with chilliness, watery discharge from the nose, etc.

° Rubeola; it seems to prevent chronic catarrhal affections, and bronchitis.

° In all eruptive fevers the *Gelseminum* may be thought of.

° Especially in the eruptive fevers of children when there is a strong tendency to convulsions at or about the time of the appearance of the eruption.

### Nervous System.

Acute, sudden, darting pains, evidently along single nerve branches, in almost any part of the body and limbs, sometimes so sudden and acute as to make me start.

° Neuralgia; absence of organic lesion, with indistinct or double periodicity.

° Hysterical epilepsy, after suppressed menses, lasting an hour or two: so severe was the spasm of the glottis that asphyxia seemed inevitable.

° Epilepsy of ten years' standing, preceded by dull feeling in the head and vertex, and some pain and fullness in the region of medulla oblongata; (marked improvement from the use of *Gelseminum*).

° Tetanus; spasmodic action entirely ceased after the third dose.

Seems strongly indicated in hydrophobia, as it relaxes all the muscles, calms the fury of nervous excitement, relaxes the glottis, and prevents spasms.

° Laryngismus stridulus.

° Coma and apoplexy, sub-arachnoid, arising from passive congestion, with nervous exhaustion.

° Hysteria in a lady of 40.

° *Cerebro-spinal meningitis*, ushered in by a severe chill, accompanied by evident congestion of the spine and brain, etc.

° Nervous chills, in which, with shivering and chattering of the teeth, there is no sensation of chilliness.

### Glandular System.
° It first arrests the secretion of glands, and afterwards increases it.

### Muscular System.
\* Intense prostration of the whole muscular system.

° Myalgia from over-exertion, lameness and stiffness for several days.

° *Acute myalgia*, accompanied with fever.

### Mucous System.
\* Catarrhal condition of all the mucous membranes, acute, with fever, or chronic when suppressed, and other disturbances appear.

---

# GERANIUM MACULATUM.
### (*Cranesbill.*)

BOTANICAL DESCRIPTION.—This plant is also known by the names of Cranesbill, Geranium, Spotted Geranium, Alum root, Crowfoot, etc. It has a perennial, horizontal, thick, rough, knobby and fleshy root, with short fibres, and sends up annually one or more erect, angular, or round, retroversely pubescent, herbaceous, dichotomous stems, from one to two feet high, and of a grayish green color. The leaves are spreading, hairy, palmate, with three, five or seven deeply cleft lobes, two leaves at each fork; the lobes are cuneiform and entire at the base, incisely serrate above. The radical-leaves are on long petioles, erect and terate; the leaves at the top are opposite and subsessile, and those at the middle of the stem are opposite, petiolate, and generally reflexed. The stipules are linear or lanceolate. The flowers are large and generally purple, mostly in pairs, on unequal pedicles, sometimes umbelled at the ends of the peduncles.

OFFICINAL PREPARATIONS.—Tincture or trituration of the root.

ANALOGUES.—*Gallic acid, Tannic acid, Hamamelis, Plumbum, Ratanhia, Rheum.*

[The tincture should be made with water and alcohol, equal parts. It contains 136 grs. of Tannic acid and 120 grs. of Gallic acid in 7,000 grs. of the root.]

### (*No provings.*)

° Abnormal discharges from mucous surfaces, after the inflammation has subsided.

° Catarrhal ozœna; (used topically).

° Intestinal catarrh, chronic; (internally).

° Leucorrlœa, vaginal; (topically).

° Hæmorrhages from ulcerated surfaces.

° Gonorrhœa and gleet; (as an injection.)

° Diabetes and Bright's disease.

° Aphthous stomatitis and **mercurial salivation.**

° All morbid fluxes connected **with relaxation** and debility. (*Rafinesque.*)

° Hæmorrhage from the kidneys; **equal to Gallic** acid. (*Hale.*)

° Catarrhal secretion, profuse, **from the** mucous membrane of the fauces and posterior nares.

° Chronic diarrhœa and dysentery.

[When used for the above named conditions it must be used in material doses, generally topically as well as internally, because the drug would cause such disease by its secondary action. Its (opposite) primary **effects** would call for the high attenuations. (*Hale.*)]

---

# GNAPHALIUM POLYCEPHALUM.

### (*Cud Weed.*)

BOTANICAL DESCRIPTION.—This plant is indigenous and known by the various names of Indian Posey, Sweet Life Everlasting, White Balsam, Old-field Balsam, etc. It is herbaceous and annual, with an erect, whitish, woody and much branched *stem*, from one to two feet in height. *Leaves* alternate, sessile, linear-lanceolate, acute, entire, scabrous above, and whitish tomentose beneath. *Flowers* tubular and yellow, in heads clustered at the summit of the panicled corymbose branches, ovate-conical before expansion, then obovate, involucre imbricate, with whitish, ovate, oblong, rather obtuse scales. *Florets* of the ray, subulate—of the disc, entire. Receptacle, flat, naked, pappus pilose, scabrous capillary.

It is found in Canada and various parts of the United States, growing in old fields and on dry, barren lands, and bearing whitish yellow flowers in July and August. The leaves have a pleasant aromatic smell, and an aromatic, slightly bitter and astringent, but rather an agreeable taste. They yield their properties to alcohol and water.

OFFICINAL PREPARATIONS.—Tincture of the plant.

ANALOGUES.—*Anisum, Chamomilla, Ipecacuanha, Mercurius, Pulsatilla.*

### Head and Face.

Giddiness, especially after rising from a recumbent position.

Pain in the back of the head, of a dull, continuous character with shooting pain in the eyeballs.

Neuralgic pain, of an intermittent form, of the superior maxillary of both sides.

Dull, heavy expression of countenance; face appears bloated. Fullness about the temples.

### Mouth and Throat.

Mouth feels parched and tastes badly.

Flat, sweetish, sickening taste in the mouth.

Tongue covered with long white fur.

### Stomach and Abdomen.

Flatus of stomach, windy eructations, nausea and hiccough.

* Colic pains in various parts of the abdomen, which is sensitive to pressure, in cœcum.

Borborygmus, with much emission of flatus.

### Rectum and Stool.

Looseness of bowels, with passage of pale-colored fœces (*primary*).

Rumbling in the bowels, with stool before breakfast.

* Diarrhœic discharges in morning and during the day, with irritable temper; pains in bowels in children.

* Vomiting and purging, like cholera morbus, in the night and all next day.

Constipation for three days after the diarrhœa (*secondary*).

Copious, watery stool at night, with much prostration, nausea, pain, and rumbling in the bowels.

Dark-colored, liquid, offensive stool in the morning, afterwards pain in the bowels all day.

### Genito-Urinary Organs.

Sensation of fullness and tension in the bladder, even when just emptied.

Pain in the kidneys, with frequent but slight pain in prostate gland.

Increase of sexual passion, waking with an erection and urgent desire for an embrace (a thing which never occurred before); the desire was rather mechanical than passional.

° Irritation of the prostate gland.

### Trunk and Superior Extremities.

Feeling of debility in the arms, with rheumatic-like pains.

Pains in the chest, darting from side to side.

Numbness of the lower parts of the back, with lumbago.

Sensations of weight in the pelvis.

### Inferior Extremities.

* Intense pain along the sciatic nerve, following its larger ramifications.

Frequent cramps of the calves of the legs.

Cramps of the feet when in bed.

Rheumatic pains in the knee and ankle joints.

\* Sciatica. (*Dr. Banks, Dr. Woodbury.*)

Feeling of numbness occasionally taking the place of the sciatic
pains, making exercise very fatiguing.

---

# GOSSYPIUM HERBACEUM.

### (*Cotton Plant.*)

BOTANICAL DESCRIPTION.—A biennial or triennial herb, with a fusiform
root, giving off small radicles, and a round, pubescent, branching *stem*,
about five feet high. The *leaves* are hairy, palmate, with five sub-lanceolate,
rather acute lobes, three large and two small, lateral, a single gland on the
midvein below, half an inch from the base. *Stipules* falcate-lanceolate.
*Flowers* yellow. *Calyx* cap-shaped, obtusely fine-toothed, surrounded by
an involucel of three united and cordate leaves, deeply and incisely toothed.
*Petals* five, deciduous, with a purple spot near the base. *Style* simple,
marked with three or five furrows toward the apex. *Stigmas* three or five,
involved in cotton, somewhat plano-convex, and reniform. The parts used
in medicine are the *inner bark of the root*, and the seeds.

OFFICINAL PREPARATIONS.—Tincture of the root; infusion.

ANALOGUES.—*Asarum, Apis, Cimicifuga, Bryonia, Pulsatilla, Sepia,
Lilium, Secale, Sabina, Ustilago.*

## Head.

Stinging pain in the head, going from the forehead to the
vertex.

° Pain, first burning, then stinging, extending from both temporal bones to the middle of the frontal bones.

° Drawing pain over the eyes, with stinging pain in the pupils.

° Giddiness of the head.

## Nose.

Both nostrils swollen and inflamed, the left one most so.

## Mouth and Throat.

Tonsils much swollen, the right one most.

## Gastric.

Nausea, with accumulation of saliva in the mouth.

\* Nausea, with inclination to vomit before breakfast in the
morning. (*Williamson.*)

Taste of bad eggs, better after breakfast.

Rotating sensation in the pit of the stomach, with uneasiness, anxiety, and sighing.

Stitching in the right hypochondrium, lasting for a few minutes, and then drawing pain from both hypochondriac regions to the pit of the stomach.

° Anorexia, with uneasy, depressed feeling at the scrobiculis cordis, at the time of the menses.

### Genital Organs.

Stinging pain in both ovarian regions, and at the same time drawing toward the uterus, lasting about ten minutes at a time.

*Menses* too watery and nineteen days too late.

Soreness between the thighs and vulva, with a watery secretion.

Soft tumor between left thigh and vulva, first the size of a pea, and increasing to the size of a pigeon's egg, secreting a watery fluid, with sticking pain as if caused by a needle, worse at night.

Swelling of the outer part of the left labium, accompanied with intolerable itching; some swelling in the right labium.

The outer skin of both labia studded with innumerable pale, somewhat reddish granules.

Is said to cause miscarriage at any period of pregnancy, but sufficient proof of this is wanting.

° *Amenorrhœa; dysmenorrhœa; menorrhagia.* (*Williamson.*)

* Morning sickness, ° during the early months of pregnancy, with the following symptoms: sensitiveness over the hypogastric region; prostration of the nervous system almost to syncope; and in the morning nausea from the least motion soon after waking, with distress in the pit of the stomach; and, immediately on raising the head, retching and violent efforts to vomit; at first very little comes up, except wind, with a loud noise; soon after, saliva and some thick fluid is discharged, and, occasionally, after much retching, a little bilious matter, but rarely any ingesta; wind is often discharged from the bowels during the efforts to vomit. (*Ib.*)

° Morning vomiting, followed by faintness; she was unable to rise from the bed. (*Ib.*)

° Parturient expulsive efforts *without* pain. (?) (Secale *with* pain.)

\* *Sterility*, from uterine torpor.

\* The menstrual flow lasts about twenty-four hours, and then becomes very sparse and painful.

° Retained placenta.

° Scanty and painful or painless **menses.**

° Amenorrhœa, with anæmia, dyspeptic **symptoms, etc.**

### Extremities.

Tearing pains in the right arm and hand, and jumping pain from one finger to another.

Pale, red, papular eruption on the back of both hands, with intense itching and a watery exudation.

Crawling sensation in all the fingers, as if from worms.

Heavy feeling in both hands, better when hanging them down, and worse in the warmth of the bed.

Stinging, drawing, tearing, and burning pain in the lower extremities.

Trembling, twitching, and weary sensation in the legs.

Small, round, dark red spots, with pale red spots, around the patellæ, on the shins and ankles, itching intensely.

### Generalities.

Itching of the skin over the whole body.

General lassitude, with pains as if beaten.

General external chilliness, with internal heat.

### Characteristics.

The pains are wandering, come and go (like Pulsatilla).

The pains are generally from above downward, aggravated by motion, relieved by rest.

The itching changes to burning after scratching.

The symptoms observe alternate periods of aggravation and amelioration (like Bell. and Secale).

Sympathetic symptoms of the stomach, heart, bowels, and nervous system, arising from disturbance of the uterine functions, connected with menstruation or pregnancy.

[All the above pathogenetic symptoms, and many of the curative, as well as the characteristic indications, are taken from a report by the late Dr. Williamson, of Philadelphia. But one proving was made; others are needed to verify it.—*Hale.*]

# GYMNOCLADUS CANADENSIS.
*(American Coffee-tree.)*

BOTANICAL DESCRIPTION.—A pretty large tree, destitute of spines or prickles, with rough bark and few stout branches. Leaves unequally bipinnate. Flowers in axillary racemes. Petals white. Legume six to ten inches long and nearly two inches broad; a little curved, and of a brown color. Seeds more than half an inch in diameter. The Gymnocladus is one of the fairest trees in our Western woods, and is planted as an ornament in the gardens of Europe. A group of them stands near Paris, some of which are forty feet high. In their native air they reach even fifty and sixty feet in height, with a stem of twelve or fifteen inches in diameter; even when standing alone it does not branch out at a height of less than thirty feet; the top is formed by a few but very long branches, and is not wide, but beautifully regular. It flourishes only in the best soil, with black walnut, red elm, poplar, blue ash, honey locust, etc.; has a useful, hard wood, and bears, in some years, an abundance of large pods, containing two, three or four seeds, of a size of a walnut.

OFFICIAL PREPARATIONS.—Tincture of the seeds.

ANALOGUES.—*Agaricus, Æthusa, Belladonna, Cicuta, Hyosciamus, Lachesis, Lachnanthes, Solanum nigrum, Stramonium.*

## Mental Sphere.

Indifferent to what transpires.

Constantly forgetting.

## Head.

Fullness and pressure in and over the eyes.

Intense frontal headache, feeling as if the eyes were pushed forward.

Pain in left temple shooting through to the right side.

Intense headache, with stitches in the bowels.

Desire to lean the head on something; head feels as if bound up.

## Face and Eyes.

Sensation as of flies crawling over the right side of the face.

Face hot, swelled as in erysipelas.

Eyes feel as if pushed forward.

Burning in left orbit, and sensation as if it would be forced out.

Frequent, violent sneezing.

* Erysipelas of the face.

## Mouth and Throat.

Slightest draught of cold air sets the teeth aching.

* *Sore throat*, a dark livid redness of fauces and tonsils.

Tongue coated a bluish white.

Water in the mouth almost to vomiting.

F.21

## Stomach.

Nausea, with pain and fullness in the stomach.

Heat in the stomach, and sour, watery eructations.

Gulping of wind, nausea, dizziness, and uneasiness of the bowels.

## Abdomen.

Hot feeling in stomach and bowels after the cold chills.

Stitches and pinching pains in the bowels, disappearing after eructations.

Soreness of the abdomen.

## Stool.

Constipation.

Desire for stool, with inability.

Feeling in the abdomen as if diarrhœa would follow.

## Urinary Organs.

Frequent desire to urinate, with pressure and fullness.

Urine brown, yellow, turbid.

## Generative Organs.

Increased sexual desire.

## Larynx.

Tickling in the throat producing a cough.

Dry, racking cough in the evening (increases from morning till night).

## Chest.

Pain in right breast; pressure in the chest.

Stitches in the right breast, and on inspiration.

## Superior Extremities.

Violent pain in the left forearm, between the elbow and wrist.

Dull pain in the fingers.

Palms of the hands perspire.

## Lower Extremities.

Stinging pain in left knee joint.

Pain in left leg, from knee to ankle.

Peculiar feeling of numbness in the whole body. (Left side mostly affected.)

## Fever.

* Epidemic fevers, with typhoid character.

Cold chills and pain in the bowels.

Pulse small and quick; desire for increased heat.

22

# GUACO.

## (*Mikania Guaco.*)

DESCRIPTION.—A plant, or " *liane*," found in Central and South America
The Mikanias are climbing perennials, with opposite, commonly heart-
shaped and petioled leaves, and corymbos-panicled, flesh-colored flowers.
One species is indigenous to the United States, the M. scandens, " Climb
ing Hempweed;" flowers from July to September

OFFICINAL PREPARATIONS.—Tincture of the plant; dilutions.

ANALOGUES.—*Arsenicum* (*?*), *Baptisia* (*?*), *Mercurius* (*?*), *Phytolacca* (*?*),
*Veratrum album.*

° *Bites of venomous serpents.*

[Dr. C. Dunham gives the first account in American journals of this
plant, in the *American Homœopathic Review*, Vol. III., p. 423. He quotes
Humboldt, Forster, Schomberg, Poppig, and Tschudi, who all agree that
in South America the *Guaco* is the best remedy for the bites of poisonous
serpents. The freshly expressed juice of the plant is dropped into the
dilated wound, the surrounding parts are rubbed and covered with the
bruised leaves, and the juice at the same time taken internally. It is used
also as a prophylactic.]

° *Chancres; syphilis.*

[Turchitti states that the *Guaco*, locally applied, destroys the specific
property of the pus from a chancre, and prevents the production of a
second chancre by inoculation. He also claims for it positive curative
powers in syphilis.]

° *Cholera*, and similar maladies.

[Said to be used successfully in Mexico, Havana, Poland, and Venezuela.]

° *Cancers; obstinate ulcers.*

° Spinal and cerebro-spinal irritation.

[Dr. Elb, of Dresden. has made a proving of the *Guaco.* He refers to it
in an article on "Spinal Diseases" (*All. Hom. Zeit.*, 61, 72, *and* 23.) That
proving has never been translated, but by the kindness of Dr. C. Dunham,
I am in possession of a translation of the indications given by Dr. Elb for
the use of *Guaco* in "Spinal Diseases," which includes a portion of his
pathogenesis. After a few remarks upon the general term, spinal irritation, as embracing various conditions of congestion, anæmia, and irritation or algia, and pointing to certain remedies as corresponding in a
general way to these conditions, he desires, he says, to call attention to a
class of remedies, heroic, but not sufficiently considered in relation to
these affections. "From the symptoms produced by snake bites we cannot fail to see that serpent venom acts specifically upon the spinal marrow." He then cites and analyzes the symptoms of Lachesis, Crotalus,
and Naja tripudians, and gives the indications for each in spinal disease.
This done, he goes on as follows (*A. H. Z.*, 61, 23): "It being admitted by
homœopaths that the antidoting power of drugs resides not in their chemical properties, but must be referred to their similarity of physiological

action, we may assume that an antidote to serpent venom would produce on the healthy symptoms similar to those resulting from serpent venom.' This consideration induced him to prove *Mikania Guaco*, a noted antidote to snake bites, and he gives the symptoms in so far as they relate to the spinal cord.]

The *Guaco* produces in the nape of the neck burning, which extends to the shoulders; tearing stiffness, drawing tearing, extending to the axillæ; drawing tearing in and between the scapula, extending into the forearm; tearing, sticking tearing in the *back;* frequent fine stitches, tearing and violent drawing pain along the spine, more painful on bending; increased aching in the lumbo-sacral region and forward pressing; in connection with these spinal pains, severe aching in the occiput, which sometimes extend over the upper half of the back.

*In the upper extremities.*—Aching drawing and simple drawing pains in the deltoid muscle, with a paralyzed sensation; tearing and luxative pain in the shoulders—both of these sensations extending into the forearm; burning in the shoulder joint; tearing in the elbows and fingers.

*In the lower extremities.*—Soreness and pain as if beaten about the hip joint; drawing in the thigh; drawing and swollen feeling in the calves; very considerable heaviness in the legs, and drawing in them; tearing in the ankle joints; burning and tearing in the soles of the feet.

All the pains in the back and extremities are aggravated by motion, and mostly continue a long time.

The following very constant phenomena should not be disregarded: difficult digestion, there being no inflammatory affection; constriction of the larynx and tracheæ; deafness; heaviness of and difficulty of moving the tongue (all of these symptoms came from doses of from five to twenty drops of the tincture).

To draw from these few and not severe sensations along the medulla spinalis and in the extremities, the conclusion that *Guaco* must play an important part in the treatment of spinal affections, would be very venturesome, had I not instituted upon those indications some experiments upon the sick. The affection alone of the tongue, the muscles

of deglutition, and the larynx is to be regarded as an un-
mistakable picture of a commencing paralysis proceeding
from the medulla oblongata, as we see it frequently in a
more developed grade in apoplexy. Inasmuch as I experienced during the proving no depression of spirits, no
decrease of mental activity, and in general no debility,
but rather an excited condition, and suffered often from
headache and heat of the face, I became convinced that
the paretic conditions as well as the back pains depended
not upon a direct affection (lesion) of the medulla, but
rather upon a hyperæmia of the same; and this view is
supported by the fact that during the proving there were
clear indications of a congestion of the hemorrhoidal vessels. Moreover, the character of the affection of the extremities—the absence of numbness, formication, etc.,
the customary forerunners of paralysis—seems to indicate
that a primary affection (lesion) of the nerves, at least a
paralytic, did not exist in the parts, while, on the other
hand, the fact that most of the symptoms of the extremities originated in the point of origin of the nerves from
the medulla and extended thence to the ends of these
nerves, gave clear evidence that these phenomena were
not *local*, but dependent upon the spinal cord. On the
basis of this significance of the pathogenesy I have often
given *Guaco* in cases of spinal irritation, and in my experience it has shown itself almost " specifically " helpful
in robust, not anæmic, ruddy persons, inclined to congestions, excitable, especially in males, where the spinal disease
has not been caused by loss of fluids or depressing causes
—in persons disposed to hemorrhoids, where the pains,
with only a slight feeling of weakness in the lumbo-sacral
region, are mostly in the upper part of the vertebral
column, mostly aching, drawing or sticking in character,
very severe, with at the same time only pains in the extremities, but no paretic conditions, and the parts affected
are extremely sensitive to pressure. This condition may
be acute or chronic. We have, then, before us a real
picture of pure material stasis. If with this condition be

associated inflammatory or febrile symptoms, then, according to my experience, *Guaco* does no good, and is far inferior to Belladonna. Arterial stasis may pass on into inflammations, or, by the rupture of vessels, may terminate in apoplexy. Those in which *Guaco* is indicated incline to the latter termination. It has therefore approved itself a most excellent remedy in paralysis resulting from pressure on brain or spinal marrow, *i. e.*, apoplectic paralysis. I was led to these experiments by the already mentioned paralyzed state of the tongue in connection with most violent headache, heat and redness of the face, *i. e.*, a close resemblance to the forerunners and sequelæ of apoplexy. Frequent administration of it has taught me that this remedy is of use only after the first violent febrile storm has abated, no matter whether a soporous condition exists or not. *Guaco* developes its most eminent curative power when extravasation has caused paralysis of the tongue or of the extremities; the former is often relieved in a few hours; the latter yields to *Guaco* much more quickly than to any other remedy. But *Guaco* renders inestimable service, not only in acute but also in very old paralysis, when these have resulted from extravasations of blood and not from exudations. It is a peculiarity of its action that the paralysis of the lower extremities yields very readily while that of the upper extremities is seldom entirely cured by it. It matters not whether the paralysis be confined to one side or not.

## GUARÆA TRICHLOIDES.
### (*Ball Wood.*)

DESCRIPTION.—This is a large tree growing in the Antilles.
The following pathogenesis is from provings made by Dr. Petroz, of Spain.

OFFICINAL PREPARATIONS.—Tincture of the bark
ANALOGUES.—(?)

### Mental Sphere.

Moral anxiety, indifference, indecision, confusion of thought, fearful of losing the reason, agitation in the evening.

### Head.

Vertigo on stooping.

Turning vertigo, and vertigo on seeing objects in confusion

Immobility of the head; heaviness.

Compression; constriction; contraction.

Buzzing; sensation as if the brain were falling forward.

Headache, depressing the eyes.

Symptoms relieved or diminished by motion.

A sensation as of a blow on the head, leaving a sort of stupefaction, with diminution of the power of thought for
several days.

### Eyes.

Sensation as if the eyeballs were being pushed out.

Dilatation of the pupils.

Conjunctivitis; chemosis; swelling of the lachrymal glands.

Paralysis of the eyelids.

Objects have a greyish appearance.

° *Chemosis* where the pad was so extended and so thick that
nothing of the eye could be seen but the pupil, at the
bottom of a veritable tunnel.

### Ears.

Sensation as if stopped up, with pressure outwards.

Eruption behind the ears.

### Nose.

Coryza, with indurated excretion; heat, and ineffectual effort
to sneeze.

### Face.

Pain as if burnt; puffiness below the eyes; swellings which
suppurate.

Yellowish spots on the temples; acne rosacea.

° Lupus of an ochre-red color.

### Mouth and Throat.

Twitchings of the mouth.

Pimples, scabs, chaps on the lips and at the commissures;
swelling of the upper lip.

Compressive, corrosive pain of the teeth.

° Roughness, with caries of the palate bone.

Tongue feels cold and dry.

Tearing pain in the tongue; lancinations; paralysis of the
tongue.

Tongue is heavy, swelled, bleeding; greenish-yellow fur.

Absence of thirst, with dryness of the mouth.

Sensation of constriction and of burning heat in the throat.

Swelling of the tonsils, rendering swallowing difficult.

Throat is better on taking warm drinks, or on coughing.

### Stomach.

° Sensation as if bruised; itching; constriction.

Sensation of rupture at the præcordial region, worse after
supper.

Bitter risings, with distension and pressure at the stomach.

Vomiting of bitter, greenish matter.

### Abdomen.

Pressure in the region of the umbilicus.

° Lancination in the groins and inguinal rings.

° Pain, tensive as if contused in the abdomen walls.

### Stool.

° Ailments from flatulence.

° Chronic constipation.

Constipation during dentition.

Constipation at the anus and rectum.

° During stool, pain in the rectum.

Dysentery.

### Urinary Organs.

Inflammation of the bladder.

° Involuntary urination.

° Frequent desire to urinate in the evening.

Urine clay colored.

### Generative Organs.

*Female.*—° Itching.

Menorrhagia.

° Fœtid leucorrhœa after the menses.

° Labor pains too feeble; suppression of labor pains.

Lochia scanty.

### Chest.

* Cough; whooping cough, with bloody sputa; dry hacking
cough; cough deep, suffocating, violent, with expectoration.

The cough is accompanied with sweat, pain, excoriation and constriction of the chest; it comes on after one has cried, at the moment of falling asleep, or after taking cold; it is preceded by an itching in the throat, by an irritation in the larynx.

* Asthma of Millar; attacks of suffocation; burning respiration; sobbing respiration; intermittent constriction of the chest; the symptoms of the respiration are **more** marked on putting the hand to the throat.

° Sense of anxiety; emptiness; distension of the chest; heaviness.

° Lancinations in the right side of the chest, increased by deep inspirations.

### Back.

Weakness of the muscles.
Constricted feeling in the back; burning in the loins.
Cutting pain in the sacrum.

### Upper Extremities.

Violent shocks in the arms; cramps in the arms; burning heat in the arms; brown spots under the arms; boils on the arms; paralysis of the metacarpus; trembling of the hands; swelling of the hands.

### Lower Extremities.

Cutting pains in the legs; jerking motions.
Contraction of the feet and toes.
Red spots on the legs.

### Sleep.

Somnolence, with dreams.
Frequent waking; sad dreams full of graves.

### Fever.

* Intermittent fever, principally before noon; cold followed by heat, with sweat; shivering, with flushes of heat; horripilation in the affected parts.

° Sweat, principally when eating, or after having eaten.

° During the fever, anxiety, forgetfulness, pain in the eyes, coated tongue, desire to vomit, oppression of the chest, chest is painful.

## Skin.

° Itching eruptions; dry eruptions; eruptions of burning vesicles.

ᵛ Steatoma; hot swelling; swelling of the parts affected.

## General Symptoms.

° Weakness; chronic weakness; sensation of distension.

Lancinating and boring pains, drawing and tearing; sensation of excoriation on being touched.

° Hysterical tetanus; convulsions of children; convulsions during vomiting; cramps when touched; cramps in children.

° Paralysis subsultus.

Heat of the upper part, and coolness of the lower part.

Suppuration of the glands.

° Caries of the bones; nocturnal pain in the bones.

Cutting pain in the joints; burning heat.

Symptoms are more marked in the room, from the action of hot water, acids, after physical efforts; they are relieved on covering up warmly, and by leaving the bed.

---

# HAMAMELIS VIRGINICA.

### (*Witch Hazel.*)

DESCRIPTION.—This is an indigenous shrub, sometimes called Winter Bloom, Snapping hazel nut, Spotted Alder, etc. It consists of several crooked, branching trunks, from the same root, from one to two inches in diameter, ten or twelve feet in height, and covered with a smooth, gray and spotted bark. It is a much larger shrub than the edible hazle-nut, which has a straight trunk, not spotted, but brownish. The Hamamelis virginica grows in almost all sections of the United States, especially in damp woods, flowering from September to November, when the leaves are falling, and maturing the seeds the next summer. The bark and leaves are the parts used in medicine; they have a pleasant, aromatic odor, and a bitter, astringent taste, leaving a sense of pungency and sweetness in the mouth.

OFFICINAL PREPARATIONS.—Tincture of the bark; dilutions.

ANALOGUES.—*Æsculus, Arnica, Bovista, Collinsonia, Erigeron, Galium, Lycopus, Senecio, Trillium.*

## Head.

* Crowding fullness in the head and neck, also in forehead.

Feeling as if a bolt was passed from temple to temple, and tightly screwed.

° Passive congestion, or venous stagnation.

Fullness in the forehead, with pressing sensation in the roots of the tongue.

### Nose.

\* Epistaxis, with feeling of tightness of the bridge of the nose.

\* Profuse epistaxis, idiopathic or vicarious.

° Epistaxis of childhood, passive, venous.

° Oozing of very dark blood from the nose in a hemiplegic old man. (*Preston.*)

### Mouth.

Dryness of the mouth; tongue feels as if burnt.

Blisters on the sides of the tongue.

Tongue coated white, with flat taste.

° Bleeding from the gums.

° Burns of the tongue and lips.

° Hæmorrhage after extraction of teeth. (*Cushing.*)

### Eyes.

Painful inflammation of the eyes; excessive congestion.

° Conjunctivitis, from the burn of a flame. (*Dr. Holcombe.*)

° Conjunctivitis, from a splinter in the eye. (*Ib.*)

### Throat.

Dry, thirsting feeling of the throat, not relieved by water.

Fullness in the neck; have to sleep with the neck free of any covering.

Feeling as if something had lodged in the fauces.

\* Tonsils and fauces congested.

° Hæmorrhage from the throat and fauces.

° Varicose condition of the throat and fauces.

### Stomach.

Burning in epigastrium; sharp pains in the stomach

Nausea, from pain in the testicles.

° Hæmatemesis of black blood.

### Abdomen.

Constant distress in the umbilicus.

Burning in the epigastrium and umbilicus.

Drawing pains in the abdominal muscles.

° Hæmorrhage from portal congestion.

ⁿ Hæmorrhoidal dysentery.

° Hæmorrhage from ulceration of the bowels.

° *Painful and bleeding hæmorrhoids.*

Constipation, with dry, hard stools, coated with mucus.

Ineffectual desire for stool.

### Urinary Organs.

Scanty, high-colored urine.

\* Irritation of the urethra, followed by a discharge and ardor
urinæ.

° Hæmaturia, from passive congestion of the kidneys.

° Catarrh of the urethra, with disease of the prostate gland.

° Ardor urinæ in the female.

### Generative Organs.

(*Female.*)   \* Hemorrhage from the uterus of bright red blood,
midway between the menstrual periods.

\* Active uterine hemorrhage in a young lady.

\* Acute vaginitis, with spasmodic action and painfulness of
the vagina.

\* Prurigo of the vulva, with vaginitis and vaginismus.

° Leucorrhœa profuse and almost constant.

° Vaginal leucorrhœa, bloody.

° Ovaritis following miscarriage (left side).

° Varicose veins during pregnancy.

° Dysmenorrhœa, inflammatory or neuralgic.

° Retention of the menses, with hæmatemesis, constant constipation and varices of the legs.

° Vicarious menstruation.

° Hemorrhage, blood flows steadily, venous in character, and
without uterine pains.

° Ovaritis—pain commences in the right ovary, passes down
the broad ligaments to the uterus.

° Ovarian soreness and painfulness.

° Phlegmasia alba dolens (milk leg).

(*Male.*)   Amorous dreams, with emissions, followed by lassitude, gloomy, depressing mood, and dull pain in lumbar
region.

\* Great prostration of the animal passions, with severe neuralgic pain in testicle, suddenly changing to bowels and
stomach, causing nausea and faintness.

Drawing pains in testicles day and night, extending from the groins.

Profuse cold sweat of the scrotum at night.

° Enlargement of the right testicle, hot and painful, following gonorrhœa. (*Hale.*)

ᵓ Urethritis, with discharge of transparent mucus with pain.

ᵓ Orchitis, one of our most valuable remedies; (used locally and internally.)

° Neuralgia of the testicles.

° Varicosis of the spermatic . veins (circocele). (*Dr. D. S. Smith.*)

### Larynx.

Tickling in the larynx, with constant inclination to cough.

### Chest.

Labored inspiration; oppressive tightness of the lower part of the thorax, with inability to make a deep and full inspiration; breathing impossible in a recumbent position, and a crowding fullness in neck and head.

**Pricking** pain in the region of the heart for days, also in the superficial veins of both arms.

° **Cough**; hæmoptysis, with dull frontal headache; taste of Sulphur in the mouth.

° **Tickling** cough, with taste of blood on waking.

° Slight hacking cough, with blood-spitting.

° Hæmoptysis in consumption.

### Back.

Tearing pains across the small of the back, with fullness of the joints of the legs.

### Upper and Lower Extremities.

Pricking pains in the superficial veins of both arms.

Painful fullness of the joints of the legs, as if they would burst, which soon extends to all the joints of the body.

Severe drawing pains in flexor muscles, wrists, hands and fingers.

° Varicosis of the limbs.    ° *Phlegmasia alba dolens.*

Articular rheumatism, with swollen and painful joints.

° Phlebitis of the vessels of the extremities.

° Varicose ulcers.

# HEDEOMA PULEGIOIDES.

*(American Pennyroyal.)*

BOTANICAL DESCRIPTION.—This plant is erect, branched and hairy; its *leaves* are petioled, oblong-ovate, obscurely serrate, the floral similar; whorls few-flowered; *corolla*, bluish, pubescent, scarcely exceeding the calyx; sterile *filaments*, tipped with a little head. It is common and mostly found in open barren fields and woods; flowers from July to September; plant from six to ten inches high, with nearly the same odor and taste as the true *Pennyroyal* (Mentha pulegium.) of Europe.

[H. HISPIDA.—Erect, hairy; plant from two to five inches high; *leaves* sessile, linear, entire, the floral similar, and exceeding the flowers; *corolla* scarcely longer than the ciliate, hispid *calyx*. It is found in Illinois and southward.]

This is a well known plant growing in dry, sterile situations, especially in calcareous soils, and blossoms from June to September, rendering the air fragrant for some distance around it. It is an indigenous annual, common to all parts of the United States. It has a pleasant, aromatic smell, which, however, is very offensive to some persons, and a warm, pungent, mint-like taste. It must not be confounded with the *Mentha* pulegium, or European Pennyroyal.

OFFICINAL PREPARATIONS.—Tincture; oil; dilutions.

ANALOGUES.—*Apis, Cantharis, Caulophyllum, Copaiva, Erigeron, Pulsatilla, Sabina, Secale, Senecio, Tanacetum, Turpentine.*

## Head.

Excessive pains in the head.

Sore pain in the left temporal region.

## Eyes.

Loss of vision, everything turns black.

## Nose.

Epistaxis.

## Mouth.

Dryness of the mouth; tongue covered with a very thin white coat.

## Stomach.

\* Nausea; straining to vomit; pain or spasm in the stomach.

\* Drawing pains from the stomach to the uterus and back.

Everything taken into the stomach causes pain.

Sensation as if the stomach would come up into the mouth.

° Gastritis.

## Abdomen.

Bearing down pains; periodical pain.

Distension of the abdomen; soreness and sensitiveness.

Obstinate constipation.

° Colic-like pains from colds, diarrhœa, etc.

° Intestinal spasms of children.

### Urinary Organs.

Suppression of urine; tenesmus; painful urination

Scanty urination, with frequent and urging desire.

Cutting, burning pains in the urethra.

Urine very dark, like black tea.

### Generative Organs.

*Female.*—Excessive bearing down pain, with pressure outward from lower abdomen.

* Pains are periodical, like true labor pains, severe, aggravated by movement, and attended by sensation of weakness or paralysis of the lower limbs.

Drawing from upper sacral spine to the uterus.

* Leucorrhœa, itching and burning, yellow, excoriating.

Excessive sensitiveness to pressure over both ovaries.

° Amenorrhœa from atony of the organs.

° Spasms of the uterus.

° Congestion of the uterus and ovaries.

° False labor pains.

° Suppression of the menses, from a cold.

° Suppression of the lochia.

° Threatened miscarriage.

### Throat.

Choking sensation, as if something were rising in the throat.

### Chest.

Frequent and periodical dyspnœa and oppression of the thorax.

Labored. asthmatic breathing.

### Back and Loins.

Excessive pain in the back, with pressing downwards to the uterus.

### Extremities.

Paralytic weakness in all the limbs.

Stiffness and weakness of the joints, with soreness.

Pains; laming, aching, rheumatic pains in the limbs.

Stiffness of the knees, can hardly get up.

# HECLA LAVA.

*(The lava and scoriæ thrown out from Mount Hecla, in Iceland.)*

DESCRIPTION.—Hecla lava, according to Prof. Morris, of University College, London, has for general constituents, silica, alumina, lime, and magnesia, with some oxide of iron; sometimes it contains anorthite and other minerals.

OFFICINAL PREPARATIONS.—Triturations; dilutions from the 3×.

ANALOGUES.—*Anisum, Chamomilla, Ipecacuanha, Mercurius, Pulsatilla. Phytolacca, Phosphorus, Sulphur, Stillingia.*

### Head.

The head bones, especially the jaw bones, swelled, and became so friable that when boiled they fell in pieces (in cattle.)

\* Toothache and swelling about the jaws. (*J. G. Wilkinson.*)

Enormous exostoses of the jaws (in sheep).

The jaws and teeth are covered with a shining metallic crust (in cows).

Lumps on the jaw bones, so large as to cause dislocation and death (in horses).

The jaws were sometimes covered with large swellings, which spread, and were of loose texture, and darker in color than the bone (in cattle).

Caries of the jaw bones, under the exostoses.

° Gum abscesses from decayed teeth. ( *Wilkinson.*)

° Difficult teething, in children. (*Ib.*)

° Neuralgic pains in the cavities from which teeth had been extracted. (*Holcombe. Cure with the* 30*th.*)

° Injury to the inferior maxillary of a scrofulous girl, which produced an immense abscess, and afterward great enlargement of the maxillary bone. (*Holcombe.*)

° Destructive syphilitic ulceration of the nasal bones. (*Thompson.*)

The thigh, and particularly the shinbones swelled and bulged (in cattle).

° Myalgia, especially of the intercostal muscles. (*Cate.*)

---

# HELONIAS DIOICA.

*(False Unicorn.)*

BOTANICAL DESCRIPTION.—This plant is known to botanists, at present, as the *Chamælirium luteum.* (Wildenow, Gray.) It is the *Veratrum luteum* of Linnæus, the *Melanthium dioicum* of Walter, and *Helonios dioica* of Pursh. It is also known by the common names of *Devil's Bit, Starwort, etc.* The same popular names are applied to the *Aletris farinosa.*

It is a herbaceous perennial, with a large, somewhat bulbous, premorse *root*, from which arises a simple, very smooth, somewhat angular, *stem or scape*, one or two feet in height. The cauline leaves are lanceolate, acute, small, and at some distance from each other, without petioles; the *radical leaves* are broader, being from four to eight inches in length, by half-an-inch to an inch in width, narrow at the base, and formed into a sort of whorl at the base of the scape. The *flowers* are small, very numerous, greenish-white, and are disposed in long, terminal, spicate, nodding, diœcious racemes, resembling a plume, and which are more slender and weak on the barren plants.

*Male flowers*, with white, linear-spatulate, obtuse, one nerved petals; *stamens* rather longer than the petals. *Female flowers*, the raceme is generally few-flowered, becoming erect; *petals* linear; *stamens* very short, abortive; *ovary* ovate, sub-triangular, with the sides deeply furrowed; *stigmas* three, spreading or reflexed. *Capsule* ovate oblong, tapering to the base, three-furrowed, opening at the summit. *Seeds*, many in each cell, acute compressed.—(*Gray*).

OFFICIAL PREPARATIONS.—Tincture of the root; dilutions; triturations of the root; and of the active principle, *Helonin.*

ANALOGUES.—*Aletris farinosa, Chelone glabra, Cornus florida, China, Frasera, Ferrum, Hydrastis, Nitrate of Uranium* (?), *Phosphoric acid, Senecio, Sepia.*

### Mental Sphere.

The mind is *exceedingly* dull and inactive.

Irritable; could not endure the least contradiction, or receive any suggestions in relation to any subject; all conversation was unpleasant.

* Desires solitude: *fault finding.*

### Head.

Feeling of pressure from within upwards to the vertex, aggravated by looking steadfastly at any fixed point.

Pain in the occiput, with pulsative pain in the vertex, increased by stooping, attended by vertigo.

Pain in forehead, as if a band about an inch wide were drawn across from the temples.

### Stomach.

Wakes every morning at 5 A. M. (an unusual hour), with the lips, tongue, and fauces dry, and a bitter taste in the mouth.

Soon after taking each dose, sensations of pain, tightness and pressure were felt in the stomach, which were partially relieved by the eructation of tasteless gas.

Cramp-like pain in the stomach; motion and rumbling in the intestines, as if diarrhœa would come on.

Vomiting and purging, with a griping and burning sensation in the epigastrium, slight.

° A woman suffering with dropsy could not retain her food; the *Helonias* relieved this condition.

Burning in lower third of the abdomen.

### Stool.

Sensation as if each lump of fæces had the shape of a large Minnie bullet, which passed from the anus the big end first; the anus seemed to be much distended for an instant, then out flew a fœcal mass; the stool consisted of four lumps, which made their exit separately.

Yellow and mush-like stool.

### Urinary Organs.

\* Urine profuse and light color.

\* Pain in the kidneys, with *albuminous urine*.

° Constant aching and extreme tenderness in the region of the kidneys, especially the right; tenderness in region of the bladder; when urinating, intense, cutting, tearing pains in the urethra; very frequent desire to urinate; urine very limpid when first voided, but deposited after a time a lead-colored, flocky sediment, adhering to the vessel.

° Pain in region of the kidneys; painful stiffness of the back; much burning, scalding pain when urinating; frequent and urgent desire to urinate, with emissions of large quantities of red urine; there was present a condition of complete impotence.

° Bright's disease.

Involuntary emission of urine, after having emptied the bladder.

° Chronic albuminuria.

° Saccharine diabetes (many cases).

### Generative Organs.

*Male.*—Increase of the sexual desire and power.

Unusually strong and frequent erections at night.

23

° Impotence complete or partial.

*Female.*—Pain in the lower part of the back, through to the uterus, like inflammation, piercing, drawing (*primary*).

Breasts swollen, nipples tender and painful, and will not bear the pressure of even an ordinary dress.

Aphthous inflammation of the vagina and vulva.

Great uterine hemorrhage came and lasted through the proving.

Intense pruritus of the vulva and vagina, with curdy secretion from vulva.

Amenorrhœa marked by general atony (*secondary*).

Leucorrhœa, with general atony (*secondary*).

Congestive amenorrhœa (*primary*).

Menorrhagia from active congestion (*primary*).

° Prolapsus uteri, with ulceration, and a constant dark, fœtid, bloody discharge.

° Prolapsus uteri, dependent upon want of muscular tonicity (*secondary*).

Pain in back, with irritation of the vagina.

° Threatened abortion, especially in cases of habitual abortion.

° Profuse flooding, with profuse serous leucorrhœa at the climacteric, with much uterine and ovarian pain.

° Useful for many of the consequences of miscarriage.

° *Loss of sexual desire and power, with or without sterility.*

### Back, etc.

° Feeling of uneasiness and weight in the region of the kidneys.

° Sharp, spasmodic pain in the back, running to the crest of left ilium.

Severe, rheumatic (?) pain in right hip joint, worse during motion.

° Pains in the back, more troublesome during the night.

° Pains in the back, with lameness, stiffness, etc., located in the sacro-lumbar region.

---

# HEPATICA TRILOBA.

### (*Liverwort.*)

BOTANICAL DESCRIPTION.—The Hepatica Americana of De Candolle is the Hepatica triloba of Wildenow. This is a perennial plant, the root of which consists of numerous strong fibres. The *leaves* are all radical, on long, hairy petioles, with three ovate, obtuse or rounded entire lobes, smooth evergreen, coriaceous, cordate at base, the new ones appearing later than the flowers.

The *flowers* appear almost as soon as the snow leaves the ground in the Spring. They are single, generally blue, sometimes white and flesh color, and are nodding at first, then erect, on hairy scapes three or four inches long; by cultivation they become double; involucre simple, composed of three entire, ovate, obtuse bracts, resembling a calyx, situated a little below the flower. *Calyx* of two or three rows of petaloid sepals; *stamens* awl-shaped, *anthers* elliptic, *achenia* ovate, acute, awnless.

*Hepatica acutiloba* differs in having the leaves with three ovate and pointed lobes, or sometimes five lobes; leaves of the involucre or acutish.

OFFICINAL PREPARATIONS.—Tincture of the whole plant; dilutions and tincture-triturations.

ANALOGUES.—*Calcarea carbonica* (*?*), *Glycyrrhiza*, *Hepar sulphur* (*?*), *Phosphorus* (*?*), *Stannum* (*?*).

## Eyes.

Eyes somewhat sensitive to light; itching and swelling, slightly aggravated in the morning.

## Nose.

Bloody mucus blown from the left nostril for three or four days in succession.

Soreness at the opening into the nostrils.

## Throat.

° Free and easy expectoration; the rough, scraping irritation and tickling sensation in the throat and fauces disappears, as also the sensation about the epiglottis and larynx, as of particles of food remaining (following an attack of hæmoptysis). (*Kimball.*)

° Accumulation of thick, viscid and tenacious phlegm, inducing frequent hawking and disposition to hawk, disappears. (*Hale, Kimball.*)

---

# HYDRASTIS CANADENSIS.

### (Golden Seal.)

DESCRIPTION.— An indigenous plant found growing in shady woods, in rich soil and damp places. The root is of a beautiful yellow color, and imparts its virtues to water or alcohol.

[The Muriate of Hydrastia is a valuable preparation, especially as a topical application. The medicinal properties of the root of Hydrastis Canadensis depend upon two Alkaloids, both of which are now well settled principles in their ultimate composition and nomenclature. For some years the precipitate occurring when muriatic acid was added to an infusion of this root was collected, dried, and sold as Hydrastin, by manufacturers of the Eclectic School of Medicine — subsequently a definite examination of this substance by Dr. Mahla, of Chicago, proved it identical in its reactions and composition with the Alkaloid Berberina, obtained from the bark of Berberis Vulgaris, and now known to exist in several genera and species of five natural orders of the vegetable kingdom. Berberina and its salts are but sparingly soluble in cold water or alcohol. They dissolve to quite an extent in both liquids when heated, and separate in minute yellow crystals when cooling.

J. Dyson Perron says (*Journal of the Chemical Society,*): "Doubtless its therapeutic effects merit much careful investigation. Natural instinct has pointed out its value for the alleviation of human sufferings, to nations widely separated, and enjoying different degrees of civilization. The polished Greeks, the semi-barbarous nations of Hindoostan and China, the North American Indians and the natives of tropical Africa, have been all impressed with the medicinal value of Berberina. In the West India Islands and in American pharmacy its virtues have long been recognized, though derived from different plants, and veiled under erroneous names; certainly it holds a place in European pharmacy, but one of little prominence, yet it seems to possess properties scarcely inferior to quinine itself. I am persuaded that nature has not placed Berberina in nearly every country without some adequate purpose."

Hydrastia, the White Alkaloid of Hydrastis, was discovered by Mr. A. B. Durand, of Philadelphia, but was first prepared in a pure state by Dr. Mahla, who determined its formula. When perfectly pure it separates from its hot alcoholic solution in tasteless, white prismatic crystals of great brilliancy. It dissolves readily in acids, forming soluble, uncrystallizable salts, bitter, and of a peculiar, somewhat metallic, after-taste. It is generally used in the form of muriate. In the preparation of this salt it is not necessary to carry the practice of re-crystallization, or bleaching with animal charcoal, to a sufficient extent to insure a product purely white, as it is considered profitless. It is essential that physicians, in prescribing these Alkaloids, do not confound them, as the insoluble yellow principle (Berberina) is often sold under the improper title of Hydrastia. The therapeutic action of the two principles is widely different — Berberina having no medicinal action upon diseased mucous tissues.

SPHERE OF ACTION.—(1.) The mucous membranes generally, which it stimulates to higher secretion, erosion and ulceration. (2.) The muscular tissues, increasing their nutrition, and imparting tonicity.

OFFICINAL PREPARATIONS.—Tincture of the root; dilutions; triturations of Hydrastin, and Muriate of Hydrastia.

ANALOGUES.—*Aletris farinosa, Ammonium muriaticum, Berberis vulg., Coptis, China, Cornus florida, Helonias, Iodine, Kali hydrojodicum, Mercurius jodatus, Nitric acid, Muriatic acid, Phytolacca.*

## Head.

\* Dull, heavy frontal headache.

\* Constant dull headache, with pain in the hypogastrium and small of the back of a dull, aching character.

Sharp, cutting pain through the temples, with dimness of vision.

Feeling as if intoxicated.

° Headache of a nervous, gastric character, almost constant.

° Myalgic headache, in the integuments of the scalp and muscles of the neck.

## Face.

Flushes of heat, followed by an erysipelatous eruption; mouth, lips and nose very much swollen, and pimples around the mouth and chin.

Eruption similar to all stages of small-pox.

Erysipelatous rash on the face, neck, etc.

° Pale face, with worn, weary expression.

## Nose.

\* Constant discharge of thick, white mucus, with frontal headache.

\* Secretions so profuse as to be removed in long tenacious shreds or pieces.

\* Stuffed up, smarting sensation in posterior nares, with discharge of thin, clear mucus.

\* Sharp, raw, excoriating feeling in both nares, with constant inclination to blow the nose, with hoarseness.

ᵛ Fluent coryza, followed by thick catarrhal discharge.

ʻOzæna, with ulceration, bloody or mixed purulent discharge; (applied with a douche or syringe.)

## Eyes.

\* Mucous membrane of the eyelids much congested; discharge of large quantities of thick, white mucus.

\* Profuse secretion of tears; smarting of the eyes; burning of the eyes and lids.

\* Catarrhal inflammation.

° Acute conjunctivitis, with or without ulceration.

ᶜ Scrofulous ophthalmia; (used as a collyrium, and giving the anti-psorics internally, hastens the cure.)  (*Hale.*)

° Opacity of the cornea.

## Ears.

Roaring in the ears, like cog-wheels, or the drumming of a partridge.

° Otorrhœa, with thick mucus discharge.

ᶜ Tinnitus aurium, from catarrh of the inner ear.

° Many diseases of the outer canal of the ear, with bad discharges; (used as an injection.)

## Mouth.

Mouth sticky, with yellow coat on the tongue.

Aphthæ on the mucous membrane of the lips and mouth.

Taste as of pepper in the mouth.

Excessive secretion of sticky, tenacious mucus from the buccal cavity.

Tongue seems large, and marked by the teeth.

° Stomatitis of children, with weakness.

° Stomatitis materna, with general debility; (used as a wash;) gr. × of the muriate to ℥ iv of water.)

° Mercurial salivation, an excellent topical application, after chlorate of potassa. (*Hale.*)

° Cancerous affections of the tongue.

## Fauces, Throat, etc.

Sticky mucus in the fauces, with bad taste.

\* Hawking up of tenacious, yellow or white mucus, with rawness of the fauces.

° Ulcerated sore throat from salivation by mercury.

° Sore throat from gastric derangements.

° Ulceration of the mucous membranes of fauces and throat.

° Diphtheritic exudations (?). Probably pseudo-membranes or tenacious mucus secretions, resembling diphtheria, accompanied or not by ulceration. It is not a remedy for true diphtheria. (*Hale.*)

° Chronic catarrhal affections of the throat.

## Gastric Symptoms.

Eructations of sour fluid.

\* Faint feeling at the stomach, preceded by a dull aching pain.

Burning pain in the umbilical region, with faintness.

Cutting pain in the stomach, which is acute and distressing.

Great sense of sinking and prostration at the epigastrium, with violent and long continued palpitation of the heart.

Painless gurgling in the stomach.

` Chronic inflammation of the stomach.

° Indigestion from an atonic state of the stomach.

° Indigestion, with acidity, and general weakness.

° Chronic gastric catarrh, the most general cause of so-called chronic dyspepsia. (*Hale.*)

° Cancer of the stomach. (?)

° Chronic ulceration of the mucous membrane of the stomach.

° Gastralgia and dyspepsia, followed by an epigastric tumor, supposed to be scirrous. (*Dr. Le Brunne.*)

### Liver.

Torpor of the liver, with pale, scanty stools.

° Catarrhal inflammation of the mucous linings of the gall bladder, biliary ducts, etc.

° Jaundice from structural disease of the liver.

### Abdomen and Stool.

\* Severe cutting pain in the hypogastric region, extending into the testicle, occurring after stool, with faint feeling.

Dull pains in the hypogastrium and small of the back worse from moving, with rumbling in the bowels.

\* Constant dull, aching pain in the stomach, with faintness.

\* Sharp pain in the region of the spleen, with constant dull pain in stomach and bowels, with hot, burning sensation.

\* Sharp pain in the region of the coecum.

\* Griping, with profuse light-colored diarrhœa.

\* Griping, with light acrid stools.

\* Intestinal catarrh, followed by ulceration.

° Flatulent colic, accompanied by faintness.

° Chronic catarrhal enteritis.

° Soft stool, followed by severe cutting pain in the hypogastrium, with dull aching in the testicles, with faint feeling.

Soft stool, with great rumbling in the bowels.

Obstinate relaxation of the bowels.

Tenesmus, with acrid, greenish stools.

Profuse light-colored diarrhœa, with griping.

° *Constipation*—"A precious remedy, far superior to **Nux** vomica." (*Hughes.*)

° *Constipation, with piles.*

° Constipation following rheumatic fever.
° Constipation attended with dyspepsia and hemorrhoids.
° Fissures of the anus.
° Excoriation of the anus.

### Urinary Organs.

\* Urine smells decomposed.
Dull aching sensation in the region of the kidneys.
Urine increased and neutral.
° Cystitis, chronic.
° Chronic catarrh of the bladder, with thick, ropy mucus sediment in urine. (This disease can be cured promptly by the use of daily injections of a weak infusion of Hydrastis, (or the muriate; gr. x to water 3 viii,) first drawing off the urine with a catheter. A high potency should be given internally at the same time.) (*Hale.*)

### Generative Organs.

*Male.*—° *Gonorrhœa*, in the second stages, after the inflammation has subsided, and the discharge is thick and yellow; use also an injection of the *Muriates.*
° Gleet, with obstinate, thick discharge; (use as above.)
° Debility following spermatorrhœa.
*Women.*—° *Tenacious viscid leucorrhœa, uterine or vaginal.*
° *Ulceration of the os, cervix, and vagina.*
° Uterine diseases, with sympathetic affections of the digestive organs.
° Cancer of the mammæ (palliative in many cases); use topically and internally.

[Injections of an infusion of the root, or the Muriate, are better than the tincture in water (1 dr. to aqua 8 oz.) For ulceration or erosion I prefer to apply with a brush or on cotton, or a solution of the muriate of Hydrastia in glycerine, gr. v. or x. to 1 oz.—*Hale.*]

### Larynx, Chest, etc.

Bronchial catarrh, with debility, loss of appetite, etc.
° Catarrhal cough, rough, harsh and rattling, day and night.
Constant tickling of the larynx, with harsh, dry cough.
° Thoracic or intercostal myalgia.

### Back and Neck.

Great soreness and lameness of the muscles of the neck.
Flushes of heat on the face, neck and hands.

Dull aching sensation in lumbar region.

### Back and Upper Extremities.

* Pain in the small of the back.

Aching in the lower region, with weariness in the arms.

"Crick" in the right elbow, also in the phalanges of the left hand, on waking at night, and quite painful.

Sharp cutting pains in the elbows and biceps muscles, with feeling of contusion and lameness.

Rheumatic pains in elbows, forearms, right shoulder, and first finger of left hand.

Intense aching pain in the small of the back.

### Lower Extremities.

Legs feel very weak, and ache.

Severe pain in right knee, lasting all day, worse on walking.

Dull aching in the loins.

Aching in the sole of the left foot.

° Irritable and indolent ulcers on the legs.

° Scrofulous ulcers on the leg and foot.

### Fever.

Heat of the skin, with flushes of heat on the face and neck, and intense itching in various parts of the body.

Pulse slow and labored, fifty-two; with palpitation of the heart.

Chilliness, with aching in the back and limbs.

° Quotidian fevers, with gastric disturbance; jaundice.

° Debility from gastric, bilious and typhoid fevers.

### Skin.

Erysipelatoid rash on the face, neck, palms of the hands, joints of the fingers and wrist, with burning heat and exfoliation of the skin.

Eruption like varioloid on the face.

Eruptions dependent on debility.

° Infantile intertrigo. (use internally and topically.)

° All stages of small-pox, as a wash. ( *Wilkinson.*)

---

# HYDROPHYLLUM VIRGINICUM.

### (*Water-leaf.*)

DESCRIPTION.—A smooth plant, one to two feet high; *leaves* pinnately divided, large and petioled; *flowers* in dense clusters, *blue.* *Calyx* five-parted; *corolla* bell-shaped. It grows in damp, rich woods, all over the United States.

OFFICINAL PREPARATIONS.—Tincture of the fresh leaves.

ANALOGUES.—*Rhus* (*?*), *Cypripedium* (*?*), *Pulsatilla*, *Euphorbia*.

### Symptoms.

* Inflammation of the eyes and eyelids. (*Hoyt.*)

(*See Therapeutics, Vol. II.*)

---

# HYPOPHOSPHITE OF LIME.

### (*Calcis Hypophosphis.*)

Hypophosphite of Lime is a white salt, with a pearly, margarin-like lustre, and crystalizes in flattened prisms. Its composition, according to Wurtz, is $CaO + 2HO\ PO$, the water being essential to the salt. It is soluble in six parts of cold water, and in not much less of boiling water; soluble, slightly, in dilute alcohol; insoluble in strong alcohol.—*Sp.gr.* 835.

OFFICINAL PREPARATIONS.—Triturations.

ANALOGUES.—*Calcarea carbonica, Calcarea phosphorica, Kali carbonicum, Lycopodium, Phosphorus, Phosphoric acid, Rumex, Sanguinaria, Sulphur.*

### Generalities.

A well marked increase of nervous force.

Remarkable sensation of health and strength.

* Nervous prostration, with depression of spirits.

* Cerebral congestion—tendency to (in scrofulous children).

° Phthisis pulmonalis, in the first and second stages.

° Palliates phthisis, even in last stage.

° Night sweats from any debilitating disease.

Calm and profound sleep (in consumption).

The quality and color of the urine improves.

* In *large* doses tend to *cause* the development of the pulmonary inflammation unhappily so frequent and fatal among consumptives. (*Dr. Churchill.*)

Plethora, with tendency to hemorrhages. (*Ib.*)

Hæmorrhoids bleed for the first time, or recommence under its excessive use. (*Ib.*)

Profuse epistaxis. (*primary.*)

Pulmonary hemorrhage. (*do.*)

Profuse and too frequent menses. (*do.*)

° Scanty and delaying menses. (*secondary.*)

° The thoracic pains of consumptives. (*do.*)

° Expectoration and night sweats diminish. (*do.*)

### Head.

° Incipient tubercular meningitis in children, with the following symptoms: Cough for several months; cough dry and recurring in paroxysms; loss of appetite and flesh, and depression of spirits; can scarcely walk, required to be held constantly; complains much of the head, says that it pains her in front; disposition capricious and variable, changes suddenly from sadness to laughter, often bursts into fits of violent weeping; perspires very freely, especially about the head and neck; she sleeps badly at night, wakes with a start, suddenly, uttering piercing cries, after which she relapses into a species of syncope, becomes quite pale and cold, face pale and sad; eyes preternaturally large and deep set, with a haggard wild stare, pupils much dilated; skin alternately burning and hot then cold. (Several cases cured in from ten to twenty days with one-half grain four times a day.) (*Churchill. Hale.*)

° *Hydrocephaloid diseases* in children, when the symptoms call for Cal. c. and Phos. ac.

° Hydrocephaloid disease in a child after pneumonia, with great prostration, pulse feeble and too frequent to be counted; unconscious of all surrounding objects; constant moaning; arms constantly sawing the air; occasional muscular spasms; eyes either strongly drawn to one side, or strabismus; eyes open, but no evidence of seeing; pupils alternately contracted and dilated. (Cured by 1-20 gr. every two hours; recovery was slow.) (*Dr. Gibbs.*)

### Face.

\* Face pale, wan and emaciated.

### Eyes.

\* Eyes dull and lustreless.

(See, also, cases under " Head.")

### Nose.

Abundant epistaxis in healthy persons.

Nose thin and pinched.

° Unhealthy discharges from the nose.

° Ulceration of the nasal cavities in tuberculous children, or from catarrh.

### Appetite.

\* Appetite and digestion greatly increased.

### Abdomen, etc.

Pains in the abdomen from weakness.

° Swelling of the abdomen in strumous children.

° Mesenteric tuberculosis.

° Chronic diarrhœa, undigested.

° Diarrhœa in phthisis pulmonalis.

\* Hæmorrhoids, bleeding profusely.

### Sexual Organs.

Increases the reproductive power.

\* Menses too profuse, high colored and frequent.

° Scanty and delaying menses.

° Chronic, irritating leucorrhœa.

° Leucorrhœa in young children.

### Respiratory Organs.

° *Cough* of a child, several months, dry and recurring in paroxysms; loss of appetite, flesh, and depression of spirits.

ugh associated with tubercular meningitis.

° Cough in phthisis pulmonalis.

\* Hæmoptysis of one day's duration.

° *Pulmonary consumption;* the strength increases, cough, sweat, and hectic diminish, the tubercles are absorbed and disappear, leaving no trace. (in some cases. *Hale.*)

° The pains in the chest which many consumptive patients feel so acutely, cease or very considerably diminish in a few days.

\* *A state simulating the development of that pulmonary inflammation unhappily so frequent and fatal among consumptives.*

° Acute ulceration of the lungs after pneumonia.

### Back.

Pains down the back in the muscles and ligaments.

° Spinal curvature in its incipient stage, from anæmia, in strumous children.

° Ulceration of the vertebræ.

° Psoas abscesses, with great debility and anæmia.

### Extremities.

Increased circulation of blood in the limbs.

Fullness of the blood-vessels of the hands and feet.

* *Habitual coldness of the extremities;* (a characteristic indication for this remedy in all conditions of debility from exhausting discharges and in tuberculosis.) (*Hale.*)

° Torpid and extensive abscesses on the lower limbs, with profuse suppuration.

---

# HYPOPHOSPHITE OF POTASH.

### (*Kali Hypophos.*)

Hypophosphite of Potassa is a white, deliquescent salt, opaque, very soluble in water and alcohol. Its greater tendency to absorb moisture renders it less eligible for prescription than the lime salt. Its composition is $KO + 2HO\ PO$.

OFFICINAL PREPARATIONS. — Aqueous solution 10 grs. to gtts. 100; aqueous dilutions to the 3°, then alcoholic.

ANALOGUES. — *Calcarea carbonica, Calcarea phosphorica, Kali carbonicum, Phosphorus, Phosphoric acid, Iodide of Potassa, Rumex, Sanguinaria, Sulphur.*

### (*No provings.*)
### Special Indications.

* Melancholy and hypochondria.

° Great debility, *especially when attended by marasmus,* and wasting of *muscular* tissue.

* Muscular debility, with myalgia and loss of muscular tonicity.

° Extreme prostration from profuse expectoration.

° Under its use the cough reappears, when it has ceased from debility.

° Deep thoracic pains; shortness of breath; muscular and arthritic pains in the limbs, the result of excessive *tea-drinking* and want of phosphatic food.

* A painful feeling in the anterior part of the thorax.

° *Asthmatic difficulties* occurring in phthisis or chronic bronchitis, always with great muscular debility (many cases).

° Chronic bronchitis, with scanty, tough expectoration.

° Chronic pneumonia, with myalgic pains.

° Useful in all cases of loss of the *phosphates,* namely, from long lactation; leucocythæmia and general anæmia; dentition of strumous children; catarrhal and leucorrhœal discharges; all inordinate secretions of pus; dyspepsia.

° Pleurodynia, from muscular debility.

° Ailments from nursing; pain and stitches in the back, chest, and abdomen; dimness of vision; nausea at the sight of food; despondency and a painful sense of dragging in left breast; (cured by one grain three times a day.) (*Taylor.*)

° Obstinate *chronic bronchitis*, with *thick, fœtid expectoration.* (*Sherwood.*)

° *Oxaluria*, with dyspepsia, increased density of urine, despondency, impoverished blood, emaciation, and an abundance of crystals of oxalate of lime in the urine. (*Ib.*)

° Diseases of children, characterized by debility, fretfulness, diarrhœa, want of firmness in the bones, non-appearance of the teeth, and delayed closing of the fontanelles; relieved promptly by the 2d dilution, five drops in milk, three times a day. (*Hale.*)

° *Ailments from excessive tea-drinking:* shooting pains about the chest and scapulæ, tenderness on the hypochondrium, bilious vomiting, constipation, painful flatulence, despondency, aversion to food, palpitation of the heart, etc.; (one grain, three times a day, cures nearly all cases. (*Ib.*)

° *Anæmia;* pains through the chest and limbs; palpitation; short breathing; giddy on rising in the morning; can scarcely dress herself; pulse 60, slow and weak; countenance pale; catamenia irregular; (removes these symptoms in a week or two generally).

° Great debility and nervous prostration after parturition, with non-appearance of, or scanty milk, cold and damp skin.

° Hydrocephaloid disease in debilitated, emaciated, poorly nourished children.

° Incipient tubercular meningitis in thin, pale children.

° Chronic myalgia — commonly called "**chronic muscular rheumatism.**"

# IBERIS AMARA.

### (*Bitter Candy-tuft.*)

DESCRIPTION.—This plant has a herbaceous *stem*, about a foot in height; *leaves* lanceolate, acute, somewhat toothed; *flowers* white, in corymbs, becoming racemes. *Silicles* obcordate, narrowly emarginate; cells one seeded. A small annual, common to Europe, indigenous to England Cultivated in gardens in this country.

OFFICINAL PREPARATIONS.—Tincture of the seeds; dilutions.

ANALOGUES.—*Amygdalis amara, Belladonna, Cactus grand., Digitalis, etc.*

## Mental Sphere.

Feels sad, down-hearted, oppressed, with desire to sigh.

A peculiar inability to fix the mind on any one thing.

Very *irritable*, with dullness of mind and lack of memory; forgets what is said in the lecture in a moment, unless the mind is concentrated on it.

Feels as if frightened; an indefinable dread, with trembling.

An excited, frightened feeling, with cold sweat on the face.

## Head.

Increased fullness (sensation of) in the neck and head, with increased action of the heart.

Heat, and fullness in neck and head, with flushed face, and cold feet and hands.

Pain in right side of the head.

Frontal headache on rising in the morning.

Severe frontal headache, with nausea and loss of appetite.

Heaviness of the head, with roaring in the ears.

Dull pain in the head, with vertigo and feverish chilliness.

Vertigo when rising in the morning; had to lie down.

Feeling of lightness and giddiness of the head.

Vertigo when making any exertion, with slight nausea.

Vertigo when standing, worse on stooping.

*Vertigo* in back part of head, as if the occiput were turning around.

## Face.

Flushed, hot face and red eyes, with the palpitations.

Cold sweat on face, with fearfulness.

## Eyes.

Feeling in the eyes as if being forced *outward*.

Eyes red, with flushed face.

Flashes before the eyes, with dull headache and palpitation of
the heart.

### Ears.

Roaring in the ears, with heaviness of the head, slight nausea,
and palpitation of the heart.

Dullness of hearing and comprehension.

### Throat.

Dryness of throat, as if filled with dust.

Throat feels as if both tonsils were enlarged.

*Constant hawking up of thick, viscid, stringy mucus, until
after a meal.*

Choking sensation in throat, with fullness and heat.

Choking sensation just above cricoid cartilage.

Constrictive sensation in the throat, with stabbing pains in the
heart, dyspnœa and palpitation.

### Gastric Symptoms.

Loss of appetite, with feeling of indigestion.

Sour eructations after eating, for hours.

Nausea, with cold, chilly feelings over the body.

Fullness and oppression on the right hypochondriac region.

Pain in region of liver, with clay-colored stool.

### Intestinal Symptoms.

Tenderness of the bowels, with thin, whitish stool.

Large, white or clay-colored stools.

Fullness and distension of the bowels.

Clay-colored stools, about ten minutes apart.

### Urinary Organs.

Frequent but scanty urination.

Excessive evacuations of urine.

### Respiratory Organs.

Dryness in throat and larynx, with hawking up of thin,
stringy mucus, for many hours; (eating removes this
symptom.)

Tickling sensation in the throat, with expectoration of stringy
mucus.

Tightness and constrictive feeling in the larynx.

Respirations more frequent and labored; dullness of hearing.

F.23

Fullness in the chest, with fullness and heat in head and neck, and flushed face.

*Dyspnœa*, and palpitation, on going up stairs.

Constant desire to draw a long breath, without relief.

Slight pain under sternum at articulation of *third* rib.

Feeling of weight and pressure under the sternum, with sharp pains in the chest (cardiac region).

Fullness and constriction under the sternum, with lancinating pains through the chest.

Continual feeling of weight and anxiety in the chest.

### Heart and Pulse.

Increase of heart's action from seventy-two to eighty-eight (in fifteen minutes).

A wavy, tremulous sensation in the radial artery, felt by the finger, with pulse intermitting every third beat, and easily compressible; pulse has peculiar double beats, which seemed to run into each other, but full, soft, and easily compressed.

*Palpitation of the heart on slight exertion*, as when putting down a window (never had it before).

*Palpitation, with vertigo and choking in the throat* after walking, and on entering the house felt *faint;* a tingling and numbness commencing in fingers of left hand and gradually extending up *left* arm, *with* pulse irregular, tremulous, not well defined; also, a dull, heavy aching in left arm (no perceptible palpitation, however).

Much pain over the base of the heart, with dull, heavy pain in left arm, and tingling and numbness in the tips of the fingers.

\* *Palpitation*, plainly visible on the whole chest, aggravated by walking, passing off on sitting still, but renewed by the slightest exertion. (*English physicians.*)

Walking causes indescribable sensations under the sternum, under articulation of third rib.

*Sensation of weight and pressure in the region of the heart, with occasional sharp, stinging pains in that region,* passing from before backwards, lasting but a short time, attended by acceleration of heart's action from seventy to ninety-six.

The pulse rises from sixty to ninety-four in fifteen minutes after taking the drug, with slight pains in the region of the heart.

Pains darting through the heart at night in bed, worse when lying on left side.

Pains of a dull, dragging character in region of the heart, not relieved by any position, nor by pressure with the hand.

Sharp, sticking pain in the region of the heart, with constrictive sensation in throat; eyes red and face flushed.

On turning on *left* side at night, a sharp, sticking pain is felt, as if a needle were crosswise in the ventricles and pricked at each contraction.

\* *Palpitation*, with marked increase of the *force* of the apex-beat, and irregular and jerking pulse, with a peculiar thrill under the finger. (*Hale*.)

Strong palpitation, with forcible impulse; the hand placed on the heart was visibly moved.

Palpitation when going up stairs (he was obliged to lie down), with *dyspnœa* and weak feeling.

Constant dull pain in the heart, worse when lying down.

Coughing, laughing, or slight exertion causes distressing palpitation, with increase of dull pain.

In one prover the cardiac symptoms lasted all day and night, and continued three days.

The attacks of palpitation and other cardiac symptoms occur within from five to fifteen minutes after each dose of the drug, and frequently pass away altogether within an hour.

### Physical Signs.

1. During the first part of the proving (Dodge's), no abnormal sounds discoverable on auscultation.

2. About the middle of the proving, with the full intermittently-irregular pulse, auscultation revealed great excitement of the contractions at intervals of three or four beats, after which there was a much longer interval than usual before another pulsation.

3. Near the end of the proving, the sounds of the heart were

found to be increased in intensity, especially on the region of the semi-lunar valves.

During the whole of the proving (Sabin's), the *force* of the apex-beat was visibly increased, and the heart impulse visibly raised the hand when placed on the chest, and the pulse was hard and jerking, intermitting every third beat; rising from seventy to ninety.

Heart's action *apparently* weakened for the first few moments after taking the drug, but in ten minutes the pulse rose to one hundred, full and strong, but somewhat irregular

Heart's action weak and fluttering, with small, weak pulse.

### Extremities.

Trembling of lower extremities after exercise.

Dull aching in left arm, as if he had slept upon it all night.

Rheumatic pains in right shoulder.

### Fever.

Feverish chilliness.

Quickly passing febrile paroxysms.

### Conditions.

Cardiac symptoms better in afternoon, worse at night.

*Worse* in warm room. *Better* in open air.

### Sleep.

Sleep at night disturbed by all sorts of dreams—(unusual, as I never dream).

Restless and continually turning in bed, with ludicrous dreams.

Very restless night, with horrid dreams.

Nervous and irritable on rising in morning.

### Generalities.

Feels weary, with desire to lie down.

Feeling of nervous excitement in whole system.

Feeling of inability to move even a finger.

A feeling of lameness and soreness throughout the whole body, as from a cold.

Trembling sensation all over, so that he had to lie down.

Desire for stimulants.

Great weakness and debility.

Looks as if he had been ill a good while.

[The *Iberis* was proven by students of Hahnemann College under my own directions. It will doubtless become a valuable cardiac remedy.—*Hale.*]

# ILEX OPACA.

*(American Holly.)*

DESCRIPTION.—A tree, from twenty to forty feet in height, having *leaves* which are alternate, coriaceous, evergreen, smooth, shining, flat, oval, acute at the end, and the wavy margins armed with strong, scattered, spiny teeth. The flowers are small, greenish-white, and are scattered in clusters along the base of the young branches. *Berries* red, as large as a whortle-berry, and of an acrid, bitter taste. [The European Holly, *I. aquifolia*, is similar in appearance.]

OFFICINAL PREPARATIONS.—Tincture of the leaves and berries.

ANALOGUES.—(?)

*(No provings.)*

° Intermittent fever, jaundice, pleuritis, catarrh, enlargement of the spleen, rheumatism, (periostitis I. aquifolia).

*(See Therapeutics.)*

# IODIDE OF ARSENIC.

*(Arsenici Iodium.)*

PHARMACOLOGY.—Gently heat in a tubulated retort placed in a sand bath, a mixture of one part finely pulverized metalic arsenic and five parts iodine. The iodide is afterwards to be re-sublimed, to separate the excess of arsenic. This forms an orange-red volatile solid, which is dissolved by water, and entirely volatilized by heat.

OFFICINAL PREPARATIONS.—Triturations; aqueous solutions.

ANALOGUES.—*Arsenicum, Arum triphyllum, Nitric acid, etc.*

### Head.

Vertigo.

Dullness of the head, with dull pain in the left malar bone, and occasional slight frontal headache the entire morning.

An exceedingly sharp pain in the forehead and both ears.

Severe frontal headache, with dullness of the entire head in forenoon, with stiffness and soreness of left side of neck; worse on moving the head.

° Chronic, obstinate, scaly eruptions on the scalp. (*Hale.*)

### Face.

Erythematous redness of the face.

### Eyes.

Puffiness of the lower eyelids.

An uneasy sensation of tension or stiffness around the eyes.

Weakness of the eyes with burning pain—a feeling as if lachrymation would set in.

° **Chronic** strumous ophthalmia, with ulceration. (*Ib.*)

### Nose.

* Thin, watery, irritating discharge from the nose, from the anterior and posterior nares.
* Fluent, acrid coryza, with paroxysms of sneezing --- worse in the open air.
* Soreness, rawness and scabbiness in the nostrils.
° Acute and chronic catarrh, with ulceration and inflammation of the nasal passages and frontal sinuses.
° *Hay-fever;* the most effectual remedy after Gelseminum. (*Hale.*)

### Ears.

Sharp pain in both ears, especially in left ear, when riding in a sharp cold wind.

° Chronic otorrhœa, with corrosive sanious discharge. (*Ib.*)

### Mouth, Tongue.

Intermittent pain in front right upper molar tooth.

White tongue, with edges and tip of a florid, red hue.

Salivation, with acrid saliva.

° Diphtheria maligna.

° Phagedenic ulceration of the fauces and tonsils.

### Stomach and Abdomen.

Severe, burning, lancinating pains in the stomach, with heat of mouth and fauces.

The abdomen is hard and distended with flatus, which is constantly discharged.

Severe, cutting pains in the abdomen, as if he would have a stool; he had no stool, but large quantities of wind escaped; then pains are partially relieved by an escape of flatus, and by the application of warmth to the abdomen. (8 A. M.)

Sharp, cutting pains in the abdomen (at 9 A. M.) which warned him to go to stool; the pains became excruciating, embracing the entire abdomen, and obliging him to bend almost double; after a great deal of straining he passed a large, soft stool, which afforded him some relief. (*Dr. Blakeley.*)

[This is the kind of colic cured by *Dioscorea.* (*Hale.*)]

° "The most serviceable remedy we have in the diarrhœa of phthisis." (*Watson.*)

° *Chronic diarrhœa, with intestinal ulceration*—in cases of soldiers returned from the army. (*Hale.*)

### Back.

Stiffness and soreness of left side of neck; worse when moving.

Soreness of the back, especially of back of neck, as if beaten.

Burning heat in the back (lumbar region), as if the clothes were on fire.

Itching, especially on the back.

### Extremities.

Itching of back of left hand, followed by stinging-itching of back of right hand.

Peculiar chilliness of left thigh, followed by formication and weight in left foot; the clothes when extending the left limb, feel cold; the formication and weight extended to right foot—was partially relieved by walking; the chilliness disappeared from warmth.

Formication on exterior border of left foot, followed by burning in left instep.

Formicating prickling on left ankle, also on right ankle.

Tired, weary feeling in calves of both legs, while kneeling.

Dull, heavy soreness of calf of left leg, afterwards embracing the entire leg; disappearing during active motion, returning when at rest.

Heaviness of the legs, with general weariness.

### Chest and Heart.

\* Tightness of the chest, with short dry cough.

° Asthmatic complaints; cardiac asthma.

Anxiety in the region of the præcordia. (*Wilson.*)

° Palpitations; in hypertrophy of the heart. (*Hale.*)

### Skin.

Persistent itching all over the body—especially the back.

Formicating, prickling itching on skin of body and extremities.

\* *Erythema*—especially in the face.

\* Dry, scaly, burning, itching eruptions on various parts of the body. (*Hale.*)

' Lepra, impetigo; diseases resembling cancer. (*Thompson.*)

' *Obstinate chronic eruptions,* psoriasis versicolor; tinea furfurans; pityriasis. In the *3d trit.* will often give better results than any other preparation of *Arsenicum.* (*Ib.*)

### Fever.

\* Hard, full pulse, with puffiness of the lower lids and face; thick, white tongue, with red tip and edges.

° Febrile movements attending chronic, irritable eruptions.

---

# IODIDE OF BARIUM.

### (*Baric Iodide.*)

PHARMACOLOGY.—This compound may be formed by double decomposition, by adding native carbonate of baryta in powder to a boiling solution of iodide of iron. Iodide of Barium crystalizes in small, colorless needles, which deliquesce *slightly,* and are very soluble in water. The solution promptly undergoes decomposition by exposure to *air,* carbonate of baryta being precipitated, and iodine set free, which colors the solution.

OFFICIAL PREPARATIONS. — Tincture (made by adding one hundred grs. to one thousand drops of aqua distillata, and kept in colored glass bottles, hermetically sealed); triturations (with dry, pure sugar of milk, and kept like the tincture).

### (*No provings.*)

° All scrofulous, glandular enlargements. (*Lugol.*)

° Chronic enlargements and indurations of the tonsils. (*Hale.*)

° Ovarian tumors—in strumous subjects.

° Swellings of the lymphatic glands; it often prevents suppuration.

° Scrofulous ophthalmia; especially swellings of the meibomian glands.

° Obscure brain affections in old persons. (?)

° Old swellings and indurations of the testicles.

### (*See Therapeutics, Vol. II.*)

---

# IODIDE OF LEAD.

### (*Plumbi Iodium.*)

PHARMACOLOGY.—Dissolve one part Nitrate of lead in twenty parts distilled water, and then mix with solution of one part iodide of potassium and eight parts of water; allow the precipitate to subside, throw it on a filter, wash it well with cold water, and dry with a gentle heat. The product will be one and two-fifths parts. Acetate of lead cannot be substi tuted for the nitrate, as the acetate of potassium that results is a solvent of Iodide of Lead.

The Iodide of Lead is an odorless, fine yellow powder, without taste, soluble in 1.990 parts of cold and 1.330 parts of boiling water. The solutions are colorless, the hot one depositing, as it cools, large brilliant golden scales, soluble in 4500 parts 80% cold alcohol, a trifle less of hot alcohol, forming a pale straw-colored solution.

OFFICINAL PREPARATIONS.—Triturations only.

ANALOGUES.—*Kali bichromicum, Mercur. iod., Phytolacca, Conium, Lachesis, Apis, etc.*

° Enlargement of the tonsils.

° *Diphtheria.*

° Amenorrhœa from atrophy of the ovaries.

---

# IRIS VERSICOLOR.

## (*Blue Flag.*)

DESCRIPTION.—An indigenous plant, with a fleshy, horizontal, fibrous root, or rhizoma. It is common throughout the United States, growing in moist places, and presenting *blue* or *purple flowers* from May to July. The root resembles that of Acorus calamus (sweet-flag). It has a peculiar odor, augmented by rubbing or pulverizing, and a disagreeable taste, with persistent acridity.

The active principle is an oleo-resin, named *Iridin* (or *Irisin*).

SPHERE OF ACTION.—The gastro-intestinal mucous membrane, and, by reflex action, the head and liver.

OFFICINAL PREPARATIONS.—Tincture of the fresh root; *Iridin* (*Irisin*) and triturations.

ANALOGUES.—*Antimonium crudum, Arsenicum, Colchicum, Eupatorium perfoliatum, Euphorbia corollata, Ipecacuanha, Juglans cinerea, Leptandra, Mercurius, Pulsatilla, Podophyllum, Phytolacca, Robinia, Sanguinaria, Veratrum album.*

### Sensorium.

* Despondency; low spirits; easily vexed.

Confusion of mind, with great mental depression.

### Head.

* Dull, heavy headache in the forehead, with nausea.

* Shooting pains in the temples, generally the right, with constrictive feeling in the scalp.

* Severe pain in the occiput, more on the right side.

* Violent, stunning headache, with facial neuralgia, followed by copious limpid urine and vomiting.

° Sick headache of a gastric or hepatic origin.

° Neuralgia, facial or cephalic, with nausea and vomiting.

° Habitual headache; a violent throbbing on either side of frontal protuberance, worse in the evening or after exer- tion. ( *Wesselhœft*.)

° Sick headache every Sunday regularly. (*Hale*.)

The headache is aggravated by *rest*, but relieved by continued motions. (*Rhus*.)

° Pustular eruptions on the scalp in children.

### Eyes.

Redness of the conjunctiva, as if from a cold.

Eyes feel dull, with pain over left superciliary ridge.

Severe burning pain in internal canthus, with effusion of tears.

Eyes sunken, with blueness around the eyes.

° Chronic inflammation of the eyelids. (*Kitchen*.)

### Ears.

Singing and buzzing in the ears.

### Face.

* Facial neuralgia, involving the supra and infra-orbital and the superior maxillary and inferior dental nerves; begins after breakfast every morning with stupid headache and lasts several hours. (*Holcombe*.)

* Pustular eruptions on the face, around nose, lips and cheeks, secreting a sanious, irritating matter.

° Tinea capitis; crustea lactea; porrigo; eczema of the face.

### Mouth, Fauces, etc.

Greasy feeling over tongue and gums on rising in the morning.

Feeling of rawness in the mouth.

* Back part of the mouth and fauces feels on fire.

* Constant discharge of saliva, *not* fœtid.

* Ulcers on the mucous membrane of the cheeks.

° Stomatitis, with painful burning in the mouth and fauces.

Teeth feel sore and elongated, with dull aching.

° Salivation following diphtheria, with swelling of the parotids.

### Gastric Symptoms.

* Loss of appetite, with nausea and empty eructations.

* Constant nausea and vomiting of watery and *sour* fluids.

Aching in the stomach before breakfast and after drinking cold water.

Great burning distress in the epigastric region (pancreas?).

\* Colic-like pains every few minutes in epigastric region.

Vomiting, with pain in the stomach, *with diarrhœa.*

° Bilious vomiting, with great heat of the head and perspiration.

\* Severe shocks of pain in umbilical region, passing upwards to epigastric region, with nausea, straining and belching of wind.

° *Vomiting of ingesta; of acid matters; of bile; of soured milk in children.*

° Increase of (*primary*) or deficiency (*secondary*) of pancreatic juice; it caused, in a cat, intense congestion and rupture of the minute vessels of the pancreas. (*Burt.*)

° Chronic indigestion of *milk;* it sours and is vomited. (*Hale.*)

### Liver.

\* Pain in the right hypochondria, worse on motion.

Pain above the crest of the ilium, on both sides, first on right.

Crampy pains in the right lumbar region.

Cutting pains in the region of the liver.

° Acute and chronic disorders of the liver.

° Increase of bile (*primary*), then deficiency of (*secondary*), with jaundice.

### Abdomen, Stool, etc.

\* Rumbling and cutting pain in lower part of the abdomen, relieved by flatus.

\* Colic, obliging him to bend forward for relief.

\* Diarrhœa with slight pain, with rumbling and cutting in the lower part of the abdomen.

Constipation, succeeded by thin, watery diarrhœa.

\* Copious watery stool, with or without tenesmus.

Stool tinged with green, copious, watery, mixed with undigested food.

\* Stool of blood and mucus, with great tenderness, and a sensation as if the anus was on fire.

Swelling of the stomach and abdomen.

Great smarting and burning of anus after every stool.

\* *Autumnal bilious diarrhœa and cholera morbus.*

Severe intermittent colic in umbilical region, with soft, mushy, *sour* stools.

° A grumbling bellyache, with stools twice a day, scanty; with mucus, fluid fæces, offensive, putrid odors, and discharge of very fœtid wind of a coppery odor. (*Kitchen.*)

° Periodical night-diarrhœas, with pain and green discharges. (*Ib.*)

° *Cholera infantum,* with profuse sour discharges from stomach and bowels, and pain in head.

° Asiatic cholera, with rice-water discharges, cramps, etc. (*Dr. Lade, of England.*)

### Urinary Organs.
Sharp, cutting pain in the urethra on urinating.

Urine copious; strong, disagreeable smell of the urine.

Dark-red urine, with burning in the urethra.

\* *Nocturnal emissions, with amorous dreams.*

° Gonorrhœa; syphilis, mercurial syphilis. (*Eclectic.*)

° Spermatorrhœa. (?)

### Genital Organs.
° Morning sickness during pregnancy.

° Uterine leucorrhœa; metrorrhagia.

### Larynx and Chest.
Short, dry cough, excited by a tickling in the larynx.

Pain in the left side, as though the ribs were pressing against the lungs, and unable to take a long breath.

Hoarseness, with ringing in the ears.

Soreness and rawness of the fauces.

### Back.
Constant pain in the lumbar and sacral region, aggravated by motion.

### Upper Extremities.
\* Sharp, tensive pain in the right shoulder, worse on motion, especially on raising the arm, mostly in the evening.

\* Severe pains shooting about in the phalangeal and meta-carpal-phalangeal articulations.

Rheumatism of the shoulders, wrists and hands.

### Lower Extremities.
Pain in right knee joint, worse on motion.

Violent tearing pain in right hip and knee joints, extending
to right foot, worse on motion.

Trembling and weakness of the knees.

Calves of the legs painful when walking, especially the right.

Pain in lower extremities and cramps in calves of legs, with
nausea and retchings.

### Nervous System.

Nervous, irritable, with prostration of the whole system.

### Skin.

\* Pustular eruption on the *scalp, face*, and other parts of the
body.

° *Psoriasis;* irregular patches on knees, elbows, and all over
the body, covered with shining scales, edges slightly
raised and irregular; (cured in fifteen days with *Iris ix.*)
(*Dr. Alabone, of England.*)

° *Psoriasis in relievo*, skin fissured and irritable. (*Ib.*)

° Lepra vulgaris — obstinate, on the arms. (*Ib.*)

### Sleep.

Sleepiness, with chills.

Restless every night, with bad dreams.

Amorous dreams during sleep.

### Fever.

\* Sweat over the whole body, particularly in the groin.

\* Heat followed by chill, with cold hands and feet.

Dry, hot skin; hands hot and dry.

° Typhoid fever, with symptoms similar to *Baptisia*

° *Bilious fever*, after *Bryonia* or *Aconite*.

## ᵀUGLANS CINEREA.

### (*Butternut.*)

BOTANICAL DESCRIPTION.—This is an indigenous forest tree, known in
different sections of the country by the various names of *Butternut, Oilnut,
and White Walnut*. In favorable situations it attains a great size, rising
sometimes fifty feet in height, with a trunk three or four feet in diameter
at the distance of five feet from the ground. The stem divides at a small
distance from the ground into numerous horizontal branches, which spread
widely and form a large tufted head, giving to the tree a peculiar aspect.
The young branches are smooth and of a grayish color, which has
given origin to the specific name of the plant. The leaves are very long,

and consist of seven or eight pairs of sessile leaflets, and a single petiolate leaflet at the extremity. These are two or three inches in length, oblong-lanceolate, rounded at the base, acuminate, finely serrate and somewhat downy. The male and female flowers are distinct upon the same tree. The former are in large aments, four or five inches long, hanging down from the sides of the shoots of the preceding year's growth, near their extremity. The fertile flowers are at the end of the shoots of the same spring. The germ is surmounted by two, large, feathery, rose-colored stigmas. The fruit is sometimes single, suspended by a thin, pliable peduncle; sometimes several are attached to the sides and extremity of the same peduncles. The drupe is oblong-oval with a terminal projection, hairy, viscid, green in the immature state, but brown when ripe. It contains a hard, dark-colored, oblong pointed nut, with a rough, deeply and irregularly furrowed surface. The kernel is thick, oily, and pleasant to the taste.

HISTORY.—The Butternut grows in Upper and Lower Canada, and throughout the whole Northern, Eastern, and Western United States. In the Middle States the flowers appear in May, and the fruit ripens in September.

The bark is used in dyeing wool a dark-brown color, though inferior for this purpose to that of the Black Walnut. It is said, when applied to the skin, to have a rubefacient effect. The inner bark is the medicinal portion, and that of the root being considered most efficient, is directed by the National Pharmacopœia. It should be collected in May or June.

OFFICINAL PREPARATIONS—Tincture of the inner bark (or leaves); triturations of *Juglandin*.

ANALOGUES.—*Bryonia, Colocynth, Ptelea, Croton tig., Podophyllum, Iris, Sulphur, Rhus.*

## Sensorium.

Depression of spirits; mind depressed.
Vertigo, with faintness.

## Head.

Dull headache on rising, passing off on getting up.
Fullness of the head at night.
° Eruptions on the *scalp.*

## Eyes.

Inflammation, with pustules on the lids and around the eyes.

## Ears.

Pain on swallowing, which is deep, drawing, tickling.

## Nose.

Coryza from the left nostril.
Dryness of the nose.

## Face.

Erythematous redness.

### Mouth, Teeth and Throat.

Sore throat, with dry lips and mouth moist.

Tip of the tongue is sore, with dryness of the fauces.

\* Throat feels swollen, with pain on the right side.

° Chronic inflammation of the throat, with general debility. (*Horton.*)

### Appetite, Taste, etc.

Loss of appetite, with coppery taste.

### Gastric Symptoms.

Nausea in the morning; vomiting, retching, with colic.

° Indigestion, with gastric irritability; flatulence.

### Stomach.

Sinking sensation at the stomach, and boring in the stomach.

### Abdomen.

Deep-seated pain on left side near the kidneys.

Pain in the epigastrium.

Heat and pain in epigastrium.

Flatulence and aching in the abdomen after dinner.

Irritation and inflammation of the mucous membrane of the bowels, followed by dysentery.

### Stool.

Loose stool which smells like onions.

Tenesmus and burning after stool (*primary*).

° Constipation preceded by diarrhœa (*secondary*).

° Colic, very severe and prostrating, with purging.

° Diarrhœa of soldiers in camps. (*Neidhard.*)

### Larynx and Trachea.

Rattling in bronchia on coughing, without expectoration.

Expectoration of very tenacious mucous and musty sputa.

### Chest and Respiration.

Pain on the left side, worse on pressure.

Great oppression in the chest, with cutting pains in the lungs.

Congestion of the lungs.

Stitching pain under the right scapula.

° Scrofulous consumption, with great emaciation. (*Small.*)

### Back.

Aching pain in small of the back on stooping.

Aching pain in the lumbar vertebræ.

Shooting pain in the lumbar region.

## Upper Extremities.

Aching pains in arms and wrists, as if sprained.

Great pain in right axilla, extending down the arms, along the course of the nerves.

Aching in right shoulder.

## Lower Extremities.

Heat on inner side of the thigh, and in the feet, with cramp like pain in left hip at night.

## Skin.

* A peculiar exanthematous eruption, very much resembling the flush of scarlet fever.

* Erysipelatous inflammation of the skin of the body and extremities.

* Erythematous redness of the face.

* Eruption resembling eczema simplex. (*Dr. Martin.*)

* Pustular eruptions.

[Dr. A. E. Horton, of East Poultney. Vermont, claims to have extensive experience with *Juglans* in acute and chronic skin diseases. He claims that it is curative and homœopathic to the " whole range of skin diseases, from simple erythema to pemphigus." In the second edition of New Remedies, and in the journals since, he has reported many cases of *pustular, vesicular, erythematous,* and ulcers; also, other lesions of the skin cured promptly with the tincture and dilutions, or triturations of *Juglandin.* He mentions its successful use in nearly all cutaneous eruptions. The internal administration is aided by a lotion of the same medicine.]

[Dr. Small, of Chicago, reports a case of *noli me tangere* on the nose and mouth, cured by a cold infusion of the leaves; also, cases of scrofula and scrofulous swelling of the glands.]

---

# JUNIPERIS COMMUNIS.

### (*Juniper.*)

DESCRIPTION.—This is a small evergreen shrub, never attaining the height of a tree, with many very close branches, the extremities of which are smooth and angular. Juniper is common to Europe and this country, growing in dry woods and hills, and flowering in May. The fruit, or berries, are the officinal parts; those which are imported from the southern parts of Europe are the best. The American berries possess less virtue, and are seldom employed. Juniper berries are about the size of currants, of a purplish-black color, shrunken, marked at the top with a tri-radiate groove, and at the base with bracteal scales; they contain three seeds. Their odor is peculiar, terebinthinate, and aromatic, and their taste tere-

binthinate and sweetish, succeeded by some bitterness. These qualities are
due to an essential oil, which may be obtained by distillation with water.
They yield their properties to hot water or alcohol.

OFFICINAL PREPARATIONS.—(1) Tincture of the berries; (2) dilutions
from the Oil of Juniper. (Infusion of the berries.) [If the *Juniperus
Virginiana* is used, the tincture must be made from the leaves and terminal
twigs, as it is prepared from the Juniperus *Sabina*.]

ANALOGUES.—*Apis, Barosma, Cannabis, Copaiva, Cubebs, Equisetum,
Galium, Sabina, Terebinth.*

Great flow of limpid urine of low specific gravity.

° Scanty, dark, scalding urine, with pain in the bladder and
   kidneys.

° Gonorrhœa, gleet, leucorrhœa, cystorrhœa.

° *Dropsy,* not caused by organic disease; (a palliative in incur
   able dropsy.)

(*See Therapeutics, Vol. II.*)

-----

# KAOLIN.

### (*Silicate of Alumina.*)

DESCRIPTION.—Kaolin is "Porcelain clay." It is composed of Silica
and Alumina from decomposing feldspar. It is found native in Europe,
in the form of a clay, from which smoking-pipes are made.

OFFICINAL PREPARATIONS.—Triturations to 3d ×; dilutions.

ANALOGUES.—*Bromine* (?), *Hepar sulph.* (?), *Iodine* (?), *Kali bich.* (?),
*Spongia* (?), *Sanguinaria* (?).

(*No Provings.*)

° *Pseudo - membranous croup* — used successfully by Dr.
   Landsmann, of Vienna, Dr. Parker, of Philadelphia, and
   Dr. W. S. Searle, of New York.

(*See Therapeutics, Vol. II.*)

-----

# KINO.

### (*Pterocorpus Marsupia.*)

DESCRIPTION.—Called by the natives "red-gum." It is a juice which
exudes from the trunk of a tree growing in Australia and other portions
of the tropics. It comes in the form of a laminated, friable mass, which,
when reduced to powder, is of a brownish purple color.

OFFICINAL PREPARATIONS.—Triturations or tincture, made by macerating one part in nine of alcohol; dilutions.

ANALOGUES.—*Alum, Geranium mac., Gallic acid, Tannin, Rhatany, Nux. Nitric acid, Sulphuric acid. etc.*

*(Fragmentary Proving.)*

Colicky pain toward evening and all the next day, with bearing-down and inclination to stool, but without evacuation.

Colic pains, with bearing-down in the lower bowel; the pain was relieved by lying flat on the face; in the morning a hard, dry evacuation was passed, with a little blood at the end of the passage.

For four or five days after this the bowels were obstinately constipated, the latter terminating in sickness and diarrhœa, with extreme giddiness and debility; (relieved by Ipecac.)

Evacuations hard, with sensation of turgescence of the mucous lining of the bowels; slight bearing-down, with frequent desire for an evacuation.

Nausea, headache, great amount of flatulent distension, appetite decreased.

Mucous lining of the bowels irritable, with evacuations tending to diarrhœa, with bearing-down and rapid action of the bowels.

\* *Chronic dysentery.*

\* Constipation, following dysentery.

---

# LACHNANTHES TINCTORIA.
### *(Spirit-weed.)*

BOTANICAL DESCRIPTION.—*Perianth* woolly outside; six-parted down to the adherent ovary. *Stamens* three, opposite the three larger or inner divisions; *filaments* long, exserted; *anthers* linear, fixed by the middle. *Style* thread-like, exserted, declined; *pod* globular; *seeds* few on each fleshy placenta, flat and rounded, fixed by the middle. Herb with a red, fibrous, perennial *root*, equitant, sword-shaped leaves, clustered at the base and scattered on the stem, which is hairy at the top and terminated by a dense compound cyme of dingy yellow and loosely woolly *flowers*. Grows chiefly in sandy swamps, southward near the coast, but has been seen in Rhode Island and New Jersey.

OFFICINAL PREPARATIONS.—Tincture of the leaves and root; dilutions.

ANALOGUES.—*Æthusa, Agaricus, Belladonna, Cicuta, Crotalus, Cimicifuga, Cannabis indica, Gelseminum, Glonoine, Gymnocladus, Hyosciamus, Lachesis, Opium, Platina, Phosphorus, Sanguinaria, Stramonium.*

25

## Mental Sphere.

Ill-humored, and sleepy, whining mood, with the headache.

Great loquacity, afterwards stupid and irritable.

° Delirium during pneumonia, with circumscribed red cheeks, worse from one to two A. M.

## Head.

Giddiness in the head, with sensation of heat in the chest and around the heart.

Sensation as if the vertex was enlarged and was driven upwards.

Headache pressing the eyes outward (*Sepia, Cimicifuga*).

Head feels enlarged, and as if split open with a wedge from the outside to within; the body is icy cold, she cannot get warm; the whole face becomes yellow; the head burns like fire, with much thirst; during the cold sensation the face is moist and sticks.

Tearing in the forehead, from left to right.

A continuous stitch in the left forehead from within to without, leaves after a few minutes a pressing pain, and extends over the whole forehead, pressing from within outwards.

Sensation as if the hair was standing on end, with soreness of scalp.

## Eyes.

Obscuration of sight, if he looks on anything fixedly he sees gray fixed rings.

While reading in the forenoon, a large yellow spot as large as a hand on the paper, which follows as he reads.

Looking at an object for some time, it becomes dark before his eyes. (*Gels., Calabar, Chloral.*)

Pupils very much enlarged, with brilliant eyes.

If he suddenly moves his head it becomes dark before his eyes. (*Gels.*)

° Brilliant eyes, red face, and delirium during pneumonia.

Compression of the left eyeball from below upwards.

Pressing in the eyes, with secretion of white mucus.

When closing the eyes the upper eyelids twitch visibly; when he closes them tight it grows worse.

Redness on the left upper eyelid, covered with little vesicles; they itch a great deal.

## Ears.

Tearing in the left ear, and in the right (frequent symptom).

Crawling sensation in the ears.

° Almost complete deafness, in pneumonia nervosa.

## Nose.

Nose bleeds profusely — blood pale.

## Face.

Tearing pressure in the left cheek, toward the eye, as if the eye should be pressed out.

Tearing from the right side of forehead into the cheek.

° Circumscribed redness of the face in the morning, with violent delirium and brilliant eyes in pneumonia nervosa.

## Mouth.

Pain in all the teeth from warm drinks.

Sensation as if the upper incisors and eye-teeth have broken loose, with sensation of soreness, worse when touching them with the tongue and when closing them.

All the teeth pain, feel loose and too long, worse in bed.

Saliva of tough mucus.

## Throat.

Roughness and swelling, with pricking when swallowing; continually increasing dryness of the throat, with sleeplessness, followed by hoarseness.

° Great dryness in the throat, especially on awakening during the night, with much coughing (in a patient who had an ulcerated sore throat).

° Sore throat, with short cough.

° *Diphtheria*, with stiffness of the neck; head drawn to one side.

## Appetite and Taste.

Aversion to meat.

The headache in the forehead is better after supper.

## Stomach.

Rising of sweetish water, with nausea.

Sudden sensation of squalmishness in the stomach.

Fullness in the pit of the stomach, with borborygmus.

## Abdomen.

Twirling and twisting sensation in the upper part of the abdomen.

Fermentation and rumbling in the abdomen almost constant.

° Much flatulency in the abdomen during pneumonia nervosa.

Cutting in the upper part of the abdomen, from the left to the right side.

Cutting in the right side of the abdomen.

Sensation of heat through the abdomen; feels as if the bowels would be moved.

### Stool and Anus.

Frequent desire to evacuate, without result.

Evacuation as usual, but with much discharge of flatulency and purging; after the passage the sensation of heat in the abdomen becomes less.

Continuous stitch in the anus.

### Urinary Organs.

Pressing on the bladder when urinating.

### Generative Organs.

(*Male.*)  Violent burning, tingling and itching of the scrotum and around it.

Perspiration and itching of the scrotum and penis.

### Larynx and Trachea.

° Hoarseness; dry cough from irritation of the throat, worse in bed.

Burning in the right side of the larynx.

### Chest.

° Cough dry as if it came from the larynx; expectoration is streaked with blood, with severe pain in the chest, in pneumonia nervosa.

When inhaling, deep pressing pain under the short ribs near the spine.

Stitches like knives in the region of the left clavicle, previously stitches like knives in the right chest.

She feels hot and oppressed in the chest, with mild perspiration all over.

### Heart.

Stitches like knives following one another in quick succession in the right side of the chest, below the mammæ, while at rest and when moving.

Boiling and bubbling in the chest and region of the heart; it rises to the head and he becomes giddy; he breaks out with a prespiration.

Sensation of heat in the region of the heart, going and coming.

### Back.

Sensation as if sprained in the neck when turning or moving the head backwards.

Pressing pain under the short ribs near the right side of the spine, deep inside when taking a deep inspiration.

Burning in the region of the left kidney, deep, extending toward the right side.

Burning in the sacrum and immediately above.

Stinging, as from the sting of a bee, on the inner corner of left shoulder-blade.

Stiffness of the neck following a pain in the occiput.

Sensation of pain and stiffness of the neck, which extends over the whole head down to the nose.

° *Wry neck*, especially in diptheria. (*Lippe.*)

### Upper Extremities.

Tearing in the upper part of the arm, beginning at the elbow joint and running up into the shoulder.

Tearing in both elbow joints, at times upwards and then downwards, frequently through the whole day.

\* Burning of the palms of the hands and soles of the feet.

Tearing in the knuckles of the middle fingers of the right hand.

### Lower Extremities.

Tearing in the right ischium.

Small pimples around the left gluteus muscle, which discharge a watery fluid when they are scratched open.

Itching, burning, stinging inside of the right thigh.

Burning, stinging pain above the left knee.

Burning and pressing on the right knee, which becomes red as scarlet.

Tingling in the lower extremities and feet.

Cramps in the calves of the legs and feet.

Tearing in the right big toe awaking him from his sleep.

Twitching of the muscles in various parts of the body.

[The hogs (except the black ones) which eat the roots and leaves of this plant, lose their hoofs, which fall off (from ulceration ?) (*Darwin.*)]

## Sleep.

Restless sleep at night, with disturbed dreams, followed by perspiration.

Sleeplessness, with continually increasing dryness of the throat.

\* In the night, in bed, short cough, with sore throat, followed by coryza.

Awakens at 2 A. M. with a cramp pain in his breast, extending from the right to the left side.

## Fever.

Icy coldness of the body; skin is cold, damp and clammy during the coldness.

Flushes of heat alternating with chilliness.

\* Burning heat, with redness of the face, more on the right side, followed by circumscribed redness of the cheeks.

Evening fever, worse from 6 to 12, with redness of the face.

° Fever, with delirium, circumscribed redness of the cheeks, and brilliant eyes in pneumonia.

Pulse 74, some beats fast, some slow.

° Pulse 110, small, thin, hard (pneumonia).

° Perspiration, with dizziness in the head and boiling and bubbling in the cheeks and region of the heart.

° Pneumonia nervosa and typhus fever.

---

# LAPIS ALBUS.
### (*Silico-Fluoride of Calcium.*)

This fancy name, Lapis Albus, is given by Dr. Grauvogl, to an unnamed species of gneiss, which he first found held in suspension in the waters of the mineral springs of Gastein, Germany.

These springs start from the foot of the Tauern mountains, and flow down ward into the valley of Achen, over formations of Gneiss.

The substance proved, was a trituration of this solid Gneiss rock.

Dr. Grauvogl calls it a white primitive calcium gneiss; the late Dr. Bellows, of Boston, in 1867, before Grauvogl's discovery, arrived at the same conclusion as to the poisonous effects of this rock, based on observations made in Derbyshire, England. He calls it a *Silico-Fluoride of Calcium*, the analysis of which is, Calcium, fourteen parts; Fluorine, fifty-five parts; Silicium (silex), fifteen parts; water, fifteen parts. "It is a dry, white, glimmering, impalpable salt."

Officinal Preparations.—Until a careful scientific analysis of the rock used by Grauvogl is made, we must only consider as officinal, tritu rations of the Gneiss from the springs of Gastein, Germany.

ANALOGUES.—*Arsenicum, Conium, Cundurangu, Silica.*

(None but fragmentary provings, made by Grauvogl, with the sixth trituration.)

" *Burning, stinging pains in the cardia and pyloris; in the female breast and uterus;* sometimes the pains were of considerable intensity." (*Grauvogl.*)

The waters containing this gneiss, when drank for some time, rendered cancerous sores, as well as other ulcers, decidedly worse.

" After drinking the water for seven weeks, my thyroid gland began to swell." (*Ib.*)

The inhabitants of the Achen valley, along the river, have thick necks and goitres of immense size.

° Carcinoma of the cheek in a woman fifty years of age. (It had produced an opening as large as a silver dollar; this hole gradually filled up, the complexion of the patient entirely changed, she obtained a healthy color, instead of her previous yellowish and cachectic appearance.) (*Ib.*)

° Many cases of pronounced cancer. (*Ib.*)

° Scrofulous affections, abscesses and sores. (*Ib.*)

° All affections of the glands and lymphatics. (*Ib.*)

° Glandular tumors, where physiologically no glands are usually found. (*Ib.*)

° Tuberculosis, unbroken carcinoma, scrofulous. (*Ib.*)

° Fluor albus. (*Ib.*)

° Five cases of uterine carcinoma (so pronounced by allopaths) permanently cured (these cases were reported to *Dr. Von Grauvogl*).

" I have not yet seen an open cancer cured by this remedy."

" It must not be given to persons who have suffered previously from intermittents, or other malarious diseases, as it engenders relapses of those diseases." (*Ib.*)

° *Goitre, cretinism, and scrofulous diseases,* caused by the waters in Derbyshire, England, which contain Fluorine, Lime and Silex. " I have used this salt, Silico-Fluoride of Calcium, in at least ten complicated cases of scrofulosis, with good result." (*Dr. Bellows.*)

" More than fifty physicians have reported to me many interesting cases of tumors, and other scrofulous diseases, cured by this salt." (*Ib.*)

Some of the mineral springs of California, containing particles of gneiss in suspension, have considerable reputation for the cure of cancers and obstinate ulcers. (*Hale.*)

---

# LEPTANDRA VIRGINICA.

(*Black Root—"Culver's Physic."*)

DESCRIPTION.—This is the Veronica virginica of Linnæus. It is an indigenous, perennial plant, with a simple, straight, smooth, herbaceous *stem*, from two to five feet high. The *leaves* are whorled in fours to sevens; short petioled, lanceolate, acuminate, finely serrate. The *flowers* are white, numerous, nearly sessile, in long, terminal, and verticillate, sub-terminal spikes. It grows in rich, moist places, thickets, and flowers in July. The *root* is perennial, horizontal, woody, about as thick as the finger, six to twelve inches long; black externally, brownish internally, with many long, slender, black fibres. It should be gathered in the fall of the second year. It has a bitter, nauseous taste. The active principle, *Leptandrin*, is a jet-black, resinous substance, resembling pure asphaltum; or, of a greyish-brown color, with a peculiar, faint cyanic smell and taste; somewhat bitter, nauseous and disagreeable. When powdered, it has a black, glistening, soot-like appearance, and coalesces in a warm and moist air. It is soluble in water and alcohol.

OFFICINAL PREPARATIONS.—Tincture of the root; dilutions; triturations of the dry root; *Leptandrin*, and its triturations.

ANALOGUES.—*Arsenicum, Baptisia, Carbo vegetabilis, China, Iris versicolor, Mercurius, Myrica cerifera, Nitric acid, Podophyllum*

## Sensorium.

° Gloomy; desponding; drowsiness, attending hepatic derangements.

## Head.

* Constant, dull, frontal headache, worse in the temples, with aching sensation in the umbilicus.

* Dull, frontal headache, with neuralgic pains in the right temple.

° Bilious headache, with constipation, bitter taste, indigestion, etc.

## Eyes.

* Smarting and aching with or without secretion of tears.

## Mouth and Throat.

* Tongue coated yellow along the centre, with pain in the submaxillary glands.

### Gastric Symptoms.

Nausea, with deathly faintness on rising in the night.

Nausea followed by vomiting and diarrhœa.

<sup>c</sup> Dyspepsia from disorder of the liver and stomach.

### Stomach.

\* Constant distress in lower part of the epigastrium.

Constant, burning, aching sensation in the stomach and liver, worse after drinking water.

\* Great distress in the stomach and small intestines, with immediate desire for stool.

\* Weak, sinking sensation at the pit of the stomach.

### Liver.

\* Dull aching in the whole of the liver, pain worse near the gall bladder.

\* Constant, dull burning distress in the epigastric and hypochondriac regions.

\* Great distress in the region of the liver following profuse, black, undigested stool.

\* Great burning distress in the back part of the liver and in the spine.

\* Pain in the right shoulder and arm.

° *Jaundice, with clay-colored stools.*

° Functional derangement of the liver.

\* Yellow coated tongue, with vomiting of bile, shooting or aching pains in the region of the liver, and black evacuations.

° Chronic congestion and other chronic disorders of the liver.

*Leptandra* causes black, tarry, bilious stools (*primary*), followed by clay-colored stools with jaundice (*secondary*)

### Abdomen.

\* Constant, dull, aching distress in the umbilical region.

\* Great distress in the whole of the bowels, with rumbling and desire for stool.

\* Rumbling and distress in the hypogastric region, with a profuse, *black, fœtid stool*, with pains in the bowels

Pains aggravated by drinking cold water.

Pain in the left inguinal region.

° Bilious colic, or a tendency to it.

° Chronic abdominal complaints caused by derangements of the portal system.

### Stool.

Hard, black, and lumpy evacuations.

* Stool soft and mushy, with *weak* feeling in the bowels.

* Distress in the hypogastrium, with profuse, black, fœtid stool.

* Watery stool with mucus, followed by severe cutting pains in the smaller intestines.

* Copious tar-like evacuations.

* Diarrhœa from chronic irritation of the mucous membrane.

° Diarrhœa dependent on hepatic derangement.

Diarrhœa, with great debility, sallow skin, and emaciation.

° Camp-diarrhœa in soldiers, from exposure, improper diet, etc.

° Chronic ulceration of the intestines, with hepatic disorder.

° Diarrhœa; stools of greenish, muddy or dirty water; profuse, "like water running from a spout;" coming on in morning as soon as he moves; aggravated by meat, vegetables, and walking; before stool, rumbling, after stool, weak, faint, purging feeling at stomach; dull aching across umbilical region all the time; canine hunger, no thirst. (Cured in four days.) (*Dr. R. R. Williams.*)

### Urine.

Urine very red (neutral), with dull, aching pain in lumbar region.

° Dropsy from hepatic derangement.

### Generative Organs.

° Suppressed or retarded menses from disease of the liver.

### Thorax.

Soreness in the cardiac region.

### Back.

Sore and lame feeling in the small of the back.

### Fever.

Pulse diminished in frequency.

Pulse slow and full.

° Infantile remittents, with black and tarry, or white fœtid stools.

### Skin.

* Hot and dry skin in bilious fevers.

### Upper Extremities.

Both wrists are lame and ache severely.

° Pain in the left shoulder and arm.

Chilly sensation at the shoulder and down the arm.

### Lower Extremities.

Feet and legs cold and numb.

### General Symptoms.

Languid, tired feeling, with great prostration.

Physical and mental depression, with vertigo and drowsiness.

---

# LILIUM TIGRINUM.*

### (Tiger-Spotted Lily.)

DESCRIPTION.—The Tiger Lily is a well-known, showy, orange-colored coarse-flowered garden plant, very abundant in cultivation, and is a native of China and Japan. The *stem* is from four to six feet high, unbranched and woolly. *Leaves* scattered, sessile, three-veined, the upper cordate-ovate. The *axils* bulbiferous. *Flowers* large, in a pyramid, at the summit of the stem, dark orange-colored, with black, or very deep crimson, somewhat raised spots, which give the flower the appearance of the skin of the tiger. It blooms in July and August.

OFFICINAL PREPARATIONS.—Tincture of the flowers and pollen; dilutions.

ANALOGUES.—*Agaricus, Belladonna, Cimicifuga, Cactus, Helonias, Murex, Podophyllum, Platina, Sepia.*

### Mind and Disposition.

*Female.*—Great depression of spirits, with fearfulness and apprehension of an impending fatal internal disease, or that it was already preying upon her; constant inclination to weep (very marked): blurred vision, all objects appearing very indistinct.

Despondent and gloomy, with loss of memory and great difficulty in expressing her thoughts, often selecting wrong words, but in making the correction would as often take other words quite as inappropriate; great fear and dread of insanity.

Does not want to be pleased, and don't want to talk, but wants to sleep, and, during sleep, very unpleasant dreams.

*From the exhaustive resumé of Dr. Paine, in *American Observer* and N. Y. Transactions for 1872. (*Hale.*)

Wild feeling in the head, with confusion of ideas; pressure and a crazy feeling on the top of the head, rendering her incapable of recording her own symptoms; fear of insanity, and that, should she become insane, there would be no one to take care of her; worse at night, but better in the morning.

Opposite mental states; she feels nervous and irritable, and yet she feels jolly.

Cannot think; acts without thought; keeps walking fast, as if by instinct; feels hurried, does not know why; is forgetful; cannot decide for herself; must depend upon others.

Both the social and moral conditions were profoundly affected; dislikes to be alone, though formerly she preferred it, but has no dread of being alone; sexual desires strong, though formerly weak; can repress the desire by keeping very busy, but as soon as occupation ceases the desire returns in full force.

*Male.*—Irritable in the evening, with disagreeable dreams at night, and unrefreshing sleep.

Obtuseness of intellect, with inability to find the right words with which to express his thoughts; forgets what he is about to say; vertigo, especially when walking; a feeling as if intoxicated; staggering forward.

Makes mistakes when speaking, using wrong words, with fullness and heaviness in the forehead, especially the left side; dim sight and weakness of the lower limbs, as if unable to support the body.

In half-waking dreams, occurrences which took place in quick succession seemed to be at very long intervals; for example, when his son got up to urinate, the intervals between getting up, urinating and going to bed again seemed very long.

Great apprehensiveness of the prover that he had mistaken the nature of his heart symptoms, and that instead of medicinal symptoms he **was suffering from organic disease of the heart.**

### Head.

Intense, blinding headache in the forehead, commencing between five and six o'clock P. M., continued two hours, then changed to the back part of the head and extended down the neck, leaving a strange muddled feeling about the head, with general weakness and desire to lie down.

Heavy feeling in the head, with morning diarrhœa, griping in the bowels, nausea and abundant saliva.

Pain all over the head, with a heavy sensation as if too full of blood; congested feeling as if blood would issue when blowing the nose; must support the head with the hands; worse when walking in the open air; better at sunset.

Pressing sensation of fullness in the temporal region, with a bursting sensation; a feeling as if the contents of the skull would issue through the ears and surrounding parts, relieved by pressure with the hands.

Frontal, stinging, burning headache, with a sensation as if a rubber band were stretched over the head; the head feeling so muddled that he could not lecture, could not concentrate his thoughts, but self-possession was regained as he went on.

Headache in the morning on waking, which gradually increased, when at noon it became very severe, passing from the forehead and temple to the protuberances of the occiput, dull, pressive and heavy, continuing through the afternoon, evening and night, with irritability of temper.

Dull headache; the pain moved continually from the sinciput to the occiput of the left side, but seemed at last to concentrate in the left temple, with frequent urination.

Headaches gradually diminish, though they maintain usual character of evening aggravation; at the end of ten days only slight tenderness on the left side of the head, forehead and temple remained.

° Suspended the recurrence of sick headaches (to which the prover had been accustomed) during the whole course of the proving, and for some time longer.

\* *Headaches;* especially those depending on uterine disorders.

*Scalp.*—Fine, rash-like eruption about the forehead, and around the border of the hair, with much itching.

### Eyes and Sight.

*Eyes.*—Intense pain in both eyes, extending backward into the head, with great dimness of sight.

Right eye very sensitive to gaslight, with intolerable burning pain subsequently extending to the left eye, and continuing for several days.

Burning in the eyes after reading or writing, and feeling of great general weakness.

*Sight.*—Blur before the eyes after a night made restless by lascivious dreams and seminal emissions toward morning, attended by difficulty in keeping the mind fixed upon the subject under consideration, selecting wrong words with which to express his ideas.

Blurred vision, cannot see objects distinctly, with loss of appetite, aversion to coffee, nausea when thinking about it; frequent desire to pass urine, but in small quantities; faint in a warm room and when standing, with cold perspiration on the back of the hands and feet; fearfulness and apprehension of some impending evil.

Dimness of sight, with intense pain in both eyes, extending into the head; shooting pain in the right temple, passing over to the left; crampy pains in the left mammæ and fingers, and pressing pain in the right arm and wrist, beginning at seven o'clock p. m., and continuing through the night.

*Muscæ volitantes* at various times.

Eyesight, which was always weak, hypermetropic, wearing 1-14 glasses, is now much worse; this aggravation continued for more than four weeks, when the eyes had returned to their natural condition with this improvement; whereas formerly she had a habit of turning the head toward the left when reading, in order to see the whole of a letter, for example, s p d and f u, when looking straight forward, could see only the straight part of the letter and not the curve; now can see the whole letter distinctly without looking sideways.

### Ears.

Rushing sound in both ears.

### Nose.

Frequent sneezing at ten o'clock P. M., relieving a severe, burning headache, and pain in the eyes.

Sensation as if blood would issue from the nose when blowing it, with feeling of fullness and heaviness of the head.

Heat and fullness of the face and head.

The left cheek bright and red hot in the morning on awakening.

### Mouth and Throat.

Hawking mucus from the throat, with constant disposition to vomit.

* Hawking of mucus, with constant nausea.

### Taste and Appetite.

*Taste.*—Taste of blood in the mouth, with severe congestion of the chest; weak beating of the heart.

Great craving for meat, and the more pronounced the symptoms the greater the desire.

Voracious hunger, seemingly in the back, extending along the vertebral column, and up to the occiput, not appeased by eating.

Loss of appetite, and aversion to bread particularly, continuing for three weeks after the last dose of the drug, with depression of spirits; disposition to weep; pressing in the rectum (from *prolapsus uteri?*); cold chills in the back, particularly after going to bed, with hot flushes toward morning.

° *Loss of appetite cured.*

*Thirst.*—Great thirst, drinking often and much.

### Gastric Symptoms.

Frequent eructations, with great distention of the stomach, and escape of flatus from the rectum [constant during the proving].

Constant nausea, with the sensation as of a lump in the stomach, which moved down at every attempt to swallow, but immediately returned.

Nausea, with pain in the back; aversion to food; depression of spirits, and disposition to weep.

Sweetish nausea, no desire to vomit, with feeling of fullness of the abdomen after eating very little; eating does not increase the nausea; nausea and full feeling in the abdomen subside after discontinuing medicine two days.

### Stomach.

Hollow, empty sensation in the stomach and bowels.

Great distention of the stomach and abdomen, with flatulent movements, relieved by passing wind up and down.

### Abdomen.

Bloated feeling of the bowels after a meal, continuing after a diarrhœic discharge.

Griping pain in the abdomen, commencing at from three to five o'clock P. M., increasing till late in the evening, and ending with a free bilious evacuation, which evacuation was followed by smarting in the rectum.

Griping pain in the abdomen after each morning diarrhœic discharge, with nausea, abundant saliva and heavy feeling in the head.

Weak, tremulous sensation of the bowels, extending to the rectum, continuing through the night.

Dragging down sensation of the whole abdominal contents, extending to the organs of the chest, greatly feeling the need of support.

Sensation as if the bowels were greatly bloated, but they are not so.

Constant burning pain across the lower part of the abdomen from groin to groin.

Pressure downward and backward against the rectum, aggravated by standing; relieved by walking in the open air or riding.

### Stool.

*Dark colored and very offensive stools in the morning on rising, followed by smarting and burning sensation, extending from the rectum high up into the abdomen, continuing for several hours.*

During the day time a stool every half hour, lumpy, small and diarrhœic, with escape of flatus; constant tenesmus and a feeling as though she could sit on the stool forever, with burning in the urethra.

Abdominal muscles unbearably sore just before stool, but less so during stool.

Tenesmus and great desire to go to stool, but every effort resulted in the voiding of a little urine only.

### Urinary Organs.

Frequent desire to urinate in the latter part of the night and early morning, with acrid smarting sensation after every discharge. (The acrid, smarting sensation always occurs after, and not during the flow.)

Urine milky in appearance when first discharged, but on cooling, deposits a thick, reddish sediment.

Urine scanty, milky, thick and roily in appearance when cool, with frequent desire to pass it, every passage is followed by smarting and burning in the urethra.

The urinary tenesmus and smarting after every passage, together with the morning diarrhœa, and acrid smarting in the rectum, continued to recur for more than six weeks after the last dose of the drug was taken.

A feeling of irritation in the bladder, with inclination to urinate, but can control the desire by an effort of the will.

Frequent desire to urinate through the day, with smarting in the urethra; if the desire is not immediately attended to, a feeling of congestion of the chest ensues (male).

### Reproductive Organs.

*Vagina.*—Itching and smarting of the labia, with great uneasiness of the parts.

Smarting and feeling of irritation of the labia, with great heat, as though the parts were inflamed, and sharp, incisive pains extending upward into the vagina.

Great tenderness to touch, of the whole sexual organs.

Pressure and weight low down in the vagina.

Pressure in the vagina and pain at the top of the sacrum extending to the hips.

*Uterus.*—Pain in the sacrum, with a sensation of weight and downward pressure in the lower part of the abdomen

26

(pelvis?), which continued for six days, very severe; worse when standing.

Bearing down in the lower part of the abdomen for more than twenty days, with constant nausea; a sensation as of a lump in the centre of the chest which moved downward by empty swallowing, but immediately returned; severe pressure in the rectum and at the anus, and a constant desire to go to stool, but with every effort to evacuate the bowels, a little urine only was discharged; sensation as if a hard body were pressing backward and downward against the rectum and anus (in the provers), standing aggravated and increased the desire to go to stool.

Great weight and pressure in the region of the uterus, with downward pressure, as though the whole contents of the abdomen would pass out through the vagina.

Great bearing down in the uterine region, with a sensation when on the feet as though the whole pelvic contents would issue from the vagina if not prevented by hard pressure with the hand against the vulva, which there was a constant and uncontrollable inclination to do.

Severe dragging down sensation in the whole sexual organs, with a feeling as though the whole internal parts were being pulled downward from the breasts and umbilical regions, through the vagina, and an uncontrollable desire to press the hands against the vulva to prevent the parts from escaping, with irritability of temper, anxiety and dread of impending evil (constant throughout the proving).

Severe neuralgic pains in the uterus, could not bear to be touched or moved, nor even the weight of the bed clothes; the slightest jar of the bed was torture. This condition continued an hour and a half, and suddenly passed off without leaving any lameness of the parts. On examination the uterus was found to be in an anteverted position.

*Anteversion of the uterus was found to be present in three provers, and resting a diagnosis upon well proved subjective symptoms, there can be little doubt that this condition of the uterus existed in a fourth case, though, owing to extreme sensitiveness of the prover, it was not verified by touch.*

\* *Prolapsis uteri; anteversion; retroversion; uterine inflammation, sub-acute; endo-cervicitis.*

*Leucorrhœa.*—Thin, acrid leucorrhœa, which from leaving a brown stain upon the linen was mistaken for a return of menstruation, though the menses had ceased but a week before; the leucorrhœal discharge attended and followed severe bearing down pains in the uterine region; the bearing down pains, four days later, culminated in severe labor-like pains simulating those of an imminent miscarriage, worse in the afternoon till midnight, then better till the next afternoon, when all the symptoms of the previous day returned; the leucorrhœa becoming more acrid and excoriating, producing a rash-like eruption and swelling of the labia.

Bright yellow leucorrhœa, excoriating the whole perinæum, with scanty menstruation, not one-fourth part as much as usual.

Profuse acrid leucorrhœa following immediately the cessation of the menstrual flow.

*Ovaries.*—Dull, drawing pain in the left ovarian region, relieved by gentle pressure on the part with the hand.

Great tenderness from pressure over the left ovarian region, with darting pains extending to the groin of that side, and the pubes in front, and frequent desire to pass urine, which was small in quantity, and followed by an acrid, smarting sensation in the urethra, continuing for several minutes.

Continued stinging sensation in the left ovarian region, with a sensation of fullness and voluptuous itching in the vagina.

Pains mostly in the right ovary, but some days later it was most severe in the left, extended down the anterior and internal side of the left thigh, with aggravation by walking, seeming, when one step was made, that another could not be taken; nevertheless, a feeling of restlessness compelled her to extend and flex the limb as in walking; this

disposition she could not resist, though she knew the effort
would be followed by greater pain; the *effort*, rather than
the *act* of moving the limbs, seemed to aggravate the pains.
She could not decide which pelvic pain was worse, that in
the back or that in the front.

*Burning pain* in both ovaries in the morning, with burning
higher in the abdomen, and four loose, dark stools before
eleven o'clock A. M. ; stools very urgent, could scarcely
wait.

Gnawing pain in the right ovarian region, with a dragging
sensation, aggravated by walking, and a sensation as if
something were shaking loose in that region whenever the
right foot was planted heavily upon the floor or ground
as in walking; also gnawing pain in the back, worse in
bed, and continuing all night.

* Sub-acute and chronic ovaritis, and neuralgia of the ovaries.
(*Hale.*)

*Catamenia.*—Menstruation came on at the usual time, normal
in quantity, and continued to flow as long as she kept
mo  ng about, but ceased to flow whenever she ceased
wa   g.

Menstruation returned [hemorrhage?] after having been absent two years in the case of a person who had passed her
climacteric.

Menstruation returned in two weeks, slight in quantity, dark
in color, thick, with odor like that of the lochial discharge.

Menstruation too scanty, not one-fourth part as much as usual,
followed by profuse bright yellow leucorrhœa, so acrid as
to excoriate the perinæum.

### Sexual Instinct.

*Female.*—Voluptuous itching in the vagina, with feeling of
fullness of the parts.

Sexual desire strong, though formerly not so; can repress it
by keeping very busy, but as soon as occupation ceases
the desire returns in full force.

*Male.*—Sexual desire, which has been dormant for years,
roused into activity.

Lascivious dreams, with seminal emissions toward morning,

followed by weakness and a feeling of irritability, and great difficulty in keeping his mind fixed upon the subject under consideration, frequently selecting wrong words to express his idea.

*Mamma.*—Severe cutting pains in the left mammary gland, extending through to the left shoulder-blade, aggravated by lying on the left side (constant throughout the proving).

Sharp, cutting pains in both mammary glands, extending from the left mamma through to the left shoulder-blade and to the spine.

° *Clinical.*—In several cases of delayed post-partum recoveries, the *Lilium* has accomplished all that could be desired. When the uterus is slow in returning to its normal condition; the lochial discharge continues too long, is profuse and excoriating; pain in the back and hips, bearing down and dragging from high up, when in an upright position or at stool, as if the whole pelvic organs would escape through the vagina if not prevented by firm pressure with the hand against the vulva; painful smarting in the urethra after passing urine; constipation, with itching, painful hemorrhoids, or morning diarrhœa; fears the presence of an internal disease from which she never will recover, and dreads insanity. *Lilium tigrinum* 30 effected a prompt change for the better. (*Paine.*)

### Respiratory Organs.

*Larynx and bronchia.*—Cough dry and hard, coming in single coughs.

*Respiration.*—Oppressed breathing, with oppression in the lower part of the chest, aggravated about four o'clock in the morning.

Desire to take a long breath frequently, and sighing, which appeared to come from the lower part of the abdomen.

Out of breath when ascending, obliging her to stop; seemed as if it proceeded from the heart.

Oppressive heat and congestive feeling of the chest; a kind of ebullition, worse in the evening, must go into the fresh air for relief, **but going into** the fresh air increases the headache.

Feeling of compression of the chest and great weight; a feeling as if the chest had too much blood in it, producing **a** choked, suffocated sensation, that might be relieved **by** letting out the blood; slight relief from sighing.

### Chest and Heart.

*Chest.*—Sharp twinges, followed by a dull, drawing sensation in the left side of the chest, extending upward to the clavicle.

Hot, congested feeling in the chest; generally chilly feeling, and chills, especially in the face.

*Heart.*—Thirteenth day after commencing the proving, heart symptoms appeared; sudden fluttering of the heart, after walking, felt less when very busy.

Hurried, forcing feeling about the apex of the heart, with fluttering and general faint feeling; could do nothing, obliged to put aside her work; relieved by sitting still.

Sharp and quick pain in the left side of the chest, with fluttering of the heart.

*Sensation as if the heart were squeezed in a vise, as if the blood had all gone to the heart, producing a feeling as if the prover must bend double; inability to walk straight.*

Heavy feeling, as if the blood were shut up in the heart; pulse small and weak; a sensation as if blood did not reach the radial artery in sufficient quantity.

Weak beating of the heart, with severe congestion of the chest; bloody taste in the mouth; severe left-sided headache; dizziness; feeling of faintness; blur before the eyes, and fear of falling.

Awakened from sleep at night with a distressing, pressive pain in the region of the heart and palpitation.

Constant pain in the region of the heart, increased by bending forward, stooping, or on lying down.

Heaviness and pressure in the region of the heart, almost unbearable after eating.

Fluttering or palpitation of the heart; cold hands and feet, covered with cold perspiration.

Violent beating of the heart, and throbbing of the carotids, preventing sleep when lying on either side.

Heaviness in the region of the heart, and palpitation when lying on the left side; worse at night and when lying down.

The heart symptoms were all worse at night, and there was great fearfulness that he had mistaken his case, and that he was really suffering from an organic disease of the heart instead of medicinal symptoms, though he had never had such symptoms before.

*Arteries.*—Conscious pulsations over the whole body, and out-pressing sensation in the hand and arms, as though the blood would burst through the vessels

### Back.

*Cervical.*—Drawing sensation in the muscles of the neck, left shoulder, and stitching pains in the left mammary gland, increasing after two o'clock P. M.

*Dorsal.*—Pain in the dorsal vertebræ, as if the back would break.

*Lumbar.*—Sharp pain in the lumbar region, extending over the right hip to the umbilical region, ameliorated by rubbing.

Steady pain in the small of the back, spreading from the spine both ways toward the kidneys, continuing all day after a restless night.

*Sacral.*—Pain in the sacrum.

*Coccygeal.*—Sensation of pulling upward from the tip of the os coccygis.

### Upper Extremities.

*Fore arms.*—Pressing pain in the right arm and wrist, with cramps in the fingers.

*Hands.*—Burning heat in the palms of the hands and soles of the feet, extending up the limbs, with constant searching for a cool place, aggravated at night.

Cold hands and feet, with profuse, cold and clammy perspiration, keeping the hands and feet constantly wet.

Stiffness of the fingers, almost like paralysis; great difficulty in holding and guiding the pencil to write.

### Lower Extremities.

Boring pain in the right hip joint; stiff feeling of the muscles of the thigh, and pain in the ankle, going down to the toes.

Stitches coming and going throughout the day in the right hip joint; with chilliness and headache, increased as the evening advanced.

Severe drawing pain in the right hip, extending down the outside of the thigh, relieved by moving the limb from place to place.

Pain in the left thigh, aggravated by walking, yet the pain was so much worse after having ceased to walk, she was impelled again, though she knew after doing so she would be worse again.

Aching of the legs; with inability to keep them still in bed; worse when giving up control of herself, as when trying to sleep.

Severe pain in the ankle joints and second joint of the fingers, making the motion of a carriage very painful; bruised feeling in the soles of the feet, and great muscular soreness, making pressure of the clothes painful.

### Fever.

Chills in face, extending downward, with a more general chilly feeling than in cold weather, at the chest.

Chills running from the face downward, with constriction of the chest, as if too narrow or too much crowded with blood, and burning heat over the body the whole night, with queer, half-waking dreams.

Great heat and general lassitude in the afternoon, with throbbing pulsations over the whole body, and out-pressing sensation in the hands and arms, as though the blood would burst through the veins.

### Sleep.

Inability to sleep, with wild feeling in the head, as if she would be crazy.

Inability to sleep for a long time, eyes wide open; at length went to sleep lying on the back with the knees drawn up.

Sleep unrefreshing, broken by disagreeable dreams, with great irritability in the evening.

### General Symptoms.

Some of the pains are ameliorated by change of position, while others are aggravated.

Symptoms return every day from five to six o'clock P. M., gradually increase through the night, and abate at about eight o'clock A. M. [Constant throughout the proving.]

In some cases the uterine symptoms are better after riding, and exercise in the open air.

With some of the provers, the symptoms of the reproductive organs were more clearly defined on the left side, while with others more on the right, but *generally* more on the left.

The pains occupy small spots, as if produced by hand pressure with the ends of the fingers. (Compare Oxalic acid.)

After the symptoms have entirely disappeared, they return again very suddenly in the same order, without any apparent provocation.

The muscles of the whole body feel sore and bruised, rendering stepping, the motion of a carriage, and even the pressure of the clothes very painful.

Convulsive contractions of almost all the muscles of the body, and a feeling as if she would be crazy if she did not hold tightly upon herself.

Most of the symptoms better when walking out of doors in the open air, when the cool air strikes the uncovered head and face, and worse in a close, hot room.

### Characteristics.

All the symptoms return again and again, after having disappeared, but diminished in degree at each successive return.

The social and moral conditions are profoundly affected, generally changed to their opposites, though in some instances they seem very contradictory.

The symptoms connected with the female reproductive organs, and the consecutive moral conditions, are very pronounced and peculiar; the ovaries are the seat and origin of peculiar sharp and burning pains; backache; dragging, bearing down sensation in the uterine region, seeming to drag even from the thorax and shoulders, and, at the same time, pressure on the rectum and bladder producing a constant desire to evacuate these viscera, as in cases of prolapsus uteri, were very marked and persistent, and physical exploration showed that the uterus was actually prolapsed and anteverted.

---

# LITHIUM CARBONICUM.

### (*Lithiæ Carbonas.*)

PHARMACOLOGY.—This is a white powder, sparingly soluble in water, and having a feeble alkaline reaction. It dissolves with effervescence in dilute sulphuric acid, and forms a freely soluble salt. It imparts to the flame of burning alcohol a carmine red color.

OFFICINAL PREPARATIONS.—Triturations to the 3d.

ANALOGUES.—*Lach. Graph. Lyc.* (?)

### Mental Sphere.

Disposition to weep about his lonesome condition.

° The whole night anxiety and feeling of helplessness.

Difficulty in remembering names.

### Head.

° Heaviness in the sinciput, especially in the frontal eminence.

Toward evening, pain and heaviness over the brows, with restlessness in the stomach, unchanged by eating supper and by walking out, continuing until he goes to sleep.

Fullness in the right temple the whole afternoon.

Pressure in both temples from without inwards, with a pressing pain in the middle of the chest, extending outwards and toward both sides, in the region of the fourth rib.

° Tearing, sticking headache on the right side, worse on assuming the erect position and on motion, better during repose.

Early on awaking, violent headache in vertex and temples (after sudden cessation of the menses), second and third day; less on the fourth and fifth days, but on the sixth day, in the afternoon, again very severe in the left eye, temple and small spot in the occiput; in the temple and vertex very severe, with nausea.

Heavy weight upon the vertex, with **pressure** upon the left temple; the whole head is as if **too large**; at the same time it feels as if it were violently squeezed in a small spot, which greatly increases the nausea; could hardly keep the eyes open; they pained as if sore from morning till noon; when looking at anything the headache grows worse; she can't continue lying down; it pains everywhere; somewhat better when sitting, relieved by going out.

° Headache relieved or ceases while eating, but returns afterwards.

### Eyes.

On the second day of the menses, after being obliged to get up from reading and go into the open air, she noticed on taking up the book again, an uncertainty of vision and an entire invisibility of the right half of whatever she looked upon; if two short words occurred in succession, the one toward the right hand was invisible; both eyes similar in this respect.

Pains internally in the globe of the right eye, above the external canthus.

° Pains in the eyes, as if little grains of sand were in them.

Feeling of dryness in the eyes, although they were moist, worse in the left.

Throbbing, drawing pain about the right eye, around, outside, above and deep in the orbit.

### Ears.

Pain behind the left ear, in the bone, extending toward the neck

ᶜ Earache, left side, from the throat, with prosopalgia.

### Nose.

Obstruction of the nose.

Constant discharge of mucus in the evening.

Dropping from the nose in the open air.

° Nose red, swollen and dry.

° Nose, especially on the right side, somewhat swollen, red, sore internally—shining crusts form in it; it is dry and as if inflamed; (at the same time frequent urinating at night, disturbing the sleep.) (*Hering.*)

## Mouth and Throat.

Toothache in the right lower back tooth, again in the left.

Teeth seem dull, numb and loose, so that she cannot bite.

Pains are more violent on the left than on the right side.

° In the evening sore throat on the right side.

° Sore throat extending into the ear, and from ear to throat.

° Hawking up of mucus in large quantities.

## Stomach.

° Nausea, with gnawing in the stomach, fullness of the temples and headache.

° Acidity of the stomach relieved quickly by *Lithium*.

Cannot bear the slightest pressure on the stomach.

° When eating, *the gnawing in the stomach goes away.*(*Lach.*)

Good appetite, with gnawing in the stomach.

## Hypochondria.

° Violent pain in the hepatic region, between ilium and the ribs.

Sticking pain in the left hypochondrium.

Pressure in the hepatic region and gentle pressing pain in the right side of the forehead; later over the eyes; the forehead pain extends to the left side, with nausea.

## Abdomen.

Abdomen feels swollen and as if distended with wind.

Violent pain across the abdomen, upper part.

Pain in the left abdominal ring, like a pressing from within outwards, with confusion of the head and dull pressure from without inwards in both temples.

## Urinary Organs.

Sensitive pain and sharp pressure in the vesical region, more on the right side soon after passing water.

° Tenesmus (vesical) after micturition.

Pain in the region of the neck of the bladder.

Before passing water, flashes of pain in the region of the bladder, inferiorly, more toward the right; after urinating, pains extending into the spermatic cord, more on the left.

° Quick, strong tenesmus, with sensitive pain in the middle of the urethra.

° Frequent and copious urination.

On rising to urinate, *a pressing in the region of the heart,* which did not cease until after urination.

Turbid urine, with much mucus deposit.

Urine scanty and dark, very acrid; it pains when being passed, which is difficult.

\* Very frequent urination, disturbing in sleep.

Dark reddish brown deposit in the urine.

### Stool and Anus.

Soft stools early in the morning.

° At night diarrhœa, which is very offensive.

Diarrhœa immediately after drinking chocolate.

Discharge of flatus in the evening, which is offensive.

° Soft abundant stool in the morning; it had for a long time been hard and difficult.

Violent, painful, dull stitch in the perineum near the anus, from above downwards, from within outwards; when walking, being sharp, quick, short, itching in the anus in the evening.

### Generative Organs.

(*Female.*) Menses suddenly cease and headache comes on.

Menses four days later and diminished.

When taken before the menses, the symptoms were most violent on the left side; when taken after the menses, on the right side.

(*Male.*) \* Burning in the urethra.

° Pains on the right side in the urethra and through spermatic cord into the testicle.

Voluptuous titillation in the urethra at night on waking.

Erection after urinating at night.

Pains in testes, and when sitting, with stitches in the penis.

### Thorax.

° On inspiration, the air feels so cold that it seems to be felt unpleasantly, even in the lungs, in heart disease.

Pressive pain in the middle of the chest, from within outwards toward both sides.

Violent cough late in the evening, while lying down, compelling to rise, without expectoration; the irritation which provokes the cough is in a little spot posteriorly and

inferiorly in the throat; cough consists of very quick
shocks, which do not seem to come out of the chest, but
out of the throat, and to be very violent and prostrating
in short paroxysms.

Constriction of the chest when walking out, after breakfast,
then expectoration of mucus in great quantity brought up
by hawking; the mucus seems to come from the middle
of the sternum.

### Heart.

Pains in the region of the heart, throbbing, like a dull stitch.

As she bent forward over the bed, in the morning after rising,
a very violent pain in the region of the heart.

Pressure in the region of the heart on rising to urinate, passing away after urination.

° Rheumatic soreness in the region of the heart.

° Pains in the heart before and at the time of the commencement of the menses.

° Often, in deficiencies of the valves especially after mental
agitation of a vexatious character, to which she is very
subject, a trembling and fluttering of the heart, distress-
ingly painful in the heart and as far as between the shoulders; it extends upward also into the head where it is felt
as an equally painful throbbing; at the same time the air,
on inspiration, seems so cold that it is felt unpleasantly
cold even in the lungs. (*Neidhard.*)

### Back.

Pain and weakness in the sacrum.

Feeling of prostration in the sacrum at night.

In the morning, on rising, a feeling of soreness on the right
side near the spine, below the loins, upon a spot not
larger than the point of the finger, sensitive to pressure,
lasting all day.

### Upper Extremities.

Pain on the anterior side of the right shoulder joint, near the
point of insertion of the pectoralis major muscle on the
margin of the same.

Burning stitch in the ball of the hand.

Itching, throbbing, very sensitive pains in all the fingers, especially in the second and third fingers of the left hand, as if it were in and upon the bones, extending from the hand to the end of the fingers, only during repose; it ceases upon pressure, when grasping and during motion.

Left middle finger very painful, through and through.

Soreness at the margin of the nail, redness and pain, more at the external angle, first of the left thumb, then of the right fourth finger, then of several fingers of the left hand, then of the right middle finger, lasting several weeks.

### Lower Extremities.

Itching, burning pain in a small spot on the right hip, then on the thigh, then on the little toe; all on the external aspect of the limb.

Itching, burning pain internally on the left thigh, and at the left knee.

Occasional rheumatic pains in the lower extremities.

Great weakness of the knees, with pain, especially on going up stairs.

° Painfulness of the feet, ankles, metatarsus, all the toes, especially at the border of the foot and the sole as if it were gouty.

Ankle joints pain when walking, first the right then the left.

Itching, burning of the feet.

A paralytic stiffness in all the limbs and in the whole body.

Prostration of the whole body, especially in the knee joints and in the sacrum.

Over the whole body, as if beaten, stiff and sore in all the bones, joints and muscles.

### Sleep.

Anxious and restless at night.

Voluptuous dreams, tenesmus (vesical,) and erection which subsides after urination, on awakening.

Offensive diarrhœa awakening from sleep.

Sleep disturbed by the pains in the feet and sacrum.

### Fever.

Coldness of the feet, especially of the soles, then sudden heat beginning in the soles of the feet and extending over the whole body.

General feeling of heat in the body; sweat on the back of the hands and very copious sweat.

[No skin symptoms of importance.]

---

# LOBELIA CARDINALIS.

### (Cardinal Flower.)

DESCRIPTION.—This is a tall, smooth plant, with oblong, lanceolate leaves, slightly toothed. The flowers are *deep red, large, and very showy*, in an elongated raceme, rather one-sided. It grows in wet places, all over the United States, flowering from July to October. There are twelve or more species of the Lobelia found in this country. This pathogenesis is from a proving by Dr. Samuel R. Dubs.

OFFICINAL PREPARATIONS.—Tincture of the plant when mature.

ANALOGUES.—(?) *Lobelia cerulea* (?)

### Mind.

Disposition to sing while walking.

### Head.

Headache, dull and distressing, with fullness in the forehead and base of the occiput; the latter was peculiarly painful; the pain increased by motion on shaking the head.

Hot sweat on the forehead; throbbing in that portion, and low in the occiput, with stiffness in the nape of the neck.

Head feels light, with dull pain in the forehead and occiput.

### Face.

Dryness of the *nose*, with fullness, followed by sneezing.

Dull pains in the upper maxillary bones of each side, with aching in the molar teeth.

### Mouth and Throat.

Unpleasant taste in the mouth in the morning.

Burning, stinging in the mouth and fauces.

*Tongue* raw, sore, very red, especially at its tip, and a painful blister on that part.

Soreness of the fauces, with burning and pricking, extending down to the pharynx and œsophagus.

Throat sore and dry, with disposition to swallow and to hawk up phlegm.

Raw and distressed feeling in the throat, extending down to the epigastrium.

F.26

### Eyes.

Soreness in the eyes, with smarting and slight watering, with repugnance to lamp light.

The eyes feel sore on closing them; with lachrymation.

### Stomach.

Dull, heavy pain in the epigastrium, with sensation of a weight, or load there.

Dull, distressing pain about three inches below, and a little to the left of the epigastrium.

Some nausea, with the distress at the epigastrium.

Sticking pains in the stomach, with heaviness there.

Loss of appetite, and much thirst.

Dryness and rawness from the mouth to the stomach

### Abdomen.

Sticking pain in the left hypochondrium, which came on so suddenly and so violently as to cause me to cry out; the pain was relieved by light pressure on the spot.

° Used as a vermifuge by the Choctaw Indians.

Bowels loose, stools at first thin, then consistent.

### Chest.

Severe stitch in the left side of the chest, which compelled me to press with the hand to moderate it; it nearly took my breath.

Oppression of breathing, with dull and distressing pain under the lower part of the sternum, with the same feeling on each side; *relieved* by beating lightly on the part, with the hand (lasting ten minutes).

Oppression of breathing, with sticking pains on taking a long breath.

Pricking pains in the left lung (side), coming on several times a day, lasting several minutes.

### Back.

Weakness, as from a sprain, across the kidneys, with general languor.

### Extremities.

Pricking as from needles, in the calf of left leg, sole of left foot and heel.

Great debility of the lower extremities; the knees seem to bend under the weight of the body.

27

## Generalities.

General debility, languor, with loss of appetite, and distress
in the stomach.

---

## LOBELIA CERULEA.

*(Blue Lobelia.)*

DESCRIPTION.—This is named by Gray the *L. syphilitica*, because of the
reputation (baseless) which this plant once possessed. A common name
is the "Great Lobelia." It has a somewhat hairy *stem*, leafy to the top,
one to three feet high. *Leaves*, thin, ovate, acute at both ends, two to six
inches long, irregularly serrate. *Flowers, light blue*, rarely white, crowded
in a long spike. It is common in low grounds, flowering in August and
September.

OFFICINAL PREPARATIONS.—Tincture of the leaves; dilutions.

ANALOGUES.—*Cistus (?) Hepar sulph (?) Hydrastis (?)*

## Mind.

* Great depression of spirits; unhappy state of mind, always
associated with "pain about and under (not below) the
short ribs, in the back, on the left side, and extending
outward nearly to the left side; this embraces the posterior aspect of the region of the spleen." (*Dr. Jacob
Jeanes.*)

Frequent mistakes in writing and spelling, with aching and
confusion in the head.

## Head.

Pain on the left side of the head over the coronal suture.

Pains in the head and left arm, and a similar one in the same
part of right arm.

Face flushed and headache after dinner, with drowsiness and
lassitude, but inability to sleep when lying down; somewhat better going into the open air; restless sleep, with
frequent wakings through the night; headache continuing
until daylight.

Confused feeling, with slight aching in the head immediately.

A dull, aching pain in the forehead, over the centre, lasting,
with slight intermissions, until the evening, increased by
reading or writing.

Slight aching pain from the back of the head down the nape
of the neck.

Oppression in the forehead over the eyes; dizziness, particularly in moving about, lasting three hours.

### Eyes.

Drawing sensation under the right eye, with pain in both mastoid processes, first felt and worse in the right one.

Soreness of the eyeballs from turning them; boring pain in the right orbit.

Itching of internal canthus of left eye.

Burning in right eye; itching in external canthus; soreness of the tarsi of the right eyelid; feeling of a foreign body under the upper lid of the right eye, with smarting and burning.

Heaviness over the eyes, like a weight, but no pain.

Oppression over the eyelids and slight drowsiness.

Slight aching over the eyes, particularly left eye.

### Nose.

Itching and tingling feeling in the left nostril, as if about to sneeze.

A feeling of dryness and sensitiveness of the nostrils, so that the inhalation of air of a moderate temperature (supposed 60 degrees) creates a slightly painful feeling in two hours, also second day.

Frequent sneezing, with copious discharge of thick mucus from both nostrils.

A dull aching pain over the root of the nose, in the centre, lasting until evening.

### Face and Lips.

Sensation of dropping under the left cheek bone.

Flushed face with heat when lying down.

Drawing pain in right cheek bone.

Constrictive feeling of mouth and tongue, especially at left commissure of the jaws, afterwards toward the root of the tongue.

Perfect dryness of the lips.

### Jaws and Teeth.

Constrictive feeling at left commissure of the jaws.

Frequent shooting pains through the teeth on the right side.

**Mouth anu Throat.**

Sensation of a lump in the upper portion of the œsophagus; dryness of the left half of the palate.

Bleeding of the gums, with putrid taste.

Pain in the region of left tonsil immediately, also pain in region of right tonsil.

Great soreness, rawness, pricking dryness of the lower surface of the palate, extending forward through the whole mouth.

Thick mucus secretion in the throat, with diminution of the very unpleasant feeling of constriction, rawness, dryness and soreness of throat; the soreness of palate and the astringent feeling in the left side of the mouth, though abated after the mucus secretion at noon, still continues to be felt after eleven hours.

A renewed secretion of thick mucus in thirty-six hours, apparently on the superior surface of the palate, removed by snuffling and hawking, with still further diminution of the soreness of the throat.

Much tickling about the top of the larynx, with disposition to hacking cough; dryness in back part of throat.

Throat moist, showing red, elevated spots.

Increased secretion of mucus from the throat.

° Catarrhal inflammation of posterior nares and fauces. (*Hale.*)

**Gastric Symptoms.**

Violent pain in stomach followed with copious eructations of watery fluid; morning hoarseness connected with the state of the stomach; dyspeptic symptoms continue, but they are much lighter.

Sinking feeling in the stomach followed by borborygmi below the epigastrium, directly after dinner.

° Acid eructations from 5 to 6 p. m. (*Williamson.*)

**Hypochondria and Abdomen.**

Pain in left hypochondria.

Pain from jolting, in the stomach and both hypochondria.

Pain in region of left kidney.

**Urine.**

Increased quantity of urine, with *free* discharge.

Pain in bladder, caused by retaining urine; when evacuated

of a deep amber color; itching and smarting in the fore
part of the urethra.

### Stool and Anus.

Loose evacuations from the bowels.

Copious evacuations of watery stool, with tenesmus and soreness in the anus.

Ineffectual effort at stool, with free eructations of tasteless
wind on rising from bed.

Pains in the abdomen, most below the umbilicus, followed by
diarrhœal stools in the afternoon and evening.

### Chest.

Pain in left side of chest near the axilla, with aching in left
shoulder and arm.

° Oppression in the lower part of the chest, as if the breath did
not reach there; *distress in the region of the heart*, and
audible " knocking " respiration (like the sound of an axe
in chopping wood); pain under the short ribs, and dry
cough. (*Neidhard*.)

° Dry hacking cough of four weeks' duration, extremely troublesome day and night, and pain in the right side about the
junction of the sixth rib with its cartilage, of a year's
duration; dryness of the back part of the throat. (*Ib*.)

Difficulty in breathing.

### Neck, Back and Loins.

Stiffness of the nape (worse in left side), from looking up.

Rheumatic pain along the right collar bone in the evening.

Flashing of heat in the back and shoulders.

Stitching pain in right back, passing from eighth rib downwards; pains between shoulders and in neck both sides.

Cutting pains in the back under the false ribs, cutting forwards
and upwards.

Slight aching pain in the nape of the neck.

* A pain commencing at the right side of the small of the
back, then going down to the os ischium, which is very
sore to touch. (*Neidhard*.)

* Great rigidity of the spine; least motion exceedingly painful; the pain goes from the right to the left side of the
back, and shoots down the legs. (*Ib*.)

° Pain in the eighth dorsal vertebræ, and in the back under
    the short ribs; the pain is increased by movement and
    deep inspiration.   (*Ib.*)

Pain, heavy, aching, in the back under the false ribs, worse at
    night in bed, increased to a cutting pain by deep inspira-
    tion and by turning in bed.

**Painful** weakness of the loins when standing.

### Upper Extremities.

**Heavy** pain in radial muscles of left arm.

**Aching** in left shoulder and fingers whilst writing.

**Stiff**, numb feeling in palm of right hand.

### Lower Extremities.

Pricking and stinging pain in soles of both feet, as if asleep.

Stitching pain in left tibia.

Pain in heel of left foot.

---

# LOBELIA INFLATA.
### (*Indian Tobacco.*)

BOTANICAL DESCRIPTION.—This plant is generally known as wild or
*Indian Tobacco*, and is an annual or biennial indigenous plant, more commonly the latter, with a fibrous, yellowish white *root*, and an erect, angular,
very hairy *stem;* in the full-sized plant, much branched, and from six
inches to three feet in height. The *leaves* are alternate, scattered, sessile,
ovate-lanceolate, serrate, veiny, hairy. The *flowers* are small, numerous,
pale-blue, on short peduncles, each originating from the axil of a small
leaf. The *calyx* consists of five subulate segments. The *corolla* is tubular,
small, slit on the upper side and ventricose at the base; the limbs bilabiate;
tube prismatic; segments spreading and acute, two upper ones lanceolate,
two lower ones oval; *anthers* united into an oblong, curved body, purple;
*filaments* white; *style* filiform; *stigma* curved, two-lobed, and enclosed by
the anthers; *capsule*, two celled, ovoid, inflated, striated, ten-angled and
crowned, with the persistent calyx. *Seeds*, numerous, small, oblong,
brown.

OFFICINAL PREPARATIONS. — Tincture of the whole plant or seeds ;
triturations of the seeds; dilutions.

ANALOGUES. — *Aconite, Euphorbia, Ipecacuanha, Lachesis* (?) *Squilla,
Tabacum, Tartar emeticus, Veratrum album, Veratrum viride.*

### Sensorium.

**Great** dejection with exhaustion, and sobbing.

* **Fear** of death, with difficulty of respiration.

* **Great** mental depression.

Insensibility and loss of consciousness.

### Head.

Vertigo, with nausea; pain in the head and trembling; agitation of body.

\* Pressive pain in the occiput, with dull heavy pain around forehead, from one temple to the other.

Sudden shocks through the head.

Chilliness of the left side of the head, with feeling as if the hair would rise on end.

\* Pressive headache at the occiput, left side; worse at night and on motion.

Continual, periodic headache in the afternoon ; and in the evening till midnight.

### Eyes.

Pressing pain in the eyeballs, with intense itching.

Intense smarting of the inside of the lids.

Hemiopia.

° Conjunctivitis (used as a collyrium).

Weakness of eyes, as if from weariness (1)

### Ears.

Shooting pain extending into the left ear, from a painful **spot** in the throat.

### Face.

Heat of the face accompanying the nausea.

Chilly feeling in the left cheek extending to the ear.

Circumscribed redness on one cheek.

### Mouth.

Taste as of corrosive sublimate.

Profuse flow of clammy saliva; a tenacious **mucus**.

Mouth dry with white coated tongue, etc.

### Throat.

Burning dryness of the throat.

Frequent hawking, from tough mucus in the throat.

Prickling in the throat, with eructations and burning sensation rising up from the stomach.

\* Sensation as if the œsophagus contracted itself from below upwards.

Feeling of pressure in the whole course of the œsophagus, with

a vermicular motion, most strongly felt below the larynx
and in the epigastrium.

Epigastrium and a spot below the larynx are most sensitive
points.

Prickling in the throat, with desire to vomit.

* Sensation as of a lump in the pit of the throat. (*Lachesis.*)

### Appetite and Stomach.

* Loss of appetite, with acrid, burning taste in the mouth.

* Acidity of the stomach, with a constrictive feeling in the pit
of the stomach.

* Flatulent eructations, with acidity and heat of the stomach

* Incessant and violent nausea, with pain, heat and oppression
accompanying the affection of the respiratory organs.

Nausea and vomiting, with prostration of strength.

Vomiting of food after eating it warm.

° Dyspepsia, heartburn and running of water from the mouth.

Paroxysms of a feeling of pressure on the pit of the stomach.

Violent, painful constriction in the cardiac region.

° Gastralgia biliosa; paroxysms of excruciating pain, and feeling as of a heavy load in stomach.

° Gastralgia simplex; the pain extends up into the chest and
causes dysphagia.

* Sense of weakness and oppression at the epigastrium, with
oppression in the chest.

Inflammation of the stomach and bowels.

Burning pain in the stomach, toward the back, as if the part
nearest the spine was inflamed.

* Dyspepsia, with a sensation of *excessive weakness* at the
stomach, extending up into the chest and down to the
umbilicus, always attended with oppression at the chest.
(*Dr. Jeanes,*) (also *Baptisia—Hale.*)

### Abdomen.

Pain in the right hypochondrium, with distension of the abdomen and shortness of breath.

Flatulent rumbling in the abdomen, with pain, worse after
eating.

Sensation as if diarrhœa would occur.

Griping and drawing pain in the abdomen.

<sup>e</sup> Intussusception of the bowels. (*Marcy & Hunt.*)
<sup>o</sup> Incarcerated hernia. (*Eberle.*)

### Stool.

Papescent stools; whitish, soft stools.
Scraping sensation during stool, with discharge of black blood.
<sup>o</sup> Copious hemorrhage from the hemorrhoidal vessels.

### Urine.

Increased secretion of urine, or urine diminished.
Sticking pain in the region of the right kidney.
Urine easily decomposed, depositing a pink sediment and small brown crystals. (*Noac.*)

### Sexual Organs.

*Male.*—Aching pain in the urethra, with smarting of the prepuce.
Pressure and feeling of weight on the genital organs.
*Female.*— Uterine hemorrhage.
Violent pain in the sacrum, with fever.
Supervening suppression of the menses during fever.
<sup>o</sup> Menses suppressed, with pain in the right shoulder.
<sup>o</sup> Suppressed menses in consumptive persons.
<sup>o</sup> Rigidity of the os and perinæum during labor.

### Larynx.

Frequent, short, dry cough, from tickling in the larynx, and sensations of a foreign body in the throat, impeding breathing and swallowing.
Violent, racking cough in paroxysms, with expectoration of ropy mucus.
<sup>o</sup> *Croup*—spasmodic—a very efficient remedy.
<sup>o</sup> Whooping cough; bronchitis; spasmodic coughs.

### Chest.

\* Tightness of the chest, with laborious breathing and a sense of oppression causing a deep breath to be taken.
\* Deep inspiration relieves the pressive pain in the epigastrium.
\* Short and slow inspiration, with desire to cough.
<sup>o</sup> Chronic dyspepsia, with sensation of a lump in the pit of the throat and oppression of the *chest.*
<sup>o</sup> Paroxysmal asthma, with pain in the chest.
Pain in the chest from deep inspiration.

Feeling of drawing in the left breast from the nipple to the
axilla.

* Angina pectoris, with pain extending to the shoulder and arms.

° *Constant dyspnœa*, aggravated by the slightest exertion and
increased by the shortest exposure to cold.

* Sensation of weakness and pressure on the epigastrium,
rising from thence to the heart, with or without heartburn.

* Feeling as of a lump or quantity of mucus, and also a sense
of pressure in the larynx.

Weakness and oppression in the epigastrium, with oppression
of the heart.

° *Paroxysmal asthma, chronic, very distressing*, often cured
by *Lobelia*, and nearly always palliated. (Dose 5 to 10
drops every hour or two.)

° *Spasmodic asthma ;* the most aggravated attacks sometimes
yield quickly to small doses of the tincture. (*Jeanes.*)

### Back.

Burning and cutting in the lower part of the spine.

Rheumatic pains between the scapula.

Painfulness of nape of the neck and dorsal region.

Violent spasmodic pain in the posterior iliac regions.

### Upper Extremities.

Rheumatic feeling in the right shoulder joint.

Pain only when touched, in the muscles of the right arm.

Paralytic feeling in the left arm.

Severe rheumatic pain in the right elbow joint.

### Lower Extremities.

Pressing pain in the middle part of the thigh, with constrictive feeling of the head.

* Inflammatory rheumatism of the right knee, with tearing
pains in the fibula.

Weariness of the limbs, with cramp-like feelings in the gas-
trocnemius.

Prickling sensations through the whole body.

Cramps in the calves.

### Fever.

* Fever and ague, with chill in the middle of the day, followed

by heat and sweat, which lasts until next morning.
Sensation of heat and shuddering in the daytime.
° *Intermittent fevers* (quotidian).

### Skin.

Eruptions between the fingers, on the dorsa of the hands and
on the fore arms of small vesicles, with tingling itching.
(*Teste.*)
Prickling itching of the skin all over the body.

### Sleep.

Restless sleep, with anxious and sad dreams.

---

# LYCOPUS VIRGINICUS.
### (*Bugle Weed.*)

BOTANICAL **DESCRIPTION.**—This plant, also known as *Paul's Betony* and
*Water Horehound*, **is an indigen**ous, perennial herb, with a fibrous root,
and **a** smooth, **straight, obtusely** four-angled *stem*, with the sides concave,
producing **slender runners from** the base, and from ten to twenty inches in
height. The *leaves* **are** opposite, oblong, or ovate-lanceolate, toothed,
entire toward the base, **with** glandular dots underneath. The *flowers* are
very small, purplish, **in** dense, axillary whorls; at the base of each flower
are two small subulate bracts. Corolla campanulate, four-cleft, the tube
as long as the calyx, upper segment broadest, emarginate. *Calyx* tubular,
four-cleft, longer than the achenia; *stamens* two, distant, diverging, simple;
*anthers* erect, bilobed; *ovary* superior, four-angled; *style* straight, slender;
*stigma* bilobate; *achenia* four, smooth, abovate, obliquely truncate at apex,
compressed, margins thickened.

"Bugle weed is found growing in almost all parts of the United States,
in moist and shady situations, flowering in June and August. It has a
peculiar, balsamic, terebinthinate odor, and a disagreeable, slightly bitter
taste; it imparts its properties to boiling water in infusions. The whole
herb is officinal. It has not been analyzed, but probably its virtues
depend upon a volatile oil and tannic acid." An analysis of this plant
made by Tilden & Co., gives 40 parts of Tannin to 7,000 organic and inor-
ganic matters, also "a bitter principle, soluble in ether, 24 parts," and a
"peculiar principle, insoluble in ether, 696 parts."

In the following pathogenesis, the symptoms noted only in proving
mother tincture are marked (1); those belonging only to the 200th (2);
those common to both are unmarked. Doubtful symptoms are marked
with a note of interrogation. Of the 202 symptoms recorded, 132 belong
to the mother tincture, 41 to the 200th dilution, and 29 are common to
both (*Dr. Morrison, of England.*)

The symptoms thus marked with numerals are from the provings of Dr.
Morrison, of England. All the rest are from my own provings and clinical
experience.—*Hale.*

OFFICINAL PREPARATIONS.—Tincture of the whole plant; dilutions.

ANALOGUES.—*Digitalis, Iberis, Acid hydrocyanic, Prunus virginiana, Laurocerasus, Spigelia, Sanguinaria, Cactus.*

## Mental Sphere.

° Stupid, with lack of expression during menstrual flow.

° Mind wanders from one thing to another.

One of the mildest and best narcotics. (*Rafinesque.*)

° General wakefulness and morbid vigilance.

Obtusion of intellect (1).

Increased mental and physical activity (1).

Difficulty in concentrating attention and thought (2)

Restless activity, ready for any amount of work (1).

## Head.

Pressing-out sensation in the frontal and temporal regions.

Pains in frontal eminences, passing from left to right, and back to left.

Oppressed feeling in brain (1).

Dull aching through the sinciput.

Pressive frontal headache.

Oppressed feeling in cerebellum (1).

Giddiness, with tendencies to right and forward.

Persistent giddiness, while sitting.

Acute pain in left temple, passing to right.

Aching in left maxillary articulation and left wrist (1).

Acute pain in left frontal eminence, with **sensation** of compression of brain (1).

Severe aching through occiput (1).

Dull, oppressive general headache.

Severe, general headache, with giddiness.

Acute darting from left temporal to malar bone, with sensation as if brain were compressed, followed by irritation of scalp over the line of pain (1).

Persistent giddiness, commencing in open air, continuing while sitting.

Giddiness, while sitting, with constriction of larynx.

Aching in one spot, changing from left to right of occipital protuberance (1).

Fronto-occipital headache, from three to seven P. M. (1).

Frontal headache, subsequently passing to occiput, three to six P. M. (1).

Giddiness, with strong tendency to the right.

Neuraloid pain in the right supra-orbital region (1).

Pressing-out sensation above right frontal eminence (2).

Acute pain in right temple, passing to left frontal eminence, and returning to right temple (2).

Neuraloid pain in both temples, worse during evening (2)

Sensation of heavy pressure on parietal protuberances, moving upward to middle line (2).

Darting pains in lower half of forehead (2).

Subacute pain above left frontal eminence, passing to right lower molars (2).

Darting pain in left temple, succeeded by steady aching (2).

Acute pain at seventh cervical vertebra (1).

Nearly all symptoms shortly return with considerable severity

### Eyes.

° Protrusion of the eyes, with tumultuous action of the heart.

° Pain in the forehead and temples relieved by nausea.

Painful pressure in the eyeballs.

° Exophthalmus from cardiac disease.

### Mouth and Teeth.

Parched feeling in upper lip (1).

Aching in lower molars; passing from right to left.

Acute pain in the right lower molars, passing to right temple, left lower molars, left temple, and returning to right lower molars.

Continuous aching in left lower molars (1).

Pain passes from lower molars to lumbar and mid-dorsal regions, returning to left lower molars (1).

Pain in left lower molars, passing to left upper bicuspides (1)

Slight achings in left lower, left upper, and then in right upper molars (decayed) (2).

Pains in left lower molars, transferred to right.

### Throat.

Sensation of rawness at back and right of palate.

Slight burning in palate (1).

Subacute pain in pharynx, increased by deglutition (1).

Sensation of rawness, with swelling (which subsequently disappeared) like a hardened gland, to back of right palate.(2.)

Irritation in fauces, inciting to cough (2).

### Stomach and Bowels.

° Indigestion, with pain and distress in epigastric region.

° Gastritis; enteritis; dysentery and diarrhœa.

\* Circumscribed pain and compression in the region of the stomach.

° Constipation for six or seven days, stools dry and clog-like.

\* Diarrhœa—(in phthisis,) with griping and rumbling.

Strong bearing down in left inguinal canal, as if hernia would protrude, while sitting ; with acute pain on walking ; relieved by upward pressure on external ring (1).

Bearing down in right inguinal canal ; with subacute pain when walking; relieved by continued pressure on exterternal ring; with severe loin pain, especially to right of spine (1).

Aching in both inguinal canals, on rising from bed, increased by walking ; relieved by upward pressure on external rings (1).

Continuous aching along both inguinal canals, most marked on right side, increased by walking (1).

Acute pain down right inguinal canal, while sitting (1).

Tenderness down right inguinal canal (1).

Aching down right inguinal canal, while sitting (1).

Pressive aching down left inguinal canal, relieved by upward pressure (1).

Severe aching down spine, somewhat relieved by friction, passing off after rising (1).

° Excessive flatulence, which aggravates the palpitations.

Faintness, with slight nausea, while walking in open air.

Agreeable sensation of warmth to left of epigastrium (2).

Eructations, with distinct flavor of the drug (2).

Fæces papescent or watery, with succeeding constipation (1).

Bowels act more freely; relaxed; fæces light colored (1).

Fæces slimy, of a peculiarly shining dark-brown (1).

Fæces slimy, of a peculiar greyish-brown, as if mixed with ashes (1).

° **Diarrhœa** in jaundice, from weakened heart. (*Hale.*)

Fæces of a dark shining brown; odor strong (1).

Fæces offensive, slimy, dark shining brown, gushing out (1)

Excessive flatulent rumblings, on awaking (1).

Fæces half solid, with straining; half slimy, gushing out (1).

Fæces slimy, of a shining yellow; offensive (1).

Fæces partly solid and natural, partly slimy, dark-brown, offensive (1).

Constipation; fæces hard, scanty, dark, passed with straining and consequent bleeding (2).

Constipation succeeded by softer and freer motions, of the peculiar shining yellowish-brown previously noted (2).

### Generative Organs.

*Female.*—° Menses last from half an hour to six hours, intermitting for ten or twelve days.

° Puffing of the parts on and around the pubes and vulva, dilated condition of the vagina.

° Vagina very hot, os uteri engorged and swollen.

° When the heart's action was tumultuous the puffing (œdema) of the pubis was gone.

° Menorrhagia and metrorrhagia.

*Male.*—Sharp darting pains through left testicle (epididymis); passing to right testicle; leaving dull achings (1).

Acute aching in left testicle, with occasional darting **pains,** changing to right, and again to left testicle (1).

Acute pain, from left kidney down left inguinal **canal (1).**

The **pains** in left testicle cause **an** aching along left **inguinal** canal, extend to right testicle, **and** at times very severe **(1).**

Pain first in left, then in right, then in both testicles; **recur.** ring the whole evening (1).

### Urinary Organs.

\* Urine scanty, thick and muddy, with œdema of the feet.

Dull pain in left lumbar region—the bladder *feels* distended when empty.

Urine exhibits excess of mucus, with epithelium scales and minute crystals (1).

Urine shows less deposit, with di. sp. gr. (1007–1010.)

Urine contains scattered mucus and epithelial scales, abundance of spermatozoa, and oxalate of lime crystals; sp. gr. 1004—1006 (normal 1016—1018 (1).

Urine exhibits slight deposits of mucus; sp. gr. 1015 (2).

° *Diabetes mellitus;* several cases of great severity. (*See Therapeutics.*)

### Larynx and Cough.

° It quiets cough and irritation of the lungs.

° It lessens arterial action in fevers and plethora.

° An excellent remedy for hæmoptysis in phthisis.

° It is an excellent substitute for Digitalis or bleeding. (*Ib.*)

Sense of constriction in larynx.

Dyspnœa, as if from bronchial catarrh (2).

Cough, with slight pale expectoration, wheezing, and hot achings beneath right scapula (2).

Increased bronchial, with increased faucial irritation, and in- creased cough (2).

Unpleasant, sweetish expectoration, at times difficult (2).

Slight nasal catarrh, with sneezing (2).

° Cough and expectoration checked by repetition of medicine (2).

### Chest.

Subacute pain below and to outer side of left nipple (apex region).

Rheumatoid aching in right scapular muscles.

Pleurodynia (?) from third to seventh left interspace, with spasmodic contraction of intercostal muscles, increased by lying on right side (1).

Subacute superficial pain at third left interspace, becoming acute on moving (1).

Spasms of right intercostal muscles (?) on awaking (1).

Pleurodynia (?) below fifth right costal cartilage, passing to left and then returning to right side, on awaking (1).

Sense of constriction across lower half of thorax, impeding respiration, with subacute pain, increased by lying on right side, on awaking (1).

Intercostal pains, worse from lying on right side, with re- peated darting pains at apex (1).

Acute pain in left axilla, extending down edges of pectoral muscles to thorax, passing to base and apex of heart (1).

Acute pain in intercostal muscles, over base of heart (1).

Severe pain at insertion of right pectoral muscles, becoming more acute on inspiring deeply (1).

Pain on right side of thorax, passing to apex region, then to right axilla, and down pectoral muscles to former spot, again to apex region, and returning to right side (1).

Oppression of respiration (1).

Rheumatoid aching over apex, then above right nipple, then from third to sixth left interspaces inclusive, with pain in apex (2).

Achings in chest increase toward sunset (2).

Subacute achings over apex and above right nipple, with dull temporal headaches (2).

Achings generally increase in severity toward sunset (2).

Sensations of heat, first under right scapula, then in centre of left lung, and again beneath right scapula (?) (2).

Agreeable sensation of warmth, first to left of epigastrium, then in apex region, then at base of heart (2).

Occasional pains in chest.

Hot sensations recur, especially beneath right scapula

Oppressed respiration, with sighing (2).

Subscapular aching (2).

Shifting rheumatoid achings (2).

### Heart and Pulse.

*Constricting pain* and tenderness around the heart.

° Action of the heart, tumultuous and forcible, (when eyes seemed protruded) it could be heard several feet from the bed. (In a case of exophthalmus.)

First sound of the heart displaced by a blowing sound of mitral regurgitations.

*Stitch-like* pain in the cardia—also a *throbbing* pain. Pulse 58—irregular.

° *Cough with hæmoptysis*, feeble, quick, irregular action of the heart; (if it does not cure consumption it is a very valuable palliative.) (*Hale.*)

° It renders the beat of the heart slower, fuller and more regular.

Beats of the heart more distinct on right side of sternum.

28

° Palpitation in cardiac hypertrophy, with dilatation. (*Hale.*)
° Palpitation from nervous irritation, with plethora. (*Ib.*)
° Aneurism of the large vessels near the heart. (*Ib.*)
° It lessens the irritation, anxiety and suffering, and palliates organic disease of the heart. (*Ib.*)
A sensation of pressing outward in the cardiac region—not painful.
Subacute pain at apex of heart (1).
Cardiac oppression, lasting an hour (1).
Marked cardiac oppression (1).
Quickened pulse, with distinct intermissions (1).
Sighing and yawning (1).
Cardiac depression, with dull heavy beating.
On waking, frequent intermissions (1).
Cardiac action first steadied by drug, then rendered intermittent (1).
Pulse irregular and intermittent, especially when lying, quickened at each inspiration.
Cardiac distress, most marked at apex (1).
Pulse about 72, lying, sitting, and standing, quickened at each inspiration (1).
"Cardiac pulsation scarcely perceptible to touch."
Subacute pain, extending from apex to third lower interspace (1).
Acute pain at apex, with contraction of intercostal muscles, increased by lying on right side, from 6:30 to 10 A. M. (1).
Pulse 68, with oppressed cardiac action (1).
Palpitation on slight exertion (1).
On awaking, labored cardiac action (1).
Left-sided pains predominate.
Subacute pain at apex of heart, moving to fourth left interspace (1).
Pulse immediately steadied by a full dose of the drug, subsequently becoming jerking (1).
Pulse subsequently becomes quickened, feeble, irregular (1).
"Heart sounds indistinct, systolic running into diastolic" (1).
"Heart-sickness," not relieved by food (1).

Cardiac pains, with general debility (1).

Acute darting pains, at apex of heart (1).

Acute pain at apex, not relieved by pressure, driven by friction to left subscapular region, then passing to mid-dorsal region (1).

Acute pain at apex, with cardiac distress (1).

Pulse scarcely perceptible, irregular (1).

" Pulse extremely variable, both as to time and volume, at first almost imperceptible, not intermittent " (1).

" Cardiac pulsation much stronger than the pulse indications would lead one to expect " (1).

" Impulse feeble, heart sounds very weak, action irregular in force and rhythm " (1).

" Pulse feeble, compressible, irregular in force and rhythm " (1).

Marked cardiac depression, causing slight faintness on quickly ascending a few stairs (1).

Faint feeling returns later on quietly ascending (1).

Cardiac action barely perceptible, with moderately strong and less compressible pulse (1).

Pulse compressible, irritable, varying greatly in force and rhythm, with frequent intermissions (1).

Pulse less compressible, irregular and intermittent (1).

Cardiac depression, causing faintness (1).

Cardiac depression, succeeded by cardiac oppression, with quickened pulse (1).

Subacute pains both at apex and base of heart (1).

Pulse irregular in rhythm, extremely compressible.

On lying down, palpitation, with shortened systole and lengthened interval (2).

Cardiac depression, with intermittent pulse (2).

Pulse irregular and intermittent (2).

Acute darting pains in heart, with complete intermissions (2).

## Neck.

Acute pain in nape of neck (cervical muscles) (1).

Temporal pain, transferred to cerebellum, and again to temples (1).

Congestive pain in nape of neck (1).

Stiffness of left cervical muscles, interfering with movement of head.

### Back.

Acute flying pains to right of mid-dorsal region (1).

Continuous lumbar pain, not increased by stooping, increased by walking (1).

Aching across lower dorsal region (1).

Aching (like lumbago) across loins.

Rheumatoid pains in lumbar region (1).

Acute rheumatoid loin pain, extending to lower dorsal region (1).

Continuous lumbar and dorsal pain. most severe toward left side (1).

### Upper Limbs.

Unsteadiness of hands, rendering writing somewhat difficult.

Return of tremulous feeling in hands, while writing, lasting several minutes (1).

Rheumatoid pains, especially left (1).

Acute pains, especially in left wrist (1)

Darting pains through right wrist (1).

Pricklings (urticaria?) in lower forearm, hypogastrium, etc., returning to left forearm (1).

Troublesome urticaria, specially affecting left forearm and right leg (?) (1).

Frequent rheumatoid pains in left forearm, left wrist, left hand, and right forearm and wrist (1).

Flying rheumatoid pains (2).

Erratic rheumatoid pains in left wrist, right calf, right subclavicular region, and returning to left wrist (2).

Darting pains in left thumb (1).

### Lower Limbs.

Acute rheumatoid pain from left knee to ankle; quickly settling in loins (1).

Rheumatoid pain in calves of legs, especially left (1).

Return of acute pains in left leg, extending up thigh, on exertion (1).

Pains are transferred from left calf and leg to right (1).

Occasional pains in legs, especially left (1).

Rheumatoid pains, especially left leg and forearm (1).

Sharp aching in right leg, not relieved by friction (1).

Sharp aching down right tibia, causing lameness; not relieved by friction (1).

Acute pain in inner muscles of left calf, with straining and lameness (1).

Aching down flexor muscles of right thigh, extending to knee and calf of leg; then to left knee and calf; then returning to right thigh and knee; with slight lameness (1).

Achings down both thighs, with weakness in walking (1).

Irritation (urticaria?) in right leg, right forearm, back, etc. (1).

Subacute pain down muscles of left calf (1).

Acute pain down anterior muscles_of right thigh, causing lameness; subsequently, down both thighs (1).

Achings, passing from left wrist to right knee, left tibia anteriorly, lower dorsal region, left knee, and right forearm.

Rheumatoid pains pass from left wrist to right calf (2).

Erratic rheumatoid pains, affecting lower limbs (2).

### Sleep.

On *waking*, labored cardiac action.

Dreamy sleep, with early waking.

Sneezing, on awaking from sleep (2).

### Generalities.

It seems to cause abnormal action of the heart, and has cured some of the symptoms of *Exophthalmus*.

The left leg feels half an inch shorter, and sounds on the pavement as if it really were.

Rheumatoid pains, passing from left to right; returning to left side; chiefly affecting muscles and articulations; increased by movement, by cold air, and by concentrating the thought upon them. Dental pains, chiefly in decayed teeth, and usually passing from right to left, not relieved by *acon.*, *merc.*, nor by direct warmth. Sneezing, dyspnœa, cough, expectoration, wheezing, and faucial irritation, as if from bronchial catarrh. Cardiac distress, palpitation, and rheumatoid pains, increased as above; irregular and intermittent pulse; quickened, feeble, compressible pulse. Constipation, followed by full, soft motions, of a shining yellow-brown, offensive; gushing out. Faint perspiration on covered parts, while walking. Dreamy sleep and early waking. Rheumatoid achings, relieved by electrical current, not relieved by galvanic. Neuraloid pains, affecting testicles. Pains, as if herniæ would protrude, relieved by upward pressure on crural rings. Eructations, tasting of the drug. Nausea and faintness. Times of aggravation, early morning; afternoon (3 to 5 o'clock); sunset; and during evening.

Pains increase in severity toward sunset.

Sighing and yawning (1).

---

# MENISPERMUM CANADENSE.

### (*Yellow Parilla. Moonseed.*)

BOTANICAL DESCRIPTION—This is a climbing plant, growing in various parts of the United States, from the northern boundary to the Gulf of Mexico. The root, or rhizoma, is long, of a yellow color, and a very bitter taste.

OFFICINAL PREPARATIONS.—Tincture of the fresh root with strong alcohol; dilutions.

ANALOGUES.—*Aletris, Bryonia, China, Cocculus, Iris, Ignatia, Hydrastis, Nux vomica, Ptelea, Rheum.*

### Mind.

Very low spirited, but attends to business with rapidity.

Absent minded, but the thoughts were clear.

Torpor of the mental faculties, with physical languor.

Feels surly, ill-natured, and stubborn.

Quick tempered and irritable.

### Sleep.

Restless sleep with troubled and confused dreams.

Sudden starting from sleep.

Sleep well, but inclined to dream pleasant dreams.

Sleeps late and heavy in the morning.

Dreams of heavy cannonading.

Dreams of innumerable rats, which creep under my clothing.

### Head.

Dull, heavy headache, with a feeling of *fullness.*

Intense headache, with stretching, yawning and *chilliness.*

Feeling of fullness in the head at night.

Headache, restlessness, and a swollen sensation in the eyes at night.

Headache, with pressure from within outwards, in the morning.

Intense headache, feeling as though it would burst, with pain the whole length of the back.

Slight headache in upper frontal region, and through the temples.

*Headache through the temples, extending to the occipital region.*

## Eyes.

Eyes feel swollen and dry at night.

## Nose.

Nostrils feel dry, especially the left, and itches **painfully.**

Painful soreness within the nostrils.

° Thick yellow mucus, becoming scanty.

## Mouth and Throat.

Slight coating, of milky appearance on the tongue.

Very thirsty.

Tongue coated yellowish-white, with much thirst, and **hurried** respiration.

Burning sensation of the tongue.

Tongue feels raw, as if burned.

Tongue coated yellow, in morning **thicker posteriorly, with** raised papillæ.

Tongue dry and parched.

Tongue coated all over with a yellowish substance.

Throat feels dry and parched.

Mouth and throat dry.

Yellow coating on the tongue, **thickest at the base.**

*Tongue much swollen.*

Œdema of the fauces, with some **inflammation.**

*Excessive discharge of saliva.*

## Liver.

° Hypertrophy of the liver. (?)

° Results of chronic hepatitis. (?)

° Cirrhosis and induration of the liver. (?)

## Stomach.

Slight nausea in the morning upon rising.

° Induration of the gastric glands. (?)

Increased appetite.

Violent vomiting and purging.

## Abdomen.

Pain in the umbilical region.

*Tenesmus, but stool natural.*

Loose, frequent stool.

## Urinary Organs.

Urine high-colored, scanty, and hot (*secondary*).

Urine thirty-four ounces, white, with cloud in bottom (*primary*).

Urine yellow and cloudy, voided thirty ounces (*primary*).

Urine dark yellow and scanty (*secondary*).

Profuse flow of urine (*primary*).

° *Dropsy*, with great debility.

## Skin.

Sensation of itching over the whole surface of the body, *aggravated by warmth.*

Pimples on the face.

Itching of surface, the pimples bleed easily.

° *Syphilis* (tertiary). (?)

° Chronic herpetic eruptions.

## Upper Extremities.

Aching in the upper arm and in the left scapula.

Drawing of the brachialis anticus.

Aching, drawing pain in the shoulder joints, in the region of the scapulæ.

Slight, jerking pains near the elbow, probably in the biceps muscle.

## Lower Extremities.

Aching, drawing pains in the muscles of the thigh.

Aching in the upper part of the left femur, and left hip joint.

Legs feel sore, as if bruised, with pain in the bones.

° Arthritic, and rheumatic complaints.

## Circulatory System.

Pulse hard and quick.

Hurried respiration.

Feverishness at night, with headache and restlessness.

### General Characteristics.

Headache and pains resemble those caused by taking large doses of quinine, and were relieved by *China* 1.

Many of the symptoms resemble those occurring in the different forms of ague.

The headache was relieved by *Bryonia*, and by walking in the open air. Nearly all the symptoms appeared to be aggravated in the morning. It exerts its influence principally on the salivary and gastric glands.

Great debility in dropsical affections.

---

# MITCHELLA REPENS.

BOTANICAL DESCRIPTION.—"This is an indigenous evergreen herb, with a perennial root, from which arises a smooth and creeping *stem*, furnished with roundish-ovate, or slightly heart-shaped, petiolate, opposite, flat, coriaceous, dark green and shining *leaves*, usually variegated with whitish lines. The *flowers* are white, often tinged with red, very fragrant, in pairs, with their ovaries united.

"*Calyx*, four-parted. *Corolla*, funnel-form, two on each double ovary; limb, four-parted, spreading, densely hairy within. *Stamens*, four, short, inserted on the *corolla*. *Style*, slender, stigmas four. *Fruit*, a dry, berry-like, double drupe, crowned with the calyx teeth of the two flowers, each containing four small seed-like bony nutlets. Some plants bear flowers with exserted stamens, and included styles; others conversely—those with included stamens and exserted styles." This plant is indigenous to the United States, growing in dry woods, among hemlock timber, and in swampy places, flowering in June and July. The leaves bear some resemblance to clover, and remain green through the winter. The fruit, a berry, is a bright scarlet, edible, but nearly tasteless, dry, and full of stony seeds, and also remains through the winter. The plant is sometimes called *Checker-berry, Winter clover, Deer-berry, Squaw vine, One-berry.* The whole plant is officinal, and imparts its virtues to boiling water and alcohol. It has not been analyzed.

OFFICINAL PREPARATIONS.—Tincture of the leaves, with strong alcohol; infusion; dilutions.

ANALOGUES.—*Asclepias inc., Caulophyllum, Cimicifuga, Chimaphila, Eupatorium purp., Helonias, Pulsatilla, Senecio, Uva ursi.*

### Mental Symptoms.

Depression of spirits.

Forgetfulness; very forgetful.

Dread of approaching death.

Perceptive faculties very dull.

### Head and Eyes.

Throbbing pain on right side of head.

Severe frontal headache just behind the superciliary ridges.

Eyes dull and heavy.  Eyes feel weak and watery.

### Ears.

Dull aching pain in right ear; burning of left ear.

### Face.

Rush of blood to the face.

### Mouth and Throat.

Pricking and burning sensation in the tongue.

Fauces feel dry and irritated.

Constriction hindering deglutition.

### Stomach.

Eructation, with burning in the stomach, and along up the œsophagus.

Dull aching pain in the epigastrium.

### Abdomen.

Distension of the bowels with expulsion of flatus.

Colic pain in the colon which is tender on pressure.

### Rectum and Stool.

Bowels costive.

Urging to stool; diarrhœic stools.

Small stool with tenesmus, expelled with difficulty.

### Urine.

* Urging to urinate; urine high color; white sediment.

* Dull aching pain over the region of the kidneys.

* Swollen and irritated condition of urethra and neck of bladder.

* Catarrh of the bladder, especially in women.   (*Hale.*)

* Dysuria accompanying uterine complaints.

A feeling of uneasiness at neck of the bladder.

Notable increase of the urinary secretion (*primary*).

### Uterus.

A powerful uterine-tonic.  (*King.*)

Cervix engorged, dark, red and swollen.

° Delayed menstruation.

° Engorgement of uterus, from lack of tone in muscular wall of the organ.

° Amenorrhœa, dysmenorrhœa and menorrhagia.
° False labor pains in last months of pregnancy.
° Slow, feeble and inefficient labor pains. (The tincture to be taken three times a day (ten drops) for two weeks before confinement.) (*Hale.*)

Breathing hurried; dry, hacking cough, from accumulation of mucus in the bronchia.

### Chest.
Burning pain over region of heart (in muscles?).
Heart beats slow and irregularly, then hurried.
Hurried breathing, dry, hacking cough, and excess of mucus in the bronchia.

### Back.
Back feels very weak, with great soreness.
Muscles of both shoulders very sore.
Pain in region of the kidneys.
Dull aching pain in small of the back
Burning in small of the back.

### Extremities.
Great pain in lower extremities.
Great pain in knee joints, relieved by motion.
Muscular soreness.
Dull burning and sore pains in all the muscles of the extremities.

---

# MYGALE LASIODORA.
### (*Cuban Spider.*)

OFFICIAL PREPARATIONS.—Triturations of the spider; tincture; dilutions.

ANALOGUES.—*Apis, Agaricus, Belladonna, Cimicifuga, Doryphora, Hyosciamus, Tarantula, etc.*

### Mind.
Felt sad all day. (*Howard.*)
Great anxiety and fear of death. (*Hale.*)
Despondency and fear of death. (*Howard.*)
Delirious and restless all night, with talk about his business. (*Ib.*)
Restless all night with ridiculous dreams. (*Ib.*)

### Head.
° Frontal headache—in chorea—vertigo.

### Face.
Face flushed and hot.

### Mouth and Throat.
*Tongue* dry and parched, or dry and brown.
° Grating of the teeth—nights.

### Gastric.
*Nausea*, with palpitation of the heart.
Excessive thirst—with the fever.

### Urinary Organs.
In the morning increased discharge of urine, with stinging
    pain in urethra.
The urine during the day was burning hot, it seemed scalding.

### Chest.
Difficult respiration, with anxiety.

### Heart.
Strong palpitation of the heart, dimness of sight, nausea, and
    general weakness.

### Back.
Pain in the back, extending around to the front.
Twitching in the muscles of the back.

### Extremities.
The local inflammation (from a bite) was very extensive, reach-
    ing from foot to knee, leaving a large violet spot which
    afterwards became greenish. (*Howard.*)
*Intense redness* in streaks, following the course of the lym-
    phatics—from the calf upward to the body, with great
    anxiety, twitching of the limbs, etc. (*Hale.*)
* Convulsive, uncontrollable movements of the arms and legs.
Pulsative, stinging pains in the foot.

### Fever.
*Severe chill*, followed by fever, with trembling of the whole
    body, excessive thirst, face flushed, *pulse* 130, tongue dry
    and brown, difficult breathing, despondency, fear of death,
    delirium.

### Generalities.
* Convulsive, uncontrollable movements of the back, arms and
    legs.

° *Chorea:* arms and **limbs in** constant motion, facial muscles distorted, could not help herself; headache, vertigo, grating the teeth nights; *quiet* during sleep; *worse* in the morning. (*Dr. Spooner.*)

° *Chorea:* jerking in left leg, facial muscles, etc. (Dr. Blake's patient improved in a short time under Mygale.)

° *Chorea*—after Cimicifuga—"the twitching was now confined to the left arm (cured by Mygale 1st)." (*Dr. Blake.*)

## MYRICA CERIFERA
### (*Bayberry.*)

DESCRIPTION.—This plant, known also by the names of *Wax-Myrtle, Wax-berry,* etc., is a branching, half-evergreen shrub, from one to twelve feet high, and covered with a grayish bark. It is found in dry woods and open fields. The bark of the root contains tannic acid and gallic acid; a volatile oil; an acrid resin, soluble in alcohol and ether; an astringent resin; myricinic acid (a peculiar principle resembling *Saponin*); salts of potassa, lime, iron, magnesia and silicic acid. Its taste is bitter, astringent, acrid and spicy. Myricin, its active principle, is a light, grayish-brown powder, with a peculiar spicy smell, and a peculiar, bitterish, astringent taste, with some persistent pungency. It is soluble in alcohol.

OFFICINAL PREPARATIONS.—Tincture of the bark of the root with dilute alcohol; dilutions. Myricin; triturations.

ANALOGUES.—*Asarum canadensis, Acidum benzoic., Berberis vulgaris, Bromine, Chimaphila, Cornus circinata, Chelidonium, Cubeba, Eryngium aquaticum, Eupatorium aromaticum, Hydrastis can., Hepar sulphur, Kali bichromicum, Lachesis, Mercurius iodatus, Spongia.*

### Mind and Disposition.
Deficient concentration of mind on any subject.

Gloomy, terribly depressed, despondent.

Indifference to everything—even to friends.

Condemned himself for imaginary faults.

Irritable, with constant desire to find fault. He thinks himself better than any one else.

### Head.
Dull, heavy aching in the forehead and temples, on waking in morning.

Pain in the head, worse when stooping or moving about.

Headache, with pain and stiffness in nape of neck.

Headache, with throbbing in the temples.

Headache in morning with aching in small of back.

Dull, heavy feeling over the eyes, followed by stricture across the nose.

Soreness of the scalp to the touch.

Pain in back part of head, right side.

Heaviness in back of head, with pressure in nose.

In the top of the head a sensation like foam rising in anything fermenting.

Chills running over the top of the head, with tightness of the scalp.

Empty feeling in the head.

Headache, with drowsiness, also with ringing in the ears.

Pressure and dull pain in forehead and vertex, with throbbing synchronous with the pulse.

### Sensorium.

Vertigo, with rush of blood to the head on stooping, followed by full, oppressive headache in right side.

Vertigo with nausea, and with yawning, and drowsiness.

### Eyes.

Dull pain in the eyes and head, with heaviness in the eyes.

Smarting in the left eye.

Eyes feel swollen, and eyelids heavy and swollen.

Yellowness of the sclerotica, with congested appearance.

Both eyes feel sore, with flushed face.

Sharp pain in left eye, it is sore and looks inflamed, in morning.

Aching in right eyeball with quivering in the eyelids.

Smarting in both eyes, with feeling as of sand in them, and difficulty of closing the lids.

Hot feeling in the eyes, they tire easily on reading.

### Ears.

Ringing in both ears, with slight vertigo· also with pressure about the head.

### Nose.

Sensation in the nose, as if he had catarrh.

Constrictive feeling across the nose.

Severe *coryza*, in the morning.

Aching, excruciating feeling in the posterior nares

Tenacious, offensive mucus in the nose.

° Fœtid, bloody ozœna.

### Face.

Pressure in the malar bones.

Yellowness of the face (jaundice).

Itching and stinging in right side of face.

Burning in the face, with sensation of fullness.

Creeping sensation, as of crawling insects on the face.

Fullness about the face and head, with throbbing.

### Mouth, Teeth, etc.

Tongue furred, with bad taste in mouth and nausea.

Tongue thickly coated, dirty white or yellowish.

Saliva increased, with heartburn.

Dryness of the mouth and fauces.

Darting pain in the articulation of jaw, right side.

The whole buccal cavity, even the roof of the mouth, was
coated with an adhesive coating, difficult to detach, *with*
offensive breath and foul taste.

° Aphthæ of the mouth.

° Tender, spongy and bleeding gums.

° Follicular stomatitis.

### Throat.

Soreness of the throat in the morning.

Sensation as of a foreign substance in the throat, requiring it
to be frequently cleared, *with* painful deglutition, *in* the
afternoon.

Constricted and **rough feeling** in the throat, it feels swollen,
with a **constant desire** to swallow.

Stringy mucus in **the throat**, detached with difficulty.

Throat and nasal **organs** filled with an offensive, tenacious
mucus, detached with difficulty.

Dry, sore feeling in the pharynx, as when one has **taken cold,**
succeeded by difficult deglutition.

Lancinating pain in right side of the throat, **near the tonsil**

° Ulceration of the fauces.

° Catarrh of throat and posterior **nares**

° Aphthous tonsillitis.

### Taste and Appetite.

Taste bitter and nauseous, *with* offensive breath.

Feeling of fullness in the digestive organs, as if food was slowly digested.

Craving, unnatural appetite, with feeling of fullness in the stomach, after a hearty meal. (*primary.*)

Complete loss of appetite, but with a feeling of fullness and repletion in the abdomen. (*secondary.*)

Strong desire for acids.

### Gastric Derangements.

Nausea followed by heavy headache.

Empty eructations, relieving the pressure in the stomach for a short time only.

Heartburn with water-brash.

### Hepatic Symptoms.

Dull pain in the region of the liver.

*Complete jaundice*, with bronze-yellow skin, loss of appetite; fullness in the stomach and abdomen; scanty, yellow, frothy urine; loose, mushy, clay-colored (or straw-colored) stools, destitute of bile, much debility, and drowsiness almost amounting to stupor.*

[This jaundice was not relieved by Podophyllum, Leptandra, Nux vomica, Arsenicum, or Mercurius dulcis, but was speedily removed by Digitalis 1-10th dil.]

* The icteric symptoms of Myrica are undoubted. Dr. Walker proved the drug under my own observation. By reference to the two provings made by him, it will be seen that during the first proving he had "drowsiness, with heavy frontal morning headache, *yellowness of the eyes, scantiness of urine, and light-colored* fæces,"—all the premonitory symptoms of jaundice. At this point the medicine was suspended, and the above symptoms *disappeared.* At the next proving the same symptoms recurred, but this time were kept up by the action of the drug until complete jaundice obtained. This jaundice, I believe, was owing to *suspended secretion*, and not *obstruction*. Had the latter condition been the cause of the jaundice, critical discharges of black, tarry matters would have been noticed, whereas, in this case, the fæces, under the action of Digitalis, gradually resumed a healthy color and appearance, and the same change occurred in the condition of the urine. Jaundice appears to be a secondary effect of Myrica: consequently when used as a curative agent in that disease, the lower attenuations will be best indicated.

(Since the above was written several cases of jaundice have been reported cured by Myrica.) (*Hale.*)

\* "Black jaundice." (*Eclectic.*)

## Stomach and Abdomen.

Distress in the stomach after dinner.

Acidity of the stomach.

Weak, sinking feeling in the epigastrium, approaching nausea, increased after eating, relieved by rapid walking.

Vomiting, with heat in the stomach.

Severe griping pains about the stomach, followed by empty eructations.

Stinging, cramp-like sensation in left præcordial region, under the ribs.

Griping pressure in stomach, extending to a place on the left of the naval.

Grumbling pain in the bowels, in the afternoon.

Griping pain in bowels at night, followed in the morning by loose stool, with tenesmus.

Colic-like pains in umbilical region, in a small spot, with accumulation of flatus, and passage of offensive flatus.

Constant, unusual rumbling in abdomen, above the navel.

Griping pain in region of umbilicus, with rumbling.

Weak, faintish feeling about the bowels, as when one has diarrhœa.

## Stool and Anus.

Loose stool after dinner, with pain and tenesmus.

Sensation as of approaching diarrhœa, followed by small, costive discharges and griping, colic-like pains.

Constant discharge of flatus when walking.

In A. M. felt as though diarrhœa would occur, followed by weakness about the bowels, with urging and pressing, without stool.

**Constipation**, after previous loose stools.

**Soft**, copious, papescent stool, attended by tenesmus and cramp like sensation in umbilical region.

Urging to stool, with no other result than the expulsion of a great amount of flatus.

Excessive flatulence in P. M., with frequent rumbling, as if diarrhœa would set in.

Stool nearly natural in consistency, but lighter colored.

29

\* Loose, light-colored stool, growing lighter-colored daily, **until** it became ash-colored and destitute of bile.

° *Chronic diarrhœa.*   ° Diarrhœa of consumptives.

### Sexual Organs.

Amorous dreams, with emission of semen (this never occurred to the prover before).

° Chronic gonorrhœa.

° Leucorrhœa, excoriating, fœtid, thick and yellowish, (of several years' duration).   Cured by injections of the infusion. (*Hale.*)

### Urinary Organs.

Sharp, plunging pain in region of the left kidney.

Difficulty of urinating; the bladder seemed to lack contractive expelling power.

Copious flow of limpid urine.   [*primary effect.*]

Urine deposits a light-colored sediment.

Urine darker than usual—grows darker every day, until it is a deep brownish-yellow.   [*secondary effect.*]

A pinkish-brown sediment in the urine.

Scanty, high-colored urine, saturated with the coloring matter of the bile.

Frothy, high-colored urine—(froth yellow).

### Respiratory Organs.

Smarting in larynx and trachea.

Dull pain in right lung, middle lobe, lasting a few minutes.

Constriction in the chest when lying on the left side in bed, with such increase of the impulse of the heart that its pulsations were audible.

Sharp pain in the region of the heart.

° Cough very much aggravated by talking.   ° Tickling cough at night on lying down.   ° Cough, with profuse expectoration.   ° Chronic bronchitis.

### Back and Neck.

Dull, aching pain in lumbar region all day.

Dull pain under both shoulder blades.

Sensation of warmth along the whole spine, **particularly** between the shoulder blades.

Pain in the back of the neck.

Dull, dragging pain in small of the back.

Pain under left scapula.

## Upper Extremities.

Lancinating pain in left axilla.

Pain (tearing) in left arm, between shoulder and elbow.

Pain in third and little finger of left hand.

Severe pain in shoulder and arm, extending to little finger.

Right arm felt lame and heavy, particularly about the wrist joint.

Dull, aching pain in *all* the extremities.

## Lower Extremities.

Soreness of the muscles of both thighs.

Trembling and aching in calves of the legs; worse in the *left*.

Sharp, shooting pain in right thigh, followed by a similar pain in left thigh.

Sharp, piercing pain at the inner side of left knee joint.

Soreness and pain in the left tendo-Achillis, worse on pressure and motion.

Severe pain midway between the knee and ankle, a little outside of the tibia; a contractive pain, with soreness to the touch, changing to a burning; worse on motion.

Pain in the hollow of the right foot.

Burning in the soles of the feet.

Bruised pain in heel of left foot.

Coldness of lower extremities, with pain from knees downward.

## Skin.

Itching and stinging sensation on the skin of the face, neck, shoulder, fore-arm, and right leg.

Persistent itching in different parts, worse near the point of insertion of the deltoid muscles, in both arms.

Itching of the face, giving way to creeping sensation, as of insects.

* Yellowness of the skin of the whole body

## Sleep.

Restless night, with tossing about.

Waking with dull frontal headache.

Waking in a gloomy state of mind, unrefreshed.

Sleep disturbed at night; bad dreams and frequent waking.

Drowsiness, *with* and *after* headache.

Falls asleep in chair, in the daytime, (an unusual occurrence.)

Dreams of enormous bugs, which attacked his head, and which he killed with much difficulty.

Sleeplessness, with exhilaration of nervous system, in evening.

### Fever, Pulse and Heart.

Warmth along the whole spine, especially between the shoulders, followed by chill, gentle perspiration, more perceptible over the dorsal vertebræ.

Chilliness upon going out of doors, *with* aching pain in the lumbar region.

Severe chill, with quivering sensation in calf of right leg.

Feverish acceleration of the pulse, attaining its height about four o'clock.

Excited, feverish feeling, alternating with chilliness, *at* ten o'clock P. M., *with* pain in the lumbar region.

Feeling of feverishness, with the pulse at 60.

Pulse 51, feeble and irregular.

Impulse of heart's action increased, but the number of pulsations diminished to sixty per minute, (ordinary pulse 75 to 80.)

Increased pulsation, and audible beating of the heart when lying in bed on left side.

° Night sweats—in phthisis.

### Generalities.

General malaise, and feeling of unfitness for duty.

General languor, with depression of spirits.

Weak, sick feeling; every kind of exertion was irksome.

Shifting pains.

General muscular lameness and soreness, affecting chiefly the lower limbs.

Staggering gait, with confusion of thought and purpose in the head.

° Great debility, with the jaundice.

### Conditions.

*Worse* by the warmth of the bed—disturbing sleep.

*Better* when moving, and in open air (gastric symptoms).

*Left* side predominantly affected.

The *headache* worse when stooping or moving.
Digitalis removed the hepatic symptoms.

---

# MYRTUS COMMUNIS.

### (*Myrtle.*)

DESCRIPTION.—The common Myrtle is well known by its shining ever green leaves, and white, sweet-scented flowers. Though extremely abundant in Italy, Southern France, Spain, etc., it is not indigenous to Europe or America, but only naturalized, having originally been brought from Western Asia. In England it is not sufficiently hardy to withstand the frosts of very severe winters. It grows well in our Southern States and South America.

[See Hering's article, Hahnemannian Monthly, vol. 7, p. 62.]

OFFICINAL PREPARATIONS.—Tincture of the leaves (and berries).

ANALOGUES.—*Bryonia, Phosphorus, etc.*

### (*No provings.*)

## Chest.

° Pain in the chest; cough, with tightness on the breast.

° Dryness in the throat; pains in the throat and chest, with expectoration of blood. (*Hbgr.*)

° Acute pain in the chest; pressing pain in the chest. (*Ib.*)

\* Stitches in the left breast, running through the shoulder blade, as they often occur in tuberculosis. Relieved when no other remedy would. (*Wahle.*)

° Hepatization of left lobe of the lung. (*Ib.*)

\* Catarrhal fever with pain in the elbows and knee-joints. (*Ib.*)

° Dry, hollow cough, from tickling in the upper anterior lobes of the left lung; worse in the morning, less tickling in the evening; great lassitude during the afternoon hours. (*Ib.*)

° Cough, with tickling in the chest. (*Pehrson.*)

° Several homœopathic physicians besides myself have used the 3d in cases like the above, with great success. (*Hering.*)

° Throbbing ache, and stitching pain in the left infra-clavicular region, extending thence through to the left shoulder blade, aggravated by making a deep inspiration, sensation of burning in the left breast. (*W. E. Paine.*)

° Stitching pain in the left chest, from the upper portion
straight through to the left shoulder blade, worse from
breathing, yawning and coughing. (*Raue.*)

"I have confirmed the above symptoms." (*McClatchey.*)

---

# NABULUS SERPENTARIA.

### (*Lion's-foot.*)

BOTANICAL DESCRIPTION.—This is an indigenous perennial herb, with a
somewhat glaucous *stem*, with rough dentate *leaves*, of which the *radical*
are palmate, the cauline with long foot-stalks, sinuate-pinnatifid, disposed
to be three-lobed, with the middle lobe three-parted, and the upper *lanceolate.* The *racemes* are terminal, somewhat panicled, short and nodding,
with an eight-cleft calyx, and twelve florets. It is about two feet high,
with purple flowers; it is common to the mountainous districts of Virginia,
North Carolina, and other sections of the United States, and flowers in
August. The *root* is thick and tuberous; the whole plant is used in medicine, the milky juice of which is probably the active agent; it is the Prenanthes serpens of Pursch.

[This plant is said by botanists to be a *variety* of the *Nabulus albus,*
which is also known by the name of Lion's-foot, as well as *White-lettuce,*
*Rattlesnake-root,* all of which are given to the Nabulus serpentaria; it is
the *Prenanthes albus* of Linnæus.]

OFFICINAL PREPARATIONS.—Tincture of the whole plant; dilutions.

ANALOGUES.—*Æthusa, Dulcamara, Eryngium, Hepar sulph., Ipecac
Pulsatilla, Sulphur.*

## Head.

Headache in frontal and vertebral region, with irritability in
connection with persisting irritation of the throat, eyelids
and skin.

Frontal pains, deep-seated, behind the right eyeball.

Sharp, neuralgic, occipital pains, with pain and feeling of stiffness in the neck, increased by turning the head; worse in
the evening.

## Eyes.

Weakness of sight; she cannot use her eyes to sew or read
without pain.

## Nose.

Right nostril sore, with catarrh.

## Throat.

Sore throat, tickling and scraping only on the left side.

### Stomach.

Acid, burning eructations in forenoon.

No appetite; prefers acids and lemons.

### Stool.

Constipation; three stools in twelve days. (*p.*)

Stool hard and painful, followed by languor and prostration. (*p.*)

° Diarrhœa—profuse—in summer.

° Dysentery, epidemic.

### Urinary Organs.

Urine diminished, and no desire to urinate.

Sharp pains in the right kidney.

### Uterus.

Sharp, throbbing pains in uterus, with discharge of a white, jelly-like matter from the vagina.

Catamenia retarded nine days.

° Uterine leucorrhœa.

### Trunk.

Dorsal pains.

Dull pains in the joints, and numbness on awakening.

### Fever.

Chilliness not removed by heat.

### Skin.

Pimples on the face itch about the nose, upper lip and cheek.

Prickling sensation over the body.

### Mental.

Depression of spirits, not deep, but persisting

Vague and sensitive presentiments.

Sensation of tipsiness.

---

# NAJA TRIPUDIANS.

### (*Virus of Cobra.*)

DESCRIPTION.—A highly venomous snake, inhabiting the East Indies. It is called the *Hooded-snake*; "serpent with the hood," etc. Its name is pronounced "*Naya*," or, as Webster spells it, "*Naia*." The bite of the *cobra de capello* is generally rapidly fatal. The virus is collected from the poison-sacs, above the fangs, as directed for Crotalus and Lachesis. One drop is triturated with one hundred grains of pure sugar of milk; the triturations are carried up to the 3d or 6th, or higher; then dilutions with strong alcohol.

OFFICINAL PREPARATIONS.—Triturations of the virus; dilutions.

ANALOGUES.—*Arsenicum, Cactus, Crotalus, Iberis, Lachesis, Mygale, Sumbul, Spigelia.*

## Mental Sphere.

Depression of spirits.

Broods over imaginary trouble.

Suicidal insanity.

[Du Chaillu, the great African traveler, says he witnessed the attempt of a native to charm this venomous serpent. In the attempt, the man was bitten. "The man suffered intensely; his body became swollen, his mind wandered, and his life was despaired of; but at last, he got better, and *though complaining of great pain about the heart,* he was soon able to go about again. A short time after, having an axe in his hand, going, as he said, to cut wood, *he suddenly split his own head in two.* He had become insane."]

Wandering of the mind.

## Head.

Waking with dull pain in head, attended by fluttering of the heart.

Heaviness over the eyes, with dryness of the throat.

° Periodic, neuralgic "sick-headache," very severe, in the *left* orbital region, extending back into the occiput; the pain was aching and throbbing about the orbit, and drawing in the occiput; vomiting occurred after the pain had lasted several hours. (*D. A. Colton.*)

* Temporo-frontal headache, accompanied with great depression of spirits, and associated with spinal pain and palpitation of the heart. (*Russell.*)

## Face and Eyes.

*Livid face.*

Eyelids of right eye swollen and livid.

Eyes fixed, pupils large, acting sluggishly to light.

## Mouth and Throat.

* Grasping at the throat, with sense of choking.

Convulsive movements of the mouth.

Clonic contraction of the sterno-mastoid muscles.

Pressure and gagging in the throat.

Rawness of the throat.

* Soreness and pricking in the left side of the throat.

* Constriction and dryness of the throat.

A constricted feeling, with dryness of the throat.

Slight pricking in left side of the pharynx.

* Pharyngo-laryngeal inflammation, with dark red color of the fauces, and spasmodic, irritable cough. (*Russell.*)

### Stomach and Abdomen.

Tearing pain in the abdomen.

Pressure as from stones in the stomach, **after** each meal.

° Dyspepsia, with foul, white or yellowish-white tongue.

### Rectum and Stool.

Sudden desire to evacuate the bowels; stool light color, watery, and discharged with great force.

Diarrhœic stools.

### Uterus.

° Violent crampy pain in region of left ovary.

° Ovarian congestive neuralgia, with violent palpitation of the heart.

### Larynx and Trachea.

Failure of the respiratory function, pulse 32.

* Constriction or irritation of the larynx, giving rise to coughing.

* Short, hoarse cough, with rawness in larynx and upper part of trachea.

### Chest and Heart.

Palpitation of the heart, with uneasy dryness of the fauces.

° Valvular disease, with loud regurgitation sounds; pulse 60, with general anasarca.

Fluttering of the heart, with rising in the throat.

A dull, warm pricking, in a multitude of points, in the right side of the chest, from fifth rib downwards, with heat extending up the bronchia into pharynx; a hard cough came on immediately, ending in expectoration of a little thick mucus.

Asthmatic constriction of chest for half an hour, with mucus expectoration.

° Dyspnœa and prostration in organic diseases of the heart.

Great pain near the heart; swelling of the whole body; wandering of the mind.

Sense of dragging and anxiety at præcordia, occurring in great grief.

° Irritating, sympathetic cough in acute stage rheumatic carditis.

Naja acts primarily upon the nervous system. Especially upon the respiratory nerves, the pneumagastric and glosso-pharyngeal. (*Dr. Russell.*)

° For this reason we should expect this medicine to be of service in the irritating, sympathetic cough which attends organic disease of the heart. (*Ib.*)

° Of the great value of *Naja* in organic disease of the heart, we are convinced by experience. (*Ib.*)

° The indications for *Naja* are the presence of an irritating, sympathetic cough, in the *acute stage of rheumatic carditis*, and afterwards, *organic changes in the valves*, giving rise to tumultuous action of the heart, violent, sudden throbbing, attended with endocardial murmur, and increased size of the organ. (*Ib.*)

---

# NITRATE OF URANIUM.

### (*Uranic Nitrate.*)

PHARMACOLOGY.—The metal *uranium* is obtained from *pitchblends;* the nitrate may be obtained by treating the metal or any of its oxides with nitric acid. It crystalizes in lemon-yellow prisms.

The solutions of this salt possess the power of lowering the refrangibility of the rays of light, which fall upon it, producing the peculiar phenomenon called fluorescence.

Efflorescent in dry and deliquescent in moist air; soluble in 0.35 parts absolute alcohol, and in 0.5 of water.

OFFICINAL PREPARATIONS.—"The best preparation is a recent aqueous solution, prepared with carefully distilled water, (*by artificial light,*) and then preserved in glass stoppered amber vials." (*Blake.*) (Triturations.) "It is an extremely acrid drug; two drops of the 1+ being sufficient to kill a full-grown cat." (*Blake.*) A trituration (by artificial light,) with coarse sugar of milk is reliable."

ANALOGUES.—*Arsenicum*, *Mercurius cor.*, *Kali bichromicum*, *Plumbum*, *Phosphorus*, *Argentum* (DR. BLAKE), *Helonias* (?), *Eupatorium purpureum* (?), *Nitric acid* (?): (HALE.)

[The following is a condensation of Dr. Blake's admirable monograph, prepared for the "Hahnemann Materia Medica," *English*, and containing my first paper on the remedy. (*Hale.*)

### Mental Symptoms.

\* Ill-temper and humor; he is cross with everybody

* General malaise; he feels cross and disagreeable.

## Head and Sensorium.

Head heavy on waking; general languor; aching at occipital protuberance, occipital and frontal headache.

Woke with occipital headache; vertigo twice in the evening.

In the evening pain shooting from right orbit to occipital protuberance.

Frontal headache for two days.

Dull aching in right temple, immediately after taking it.

Slight pain over left eye, with contracted feeling in the throat, and eructations, followed by diuresis.

Heavy, burning pain in right side of vertex; fullness of head and sensation of blood flowing to that part, before eating.

Giddy, faint, flushing of upper body during the catamenia.

Headache in the left temple, with feeling as if he had taken cold, though there had been no exposure.

Severe pain at posterior edge of right and left temporal bone, lasting from 2 to 4 P. M.

*Pathological.—Brain* never affected.

*Medulla oblongata* not once affected. (*Black.*)

*Spinal cord*, lower portion slightly congested.

## Eyes.

Pain over left eye (a characteristic symptom).

Left eyelid inflamed and agglutinated.

## Nose.

Dry coryza; left nostril stuffed.

Itching in nose; small scab in right nostril; purulent discharge from left nostril.

° Scabbing of the inner nostril—chronic. (*J. N. Blake.*)

## Face.

Acne on forehead.

## Mouth.

Small, painless ulcer on buccal aspect of left cheek, opposite left anterior upper molar, more tender in evening, lasting a week.

Copious salivation.

Red spots on hard palate, which feel raw.

## Throat.

Cutting feeling at back of fauces.

### Nausea, Vomiting.

Vomiting, with much nausea, during catamenia; no appetite.

Intermittent vomiting, with great thirst, for four days, then death.

Occasional vomiting, vomits white fluid.

[Vomiting did not appear in the animals in which *ulceration* was found.]

### Stomach.

Tasteless and putrid eructations, with excessive flatulency in stomach and bowels.

Loss of appetite during catamenia.

Very thirsty, with dislike for meat.

For two days intermittent attacks of pain, radiating from the left side of the ensiform cartilage; aggravated by fasting; slight constipation, with occasional twisting, gnawing feeling, rather lower down, relieved by food.

\* Dyspeptic feelings a quarter of an hour before dinner, with gnawing, sinking at cardiac end of stomach; but without hunger or faintness.

*Pathological.*— *Ulceration of the stomach* has been produced in three out of ten rabbits; this seems to be a specific effect, for it appears even when the drug was introduced under the skin of the leg. The ulceration was near the pyloris; even in non-ulcerated rabbits, the mucous membrane of pylorus was diseased. *Stomach:* Mucous coat thickened and softened. Hæmorrhagic spots. (?)

° *Ulceration of the stomach.* (*Dr. Drysdale, British Journal of Homœopathy*, vol. xxviii.)

° *Hæmatemesis* from gastric ulcer. (*E. F. B.*)

### Abdomen.

Woke at 2 A. M., with an urgent desire to evacuate bladder and rectum; borborygmus; small, soft stool.

Constipation, with excessive flatulency in stomach and bowels.

Sharp colic and tenesmus, raw feeling in rectum. Tight feeling around waist; pain all over abdomen.

*Pathological.*--- Ascites in animals. Ulceration of duodenum. Enteritis.

[May be useful in extensive cutaneous burns, with ulceration of duodenum. (*Blake.*)]

## Bladder and Urine.

Burning in the urethra; with very acid urine.

Desire to urinate again immediately after voiding urine.

Chlorides increased, all other constituents remain unchanged.

Micturition increased in frequency (12 times in 24 hours), preceded by pain over left eye; contracted feeling in throat, and eructations.

Sore feeling in pubic region.

Average daily quantity of urine increased by three ounces.

*Urinary tenesmus.*

[Dr. Blake, in remarking on the results of the provings, says: "The results put glycosurea quite out of the court, as a condition theoretically calling for this medicine." It did not cause the urine to contain sugar in a single instance. *In animals* it caused "kidneys *pale*. Tint of medullary layer deepened. The peri-renal tissue was infiltrated with reddish, jelly-like material. *Bladder* greatly distended, full of pale, alkaline urine, with copious flocculent deposit. Bladder full of acid, *albuminous* urine." Dr. Blake says "It ought to be useful in Bright's disease and kindred renal maladies; in contracted kidneys, with gastric disturbance; in irritable conditions of the renal plexus of the sympathetic." It seems singular that it should have cured veritable cases of "sugar diabetes," which it undoubtedly has done. It is homœopathic, however, to *diabetes* generally, as witness the following:]

° Diabetes with albuminuria. (?)

[A corpulent, temperate old man, had constantly increasing debility and emaciation; œdema of the legs; great pain and weariness in legs; crawling and formication in the limbs; clammy state of mouth and tongue; tongue coated with white fur; sensation of dryness in mouth and fauces, with intense *thirst;* severe acid dyspepsia; burning, cramps, and faintness in pit of stomach; bowels constipated, fæces pale, odorless and dry; constant desire to urinate; enormous quantities of urine (16 pints in 24 hours). Perspiration and breath have a sweet odor. Skin dry and hard, and he has night sweats. Pulse 90, small. Greatly relieved by the 1st trit., (cent.) which kept him comfortable several months. (*Hale.*)]

*Bright's disease* (?) Profuse urination—nocturnal—since six months, in a man of 40, accompanied by burning and scalding; milky at times—often straw-colored, fœtid; voids 10 or 12 pints in 24 hours; he is dispirited, morose; constipation; dry mouth; saliva tenacious; tongue coated white; good appetite, but distress after eating. A constant sensation of faintness at stomach, even after a hearty meal; debility; renal pain, etc. Cured in three weeks by Uranium nit. 2 ×. (*Hale.*)

° *Bright's disease:* Urination profuse, painful, pale, milky, with ammoniacal odor; nocturnal urination frequent; great debility; night sweats; constant pain and soreness in lumbar region; legs ache and feel heavy and weary; worse toward evening; almost complete loss of sexual power; sexual organs cold and relaxed, and sweaty; afternoon fever; great thirst; canine hunger; bloated abdomen and constipation. Cured by the 2 × trit. (*Hale.*)

° *Diabetes insipidus*, (Hysterical diuresis?) A delicate nervous female, had sudden attacks of diuresis, followed by scanty and dark colored urine, and fever. The diuresis was much relieved, and was not followed by the usual fever. (2 × trit.) (*Hale.*)

° *Diabetes:* (Sugar was found in the urine.) Constipation; distressing thirst; canine hunger; tongue red and angry; loss of sleep; all greatly improved under Uranium 2 ×. (*Dr. Lowder.*)

° *Diabetes.* In three cases of glycosurea, one was cured, and in two the sugar was reduced one-half. (*Dr. Curie of Paris.*)

° *Diabetes:* Two cases greatly improved under the 6th and 12th dil. (*Dr. Jorenet.*)

ᶜ *Diabetes:* In two cases the specific gravity decreased; in one from 1042 to 1030, in the other from 1039 to 1031; the thirst, hunger and quantity of urine decreased greatly. (*Dr. Baehr, Science of Therapeutics.*)

[Drs. Dudgeon and Miller, of England, used the Uranium nit., in five cases, unsuccessfully.]

° *Diabetes:* (Saccharine.) Five cases all improved under the medicine. (*Dr. Hughes, British Jour. of Hom., vol.* 28.)

[Dr. Drysdale has found it useful in one case (*Ib., Vol. XXV.*)]

° *Incontinence of urine* at night, and frequency during the day, in a young girl who had been troubled from infancy. Cured by the 3d and 1st. (*Dr. Cook.*)

### Cough and Chest.

Pain at lower angle of left scapula, aggravated by taking a deep inspiration.

Double hydrothorax and congestion of the lungs.

*Pathology.*—Cough, with purulent discharge from left nostril, loss of appetite and great prostration; lung infiltrated with gray tubercle; no vomica.

### Back, Kidneys and Loins.

Stiffness in the loins.

Increased frequency of micturition; twelve times in twenty-four hours.

Pressure on loins caused a rabbit to fall on left side, as if moribund, then to defecate.

### Upper and Lower Extremities.

Pain at lower angle of left scapula, aggravated by taking a deep inspiration.

White vesicles on hands and legs, with red areolæ; they burn and itch.

### General Debility and Languor.

Head heavy on waking; general languor, with aching at occipital protuberance.

Extreme languor on rising from bed, with fishy odor of urine.

Great prostration and drowsiness during the catamenia.

Debility and cold feeling, with vertigo.

° Obstinate sleeplessness—in diabetes.

### Fever.

Shivering alternately with heat at night, and great restlessness.

Prostration, somnolence, and shivering, during the day; restless at night at the menstrual period.

---

# NUPHAR LUTEA.

## (Small-flowered Yellow Pond Lily.)

BOTANICAL DESCRIPTION.—There are three species of the Nuphar in the United States, namely: Nuphar advena, Nuphar kalmiana, and Nuphar sagittæfolia. The first named has *large*, yellow flowers; the second was once designated, by Smith, Torrey, and Gray, the Nuphar lutea. Smith, a botanist, quoted by Gray, says he has never seen the Nuphar lutea in the United States. Dr. Robbins, in Wood's Botany, thinks the Nuphar kalmiana wholly distinct from the Nuphar lutea or any other species.

Appended to the "proving of Nuphar luteum," * in a note by one of the editors (probably Dr. Marcy or Dr. Metcalf), we find the following observation:

"This proving is taken from the *Journal de la Societe Gallicane*, volume III., page 129, by Dr. Pitet, who gives no description of the plant, either botanically or otherwise.   \*   \*   The species in question is the small-flowered, yellow pond lily, Nuphar luteum—not the large-flowered, common yellow lily, Nuphar advena—from which, however, it is said to be difficult to distinguish it. It is quite common in the interior of the State of New York, though less frequently found than the large species. A tincture is made from the whole plant, rhizomes, flowers, leaves, and peduncles."

The identity of this plant with any species growing in the United States, is not as well established as it ought to be; but, under the circumstances, we see no better way than to consider it the same as Nuphar kalmiana, which is described as follows:

"Floating leaves, with base lobes approximate; submerged leaves, membranous, reniform-cordate, the lobes divaricate, margin waved, apex retuse; sepals five; stigma eight: twelve-rayed, crenate, petiole slender, sub-terete; upper leaves two or three inches long, one and one-half to two and one-half inches wide; lower leaves, three to four inches in diameter. Flowers in July.

OFFICINAL PREPARATIONS.—Tincture of the root; dilutions.

ANALOGUES.—*Anacardium, Arsenicum, Agnus castus, Baryta, Camphor* (?) *Conium, Gelseminum, Podophyllum, Rumex.*

### Head.

Pressive headache in forehead and temples, ceasing in the open air.

Dull, deep, lancinating pains behind the left frontal eminence

Painful, bruising, shaking in the brain at every step, when walking.

Painful heaviness in the orbit and at the base of the brain.

### Mental.

Excessive moral sensibility.

Great impatience at the slightest contradiction.

### Eyes.

Dull pain and sensation of weight in the orbit.

Discolored (around the eyes).

### Abdomen and Stool.

Soft stool, preceded by colic.

° Diarrhœic stools, morning and evening, preceded by colic-like pains.

Yellow diarrhœa in the morning.

Smarting and burning pains at the anus, after every stool.

Stitches, as from needles, in the rectum.

F.29

° Entero-colitis, chronic.

° *Painless morning diarrhœa.*—(*Dr. Petitt, seven cases, also Drs. Shipman and Barker*).

### Urine.

Urine deposits a copious reddish sand, which adheres to the vessel.

### Generative Organs.

*Male.*—* Complete absence of sexual desire; voluptuous thoughts do not cause erection.

Severe lancinations in both testicles, with pains in extremity of penis.

° Impotency, with involuntary sexual losses—during sleep, at stool, and when urinating. (*Pettit.*)

° Spermatorrhœa, even with erections.

### Skin.

Eruption resembling psoriasis, itching violently. (?)

[See Therapeutics of New Remedies.]

---

# NYMPHÆA ODORATA.

### (*White Pond Lily.*)

BOTANICAL DESCRIPTION. — The white pond-lily has a blackish, large, fleshy perennial *root* or *rhizoma*, growing in mud where the water is from three to ten feet deep, and is often as thick as a man's arm, sending up leaves and flowers to the surface. The *petioles* are long, somewhat semi-circular, and perforated throughout by long tubes or air vessels which serve to float them. The *leaves* are floating, orbicular, sometimes almost kidney-shaped, peltate, cordate-cleft at the base, quite to the insertion of the petiole, the lobes, one each side, prolonged into an acute point, entire, reddish, with prominent veins beneath, dark, shining green above and five or six inches in diameter. The *flowers* are large white, or rose-colored, and fragrant. A western species, the *N. tuberosa*, is odorless. The *sepals* are four, lanceolate, green without, and white within. The *petals* are numerous, lanceolate, from an inch to two and a half inches long, of the most delicate texture, white, sometimes tinged with purple on the outside. *Stamens* numerous, yellow in several rows. *Filaments* dilated gradually from the inner to the outer series so as to pass insensibly into petals. *Anthers* in two longitudinal cells growing to the filaments, and opening inwardly. *Stigma* with from twelve to twenty-four rays, very much resembling abortive anthers, at first incurved, afterward spreading. The pericarp is berry-like, many-celled, many seeded.

**30**

This plant grows in ponds, marshes, and sluggish streams, flowering from June to September.

OFFICINAL PREPARATIONS.—Tincture of the fresh root; with strong alcohol.

ANALOGUES.—*Asarum, Agnus castus* (?) *Baptisia; Calendula; Eryngium, Hamamelis; Nuphar; Phytolacca* (?)

We have but one proving, which was made by Dr. Edwin Cowles, at Hahnemann Medical College, Chicago, in 1865. One object of the proving was to ascertain whether its ancient reputation, as an aphrodisiac, could be substantiated. The only noteworthy symptoms related to the urinary organs, lumbar region, and throat. It caused, apparently, some soreness of the throat, in both experiments. This proving, however, needs to be substantiated by others before its symptoms will possess much value.

### Head.

Lascivious dreams.

Feeling of dullness.

Headache, through the temples, with severe coryza.

### Throat.

Sore throat, with roughness and tingling.

Frequent desire to swallow, with painful deglutition.

### Bowels.

Pain in hypogastric region.

Pain in the bowels and back.

Thin stools, with slight burning.

### Urine.

Sensation on urinating, as if the urine had not all passed.

Increased flow of urine.

Slight involuntary passing of urine.

### Back and Lower Extremities.

Pain in the back and lower limbs.

Great weakness in the lower lumbar region.

---

# ŒNOTHERA BIENNIS.

### (*Tree Primrose.*)

BOTANICAL DESCRIPTION.—This is an indigenous, biennial plant, with an erect, rough stem, branching, from two to five feet high. The leaves are ovate-lanceolate, alternate, acute, obscurely toothed, roughly pubescent, from three to six inches long and from half-an-inch to an inch wide, those on the stem sessile, and the radicals tapering into a petiole. The flowers are numerous, pale-yellow, sessile, odorous, and are disposed in a terminal, somewhat leafy spike; they are nocturnal, open but once by night, and continue only a single day. Each flower opens about dusk, and does not close until about nine or ten o'clock the next morning.

PURSH remarks that he has frequently observed a singularity in this plant, and it might be interesting to make further inquiry into its cause. It is that, in a dark night, when no objects can be distinguished at an inconsiderable distance, this plant, when in full flower, can be seen at a great distance, having a bright white appearance, which, probably, may arise from some phosphoric properties of the flower. The bark, leaves, and twigs are the parts used; their taste is very viscid, with a subsequent slight acrimony, which last is diminished by desication. Water takes up the properties of the plant.

OFFICINAL PREPARATIONS.—Tincture of the whole plant; dilutions.
ANALOGUES.—(?)

*(No provings.)*

° *Summer diarrhœa of children.*—" Its use was attended in all cases by surprising results. In many cases where the evacuations had been for days from one to two hours apart, they became six and eight hours, after the first dose, and in some instances a single dose effected a cure. There were few instances of the disease continuing more than two or three days, the evacuations steadily decreasing in frequency. Dose one drop of the Tincture after each evacuation. (*Dr. J. S. Douglas.*)

° *Exhausting watery diarrhœa*, every two hours — after typhoid fever, cured by Œnothera Tincture, after Arsenicum, Veratrum, Mercurius, Phosphoric acid, etc., had been given for five days unavailingly. (*Ib.*)

° *Chronic diarrhœa* (every summer) in a thin, emaciated woman, cured in a week. (*Dr. Perrine.*)

° Diarrhœa after confinement, with great despondency, paleness and emaciation. (*Douglas.*)

° Chronic Diarrhœa—for twelve months—about twelve evacuations daily. (*Ib.*)

[Dr. Douglas' experience, above, was written in Feb., 1871. In June, 1872, he writes me that "up to the present time it continues to justify my early expectations of it."—*Hale.*

# ŒNANTHE CROCATA.

## (Water-hemlock.)

BOTANICAL DESCRIPTION.—"The Œnanthes are smooth aquatic plants, with compound umbels, variable involucres (often wanting), polyphyllian involucelles, white flowers on long pedicles inserted on the ray of the umbellule, hermaphrodite and sterile by abortion. They grow abundantly in the northern countries of the Old World, and some have been observed in America. The genus contains very numerous species; and, as it has been limited by botanists up to the present day, we reckon a score which have been divided into two grand sections.

Genus *Œnanthe* (Linn.), perennial species, with fasciculated tubes, such as *Œ. crocata*, which is the one now before us.

SYNONYMS.—*Œnanthe safranée. Œnanthe à suc jaune.* Breton, *Kéyuis, Pembis, Pempes* (the root having five fingers) *pum bys*, Welsh. At Nantes, *Pensagre. Navet du diable.* The flowers are white, sometimes light rose, with a fascicle of tubers; in one variety the root is white, in another reddish-purple. Without enlarging on the chemical analysis let us merely state that the plant contains amongst other matters a fixed oil, a soluble oil, a resin, a yellow coloring matter; that one may ascribe to the first three the venomous action of the plant; they exist in such abundance that in order to see them you have only to cut the root across, when the oils exude to the surface and soon lose by evaporation their aqueous parts and the highly scented volatile oil, whilst the yellow resinous juice encrusts the surface of the section.

Gray does not mention it in his botany, but it is pretty certain that it has been found in the United States. Dr. Kimball, of Sacketts Harbor, reported cases of poisoning with it, in American Observer of 1867. I have had specimens of the root sent me which clearly answered the above description. (*Hale.*)

OFFICINAL PREPARATIONS.—Tincture of the root (with strong alcohol); dilutions.

ANALOGUES.—*Cicuta, Æthusa, Agaricus, Stramonium, Acid hydrocyanic, Solanum.*

## Mind.

Disturbances of intellect; mad and furious as if drunk.

Sudden and complete loss of consciousness.

*Madness*, with convulsions—death.

He remembered nothing that had befallen him during the many days of his illness, nor what caused the sickness (in a case of poisoning).

## Sensorium.

*Violent vertigo*, with falling; vertigo with nausea, vomiting, syncope and convulsions.

## Head.

Puffs (flashes) of pungent heat on the head.

*Apoplectic conditions*, speechless and insensible, with face puffed and livid, pupils dilated, respiration laborious, limbs contracted, and tenesmus.

*Coma* after the convulsions.

## Face.

Bleeding from the *nose*.

*Eyes* turned upward.

*Pupils dilated*.

Rose colored spots on the face.

Face swollen and livid, with bloody froth issuing from the mouth and nostrils.

## Gastric Symptoms.

*Burning heat* in the throat and stomach, with disturbance of intellect; vertigo, *cardialgia*, nausea, followed by alvine evacuations.

*Obstinate vomiting*, continuing for days, not relieved by anything.

## Extremities.

Numbness and feebleness of the limbs.

Tetanic contractions of the limbs.

Rose colored spots on the face, chest and arms.

## Convulsive Symptoms.

*Epileptiform convulsions in all the cases.*

*Terrible convulsions*, followed by coma, or deep sleep.

*Convulsions* with vertigo, madness, nausea, vomiting, unconsciousness, eyeballs turned up, pupils dilated; tremblings, contractions of the lower jaw, lockjaw, trismus, contractions of the limbs.

*Sudden convulsions, trismus, biting of the tongue, followed by unconsciousness and oblivion of the circumstances.*

Convulsions with deathly syncope, coldness as if dead.

Convulsions with swollen and livid face; bloody froth from the mouth and nostrils; convulsive respirations, insensibility, feeble pulse, prostration—death.

[For cases of poisoning, pathological anatomy, etc., see Vol. II. Therapeutics.]

# OLEUM CAJUPUTI.

### (*Cajuput Oil.*)

PHARMACOLOGY.—This is the volatile oil of Melaleuca Cajuputi, a small tree of the Molucca Islands, belonging to the natural family of Myrtaceas. Its name, in the language of the natives, signifies *white tree*, and serves to indicate the white bark for which it is remarkable. The oil is obtained from its leaves by distillation. It is very fluid and transparent, has a hot, aromatic taste, followed by a sense of coolness in the mouth, and a strong but agreeable odor, which is said to resemble that of turpentine, camphor, peppermint and rose together. It is wholly soluble in alcohol.

OFFICINAL PREPARATIONS.—Triturations; tincture; dilutions.

ANALOGUES.—*Cocculus*, (?) *Valerian*, (?) *Asafœtida.* (?(

### Mind.

Can't think of anything; ideas come slowly.

Disgust for books usually used in study.

Want to walk slow and very dignified; prefer to walk alone.

### Head.

Full and dull heavy feeling all through the head.

The above feeling gradually moved and became settled in the occipital region.

° Headache relieved by a few drops rubbed on the affected locality.

Feel and walk as if had taken too much beer; can walk straight, but feel very unsteady.

Feeling of dizziness when walking.

### Face, Eyes and Ears.

Heavy feeling of the eyes, but does not feel sleepy.

Eyes look very dull; upper lids feel thick and heavy.

Rough feeling of the face; can't hurt the skin by pinching it.

° Deafness; when mixed with almond oil and applied on cotton.

### Mouth, Throat and Stomach.

A cool, not unpleasant sensation in mouth and œsophagus.

° Applied to the cavity of a carious tooth it alleviates pain.

Excessive coughing and strangulation, followed by a profuse flow of saliva.

Constant inclination to spit and hawk up large quantities of tough white mucus.

Tongue feels as if it would fill the mouth.

Sensation of paralysis in the œsophagus.

Sensation of swelling and constriction of the œsophagus.

Taste in the mouth and a feeling in the œsophagus as if had swallowed lye from wood ashes.

Œsophagus seemed to close up and leave no space for swallowing.

Appetite good, can eat anything, but don't feel natural when eating.

The eating all seems to be performed mechanically.

° Nervous vomiting, or the vomiting of hysterical persons.

° Nervous dysphagia, or spasmodic stricture of the œsophagus

° Spasmodic hiccups.

On rising from a seat, sensation as if he would vomit.

Aching in and around the bicuspids when biting anything.

### Bowels.

° Flatulent colic, particularly when produced by cold, or by the retrocession of inflammation, gouty or otherwise, of the skin or extremities.

° Choleraic diarrhœa, from sudden check of perspiration.

Rectum feels paralyzed.

### Generative Organs.

° Menses suspended or diminished, and attended with pain, when caused by a cold or check of perspiration.

### Back and Extremities.

On raising the arms, feel as if they would drop down in spite of any effort to keep them up.

Lame sensation in carpel bones of left wrist.

Arms feel like soaked wood hanging to him.

Arms feel so heavy takes all the will power to raise them.

Arms feel as if they would tremble if he would let them.

On stooping forward, stitching pains through right lumbar region.

Almost complete loss of sensibility of the outer side of the thighs and dorsal surface of the forearms and hands.

The inside of the thighs and palmar surface of the hands exceedingly sensitive to pinching.

While walking, knees feel weak, as though would certainly give out.

Knees ache, continuing nearly all night.

### Generalities.

A feeling as if just a little larger all over.

° Epilepsy; palsy; paralysis; chronic rheumatism; **hysteria**; dropsy.    ° Nervous dyspnœa.

Heat in the stomach; quick pulse and perspiration.

Trembling all over.

Frequent gaping and stretching.

Feeling as if just recovering from a hard spell of **sickness.**

A general numb feeling, especially of the face.

Voice hoarse as if had taken cold.

Sharp pain through superior part of both lungs.

---

# OLEUM JECORIS ASELLI.

### (*Cod-liver Oil.*)

DESCRIPTION.—Oleum Morrhuæ, or Cod-liver oil, is obtained from the liver of the Gadus Morrhua and other species of the Gadus.  The livers of the Cod are put into a large vessel and heated by steam applied to the outside.  The liquid is drained off, allowed to stand, and the oil is finally skimmed off as it rises to the top.  The finest brands of oil are prepared by forcing currents of steam at high pressure through the mass of livers, tearing them in this way to pieces and melting out their oil.

The oil should be perfectly limpid, yellow, thick, and free from rancidity, and possessing the peculiar fishy taste.

The *brown* and *black* oils are rancid, nauseous, disgusting, and unfit for administration.

Cod-liver oil is a very complex substance, containing, according to Dr. Jorgh, glycerine, oleic, magaric, butyric, and acetic acids; also *iodine, bromine, phosphorus, phosphoric acid.*  The *iodine* is in proportion of about *one* part in *two thousand;* or, according to Dr. Jorgh, four-hundredths of a grain in one hundred grains of the oil.

OFFICINAL PREPARATIONS.—(1) The pure *oil;* (2) *triturations* of the oil; (3) *tincture.*  (Dr. Neidhard recommends a tincture made by digesting ʒ i to ʒ 1 of strong alcohol, and dilutions from this tincture.)

[For the best methods of administration, and the size of dose, see "Therapeutics," Vol. II.]

ANALOGUES.—*Ampelopsis* (?), *Alnus* (?), *Arsenicum, Bromine, Baptisia* (?), *Calcaria, Cistus, (Glycerine,) Iodine, Phosphorus, (Hypophosphites of soda, lime, etc.,) Spongia, Sulphur.*

[The following pathogenesis is prepared from Neidhard's provings and clinical experience, and arranged by Dr. Fairbanks. All the symptoms, not otherwise credited, belong to Neidhard.]

### Mind.

Fretful temper.

Talks about himself in the third person.

° Sensation as if out of her mind.

### Head.

Dull aching pain in the forehead, also in the vertex.

Giddiness, everything turns black.

Headache in the forenoon, with vomiting and constant retching.

Steady aching pain from left to right temple.

° Dry coryza and sneezing.

° Fluent coryza, hoarseness and rawness of the chest.

° Pain from occiput to forehead, with nausea.

° Bursting headache after coughing, as if it would split open.

° Aching pain about inner part of right eyebrow, as if in the periosteum.

### Eyes.

A flow of tears when walking in the open air, worse in the left.

Heaviness over the eyes; eyelids so heavy she can hardly raise them; swelling of the lids.

Blackness and blindness before the eyes, with disposition to shut them—during chill.

° Aching pain in right eye, when using it.

° Scrofulous ophthalmia. (*Hale.*)

### Ears.

° Fetid discharge from the ears.

° Marked deafness in left ear, and abscess in the right.

### Nose.

° Dry coryza, cough and sneezing

° Bleeding of nose when stooping, with amenorrhœa.

° Chronic catarrh and ozœna. (*Hale.*)

### Face.

Flushed face; burning of the face.

A growth of thin, short hair on chin and upper lip, where she had none previous to use of Ol. Jec. (2 months.)

### Mouth.

Tongue coated yellow.

Parched feeling in mouth; constant thirst
Soreness of the tongue after using the oil.

### Throat.

Soreness in the throat.
Tickling in throat pit, after dinner, with cough. (*vvvv.*)
° *Great hoarseness.* (chronic.)
° Slight hoarseness in evening, worse next day.
° Choking and oppressed feeling when lying down.
° Chronic sore throat relieved, with expectoration of **yellow**
  mucus.

### Taste and Appetite.

Loss of appetite, could not taste milk. (*vv.* **twice verified.**)
Nausea with thirst, and loss of appetite. (*vv.*)
Vomiting with bitter acid taste.

### Stomach and Abdomen.

Great nausea and sickness of stomach. (*vvv.*)
Weight and oppression in pit of stomach. (*v.*)
Heat in region of stomach. (*v.*)
Pressive tensive pain in stomach.
Acid vomiting, and purging with pain in stomach. (*v.*)
Vomiting of bile and mucus, with bitter and acid taste—after
  a chill.
Soreness and heaviness in region of liver, worse from pressure
  or exercise. (*vvvv.*)
Beating pain in region of spleen, with bearing down pain in
  the side. (*vv.*)
Jerking, drawing pain in region of spleen, worse when breath-
  ing or coughing. (*v.*)
Spasmodic pain in umbilical region.
° Tabes mesenterica. (*Hale.*)

### Stool and Anus.

Diarrhœa in the night and early morning.
Constipation, (*vvv.*) with burning of hands and **feet** (*v.*)—**at**
  times with cold feet.

### Urinary Organs.

Urine reddish, with pink sediment.
Soreness in region of kidneys.

### Sexual Organs.

° Discharge of yellow matter from the womb, with weak back.

°°°° Menstruation obstructed, from taking cold.

° Menstruation premature or copious.

° Soreness of both ovaries; dysmenorrhea.

### Respiratory Organs.

Shortness of breath, with heavy beating of heart.   (*v.*)

Asthma continually increasing in violence.   (*v.*)

Pain in right side, above and below scapula, arresting the breath.   (*vvvv.*)

Pain in left side of chest, through to back, with cough and shortness of breath.   (*vvvv.*)

Pain at apex of (left?) scapula.

Sharp stitch in left side, (*vv.*) lasting some minutes.

Oppression and heat in chest.   (*vv.*)

Stitch in right side during a long breath, lasting all day. (*vv.*)

Rheumatic pain in region of heart, also in muscles of chest. (*vv.*)

A sudden stitch in the heart.

Oppressive anxious beating of heart.   (*v.*)

*Soreness in chest and stomach, with cough*—verified many times.

Weakness in the chest, with hard coughing spells in the morning.   (*vv.*)

Sensation of excoriation in left chest, extending to the back.   (*vvv.*)

Dry hacking cough.   (*vvv.*)

Cough all night; palpitation of heart.   (*v.*)

Tickling cough, in middle of upper chest, (trachea?) with palpitation of heart.   (*v.*)

Case 1.—Mrs. O., 36. A long-continued cough, with emaciation, loss of strength and appetite. After many other remedies had failed, there was excessive weakness, with expectoration of heavy bloody mucus. Teaspoonful doses of Oleum Jec., pure, three times a day for three months, cured.

Case 2.—Mrs. F., 30. Severe cough, following exposure to cold, damp weather, with yellowish expectoration at times. At other times, dry and hacking, after ineffectual use of Calc. Hypophos 2 ×, and other remedies. ℞ Oleum Jec. 1 × (*well shaken*). Drop doses three times a day cured in a few days.

### Back and Neck.

Soreness all around the body to the back. (*vv.*)

Weakness and dull aching in sacral region, relieved by pressure. (*vv.*)

Soreness in region of kidneys, after exercise. (*v.*)

° Soreness from back to chest.

° Sharp heavy aching pain in lower spine.

ᶜ Spinal irritation, sore to the touch

° A sensation of fluttering commences in region of sacrum, and gradually ascends to the occiput. As it rises it affects the abdomen and chest, so that she can move neither hand or foot.

Expectoration of yellow mucus. (*vvvv.*)

Expectoration of tough greenish-yellow phlegm, with saltish taste. (By continuing the oil it became white.) (*vvv.*)

Expectoration of tough thin mucus in the morning. (*vvv.*)

Expectoration of thick white phlegm, with hard cough. (*vv.*)

White expectoration, with pain in side, worse when bending side inwards.

Spitting of blood. (*v.*)

°° Pain in upper part of chest when coughing.

°° Violent cough, with retching; night and day.

°° Burning heat in left chest through to back, with **cough.**

° Loose cough, with yellowish expectoration.

° Cough on raising the arm, with stitches.

° Weakness in chest and back; more in left.

° Hæmoptysis. (Cured three cases.)

° Soreness in centre of chest, with barking cough and aching between the shoulders.

### Fever.

Flushes of heat. (*v.*)

Fever and heat over the whole body. (*vvvv.*)

Pulse very frequent, varying from 100 to 120. (*vv.*)

Great thirst; constant thirst.

Chill every evening (*v.*) for four days, with acid vomiting and diarrhœa. (Relieved by Iris.)

A creeping sensation all over the body, with a rush of blood to the heart.

A tertian intermittent **fever,** returned four times, receding two hours each **time, and** lasting two hours; chill passed down the back **and around** abdomen. Relieved by Eup. perf.

Fever for two hours in the night, followed by a violent perspiration; mainly on upper parts.

Flushes of heat with red face, heat in stomach, and fever all over to ends of toes; lasting eight or ten hours.

Perspiration every night (v.) or all the time.

Chills and hectic fever, with beating pain in spleen.

Chilly at bedtime, followed by fever, oppression and heat of the chest.

Chill at three A. M., lasting one hour, followed by fever; pulse from 100 to 120.

Chill in evening, afterwards fever and palpitation of heart.

° Cold perspiration the whole day.

Case.—Lady, age 30, spare. Was constantly chilly, feeling as if she was continually taking cold. A few drop doses of Oleum Jec. 1× cured.

### Upper Extremities.

Burning heat in the palms of the hands, mostly at night. (verified by many provings.)

Hands dry and parched, with heaviness over the eyes.

° Continued aching and sore pain in the elbow and knee joints.

### Lower Extremities.

Cold feet (ever since taking the oil).

Soreness of the feet; abscess on left thigh.

° Rheumatic pain in left foot.

° White swelling of knees; scrofulous hip disease.

### Sleep.

Wakefulness and vivid dreams from the fever and excitement.

Less sleepy than usual, with night sweats.

Sleeplessness after 3 A. M., with general prostration.

° Dreams of seeing objects in the room during sleep.

### Skin.

Boil on right side of chest.

Abscess on the left thigh.

### Generalities.

A decided increase in strength and natural health. (*vvv*)

She looked fatter and healthier in the face than before.

General lassitude and prostration of whole system. (*v.*)

She feels miserable, with great nervous irritation. (After tablespoonful doses for weeks.)

The hot air is disagreeable to him.

° It influences favorably the constitution of the blood; pale, anæmic patients become, while taking it, rosy and plethoric. (*Hale.*)

° It is especially useful in that condition of the system in which, with generally lowered tone, there is a tendency to cellular hyperplasia, to the formation of "exudations," composed of imperfectly developed cells, which, in the majority of cases, from the very beginning are incapable of development into perfect entities, having only one potential quality, that of dying. (*H. C. Wood.*)

° *Scrofulosis, i. e.*, a tendency to increase in the lymphatic glands; to multiplication of their cellular elements, and the formation (1) of *cheesy* deposits, a slow, fatty degeneration, with dessication; or, (2) a rapid, fatty change, with abundance of moisture, resulting in pus and abscesses.

° A condition of *cellular hyperplasia,* affecting the mucous membrane of the air-passages. The patient, on the slightest occasion, suffers from catarrh, until, finally, a multiplication of cells occurs so rapidly, as to fill up a greater or less number of the air vesicles of the lungs, generally those of the apex, causing one of those conditions known as "*consumption.*" (*Ib.*)

° In nearly all diseases, where we find *combined,* a condition marked by *weakness, emaciation,* and *anæmia.* (*Hale.*)

° *Diseases of the bones;* scrofulous; chronic inflammations of the joints; caries; *necroses; abscesses,* etc. (*Wood.*)

° *Defective nutrition,* especially in children, where there is pallor, loss of strength, emaciation, etc. (*Hale.*)

° *Chronic rheumatism,* in cachectic, broken down constitutions.

° *Nervous affections,* neuralgia, sciatica, lumbago, in emaciated and anæmic persons, with deficiency of animal heat. (*Ib.*)

### Conditions.

Chill passes down the back and around the abdomen.

Pains move from before backwards, and from below upwards.

Pains are worse after exercise, in either side, predominantly the left, through to the back.

Pains move from right to left, and from thence through to the back.

Cough worse when lying down, when laughing, or from a draught of air. (*C. D. Fairbanks.*)

---

## OLEUM RICINUS COMMUNIS.

### (*Castor Oil.*)

PHARMACOLOGY.—This oil is obtained from the castor oil bean, by expression. (*For description of the plant, see Ricinus Communis.*)

OFFICINAL PREPARATIONS.—Trituration with fine sugar of milk. 3 i. to ʒ i.

ANALOGUES.— (*?*).

#### (*Fragmentary provings.*)

\* Diarrhœa of *children* or adults, yellow, semi-fluid, papescent, of a peculiar fœtid odor, with some griping (*primary*).

\* Dysentery, in first stage, with frequent desire and ineffectual urging or evacuations of hard, small balls, with a little mucus and blood.

ᵒ Summer complaints of children.

ᵒ Diarrhœa from indigestion or teething, catching cold, etc.

ᵒ Chronic, obstinate diarrhœas, which have resisted all other remedies.

(*See Therapeutics, Vol. II.*)

---

## OLEUM SANTALUM.

### (*Oil of Sandalwood.*)

This is probably an oi' extracted from the wood of the *Santalum album* a tree found growing in India.

OFFICINAL PREPARATIONS.—Oil; dilutions or triturations.

ANALOGUES.—*Copaiva, Cubebs, Erigeron, Erechthites, Turpentine, etc.*

#### Urinary Organs.

ᵒ Chronic catarrhal states of the mucous membrane of the urinary organs.

ᵒ *Gonorrhœa*--after the first few days (after Cannabis and Gelseminum). (*Hale.*)

° *Gleet,* when the discharge is profuse, painless, thick and yellow or green. (*Ib.*)

° *Chronic cystitis;* mucus sediment in the urine.

[This remedy was introduced into practice by physicians in India. It is far superior to Cubebs and Copaiva, and experience has demonstrated that it is the nearest a specific for *Gonorrhœa* of any drug known. It is usually given (allopathically) in *capsules* (three a day), each containing about thirty drops, and very successfully. My own experience with the oil is that it acts best after Gelseminum and Cannabis have reduced the active inflammation. I use the 1×trit., or dilution, a dose (ten grs. or gtts.), every two or three hours. It generally cures in eight or ten days.- in uncomplicated cases. *Hale.*]

---

# OPUNTIA VULGARIS.

## (*Prickly Pear.*)

DESCRIPTION.—This (with a variety, the O. Rafinesque), is the only member of the *cactus* family, growing east of the Mississippi. It is found all over the United States, in sandy fields and on dry rocks. It is low, prostrate, spreading, pale, with flat and obovate, broad joints; the minute leaves ovate-subulate and oppressed; axils bristly, rarely with a few small spines; flowers, sulphur-yellow; berry, nearly smooth, eatable. It blooms in June, in the neighborhood of Chicago.

OFFICIAL PREPARATIONS.—Tincture of the fresh petals. (*Burdick.*) Tincture of the whole plant. (*Hale.*)

ANALOGUES.—(?)

[These symptoms are from a fragmentary proving by Dr. Burdick, of New York, from inhaling the tincture of the petals.]

Burning and smarting in the margins of the eyelids, with a feeling of contraction in the line of the eyelashes.

\* Nausea, extending from the stomach down into the bowels, with sensation as if diarrhœa would set in.

\* Excoriating, sick feeling in lower third of abdomen, with sensation as if the bowels had all settled down into the lower part of the abdomen. (*Burdick.*)

° *Diarrhœa,* stools dark, slimy, excoriating, exhausting, with nausea, and cramps in stomach and bowels.

Alternate nausea of stomach and bowels; sensation as if the contents of the lower bowels were very acrid.

Nausea, with dull heavy pain in stomach, with feeling as if cramps would set in.

Feeling of prostration and coldness.

# ORIGANUM VULGARE *

*(Marjoram.)*

BOTANICAL DESCRIPTION.—This is a perennial herb, with erect, leafy, hairy, purple, quadrangular, corymbose *stems*, from six inches to two feet in height. The flowers are numerous, of a purplish-white color, and are disposed in smooth, erect, roundish, panicled, and fasciculate spikes, and accompanied with ovate purplish bracts, longer than the calyx. Wild Marjoram is common to Europe and America. It is found in limestone regions, on dry banks, and in dry fields and woods, flowering from May to October. The whole herb is officinal, but it is seldom collected, except for the purpose of procuring its volatile oil, on which its virtues depend, and which may be separated by distillation with water. The plant has a strong, peculiar, rather agreeable balsamic odor, and a warm, bitterish, aromatic taste, which properties are imparted to alcohol, or boiling water by infusion. The Origanum Marjorana, or sweet Marjoram, possesses properties similar to the above species. It is a native of Portugal, but cultivated in our gardens, and much used in cooking as a seasoning.

OFFICINAL PREPARATIONS.—Tincture of the plant; the oil; dilutions; tincture and triturations of the oil.

ANALOGUES.—*Cantharis, Cannabis indica, Collinsonia, Hedeoma, Helonias, Platinum, Valerian.*

## Mind.

She is very quiet, full of thoughts, sad, despairing; wants to throw herself out of the window; wants to walk about all the time; impossible to rest. Everything disgusts her; desire for death; disgust for life; nothing amuses her. Cannot fix the thoughts.

Lascivious ideas, with great heat in the head.

*Dreams* lascivious, with frequent waking; wakes trembling.

Moroseness and debility one day, vivacity the next.

Sadness, followed by good humor (opposite of coffee).

* Lascivious ideas, with sexual irritation.

° Deep moroseness, with an idea that she was lost and despised. When waking from a stupor she cries out that the devil comes near her. She believes herself in hell, in chains. Considered herself crazy; has thoughts of suicide (in a hysterical girl with sexual irritation).

## Head.

Great heat of the head; when this increases, the head involuntarily turns from one side to the other.

* From the French of Dr. Gallasardin, of Lyons. *N. A. Journal of Homœopathy, Vol.* 15, *page* 62.

Headache in the temples, with lasciviousness.

Vertigo when going to bed.

Epistaxis in the morning.

### Urinary and Sexual Organs.

Frequent calls to urinate at night, waking **him.**

*Increased sexual desire.*

*Lascivious ideas and dreams.*

Itching on and about the bosom.

° Onanism in girls—under ten years.

ᶜ Masturbation, with mental weakness.

° A young girl, well every other way, masturbated **every day**
 She tried her utmost to fight those sexual inclinations,
 but in vain. (Cured by the 3d.)

° Sexual irritation, with leucorrhœa and itching of the puden-
 da in an old maid of forty years. (Cured by the 3d.)
 (*Dr. Emory.*)

° Leucorrhœa, with sexual irritation, in a woman of 35, married. She had suffered several months from powerful
 lascivious impulses, producing anxiety and aversion to
 religious duties. (*Ib.*)

° A widow had neither rest nor quiet from voluptuousness.
 (Cured by the 30th.)

° Tormenting voluptuous desires, in a girl.

° Leucorrhœa, sterility, "flatulency of the uterus."—*Diosco-
 rides.*

### General Symptoms.

Rheumatic pains in arms, legs, hands and feet, wandering
 about.

Vividly red efflorescence, and spots on skin of legs and abdomen.

No appetite, but great thirst, and pains in stomach and bowels.

Wants to run or walk in fresh air, which does her good.

---

# OXALATE OF CERIUM.

PHARMACOLOGY.—This is a salt obtained as a precipitate by adding a solution of oxalate of ammonium to a soluble salt of cerium. The form-ula, according to the old nomenclature, is $2CeO_1 C_4 O_6 + 6HO$; according to the new, $Ce_2 CO_4 + 3H_2 O$.

It is a snow-white granular powder, without smell or taste; insoluble in water, alcohol, or ether; soluble in sulphuric acid.

Owing to the insolubility of the oxalate, a nitrate has been made, and is used in the form of an effervescent salt.

This nitrate is readily soluble in both alcohol and water.

OFFICINAL PREPARATIONS.—(1) of the oxalate—triturations only; (2) of the nitrate—tincture with strong alcohol on the decimal scale.

ANALOGUES.—*Arsenicum, Bismuth, Kreosotum, Cuprum* (?) *etc.*

° Obstinate vomiting during pregnancy. (*Simpson.*)

° Morning sickness of pregnancy. (*Drs. Charlton, James, Moore*, and many others.)

° Arrests vomiting of mucus, ingesta, etc., but does not stop the nausea. (*Hale.*)

° Eruptions on the mucous membrane of the stomach, causing severe vomiting (?) (*Simpson.*)

(*See Therapeutics, Vol. II.*)

---

# PANCREATINE.

(*Inspissated pancreatic juice.*)

DESCRIPTION.—It is a grayish powder; with an odor something like rancid lard.

PHARMACOLOGY.—The pancreas are dissected and macerated in water, acidulated with hydrochloric acid, for about forty-eight hours, then separated, and the acidulated solution of pancreatine passed through a pulp filter until it is perfectly clear. To this clear solution is then added a saturated solution of chloride of sodium, and allowed to stand until the pancreatine is separated. This is carefully skimmed off and placed upon a muslin filter and allowed to drain, after which it should be washed with a less concentrated solution of chloride of sodium, and then put under the press. When the mass is nearly dry, it is rubbed with a quantity of sugar of milk and dried thoroughly without heat.

OFFICINAL PREPARATIONS—Saccharrated Pancreatine.

ANALOGUES.—*Pepsin, Iris, Pulsatilla, Ptelea, Nux vom., etc.*

° Dyspepsia; when the power of digesting fatty and starchy food is deficient.

(*See Therapeutics of Pepsin.*)

---

# PASSIFLORA INCARNATA.

(*White Passion Flower.*)

BOTANICAL DESCRIPTION.—This is a vine climbing by tendrils, with a smooth stem, *leaves* three cleft, the lobes serrate, petiole bearing two glands, *flowers* large, nearly white, with a triple, purple, and flesh-colored crown, involucre three leaved.

Grows in dry soil, in Virginia, Kentucky and southward, flowering from May to July. The fruit of this variety of Passiflora is about the size of a hen's egg, and when crushed makes a report, from whence came its name of May-pop.

There seems to be a very marked difference as to the active properties of this plant as found growing in different localities. That growing on the levees around New Orleans, is very large and rank, but utterly inactive, while that growing on the uplands is much better, and that grown on the Bayou Gross Tête seems to be the strongest.

OFFICINAL PREPARATIONS.—Tincture with dilute alcohol, from the carefully dried or fresh leaves, gathered in May, or as soon as the plant blossoms, before forming fruit; dilutions; triturations from the inspissated juice.

ANALOGUES.—*Aconite* (?), *Chloral Hydrate, Nitrate of Amyl, Gelseminum, the Bromides, Calabar Bean, Cannabis Indica.*

(*No Provings.*)

° Tetanic convulsions affecting mainly the muscles of the trunk, with predominant opisthotonos. (*Dr. L. Phares.*)

° Violent tetanus, with opisthotonos, trismus, and convulsions, in a child. (*Ib.*)

° Tetanus and trismus in horses, many cases.

° Neuralgia; sleeplessness, with great restlessness and suicidal mania.

° Erysipelas and syphilis. (?)

° Tetanus infantum. (neonatorum.)

A quiet slumber, from which the patient may be wakened up, and he will talk to you as rationally as he ever did, and immediately relapse into his slumbers.

---

# PAULLINIA SORBILES.

## (*Guarana.*)

DESCRIPTION.—*Guarana* consists of the seeds (powdered) of a tree or climbing shrub growing in Brazil; these, according to Johnson, in his "Chemistry of Common Life," are used as we do cocoa. They contain an alkaloid said to be identical with that found in tea and coffee (theine). In the Materia Medica of Trusseau and Pideaux is an account of its use in *migraine* or sick-headache. At one time it attained much popularity in Paris, in the treatment of sick-headache. It has lately been called up by Dr. Wilks, of Guy's Hospital, London. It has been used successfully by Dr. Wood, of Montreal, and Dr. Helmeken, of British Columbia. No provings have yet been made, and the following observations are given instead.

OFFICINAL PREPARATIONS.—Triturations of the seeds; tincture; dilutions.

ANALOGUES.—*Agaricus, Coffea, Cypripedium, Coca, Iris versicolor, Pulsatilla, Scutellaria, Thea, Valeriana, etc.*

° *Sick-headache* — If the attacks are frequent (several in a month), a few grains of the powder should be taken every morning, half an hour before the first meal, as a preventive; at the commencement of an attack the same dose may be repeated every quarter or half an hour until relief appears. (*Trousseau.*)

° The most violent attacks of sick-headache will sometimes yield at the end of five or ten minutes, not to return. (*Ib.*)

° Used by the natives of Brazil to relieve nervousness and weariness, as we use tea or coffee. (*Johnson.*)

° Used for the cure and prevention of bowel complaints. (*Ib.*)

° Diarrhœa of phthisis. (*Gavaelle.*)

° Cholera infantum. (*Hale.*)

° Chlorosis; paralysis; neuralgia. (*Ib.*)

° Convalescence from prostrating diseases. (*Ib.*)

° Rheumatic neuralgia. (*See Therapeutics.*)

---

# PEPSIN.

DESCRIPTION.—A peculiar albuminous body secreted by the *gastric glands*, which has the power not only of coagulating albumen, but also, with the aid of acidulated water, of redissolving it.

Prof. Lionel Beale gives the following simple method of manufacture: "Dissect off carefully the mucous membrane of a *perfectly fresh* pig's stomach, and place it on a flat board; cleanse it lightly with a sponge and water, so as to remove the particles of food and much of the mucus. Scrape it hard with an ivory knife, so as to squeeze out all the contents from the glands. The viscid mucus thus obtained contains all the pepsin with much epithelium. Spread it upon a piece of glass so as to form a very thin layer, which is to be dried at a temperature of 100° (no higher) F. over hot water. When dry, scrape from the glass, powder in a mortar, and transfer to a well-stoppered bottle."

Prof. Beale recommends the following formula for pepsin prepared by his method: "Take of the powder, five grains; strong muriatic acid, eighteen drops; water, six ounces. Macerate at a temperature of 100° for an hour; filter so as to form a perfectly clear fluid."

Pepsin, prepared by Beale's process, is odorless, nearly free from any disagreeable taste, and twenty-five times as strong as the ordinary commercial pepsin.

There are several brands of pepsin in the market, namely: Boudalt's, Hawley's, and Sheffer's. The two former are foreign, the latter American. Sheffer's is the most popular. The "Saccharated Pepsin" sold by Bœricke & Tafel, and at our Pharmacies, is a similar preparation. Whatever pepsin is used, if good effects are to be obtained from it, it should be given with acid, unless, indeed, there is reason to believe that this constituent of gastric juice is not wanting. Sheffer advises that his pepsin-solution be prepared as follows: "Take of Pepsin sixty-four grains, water five ounces, and of Hydrochloric acid (dilute) one drachm; after dissolving, add three ounces of glycerine. **Mix thoroughly and filter.**"

Alcohol **destroys the digesting power** of pepsin, and therefore "wines of pepsin" **are inferior preparations** of it. The homœopathist, and all other physicians, **should avoid all** the compound "elixirs," and other proprietary preparations, and use only the powder, or freshly prepared digestive solution. The powder, however, may be combined with an attenuated medicine in *trituration*, as I shall hereafter recommend.

In making the digestive solution, water and muriatic acid; or glycerine, water and muriatic acid, should alone be employed with the pepsin.

OFFICINAL PREPARATIONS.—(See above.)

ANALOGUES.—*Pancreatine* (?), *Muriatic acid* (?), *Lactic acid* (?).

*Pepsin*, not being in any sense a drug, but the gastric juice of some animal, is not an agent to be proven, or have any pathogenetic effects.

*Rennet*, or the dried stomach of calves, has been used from time immemorial for the purpose of coagulating milk. It has been used successfully in domestic practice, and in the hands of physicians, for the cure of *dyspepsia, dysentery, and chronic diarrhœa of undigested food,* also for *vomiting of food* in children and adults.

(*See Therapeutics.*)

# PHOSPHIDE OF ZINC.

DESCRIPTION.—Phosphide of Zinc is a black granular powder, resembling very closely Iron by hydrogen, having a strong smell of phosphorus, and tastes phosphoric. Entirely insoluble in water.

OFFICINAL PREPARATIONS.—Triturations. (Even in the 2× and 3× trit. its offensive taste and odor will prove an obstacle to its administration, but it can be disguised by prescribing it in the form of a pill. They can be very rapidly prepared if the trituration is made with equal parts of sac. lac. and pulv. gum acacia.)

ANALOGUES.—*Bromides of Potash, Ammonia, and Lithium, Conium, Gelseminum, Zinc. ox. and met.*

## Head.

˒ **Useful for the secondary effects of cerebral congestion and** apoplexy, or for the *debility, paralysis, and mental depression*—preferable to phosphorus. "My experience with this medicine has been very extensive. I have never known it to produce the least unpleasant effect, and have rarely been disappointed in obtaining the full results to be expected from Phosphorus in doses of one-tenth of a grain three times a day." (*Hammond* on Nervous Diseases.)

° Useful in passive cerebral congestion. (*Ib., Hale.*)

° Cerebral anæmia. (*Hale.*)

[It is perfectly homœpathic to the so-called hydrocephaloid disease of children, from loss of fluids, fever, etc. In the "brain-fag" of literary men, in conditions threatening paralysis of the cerebral functions, and the dreadful periodic headaches to which teachers, clergymen and others, who, from over-study, have produced cerebral anæmia, or passive congestion, with irritation. In such cases the 3 × trit. will prove efficient. *Hale.*]

### Generalities.

° *Mercurial Trembling*, with the following symptoms: Nearly all the muscles of locomotion seemed agitated by regular and spasmodic oscillations, which seemed due to the alternate contraction and relaxation of the muscles. This trembling, more marked in the upper than the lower extremities, was increased by any attempt at motion. His walk was hesitating and difficult. He could neither feed or dress himself, and he could not speak distinctly. He was emaciated and cachectic, and looked prematurely old; no appetite, painful digestion, and the generative faculties were wholly lost. He was much discouraged and attempted to commit suicide.

[Cured in twenty-one days by ⅛th grain three times a day. But these doses caused diarrhœa.] *Gazette de Hopit.*

The above case strongly resembles the symptoms of zinc, especially; also phosphorus. This remedy ought to prove useful in *Chorea.* (*Hale.*)

The chemical formula of Phosphide of Zinc is P. Z n 3., and **one grain represents little more than one-seventh of a grain of Phosphorus. Nine-tenths of a grain killed a rabbit of seven pounds weight. (*Ib.*)**

# PHYTOLACCA DECANDRA.

### (*Poke-Weed, Poke-Root.*)

BOTANICAL DESCRIPTION.—This plant is herbaceous, with a perennial root of large size, frequently exceeding a man's leg in diameter, usually branched, fleshy, fibrous, white within, easily cut or broken, and covered with a very thin brownish bark or cuticle. *Stems* annual, about an inch in diameter, and from five to nine feet in height, round, smooth and very much branched; when young, they are green, but become of a fine deep purple or scarlet when matured. *Leaves* scattered, petiolate, ovate, oblong, smooth on both sides, ribbed underneath, entire, acute, and five inches long by two or three in breadth. *Flowers* numerous, small, greenish-white, on long pedunculated racemes, opposite to the leaves, sometimes erect and sometimes drooping. *Peduncles* nearly smooth, angular, ascending; *pedicles* divaricate, sometimes branched, green-white, or purple, and two others in middle. *Calyx* whitish, consisting of five round-ovate, concave, incurved sepals. *Stamens* ten. *Ovary* green, round, depressed, ten furrowed. *Styles* ten. *Berries* in long clusters, dark-purple when ripe, round, depressed or flattened, marked with the furrows on the sides. *Cells* ten. *Seeds, ten,* solitary.

This plant is a native of the United States, growing in nearly all parts, along hedges, in neglected fields and meadows, along roadsides, moist ground, flowering from July to September. It is known by various other names, as pigeon-berry, garget, scoke, coakum, pocan. The two last names originated with the Indian tribes. This species is found not only in the United States, but in the Azores, North Africa and China. The *Phytolacca icosandra,* a much smaller species, is a native of South America, extending from Rio de Janeiro to Mexico, and is found in some of the West Indian Islands. The *Phytolacca octandra* is found in the West Indies and Mexico, where the berries are used for washing, like soap. These species possess similar properties.

OFFICINAL PREPARATIONS.—Tincture of the fresh root; tincture of the ripe berries; dilutions. Phytolaccin; triturations.

ANALOGUES.—*Arsenicum, Arum tri., Belladonna, Iris ver., Kali bich. Lachesis, Mercurius iod., Mercurius hydro., Nitric acid, Stillingia, Sanguinaria, Sulphur.*

## Mental Sphere.

Mind very gloomy and irritable.

Stupefaction, with vertigo and dimness of vision.

## Head.

Dull, steady, aching pain in the head, principally in the forehead.

One-sided pain just above the eyebrows.

Sensation as if the brain were bruised, when stepping from a high step to the ground.

Pressure in the temples and over the eyes, with nausea.

° Cephalalgia—rheumatic, syphilitic, or neuralgic.

° Syphilitic nodes of the skull.

Heaviness in the head and pressure in vertex, with vertigo.

Pain in the occiput, aggravated by walking or riding.

° Weekly attacks of sick headache.

° *Tinea capitis*; also scaly eruptions on the scalp.

### Eyes.

*Double vision*, with giddiness and headache.

Burning, smarting and itching, in the eyes, as if sand were in them, with profuse lachrymation.

Reddish-blue swelling of the lids; worse on left side, and in the morning.

An eruption (pustules) on the conjunctive.

Dull, heavy pain in eyeballs, worse from motion, light, and reading. (*Burt.*)

Dimness of sight and long-sightedness.

Catarrhal ophthalmia, with flow of tears, and photophobia. (*Neidhard.*)

Eyes brilliant and dancing, *pupil contracted*, lower lids drawn down.

Eyelids œdematous and agglutinated.

° *Granular conjunctivitis*, with circumorbital pain, soreness in the periosteum and scalp, as of rheumatic origin; it prevents the *relapses*, so common. (*Fenner, Hale.*)

° Fistula lachrymalis (?)

### Ears.

Shooting pain in the ears, when swallowing.

Sense of irritation and obstruction in eustachian tubes.

Rushing sounds in ears, with feeling as if the hearing was dull, while it is really over-sensitive.

Exaltation of the sense of hearing during the pain in the forehead.

### Nose.

An eruption (pustules) on the mucous membrane of the nose.

Feeling in nose and eyes as if a cold would come on.

* Coryza; flow of mucus from one nostril while the other is stopped.

Fluent coryza, with discharge from posterior nares.

° Syphilitic ozœna, with bloody, sanious discharge, **and** disease of the bones.

° *Noli me tangere*, and cancerous affections of the nose.

### Face.

\* Pains in the bones of the face and head, *at night*.

Paleness of the face.

Heat, with redness of the face and coldness of the feet.

Sickly look of the face ; dark yellow color of the face **and** sclerotica.

Periostitis, and nodes, of the bones of the face.

° Prosopalgia, in syphilitic and rheumatic subjects.

° Ulcers and eruptions (scaly) on the face.

### Mouth, Teeth and Tongue.

Small ulcers on the inside of the right cheek.

\* Profuse flow of saliva, tenacious, yellowish, ropy, with metallic taste.

° Irresistible inclination to bite the teeth together (in teething children).

Tongue feels rough, white-coated blisters on both sides, **and** very red tip.

° Rheumatic odontalgia, also mercurial and syphilitic.

\* Great pain in *root* of tongue, when swallowing.   (*Hale.*)

Salivation, with thick, ropy discharge.

Teeth all ache; they feel sore and elongated.

### Pharynx and Œsophagus.

\* Sore throat, swelling of the soft palate in the morning; **on** removing the mucus, throat feels better.

\* Feeling, when swallowing, as of a lump in the throat.

\* Great dryness in the throat, inducing coughing.

° Right tonsil much enlarged, dark red, burning sensation **in** the fauces and whole length of the œsophagus.

Sensation as if the trachea were being strongly grasped.

\* Dryness, soreness, dullness, and roughness of the throat, **all** the time.

° Sensation of scraping and rawness in the throat and tonsils.

° *Diphtheria*, especially with severe pains in nape of neck, **ears**, **and** root of tongue.

ᵗ Ulcers on one side of the throat, constant desire to swallow.

° Scarlet fever, with diphtheritic complications.

° Parotitis; inflammation of sub-maxillary glands.

° Inflammation of the mucous membrane of the Perophages.

[One of our most reliable remedies in non-malignant diphtheritic conditions; as the experience of many American and British homœopathists have proven.—*Hale.*

### Stomach.

\* Cutting in the pit of the stomach, which is tender to the touch.

Eructations of sour fluid, with great distress in stomach and bowels.

\* Pains in cardiac portion of stomach, aggravated by a full inspiration and by walking.

Violent pressure in the stomach on waking, disappears after rising.

\* Nausea, with severe pain in the umbilical region.

Vomiting of abundant, dark, bilious substance.

\* Vomiting and purging, with griping pains and cramps in the abdomen.

° Vomiting comes on slowly, preceded by nausea, and is excessive.

° Vomiting of food, and milk, in teething children. (*Hale.*)

Burning in the stomach, with tenderness of the bowels, heat in the rectum, and bloody stools, with tenesmus.

### Liver, Hypochondria.

\* Digging pain in right hypochondrium, in the upper and lower portions of the liver.

\* Cannot lie on the right side, on account of penetrating pain in right hypochondrium.

Violent, dull, piercing pain in left hypochondrium.

° Soreness and pain in right hypochondrium during pregnancy,

° Chronic hepatitis, with enlargement and induration.

### Abdomen.

Burning pain near the umbilicus.

Neuralgic pain in left groin.

Griping pain, followed by passage of **offensive flatus.**

Rumbling noise in the bowels.

° Chronic inflammation of the bowels.

Severe colicky pains in the bowels, with or without desire for stool.

Great distress in the umbilical and hypogastric regions.

° Burning distress in the umbilical region, with vomiting and diarrhœa.

### Stool and Anus.

\* *Constipation of long standing.*

\* Intense vomiting and purging, with prostration and cramps, as in cholera.

Copious discharge of bile from the bowels.

Stool soft, undigested, dark, lumpy.

Diarrhœa early in the morning for three mornings.

Emission of flatus relieves the pain in the bowels.

° Cholera and cholera morbus; also cholera infantum. (*Hale.*)

° *Ulceration* and fissure of the rectum.

\* *Hæmorrhoids*, permanent and obstinate.

*Bloody discharge, with heat in the rectum,* tenesmus and hæmorrhoids.

Pain shooting from the anus and lower rectum, along the perineum to the middle of the penis.

### Urinary Organs.

Urgent desire to pass water.

Copious nocturnal urination.

Weakness, dull pain and soreness in the region of the kidneys, most on the right side, attended with heat and uneasiness down the ureters.

*Chalk-like* sediment in the urine.

\* Pain in the region of the bladder, before and during urination.

\* Dark red urine, which stains the chamber a mahogany color

° Urine double in amount and clear as water.

Retention of urine.

Urine acid and *albuminous.*

° Bright's disease. (*Burt, H. N. Martin.*)

° Albuminuria, after scarlatina and diphtheria. (*Hale.*)

### Generative Organs.

*Female.*—\* *Metrorrhagia.* (*Jeanes.*)

° Menstruation too copious and too frequent.

° Violent pains in the abdomen during menstruation, in a barren woman.

° Leucorrhœa; *uterine,* thick, tenacious, and irritating. (*Hale.*)

° *Inflammation, swelling, and suppuration of the mammæ.*

° *Abscesses or fistulous ulcers of the mammæ.*

° *Nipples cracked and excoriated.*

° *Irritable mammæ* during menstruation and *lactation.* **Neu-**ralgia of the mammæ. (*Fairbanks.*)

° Ovaritis, with or without rheumatic complications.

° Tumors; schirrus, and cancer of the mammæ.

*Male.*—Complete loss of sexual desire, for two months.

Continued pain in the spermatic cords, running *up.*

° Orchitis, acute and chronic, with suppuration and fistulous ulcer.

° Syphilitic rheumatism, and syphilitic eruptions.

° Syphilis, primary and secondary.

° Chancres on the penis.

### Larynx and Trachea.

° Tickling in the left side of the larynx, with hacking cough.

Sensation of roughness and *dryness* in the larynx.

Bronchial cough, which is very dry.

° Hard cough, accompanied by scraping and tickling in the throat.

° Chronic coughs; generally hard and dry, with scraping and tickling.

° Constant coughing, with vomiting, with sensation as of an ulcerated spot in the trachea; could only expectorate (pus) by pressing on this spot. (*Marshall.*)

### Chest.

\* Aching pain in the right side of the breast, passing through to the back; worse on taking a long breath, aggravated by lying on right side.

Bruised feeling of muscles of chest and ribs.

Shocks of pain in the region of heart; as soon as the pain ceases, a similar pain appears in the *right* arm.

Respiration difficult and oppressed; mucous rale audible everywhere in the room.

° Chronic rheumatic endocarditis. (?) (*Hale.*)

° Angina pectoris, when the pain goes from the heart to the right arm. (*Ib.*)

° Fatty degeneration of the heart. (?) Fatty heart. (?)

### Back.

Pain in left lumbar region, followed by severe itching.

Pain in left shoulder blade, as if from a blow.

Sensation of weight and pressure on both shoulders.

Sensation as if a piece of cold iron were pressed on the painful shoulder-blade.

\* Hardness of the glands on the right side of the neck.

\* Stiff neck; worse on right side, and in bed, after midnight.

Dull, heavy pain in lumbar and sacral regions, worse from motion.

° Lumbago; the back is very stiff every morning.

\* Rheumatism of the left shoulder, without fever.

### Upper Extremities.

° Pain in the muscles of both arms.

Twitching of the muscles of the right arm.

° Rheumatic drawing in both fore-arms.

° Rheumatic pains in the hands; sudden pricking.

Arms ache, and ends of the fingers.

° Glandular enlargements in the axillæ.

### Lower Extremities.

\* Neuralgic pain in the outer side of both thighs and left groin.

\* Rheumatic pain in right knee, worse in open air and damp weather.

° Rheumatic pain in left limb, with sensation of shortening of tendons when walking.

Coldness of the feet, with increase of the capillary circulation about the head and face.

° Neuralgic pains in the toes.

Sticking, stinging pains in the extremities.

° Chronic rheumatism of lower extremities.

° Chronic inflammation of the knee joints.

° Sciatica; periostitis; and nodes on the tibia.

° Ulcers on the leg—syphilitic.

° Pains running from hip down the limb

**Skin.**

° Intense, chronic aching in the heels, only relieved by elevating the feet.

\* Itching of the skin, with a lichen-like eruption.

\* Boils, painful, on the back, behind the ears.

° Chronic disposition to boils. (*Searle.*)

° Squamous eruptions, pityriasis; psoriasis, etc.

° Tinea capitis; crusta lactea; lupus; ulcers, etc.

° Scarlatina, with anginous symptoms; nose and upper lip excoriated; acrid discharge from nose; delirium, and non-appearance of eruption. (*Mandeville.*)

° *Syphilitic eruptions—secondary and tertiary.* \*

\* Case of poisoning by " Phytolacca-decandra," reported to the Homœopathic State Medical Society of Kansas, May 6th, 1874, by Louis Grasmuck, M.D.

The subject was a woman, aged forty-five; occupation, keeper of boarding house; temperament, bilious, sanguine, active, hardworking, with a family of grown children, and has a good character.

She had always had good health, until about one year ago, she was attacked with rheumatism; this was followed by anasarca, and many other symptoms indicative of the "change of life." She was sick several months, but, finally, her fine constitution triumphed, and she recovered. She again resumed charge of her duties, and was, to all appearance, well, with the exception of a slight pain in the right hip joint.

A month after this, I was called to see her, and found her suffering intensely with pains in the joints, and bones of the face and head, and was informed that her sufferings were such that she had not slept any for many nights.

In addition, she was covered from the crown of her head to the soles of her feet, with an eruption, the like of which I never beheld. It began on the scalp, and spread downwards to the very toe nails. It consisted of erythematous blotches, of irregular shape, slightly elevated, of a pale red or pink color, very sore and painful, itching slightly only on desquamation, but too sore to allow of any scratching for relief, and terminating in a dark red or purple spot, taking about thirty days' time for each to pass through its various stages of eruption and desquamation, and about the same length of time to advance from the head to the feet, so that the eruption could be seen at one time in all its stages of development.

There was no accompanying fever, no swelling, except in the face, no sweats, appetite good. She wanted relief from the nightly pains in the bones of the face and head, and wanted to know what the eruption was. On examining, I found the pains proceeded from " nodes," especially on the frontal bone, and resembled very much those of periostitis. My first impression was, that I was dealing with a case of Syphilis, but a closer in spection, and my intimate acquaintance with the family, together with the "history of the case," caused me to abandon this theory, and the next one of Mercurial Cachexia also.

A vigorous cross-examination revealed the fact, that about thirty days before, she had been induced to take a "blood purifying remedy," consist-ing of a pint of whisky, with about three ounces of Poke Root in it. Of this poisonous, saturated tincture, she took a "swallow three times a day" until I was called.

I informed her that she had probably furnished the Homœopathic School of Medicine the most heroic proving of Phytolacca on record, for all of which we were duly thankful, but, nevertheless, would advise its discon tinuance.

I gave Mercurius Solubilis, 3d × trituration, which relieved the sleep lessness at once, and, finally, also the pains; but the eruption grew worse rather than better, and even invaded the conjunctiva and mucous membrane of the nose and mouth, and now, after a lapse of three months, it is in the fauces and æsophagus, having almost entirely disappeared from the external surface of the body.

A month ago, and when the eruption had partly faded, the photograph which is before you was taken. It gives but a faint conception of the case, and none whatever of the color, but such as they are, were the best I could procure. This is the second case I have met during the year. The first was a man, who took it in much smaller doses, and in this case it produced a severe rheumatism in the left shoulder; no fever, and no eruption. These cases are submitted to the society without comment. Different minds will draw different conclusions; but, differ as we may, they are of interest to all alike, and the facts are submitted for your con-sideration and digestion."

### Generalities.

Loss of all the adipose matter of the body (in animals).

Great prostration; as in collapse of cholera.

Tetanus and trismus, after the vomiting and purging.

° Swelling, inflammation, and induration of glands.

° Inflammation and swelling of the bones.

° Rheumatic and neuralgic affections (after diphtheria or scarlet fever). (*Hale.*)

Tingling and prickling sensation all over the body.

° Nightly pains in the bones and nodes.

The pains fly from one part, and go like an electric shock to another part. (*Dr. Preston.*)

The pains are always worse at night.

# PLANTAGO MAJOR.

### (*Plantain.*)

BOTANICAL DESCRIPTION.—This is a well known herb, growing in rich, moist places, in fields, by road sides, and in grass-plats. Common in Europe and America; flowering from May to October. A perennial, with a round scape rising from a fibrous root, from one to three feet in height. The *leaves* are ovate, smooth, somewhat toothed, five to seven nerved, each of which contains a strong fibre, which may be pulled out, and abruptly narrowed into a long channeled petiole. The *flowers* are white, very small, imbricated, numerous, and densely disposed on a cylindrical spike, from five to twenty inches long. Small plants are frequently found with the spikes only half an inch to two inches long, and the leaves and stalk proportionately small. *Stamens* and *styles* long; *seeds* numerous.

OFFICINAL PREPARATIONS.—Tincture of the fresh root and leaves; with strong alcohol; dilutions.

ANALOGUES.—*Arnica* (?), *Hepar* (?), *Mercurius* (?), *Phytolacca* (?).

[These symptoms are selected from the pathogenesis published by Dr F. Humphreys, (New York, 1871.) *Twelve* persons engaged in the provings. (*Hale.*)]

### Moral Symptoms.

General depression and despondency, though the weather is bright and beautiful.

Impatient and restless mood, with dull, stupid feeling in the brain; very irritable and morose temper; worse in the evening.

Feeling of great prostration, with a meditative mood, and unable to associate the mind with any external object.

Attempting to exercise the mental faculties would increase the depression and occasion rapid respiration, with a feeling of great anxiety.

Great mental anxiety, pacing backward and forward in the room; then throwing one's self on the bed and rolling from one side to the other in the greatest mental agitation; sleep with the most horrible and frightful dreams, which awaken me.

Mind inactive, with a dull, muddled feeling in the head.

### Head.

Twinges of pain in different parts of the head; now through the right temple, extending backward, then through the occiput, from ear to ear, then in other parts of the head, more or less severe.

32

Oppression deep in the head, and sense of something lying in the head from one ear to the other.

Dull, oppressed feeling through the forehead, with sometimes a deep pain extending across from the temporal bones, apparently at the base of the brain.

Pains in the head, (of a shooting character,) sometimes in the right parietal region, sometimes in the left; also in the mastoid processes.

Pretty severe pain in the left side of the head, from the forehead extending deep into the brain, coming on in paroxysms.

Pain in the left side of the head, from over the left eye back toward the occiput; somewhat sharp, but soon passing off.

An intermittent, pulsative pain at the vertex of the head, in a small spot beneath the scalp.

Itching of the *scalp*, with slight eruption on the forehead, which soon disappeared.

### Eyes.

Occasional dull, stupefying pain, deep in the orbits, worse on pressure.

Dull, aching pain, deep in right orbit, lasting only a few moments; fifteen minutes after taking the tincture.

Sharp, darting pain in the external and superior side of the orbit of the right eye.

Œdema and redness of the eyelids after rising.

Unnatural sense of dryness of the eyelids, continuing for several hours.

Severe painful stitches, first in the left, then in the right eyeball, more at the internal canthus, for an hour.

### Ears.

Pains in the head, apparently running from one ear through to the other.

Pains often in the centre of the ear, most in the left, beginning in the head.

### Nose.

Sensation across the bridge of the nose as if the nasal bones were being pressed together or pressed inward.

Frequent sneezing, with discharge of sanious mucus from left nostril.

Profuse discharge of sanious mucus from left nostril, continuing all day, then gradually diminishing and affecting the right nostril.

### Face and Lips.

Unpleasant sensation of bruised soreness and tension in the integuments of the face, on rising, especially on the forehead, above the left eye, and around it; somewhat sensitive when pressed or rubbed; continued some time.

Eruption on the face of small, reddish, rough, scaly, erythematous patches the size of a pea; on the left side of the face and most near the commissure of the lips; no decided pain or itching, but an unpleasant sense of tension.

Several papulæ around the nose, which are red, and smart when touched.

Eruptions on the lips, dry, scaly, with violent burning and tension; more the inferior one.

Lips have been livid, dark, sickly, and rough, for many days.

### Jaws and Teeth.

Aching of some decayed teeth in the lower jaw of the left side, after dinner.

Toothache in left side of the face, before and after breakfast; went off in the forenoon, and returned again after dinner, for an hour or two.

Slight toothache on rising, scarcely to be noticed, but afterward increased until noon, when it was very severe; cheek considerably swelled; constant discharge of saliva from the mouth after 12 M.

Pain was in decayed tooth, but the teeth on each side sound; teeth on each side were so elongated and sore that it was difficult to eat.

Excessive boring, digging pain, profuse flow of saliva, aggravated by walking in the cold air, and by contact; also high degree of heat, partial ease obtained only by lying down in a moderately cool room. Could not endure the pain; took Mercury 30 with relief.

Teeth of the left side elongated and sore; violent pain in the upper molars of the left side (sound teeth).

Sensitive feeling in the teeth, sort of tingling, as if in the

nerves of the front teeth of the upper jaw; these symptoms came on before going to sleep, but were not long
continued or very violent.

Soreness and cold sensation in the front incisor teeth, as if
they had been chilled by inhaling cold air.

Teeth feel elongated in the morning, and then ache from half-
past two until four P. M., each day; the pain is sharp,
stabbing, and severe, running along the course of the
superior branch of the trifacial nerve, which is sensitive
and the pain readily excited, and cannot lie on that side
of the face at night.

Toothache and dull face-ache during the morning, until after
two P. M.

Toothache gone, but swelled cheek remains. The tooth was
the second submaxillary molar of the left side.

Very rapid decay of the teeth. The filling has fallen out of
two.

° *Toothache.*—The leaf fibres of this plant have long been used
in Switzerland for toothache, in the following singular
manner. The fresh leaves of the plant are torn, and the
green thread-like fibers put into the ear of the aching side.
Curiously enough, in cases benefited by the remedy,
these fibres become black, and are then renewed, while, if
no relief is experienced, they remain green. During last
year I prepared a tincture of the whole plant, and from it
made the second decimal attenuation. About seven-tenths
of the cases of odontalgia which have come under my
treatment have been cured by the administration of this
remedy, *in about fifteen minutes!* Many other case have
been much benefited. From the wide range of usefulness in this disease, I conclude it will become useful in
other diseases. (*Dr. Reutlinger, Hale.*)

° I have for many years used the Plantago successfully in
various forms of odontalgia. I doubt not this use of the
Plantago has been confirmed by all who took part in the
proving during these intervening years. (*Humphreys.*)

**Mouth and Throat.**

Dryness of the mouth and throat.

Sensation of dryness in the fauces and pharynx.

Tongue slightly coated with a whitish coating.

Unpleasant and constrictive sensation in the pharynx, on awaking in the morning, soon passed off.

Hemorrhage from the gums.

Rawness and soreness in the pharynx in the night; this symptom continuing all the next day, in a modified degree, with dryness and tickling in the throat, inducing a dry, hacking cough.

Hoarseness, as if from dryness in the larynx, on rising in the morning.

### Gastric Symptoms.

Constant eructations in the morning, which taste strongly of sulphur; lasted all day, and during the forenoon the sulphur taste always present; taste changed in the afternoon; strong taste of carbonic acid, as much so as if a bottle of well-charged soda-water had been drank; this gas eructated in large quantities, at intervals of five to fifteen minutes, during the afternoon; the gas passed down into the bowels after supper, causing great borborygmi, and passing off with a strong odor of sulphuretted hydrogen.

Sensation of heat in the præcordia, with fullness of the abdomen in the afternoon, while walking in the open air, going off soon after sitting down.

Peculiar indescribable feeling in the region of the right cardiac orifice of the stomach; especially after eating a hearty meal, there would be a coolish, painful sensation, as if the parts were distended; symptom lasted about a week.

Faint and trembling feeling, with nausea.

### Hypochondria and Abdomen.

Slight uneasiness in epigastrium; frequent empty eructations, with slight rumbling in the bowels and occasional emissions of flatus.

Griping pain in the bowels, with nausea almost to vomiting, continued half an hour in the evening.

Severe colic pain in the left side of the abdomen, deep beneath the cartilage of the floating ribs, increased by deep inspiration, and by lying on that side.

Occasional eructations, which do not relieve the pain.

Pain during the day in the right iliac region, as if a stone was in the right inguinal canal.

Acute pain in the right hypochondria and abdominal muscles, manifest themselves, and continue in a greater or less degree during the afternoon and evening.

### Urine.

Unusually free and profuse discharge of urine.

Urine of a deep orange color; secretion increased.

Frequent micturition of colorless urine.

Nocturnal enuresis; arose twice during the night, passed each time a pint or more of light-colored urine (never before).

Passed a large quantity of very dark red urine, of a very strong odor, on rising in the morning.

Urine very profuse and light-colored, and deposits a white sediment.

Urgent desire to urinate on arising in the morning, with slight tenseness of the bladder, but passing very little urine.

Tickling, with unpleasant itching in the orifice of the urethra; came on suddenly, and lasted a few minutes in the morning, and again in the evening.

Sudden, darting, stinging pain running up the urethra while sitting.

Tenderness over the region of the bladder, on pressure.

° *In enuresis.*—" Since my attention was called to the subject, some fifteen years ago, I have used this remedy with great success, in enuresis. It is especially applicable to the nocturnal enuresis of children, particularly when depending on laxity of the sphincter vesica. In most of these cases the children usually secrete a larger quantity than normal, of a pale, watery urine, and though great pains are taken to have the bladder thoroughly emptied before retiring, yet the pressure on the weak sphincter will cause its escape before morning. It has seemed of no effect when, instead of laxity, there was paralysis of the sphincter. We think it not so useful when the urine is scanty, rather than abundant, and loaded with uric acid and its deposits. The bladder itself and the sphincter are in an irritable condition, and cause frequent micturition by night as well as by day; in this condition, while the Plantago affords no relief to adults, children frequently receive great benefit from it." (*Dr. E. W. Jones.*)

### Stool and Anus.

Unpleasant sensation of uneasiness in the bowels, and yet no stool.

Uneasiness in bowels, as if compelled, to go to stool before eating.

Looseness of the bowels, with feeling of weakness.

Loose stool every day, and sometimes twice per day, with some pain in the rectum and slight colic before stool.

Very watery stool, with very little pain or desire for stool, about ten p. m. Eructations still continuing.

Frequent discharge of stinking flatus, with uneasiness of the bowels, and followed by loose stool.

Stool at one a. m., and at daylight; stools watery at first thin, then thicker and more papescent; then thin again, and so on; also passed large quantities of wind.

Passage of some blood during an easy stool.

Partial prolapsus of the rectum during stool.

Pain in the rectum and lumbar region; stools of a normal character.

° A physician, Dr. ——, remarked at the Illinois State Medical Society that he had cured, during the season, every case of cholera infantum in his practice with the 3d of Plantago. (*Dr. Hale.*)

### Male Genital Organs.

Diminished sexual excitement all through, thus far.

Unconscious emission of semen at night whilst asleep.

### Chest.

Orgasm, or flow of blood to the chest, with sensation of heat.

Great weakness and oppression of the chest, with shortness of breath, followed by nausea, almost to vomiting.

On talking or reading aloud, obliged to stop several times in a sentence to take a breath; continued all the evening.

Difficulty of breathing, as if there were no air in the room.

Frequent, involuntary, deep breathing, approaching to yawning.

Panting breathing, on the least exercise, particularly on ascending stairs, with violent palpitation of the heart, and accelerated pulse.

Stitch in the heart after dinner.

Violent beating of the heart on ascending stairs, which lasted about five minutes.

Dull, aching, sub-cutaneous pain near the left side of the sternum; a little below its centre; worse by pressure, and also on sitting, but passing off on moving.

Sharp, darting pain in the left side, several times during the day; then in the right side; at one time a very sharp, darting pain passed up the right side; very peculiar in its character.

Sharp stitch or catching pain in the lower lobe of the left lung, on drawing a long breath at night in bed.

° I have repeatedly used an application of Plantago with prompt and decided benefit, in *erysipelatous inflammations* of the female breast. Its action has proved far more satisfactory in allaying and arresting the inflammatory process than Arnica or Hamamelis.

### Neck, Back, and Loins.

Soreness and stiffness of the neck, upon moving or turning the head, passing off after some time.

Soreness and stiffness of the sterno-cleido mastoid muscles of the right side of the neck; worse on moving the head to side affected, and relieved on moving it to opposite side; continued for ten days.

Great weakness across small of the back, extending around the body, as if the body were broken.

Sharp pain in the left side, sometimes extending to the right shoulder, then to the right side, then spreads over the upper part of the back.

Pulsative pain between the scapulæ, passing from one to the other, and from thence to the dorsum of the right arm, in the extensor muscles, darting from above toward the elbow.

Dull, aching pain in the sacrum, a little below its union with the lumbar vertebræ; worse during motion or standing.

Tenderness on pressure along the spinal column.

### Upper Extremities.

Lead-like weight and heaviness of the extremities, arms and legs. Great weariness and desire to lie down.

Aching rheumatic pains in left shoulder, going off in a few minutes.

Rheumatic pains in right shoulder, came on while sitting, lasted for an hour.

Pains in the muscles of right arm, chiefly below the elbow.

Rheumatic drawing or sticking pains in the joints of the fingers.

Itching in the commissure of the fingers of the left hand; worse at night, but more or less constant.

### Lower Extremities.

Pain and uneasiness of the loins and lower extremities.

Dull, aching pain in the right shoulder, alternating with a dull, aching pain in the right hip, which passes down the limb.

Pain in the right side and right knee-joint, continued at irregular intervals.

Drawing pains in the posterior muscles of the right thigh, with tenderness on pressure.

Sharp, shooting pain, passing from the trochanter major of the right leg into the hip joint.

Painful soreness of the left leg, below the knee, as if it had been strained.

### Skin.

The skin of the whole body is sensitive, and leaves a burning sensation when scratched.

Itching in the lower limbs, also in other parts of the body; rubbing feels grateful, but does not relieve ; when the rubbing ceases, a burning sensation is experienced.

Prickling or stinging pains in the skin of different parts of the body and limbs ; these pains are sometimes of a prickling character, as if produced by very fine needles; at others with a burning sensation, as if from nettles, never appearing in different parts of the body simultaneously, but always confined to one spot at a time; they manifest themselves chiefly in the afternoon and evening, and almost exclusively while sitting in a warm room, and seldom felt during exercise in the open air.

Eruption about the hips and thighs, particularly on the inside of the thighs; the papulæ are isolated, hard, white, and flattened; some of them have a small red point in the centre; they itch slightly on first making their appearance; when scratched, the itching becomes more violent; and a burning sensation supervenes, and deep redness is diffused through the part, which lasts about five minutes; in several hours they become more elevated and acuminated, and, finally, in about twenty-four hours, gradually disappear, without suppuration or desquamation, and others spring up. Several appeared on the wrist and between the fingers.

Papulæ exude a yellowish humor, soon forming a crust.

Soreness and slight tumefaction of the submaxillary glands on each side.

\* The hand and a portion of the face, in the case of a young lady, were red, swelled, itching violently, and in places covered with vesicles; she took pellets medicated with Plantago 1st, and applied a lotion made by a teaspoonful of the tincture to a cup of water. The relief was prompt, and a cure was effected in three days.

° It is reported to have cured cases of *poisoning with ivy*, poison shumach (Rhus ven.), where the face has been fearfully swollen and red like erysipelas. The leaves were wilted under a roller and applied to the part, with prompt relief and subsidence of the swelling.

° The Plantago is used with benefit as an application for lacerated or *incised wounds or injuries*, and especially when attended with painful swelling and tendency to erysipelatous inflammations or sphacelus.

° A young man cut his thumb through the root of the nail; it was dressed and treated by an allopathic physician for two or three weeks; it became inflamed, fearfully swollen, and was very painful. I made two prescriptions, using the Plantago externally, with the tincture, and cured it.

° The second was a young man who had his finger bitten through the first joint, so as to almost sever the end of the finger. When I first saw it, it was swollen to about the size of a hen's egg, and very much inflamed. I made two or three external applications, and cured the finger.

° A young man with a frost-bite on the top of his foot; it was badly swollen, and he was unable to walk. With about a two-ounce vial of the Plantago-wash it was cured.

° A lady, about forty-five or fifty years old, had been troubled with a milk-leg for many years. At times it would swell and be very painful. I gave her a solution of Plantago, for external applications, and it relieved her at once, and with the aid of Sepia and Rhus, internally, she remained quite comfortable until she passed from my knowledge. (*Dr. George Washburne.*)

° A lady, while dressing a codfish, thrust one of the fins into the palmer surface of the middle finger, just over the second or large joint. The wound was deep and bled profusely; but no attention was paid to it at the moment, except to bind it up with a rag. The night following, the part became excessively painful, the pain extending from the wound up to the shoulder, causing great distress. The next morning the whole hand was swelled, back and front, especially the injured finger. The arm also even swelled up to the shoulder, and there were two distinct light pinkish streaks running up the front of the arm, from the hand to the shoulder. The third day, after some fruitless applications, being almost agonized with the pain and suffering, she applied bruised plantain leaves to the part, removing them as often as they became dry. In about half-an-hour after the application, she felt so relieved that she fell asleep, and slept probably an hour the first sleep she had after the accident. In two or three days the finger was well. (*Dr. C. Cresson.*)

## Sleep.

Restless at night, with inability to sleep, frequent dreams of a gloomy character, rousing me from sleep; worse about midnight.

Some throbbing of the arteries at night, and restlessness until twelve or one in the morning.

Restless sleep, with every variety of fanciful dreams, with *grinding of the teeth.* The highest degree of restlessness at night, with the most vivid, congruous, and coherent dreams, also incoherent and disgusting dreams, all in rapid succession.

### Fever.

Some chilliness and slight headache; cold hands and feet, and ringing in the ears for some time.

Cold chill running over me, and goose-skin; fingers cold.

Sharp, transient pains in the left temple, while sitting by the furnace and after having been out.

Chilliness on rising, after being seated for three hours, with sensation of heat in the chest and erratic pains in the limbs, chest and head; these symptoms continuing from one until three o'clock, with disposition to stretch.

Dull and stupid feeling, with an inclination to stretch and yawn frequently, with oppression in the chest, and aversion to mental and physical labor.

Strong, full, and intermittent pulse, varying from 70 to 80 beats per minute in a recumbent position, and increased to from 95 to 100 in an erect position, in the evening.

Intermittent and irregular pulse.

Almost imperceptible pulse; 100 per minute, and easily compressible.

Highest degree of excitability; high fever; strong, bounding pulse; 120 per minute; sensation of great heat, with thirst; imagined the room to be very hot and close.

Unnatural heat of the head, hands, and feet, all the time; pulse 72.

° (Intermittent fever.)

It was in high repute among the ancient medical writers as a remedy for intermittents, they recommending a drink made from an infusion of the roots of the plant.

° Dr G. Washburne relates the cure of several cases made with the tincture or first dilution.

° That it will prove valuable in intermittents is quite certain. The symptomatic indications, as well as the genus of the remedy, point to its value in typhus and typhoid conditions.

---

# PODOPHYLLUM PELTATUM.

### (*Mandrake, May-Apple.*)

BOTANICAL DESCRIPTION.—Height about one foot, *stem* round, sheathed at base, dividing into two round petioles, between which is the flower. *Leaves* broadly cordate, in five to seven lobes, each lobe about six inches long, from the insertion of the petiole; two lobed and dentate at apex: barren stems, with one centrally peltate leaf. *Flower* pedunculate, drooping, white, about two inches in diameter. *Fruit* ovate, oblong, large, yellowish, with a peculiar flavor, likened by Wood to the strawberry.

It is an indigenous, perennial herb, with a long, jointed, dark brown rhizoma, or *root*, about half the size of the finger, spreading extensively in rich grounds, and giving off fibres at the joints; internally it is yellowish. The *fruit* is fleshy, one-celled, one or two inches in length, of a lemon color, with brownish spots when ripe, and covered with a large, persistent stigma. The mucilaginous pulp is edible, and esteemed as a luxury by many persons; it encloses twelve seeds, in pulpy arils.

[The variety named Podophyllum montanum, by Rafinesque, grows in the South.]

Mandrake grows throughout the United States, in low, shady situations, flowering in May and June, maturing its fruit in September and October.

The *root* is the officinal portion; the proper time for collecting it is in the latter part of October, or early part of November, soon after the ripening of the fruit.

The *fruit* possesses slightly laxative and diuretic properties, the rind and seeds being the medicinal portions.

The *leaves* are deemed poisonous, probably possessing the same properties as the root.

Podophyllin is the resin obtained from mandrake, and is very extensively used instead of the crude root. Dr. King, the eclectic, claims to have discovered and introduced this preparation to the notice of the medical profession. It is a yellowish or yellow-brown powder, insoluble in water, oil of turpentine, dilute Nitric acid, and diluted alkalies. It is said to be composed of two resins, both of which are purgative, one is soluble in alcohol only, the other in alcohol and ether. It has no alkaline or acid reaction, but forms a saponaceous compound with the alkalies. It has a bitter, nauseous and acrid taste. From four to eight grains act as an emeto-cathartic, with griping, nausea, prostration and watery stools. From two to four grains as a drastic-cathartic, with nausea and griping; even one half a grain often acts as an active cathartic.

OFFICIAL PREPARATIONS.—Tincture of the root, with strong alcohol; dilutions. Podophyllin and its triturations. (The rind of the fruit, the seeds, and the leaves, are all medicinal, the pulp of the fruit edible.)

ANALOGUES.—*Arnica, Æsculus, Bryonia, Collinsonia, Chelidonium, Helleborus niger, Iris versicolor, Lilium, Mercurius Sol., Nitric acid, Pulsatilla, Sulphur, Veratrum album.*

### Mind and Sensorium.

*Stupor*, with vomiting, purging and collapse.

\* Depression of spirits; he imagines he is going to die or be very ill.

\* Hypochondriac mood, from disorder of the liver. (*Hale*.)

### Head.

\* Morning headache, with heat in the vertex.

Pressing pain in the temples in the forenoon, with drawing in the eyes, as if strabismus would follow.

Dull, heavy pain in the forehead, with soreness over the seat of the pain.

\* Giddiness and dizziness, with the sensation of fullness over the eyes.

Morning headache, with flushed face.

Pain on the top of the head, when rising in the morning.

Stunning headache through the temples, relieved by pressure.

° Headache alternating with diarrhœa.

Vertigo while standing in the open air; with inclination to fall forward.

° Rolling of the head during difficult dentition in children (*Bell, Williamson.*)

° Perspiration of the head during sleep, with coldness of the face (while teething).

° Irritation of the brain—reflex—from disorder of the bowels

° *Bilious headache*, worse in the morning.

### Eyes.

Smarting in the lids; drawing sensation in the eyes.

Pain in the eyeballs and in the temples, with heat and throbbing of the temporal arteries.

The eyes appear inflamed in the morning.

### Mouth and Teeth.

° Grinding of the teeth at night, in children; also with rolling of the head in teething children.

Copious salivation, but without the destructive action of
mercury.

* Offensive odor from the mouth, at night, perceptible to the
patient.

° Stomatitis materna. (?)

° Chronic inflammation of the tongue; cracked, swollen and
bleeding. (*Hale.*)

* Foul, putrid taste in the mouth.

˒ Tongue full and broad, *with a pasty coat in the center.*
(*Scudder.*)

° A *red* tongue, not *bright* red; *rough*, with uniformly erect
papillæ. (*Ib.*)

° A dull, bluish color of the tongue. (*Ib.*)

### Throat.

* Sore throat, commencing on the right side and going to the
left (Lyc., Lach., left, going to right). (*Williamson.*)

Sore throat, left side, worse in the morning, especially painful
when swallowing liquids.

Soreness of the throat, extending to the ears.

* Rattling of mucus in the throat. (*Ib.*)

* Goitre. (*Williamson and Eclectics.*)

### Gastric Symptoms.

Voracious appetite and great thirst, with strong digestion. (*p.*)

* Loss of appetite, or satiety from a small quantity of food, followed by nausea and vomiting. (*s.*)

* Regurgitation of food, which is *sour*, with acid eructations;
belching of hot flatus; acidity of the stomach, and unpleasant, sickly sensation in the stomach. (*s.*)

Vomiting of food an hour after meal, with craving appetite
immediately afterward.

Vomiting of food, with putrid taste and odor.

° Gastric affections, attended by depression of spirits; heartburn; vomiting of hot, frothy mucus, etc.

[The nausea commences three or four hours after a large dose; is persistent and depressing, continuing for 24 or 36 hours, often with vomiting
of bile, and ingesta, and with purging and severe colic. (*Hale.*)]

Vomiting of dark green, bilious matter, mixed with blood, the
blood dark and coagulated.

The stomach contracts so hard and rapidly in the efforts to vomit, that the wrenching pain causes them to utter sharp screams.

* *Dyspepsia*, in its most aggravated forms.   ( *Williamson.*)
* Gastritis, acute and chronic.  (*Hale.*)
* Nausea and vomiting, with fullness in the head; the vomiting is persistent.
* *Heart-burn, and water-brash, with heat in the stomach.*
Throbbing in the epigastrium, followed by diarrhœa.
* Vomiting of thick bile and blood for eighteen hours; in acute gastritis.
* Vomiting and diarrhœa of bilious matters.
Sensation of hollowness in the pit of the stomach.
Stitches in the epigastrium, from coughing.

### Liver.

* Fullness, with pain and soreness in the right hypochondrium.
Stitches in the right hypochondrium; worse while eating.
° Chronic hepatitis, with costiveness, tenderness, and pains in the region of the liver.
Twisting pain in the right hypochondrium, with sensation of heat in the part.
Sensation of weight and dragging in the left hypochondrium.
° Congestion and enlargement of the liver; acute and chronic hepatitis.
° Congestion and torpor of the portal system.
° *Gall-stones*, with the characteristic symptoms; will expel them, if given in large doses, alone, or after large quantities of olive oil.  (*Hale.*)

[Podophyllin, *primarily*, causes increased functional activity of the liver, with large flow of bile; *secondarily*, the liver becomes torpid, and jaundice and retention of bile occurs.  (*Hale.*)]

### Abdomen.

* *Intense cramp-like colic, with retraction of the abdominal muscles*, at ten P. M. and five A. M.
Pain in the bowels, at daylight in the morning; *relieved* by external warmth; by bending forward while lying on the side, but *aggravated* by lying on the back.
Pain and rumbling in the *transverse* colon, at three o'clock A. M., followed by diarrhœa.

The pain in the bowels is first attended by *coldness*, which is followed by heat and warm perspiration.

*Heat* in the bowels, with inclination for stool.

*Faintness*, with sensation of *emptiness* in the bowels, after stool.

\* Sharp pain above the right groin, preventing motion (in the last month of pregnancy).

° *Dull, unpleasant pain or weight in the hypogastric region.* (in many diseases. *Scudder.*)

*Distension* of the abdomen, even enormous swelling (in case of fatal poisoning).

° Myalgia of the abdominal muscles; after abuse of purgatives. (*Hale.*)

° Lead-colic, with *retracted* abdomen, etc. ( *Williamson.*)

° Conditions simulating *puerperal peritonitis*, when it has been preceded by diarrhœa, or abuse of purgatives (not useful in true peritonitis). (*Hale.*)

° Tympanitic distension of the abdomen in typhoid, and in children, with diarrhœa. (*Hale.*)

### Intestinal Symptoms.

\* *Primary.*— Abundant, soft, fœcal evacuations, with colic and nausea (from laxative doses), i. e., one quarter gr. Podophyllin.

Stool earlier in the morning than usual, but natural (from small doses).

\* Frequent stool during the day, but of natural consistence.

Six soft yellow stools a day, with some griping.

\* Profuse diarrhœa, preceded by colic, worse in the morning.

\* Diarrhœa early in the morning, followed by very frequent, papescent, yellow stools, for forty-eight hours.

Evacuation of *green* stools in the morning.

Diarrhœa *immediately after eating or drinking* (also **Croton** tig).

\* Hæmorrhoids—inflamed, sore, swollen and painful.

\* *Painful diarrhœa, with screaming and grindiny of the teeth,* in children (during dentition). ( *Williamson.*)

White, slimy stools, with severe colic and nausea.

33

*Hot, watery, frequent, profuse* evacuations, attended with prostration and cramps, as in cholera.

\* *Muco-gelatinous stools,* like white of egg, after which the colic ceases, and does not return. (*Hale.*)

\* Food passes the bowels in an undigested state. (*Williamson.*)

° Evacuations which consist of *dark yellow* mucus, which smells like carrion. (*Jeanes*).

\* Frequent stools, yellow, green, watery, brown mucus, all of which may be *streaked with blood,* with strong urging— and heat and pain in the anus.

\* *Diarrhœa, with prolapsus ani at every stool.*

*After stool;* flashes of heat running up the back, cutting in the bowels, severe and painful tenesmus; great weakness and faintness and pain in the lumbar region.

*During stool;* urging in the bowels; heat and pain in the anus; sensation as if the genital organs would fall out; (in women) bearing down, as if from inactivity of the rectum; nausea; gagging; tormina, and pain in lumbar region.

*Before stool;* intense nausea; colic; rumbling in left side.

° *Diarrhœa—bilious, cholera-morbus, dysentery;* pain in the back, and sometimes vomiting ; *acute enteritis; colitis, rectitis,* etc.

*Secondary*—Constipation for two days after the purging.

\* Constipation, with headache and flatulence.

Fæces hard, dry, and voided with difficulty.

\* Constipation, *alternating with diarrhœa.*

\* Hard stool, coated with tough, yellow mucus. (*Hale.*)

° The first part of the stool large and hard, followed by fluid and wind. (*Scudder.*)

° *Chronic diarrhœa*—worse in the morning.

*Frequent chalk-like stools;* very offensive, with gagging and excessive thirst (*in children*—see Calc.c.) (*Williamson.*)

\* Clay-colored, offensive stools, with *jaundice.* (*Hale.*)

\* Descent of the rectum, from a little exertion, immediately followed by stool, or a discharge of thick, transparent mucus, sometimes of a yellow color ; and mixed with blood. (*Williamson, Hale.*)

\* Prolapsus ani, most frequently in the morning. (*Jeanes.*)
\* The anus feels very sore, sensitive and swollen.
\**Chronic, painful, hæmorrhoidal tumors*, all around the anus, some of them bleeding. (*Hale, and many others.*)
\* *Internal hæmorrhoids, with prolapsus recti.* (*Ib.*)

[For the *primary* symptoms, the best curative results are obtained with the attenuation *above* the 3d; for *secondary* symptoms the dilutions *below* the 3d.—*Hale.*]

### Urinary Organs.

\* Profuse secretion of urine (*p.*)
\* Involuntary discharge of urine, during sleep. (*Williamson*).
\* Frequent nocturnal urination, during pregnancy. (*Ib.*)
Pain in the region of the kidneys, followed by flow of urine depositing calculi sediment.
\* *Suppression and retention of urine.*
\* Diminished secretion of urine.
Scanty urine, with frequent voidings.

### Generative Organs.

*Male.*—Stitching pain above the pubis, and in the course of the spermatic cords.
° Diseases of the *prostate* gland, associated with rectum troubles. (*Hale.*)
° Gonorrhœa; gleet; syphilis (?) (*Eclectic authorities.*)
*Female.* — \* Leucorrhœa ; discharge of thick, transparent mucus.
\* Leucorrhœa, attended with constipation and bearing down in the genital organs.
\* Suppression of the menses in young females, with bearing down in the hypogastric and sacral region, with pain from motion, relieved by lying down.
° After pains, with strong bearing down and flatulency.
° Prolapsus uteri, with much aching pain in the region of left ovary, heat running down to the left thigh, in pregnancy, must lie on the stomach. (*Williamson.*)
° Prolapsus uteri or vagina, especially after confinement.
° Prolapsus recti, with violent bearing down pains; intolerable pain in her back, with profuse excoriating leucorrhœa and great ardor urinæ. (*Williamson.*)

° Chronic prolapsus, with great costiveness. (*Ib.*)

° Excessive vomiting in pregnancy and conditions arising from a congested condition of the pelvic viscera.

° Prolapsus uteri, with hypertrophy, ulceration and prolapsus. Pain in the region of the ovaries, especially the right.

° After-pains, with strong bearing down.

° *Hæmorrhoids and prolapsus recti*, after confinement.

° Ability to lie comfortably, in the early months of pregnancy, only on the stomach. (*Jeanes.*)

° *Swelling of the labia*, during pregnancy.

° Induration of the os uteri.

° Uterine diseases caused by or complicated with, or aggravated by, diseases of the rectum. (*Hale.*)

### Larynx.

° Cough, accompanying remittent fever. ( *Williamson.*)

° Dry cough; loose, hacking cough. (*Ib.*)

° Whooping cough, with costiveness and loss of appetite. (*Ib.*)

° Cough from disease of the *liver.* (*Hale.*)

### Chest

Pains in the chest, increased by taking a deep inspiration.

Snapping in the right lung, like breaking a thread, on taking a deep inspiration.

Inclination to breathe deeply; sighing and shortness of breath.

Sense of suffocation when first lying down at night.

Sensation as if the heart was ascending into the throat.

Palpitation of the heart, with a clucking sensation rising up to the throat.

° Stinging pain in the region of the heart.

° Palpitation of the heart, from physical exertion or mental emotion, in persons subject to rumbling in the ascending colon.

[No proof of the Podophyllum ever having cured any organic disease of the heart. The symptoms are probably sympathetic from gastric and hepatic irritation.—*Hale.*]

### Back.

Pain in the small of the back when walking or standing.

Pain in the lumbar region, with the sensation of coldness, worse at night, from motion.

Pain between the shoulders, with soreness, worse at night and from motion.

Pains are of a myalgic character.

° A sharply defined ache in the sacro-ischiatic formica, with tenderness on pressure. (*Scudder.*)

### Upper Extremities.

Myalgic pains in the left forearm and finger.

Weakness of the wrist, with soreness to the touch.

° Pain in the course of the ulnar nerve of both arms.

### Lower Extremities.

Pain and weakness in the left hip, increased by going up stairs.

Pains in the thighs, legs and knees, worse from standing.

° Slight paralytic weakness of the left side.

Creaking in the knee joints, from motion.

Stiffness on beginning to move.

° Severe pain and swelling of the ankle joints.

Aching of the limbs, worse at night.

Coldness of the feet.

Perspiration of the feet in the evening.

### Fever.

Chilliness when lying down or in the evening.

Chill in the morning, with pressing pain in both hypochondria.

Backache before the chill.

The shaking and sensation of coldness continues for some time after the heat commences.

° Bilious fever, either remittent or intermittent.

### Sleep.

° Restless sleep of children, with whining at night.

A feeling of fatigue on waking in the morning.

### Skin.

° Sallowness of the skin in children.

° Moisture of the skin, with preternatural warmth.

### Generalities.

' *Fullness of the superficial veins*, indicating impairment of the innervation of the sympathetic system of nerves. (*Scudder.*)

# POLYGONUM PUNCTATUM.

*(Smart-weed.)*

BOTANICAL DESCRIPTION.—This plant, sometimes called *Water-pepper,* is the *Polygonum hydropiper* of Michaux. It is an annual plant with a smooth *stem,* branched, often decumbent at base, slender-jointed, swelling above the joints, and of a reddish or greenish-brown color, sprinkled with glandular dots, and from one to two feet in height.

Polygonum punctatum is a well known, intensely acrid plant, found growing in nearly all parts of the United States, in ditches, low ground, among rubbish, and about brooks and water-courses, flowering in August and September. There are many species of Polygonum, which, although possessing similar virtues, yet differ materially in their medical potency. The whole plant is officinal, and has a biting, pungent, acrid taste, and imparts its virtues to alcohol or water. Age renders it inert, and heat impairs its medicinal qualities.

It should be collected and made into a tincture while fresh. The plant has not been analyzed.

OFFICINAL PREPARATIONS.—Tincture of the leaves with strong alcohol; dilutions.

ANALOGUES.—*Asarum, Ammonium carb., Caulophyllum, Capsicum, Pulsatilla, Senega, Senecio, Xanthoxylum.*

## Head.

Pulsative headache, with sensation of fullness.

Pain in the forehead and side of the head, extending into the orbits.

Dull headache, with dizziness.

Throbbing of the carotids, with heavy beating of the heart.

## Mouth and Throat.

Sensation of dryness and scraping in the throat.

Tongue feels as if swollen, a burning from its root to the pit of the stomach.

Abundant salivation, thin and watery, with burning in the mouth.

## Stomach.

Throbbing, cutting pain in the stomach.

Thirst for water, yet water produces nausea.

Sharp pain under the right scapula, extending into the chest and to the pit of the stomach, with heavy beating of the heart and throbbing of the carotids.

*Burning* in stomach, followed by a *cold* sensation in pit of stomach.

## Abdomen and Stool.

Copious stools, followed by a smarting sensation of the anus.

Cutting pain in lower part of the bowels, with constant urging to stool.

Straining at stool, with a mucus, jelly-like discharge.

Inefficient urging to stool, with great quantity of fœtid flatulence.

Yellowish-green stools.

\* Cutting, lancinating, griping pains, with great rumbling, as if the whole intestinal contents were in a fluid state and in violent commotion, the movement proceeding from below upwards, producing nausea and disposition to vomit, with liquid fæces, which were discharged with considerable force, with pain in the loins.

° Cholera morbus and cholera infantum. (*Dr. W. E. Paine.*)

° *Dysentery,* with burning and smarting in the rectum.

° Tympanitis; flatulent colic.

### Rectum and Anus.

\* The interior of the anus studded with itching eminences, as from corrugation without contraction; a kind of hæmorrhoidal tumor.

Slight pains in the lower intestines, rectum and anus.

° *Hæmorrhoids,* with itching and burning in the tumors.

° Pruritus ani (used as a wash).

### Urinary Organs.

Unusual and increased desire to evacuate the bladder.

\* Copious discharge of clear, light-colored urine, with rumbling, griping pains in the abdomen. (*p.*)

\* Painful cutting, and feeling of strangulation at the neck of the bladder while urinating, lasting a long time after. (*p.*)

Urine scanty and red. (*s.*)

Increased flow of urine, with irritation in neck of bladder and urethra.

Pain in sacrum and bladder *not relieved* by copious urination.

° Stranguary. ° Dysuria.

### Generative Organs.

*Male.*—Pains in *left* spermatic cord and testicle, with soreness in the testicle; followed by darting pains in *right* cord and testicle (constant symptom). (*Dr. Paine.*)

When voiding urine, pain and burning in *prostate gland.*

Itching about glans penis and orifice of urethra, and constant
     desire to urinate.

Pulsative pain in prostate gland, extending along the urethra.

*Female.*—Warmth, and a peculiar tingling sensation in the
     whole system.

\* Aching pains in the hips and loins, and a sensation of weight
     and tension within the pelvis.

° *Amenorrhœa;* many cases, cured by doses of 1 3 of the tinc-
     ture three times a day. (*Eberle.*)

° Delaying menses—six or seven days—with distress and pain,
     cured by five drop doses every four hours. (*Dr. Small.*)

### Larnyx and Trachea.

Dry cough, excited by tickling under upper part of the
     sternum, with dryness in the larynx.

### Chest and Heart.

Heavy beating of the heart and carotids, with pain under right
     scapula.

Sharp, shooting pains in region of the *heart*, extending through
     to left shoulder blade.

### Back and Neck.

Severe lameness of the muscles of the left side of the neck,
     extending to the shoulder and rendering movement painful.

### Extremities.

Burning and tingling in the whole body, more in the legs, feet,
     and forearms.

Great heat and burning of the feet, continuing one and a half
     hours, and then suddenly becoming uncomfortably cold.

Darting pains through the extremities and the small joints.

### Skin.

A scarlet eruption about three inches wide (like *zona*), around
     the waist, attended with itching, burning, and pain.

It acts as a rubefacient, when topically applied.

### Fever.

Alternate chills and heat.

### Sleep.

Restless sleep, with unpleasant, laborious and fatiguing dreams,
     and waking unrefreshed.

### Generalities.

Slight vertiginous feeling passing over the head, followed in a short time by a sensation in the arms and legs as of galvanic shocks.

*Pulsation and intermitting pains* (in shoulders, lumbar region, hypogastric region, small joints, etc.)

The pains move from place to place.

The pains reminded the prover of electrical movement, or the flashes of *aurora borealis.*

A peculiar sensation of tingling and warmth in the whole body, even to the fingers and toes.

᷇ Has a great reputation in domestic practice, as a fomentation in all internal inflammations.

° Sprains, bruises, and lameness therefrom (locally applied).

° Chronic erysipelatous inflammations (as a wash).

° Old and indolent ulcers (as a wash).

° *Epilepsy,* "A protracted case of epilepsy cured by the extract." (*B. L. Hill.*)

---

# POLYPORUS OFFICINALIS.

## (*Larch Agaric.*)

DESCRIPTION.—This is a fungus, nourished on the ABIES EXCELSA tree. The *hymenium* is concrete, with the substance or the pileus, consisting of sub-rotund pores, with their simple dissepiments.

It is acrid, irritating mucous surfaces with which it comes in contact.

OFFICINAL PREPARATIONS.—Tincture or trituration of the fungus.

ANALOGUES.—*Agaricus, Bryonia, China, Cornus, Gelseminum, Ipecacuanha, Nux vomica, Podophyllum.*

[This is a fungus growing on the Larch tree, in all countries. It was formerly called *Boletus.* These symptoms are taken from Dr. Burt's Monograph, 1868.—*Hale.*]

### Mind.

Low spirited, gloomy, desponding, irritable.

Absence of mind and loss of memory.

### Head.

* Headache, dull, frontal, with fever.

Head feels light and hollow, with deep, frontal headache and faintness.

᷇ Sick headache, from organic lesion of the liver. (*Burt.*)

° Periodical headache. (*Shepherd.*)

Tight feeling in the forehead, and headache in temples all day.

° Sick headache, every month, with chilliness along the spine.

### Face.

° Facial neuralgia, of a periodical character. ( *Wakeman.*)
° Intermittent prosopalgia—a burning pain in all the upper
teeth, left jaw and temple, commencing at twelve M., and
lasting till midnight. (*Burt.*)

### Mouth and Throat.

\* Bitter, nauseous taste in the mouth.
\* Not much thirst.
\* Tongue coated white or yellow.
Rawness and scraping in the throat.

### Gastric Symptoms.

Nausea and sometimes vomiting of bile.
Bilious temperaments; sickness of stomach; **coldness of**
stomach.
In evening, feeling as of lump in stomach.
Burning distress in region of stomach.

### Abdomen.

More or less pains in the abdominal viscera, especially the
liver.
\* Intermittent diarrhœa or dysentery.
Bowels inclined to be torpid, or loose papescent mucus stools.
Some uneasiness, and severe griping pains in bowels.
Much flatus in bowels, and feeling as if diarrhœa would set in.
Sensation as if diarrhœa would come on; then slight motion
of the bowels.
Uneasiness of the abdomen, with looseness of the bowels.
° Has a decided curative action in hepatic complaints, espe
cially *jaundice.* (*Burt.*)

### Urine.

Urine thick and high-colored, or red and scanty.
Profuse flow of urine; constant desire to urinate.

### Stool and Anus.

Loose, papescent stools, without pain.
Stools of pure mucus, or mucus and blood, and bile, with great
faintness and distress in the solar plexus, after stools from
portal congestion.
\* Lienteria; stools undigested.

Loose, yellow stool, with pain afterwards.

Desire for stool, with much flatulence.

Copious *fluid* stool, expelled with force.

° *Chronic dysentery and diarrhœa.* (*Holcombe, Wood, Burt.*)

### Fever and Chills.

\* Chill alternates with the fever several times a day.

\* Intermissions very short; almost continued fever.

\* Chill, light and short; fever, long, followed by slight perspiration.

Hectic chills and fever, in consumptives.

\* Very restless all night, with fever and aching distress in the large joints.

\* Chilliness along the spine, with frequent hot flashes of fever.

Fever all one afternoon and night.

\* Skin hot and dry, especially the palms of the hands.

Awoke at midnight, two different nights, in a profuse perspiration.

Disposition to yawn and stretch when chilly.

Slight chilliness creeps up the back, to the nape of the neck, most noticeable between the shoulders.

This was succeeded by a general feeling of chilliness, lasting for several minutes.

° Intermittent, remittent and bilious fevers. (*Burt.*)

### Back and Loins.

Great languor, with severe aching pains in the large joints and bones of the back and legs.

Great *aching distress in all the large joints.*

Severe backache; back is very stiff, can hardly rise after sitting down a few moments.

---

# POLYPORUS PINICOLA.

### (*Pine Agaric.*)

OFFICIAL PREPARATIONS.—Tincture or trituration of the *fresh* fungus.

ANALOGUES.—*Agaricus, Bryonia, China, Cornus florida, Gelseminum, Ipecacuanha, Nux vomica, Podophyllum.*

[Dr. P. H. Hale first used this medicine in intermittent fever. He got his information of its use in ague from the lumbermen of Northern Michigan, who put it in whisky and use it as a panacea for the ague. He tested it in obstinate agues in Southern Michigan, and found it quite useful.

I used it in several cases, with decided benefit, and sent the medicine to various physicians, to test its powers.

Drs. Mann, Coe, Duncan and Burt, all prescribed it in obstinate cases, and generally with good success. It has been found most useful in quotidians. It acts best in the tincture or 1 × trituration.—*Hale.*]

---

# POPULUS TREMULOIDES.
### (*American Aspen.*)

BOTANICAL DESCRIPTION.—This tree, also known as the White poplar, grows from twenty to fifty feet high, with a diameter of from eight to twelve inches. It is covered with a smooth, greenish-white bark, except on the trunk of very old trees. The *leaves* are orbicular-cordate, abruptly accuminate, dentate-serrate, smooth on both sides, pubescent at the margins, dark-green, three nerved, from two to two and a half inches long, growing on long, slender, and laterally compressed petioles, which accounts for the continued agitation of the leaves by the slightest breeze. *Aments* plumed with silken hairs, about two inches long, pendulous, appearing in April, long before the leaves. Scales cut into three or four deep linear divisions, and fringed with long hairs.

OFFICINAL PREPARATIONS.—Tincture of the inner bark and leaves with strong alcohol; dilutions; *Populin* and its triturations.

ANALOGUES.—*Arnica, China, Cornus florida, Nux vomica, Pulsatilla, Terebinthina* (*?*) *Thuja.*

### (*A Fragmentary proving.*)

### Head.

Fullness about the head, with general nervous excitement.

### Gastric.

A warm, pungent sensation in the stomach, followed by a glow of heat on the entire surface.

Nausea and vomiting, and slight purging of bilious matter.

Fever, with burning sensation in the stomach.

° Chronic dyspepsia, from gastric catarrh. (*Hale.*)

° Impaired digestion, with chronic diarrhœa. (*Eclectic.*)

° Dyspepsia, attended with torpor of the liver, or an unhealthy bilious secretion. (*Ib.*)

° As a remedy for *indigestion*, accompanied with *flatulence and acidity*, we know of no single agent more to be relied upon. (*Coe.*)

° An excellent remedy for the dyspeptic symptoms accompanying pregnancy. (*Ib.*)

° Chronic diarrhœa and dysentery. (*Ib.*)
° Jaundice.  ° Lumbricoid worms.  (*Ib.*)

### Urinary Organs.

Very copious discharge of urine.
\* Irritation of the bladder and urethra.
° Scalding of the urine. (*Eclectic.*)
° Suppression and retention of urine.  (*Ib.*)
° Paramount to all the rest (of its virtues) is its property of relieving *painful urination*, and heat and scalding of the urine, especially when these symptoms occur during pregnancy. (*Coe.*)
° In diseases of the bladder, urethra and prostate, I have found the greatest benefit from it. In several cases of *catarrh of the bladder* I have found that two or three grains (of *Populin*), four or five times a day, produced a most favorable impression. (*Paine.*)
° An old gentleman troubled with vesical catarrh and *ardor urinæ*, and chronic enlargement of the prostate, for many years, got prompt relief from two grains (of Populin), three times a day, and was cured in four months. (*Paine.*)

[I have used the 1st and 3d triturations of Populin in diseases of the prostate, and with good results. (*Hale.*)]

### Genital Organs.

° Gonorrhœa.  ° Gleet, chronic.
° Highly recommended and extensively used in many diseases of the uterus and vagina.
° *Prurigo*, from an aphthous condition of the mucous membrane of the vagina and an irritable condition of the lining membrane of the uterus. (?) (*Paine.*)
° Leucorrhœa, with *ardor urinæ* and great debility.
° *Hysteria*—depending on debility; useful after the urgent symptoms have been quelled. It tranquilizes the sympathetic disturbance from uterine excitement.

### Fever.

° *Intermittent fever.* (The bark and leaves both contain a large percentage of *Salicine.*)
° I have known many obstinate cases of ague cured by an infusion, and the tincture of the bark in whiskey. (*Hale.*)

° It is one of the most reliable remedies for the **relief of** *night sweats*. (*Eclectic*.)

° *Debility*, from exhausting fevers. (*Hale*.)

## PTELEA TRIFOLIATA.

### (*Wafer Ash*.)

**BOTANICAL DESCRIPTION.**—This plant is also known as *Wingseed, Shrubby trefoil*, and *Swamp Dogwood*. It is a shrub from six to eight feet high, with *leaves* trifoliate, and marked pellucid dots: the leaflets are sessile, ovate, short, acuminate, downy beneath when young, crenulate, or obscurely toothed; lateral ones inequilateral, terminal ones cunate at base, from three to four and a half inches long, by from one and a quarter to one and a half inches wide. The *flowers* are polygamous, greenish-white, nearly half an inch in diameter, of a disagreeable odor, and disposed in terminal corymbose cymes. *Stamens* mostly four; *style* short; fruit a two-celled samara, nearly an inch in diameter, winged all around, nearly orbicular. It is common to this country, growing mostly west of the Alleghanies, in shady, moist hedges, and edges of woods, flowering in June.

**OFFICINAL PREPARATIONS.**—Tincture from the bark with strong alcohol; dilutions; triturations from the tincture.

**ANALOGUES.**—*Arnica, Bryonia, Chelidonium, Nux vomica, Rhus.*(?)

### Mental Sphere.

*Great languor and indisposition* for either mental or physical labor.

Malaise of body and mind; desire to lie down and think of nothing at all.

Inability to concentrate the thoughts, they seem to be chasing each other through the brain.

Complete incapacity for mental exertion, with headache.

Fretful and irritable at very slight cause.

Compelled to give up any attempt at exertion in P. M.

*Performed his duties in a perfunctory manner.*

*Great mental confusion.*

Extraordinary weakness of memory; inability to read names.

Peevish, irritable feeling, and intolerance of noise.

*Marked forgetfulness*, with increased headache, and disposition to hurry when writing.

Confusion of thought, with hurriedness of manner, forgetfulness, with mistakes in writing.

Sick and faint; desire to shrink from every mental work.

Dull and stupid feeling.

Aversion to society; a wish to be let alone.

Annoyance and irritation from ordinary conversation.

## Head.

Pressive feeling at the base of the brain, with nausea, closely resembling the Ipecacuanha symptoms: "Headache, as if the brain and skull were bruised, penetrating through all the bones, down to the root of the tongue, with nausea."

Frontal headache all day, pressing from within outwards.

Pressive pain in the frontal region, extending to the root of the nose, as if a nail were driven into the brain (left side).

Piercing pain shooting through the temples, with increased headache and nausea.

Splitting headache, with nausea.

Piercing pain in the brain, with giddiness, and severe aching pain in the stomach.

Headache after dinner, aggravated by mental exertion.

Sharp, cutting pains through the front of the brain, alternated by pressure.

*Racking frontal headache*, with heat of the face and head, and great desire to hurry his business.

Heaviness in the occiput, with a gloomy feeling in the fore head.

Heavy, pressive frontal headache, worse at night, piercing from within outwards, and aggravated by stooping.

Stunning, piercing headache (a similar one was cured by Rhus).

Persistent headache, with sharp pains shooting from the frontal to the left parietal region.

Frontal headache, aggravated by moving the legs and by noise.

Sudden pressive pains in the temples; worse in the right.

Fine, neuralgic pains in the temples; worse in the right.

*Constant dull headache*, aggravated by going up stairs and by walking.

Sharp, darting pain over the left eye, extending deep into the brain.

Throbbing pains over the eye, from right to left.

Shooting pains in the head before rising in the morning.

Throbbing pain over the temples, from left to right.

Severe throbbing headache on rising, with great weakness.

Dull, frontal headache, with depression and sour stomach.

Headache, intermitting with pain in the hypogastrium, dizziness and nausea.

Pain in the left side of the head and right side of the neck.

Headache over the eyes.

Sudden pressive pain in the temples, as if they would be pressed together, or as if the right would be pressed to the left (frequently occurring during the proving).

Frontal and occipital headache; headache while reading.

Giddiness, with continued vertigo, and increased abdominal tenderness.

Giddiness of the head, when rising in the morning, and when waking, reeling as if intoxicated.

Giddiness and vertigo in the forenoon, so as to necessitate a recumbent posture.

Severe attack of vertigo, with increased headache, and aggravation of all the symptoms.

Sudden giddiness, with faintness on turning the head; vertigo aggravated by even a gradual turning of the head.

Vertigo and nausea aggravated by rising to the feet, also by walking; inability to stand without the aid of a chair.

Vertigo and confusion too severe to permit letter writing.

Sudden attack of vertigo, lasting a minute.

Everything seemed to be in a violent agitation.

### Eyes.

Twisting of the eyelids.

A shooting pain over the eyes, when startled.

Nervous twitching of the upper lip, extending to the left eye.

Nervous pain, extending from left arm to left eye.

Rolling the eyes upwards aggravated the frontal headache.

Pressure over the eyes, aggravated by lifting the eyebrows.

Heavy fullness over the eyes; pain in the eye; pupils contracted.

Painful sensitiveness to light, with irritability.

### Ears.

Ringing in the ears, with slight giddiness.

Sensitiveness to sounds; impressions of sounds last heard continue for a long time.

Intolerance of noise and of loud talking; annoyance at even ordinary conversation.

Easily startled at usual sounds

Pain in the right ear, and behind the right ear.

Intense throbbing pain in the ear, worse on motion.

Itching of the right ear, with inflammation and swelling, terminating in white blisters on a red base, discharging copiously a watery fluid.

### Face, etc.

Burning heat of cheek and face.

Heat of head and face, especially of the forehead.

Yellowish face, with dry, hot skin.

Sickly paleness of the face, especially around the eyes.

Pressure at the root of the nose.

### Mouth and Throat.

Feverishness and dryness of the lips, with thirst (*p*).

The lips cracked and sore, notwithstanding an abundance of saliva (*s*).

Burning, prickling sensation of the mouth and tongue.

Much dryness of the lips and tongue, with *hawking* of mucus from the pharynx.

Great dryness of the mouth and head.

Increased secretion of saliva of a saltish or bitter taste.

Drooling in the night, wetting the pillow.

Fine prickling sensation over the whole surface of the tongue.

Tongue coated with a yellowish fur ; the papillæ red and prominent.

Tongue dry and brownish-yellow or light brown.

Tongue swollen and furred, white.

Tongue coated yellow along the centre and base.

Tongue feeling as if scalded, or as after taking Aconite.

Tongue inflamed, but not swollen.

Dull, aching pains in all the teeth.

Teeth all feel sore, with increased secretion of saltish saliva.

Pain in the right molar teeth; first lower, then upper.

34

Teeth feeling elongated, or as if something was crowding them
    apart.
Pain when moving the jaws.
Roughness of the fauces, with nausea.
Sensation as of a foreign body in the larynx.
Slight vertigo, with a choking feeling in the pharynx (in
    evening).
Soreness and inflammation of the fauces, soft palate and uvula
    (worse on right side).
Throat ulcerated and tongue inflamed (right side).
Distressing feeling of emptiness in the œsophagus.
Slight burning in the throat and stomach, with hiccough.
Sense of obstruction in the larynx, on waking.
Great hoarseness; inability to speak aloud.

### Taste and Appetite.
Unusual hunger; craving for acid food.
* Voracious appetite; food had not its natural taste; with pain
    in epigastrium following every meal; despondency.
Appetite poor; but little appetite and no thirst.
Bread seemed tasteless; all other food tasteless or unnatural.
* Great repugnance to animal food, and to rich puddings, of
    which he is ordinarily fond.  (*Hale.*)
*Great repugnance* to butter and fatty foods; even a small
    quantity aggravated the epigastric pain.  (*Ib.*)
Disgust at the sight or smell of food, especially of roast beef.
The taste of the medicine continually returning in gusts to the
    mouth, with a feeling as if vomiting would relieve.
Very little appetite, with great repugnance to butter.
Eructations tasting of the medicine, with persistent nausea.
Eructations tasting of rotten eggs; sour eructations.
Frequent bitter taste in the mouth, with dryness.
Taste of brass on rising in the morning.
° Dyspepsia, chronic, obstinate (many cases).  (*Hale.*)

### Gastric.
Nausea and retching, with increase of frontal headache; aggra-
    vated by speaking.
Severe nausea, with efforts to vomit for two minutes.

<sup>c</sup> Sensation of goneness, or an empty feeling in the stomach after eating.

Nausea, with distress in the umbilical region, and headache.

Increased nausea, with heat of skin and profuse perspiration on the forehead, after dinner.

Nausea and vomiting, without relief from the frontal headache.

*Persistent nausea* and vomiting, with giddiness and unsteadiness of the legs; aggravated by walking.

Awakened at one A. M., by a piercing pain in the stomach, as of a weight, aggravated by motion and pressure, accompanied with eructations of a bitter fluid, with deathly nausea, confusion of head, and sweat on the forehead. (The attack lasted for hours.)

Eructations, which almost caused emesis (after stool).

Griping in the epigastric region, with dryness of the mouth, yellow-coated tongue, and a bitter taste.

Eructations of bitter fluid, with deathly nausea.

Colic, with emission of flatus and borborygmus.

<sup>c</sup> Chronic gastritis; a constant sensation of corrosion, heat and burning in stomach, with vomiting of ingesta, constipation and afternoon fever. (*P. H. Hale.*)

<sup>c</sup> All the gastric symptoms were much aggravated after meals.

### Liver, etc.

Constant feeling of weight in each hypochondria, when walking (dragging pain).

Sharp, cutting pain in right hypochondrium, aggravated by a deep inspiration (while in bed).

Occasional pains in right hypochondrium, shooting downwards.

Dull, heavy pain, apparently on the convex surface of the liver.

\* Liver perceptibly swollen and sore on pressure, causing a dull, aching pain, with stitches.

Awakened by a dull, heavy pain in the liver, relieved by lying on the right side. A feeling when lying on the left side as if the liver was dragging on its ligaments.

Heavy, aching pain in the liver, with deficient appetite.

Sharp pains in the right hypochondriac and the gastric regions,
    caused by rapid motion.
Awoke with hard, aching distress in the base of the liver.
* Hepatic and gastric symptoms, aggravated towards morning,
    awaking the prover at four o'clock.
° Jaundice, with hyperæmia of the liver.   (*Miller.*)

### Stomach and Abdomen.

Tenderness of the splenic region, with soreness on pressure.
Abdomen swollen and tender, with severe splenic pain.
Severe abdominal pains near umbilicus; worse on motion.
Sharp stitch proceeding from the umbilicus toward the spine,
    when taking a deep inspiration, with increased tenderness
    on pressure.
A faint feeling in the stomach, with sourish eructations.
A squeezing pain in the epigastrium, worse in bed, with
    swollen, but not painful abdomen.
Aching of the bowels while walking.
Throbbing, griping pains in the epigastrium, aggravated by a
    full, deep inspiration, by speaking, and by pressure,
    causing nausea.
Pain and soreness across the abdomen, and in the epigastrium,
    aggravated by standing or sitting erect, and relieved by
    stooping forward.
Rumbling and swelling in the umbilical region, with slight
    vertigo, and sweat on the forehead.
*Rumbling* and bloating *in the bowels*, with tenderness on
    pressure.
Griping, contractive pain in the stomach, moving downwards.
Griping, worse on pressure, in the bowels, with rumbling and
    bloating.
* Pressure as of a stone at the pit of the stomach, aggravated
    by light meals.
Colicky pains in the small intestines (during the evening)
Flying pains in the abdomen, with desire for stool.
Stomach feels empty, after eating; sensation of soreness.
Severe aching distress in the left hypochondrium.
Frequent drawing pains in the epigastric and umbilical region.
Stitches in the abdomen, relieved by pressure.

Pain in the epigastrium, with nausea.

Severe pains in the left iliac region, changing to the right; worse on motion.

Severe bearing-down pains in the bowels ; spasmodic and griping, or sharp and throbbing.

*Pain in the hypogastrium* and bladder, with headache, intermitting during the paroxysms.

*Retraction of the abdomen,* with pulsations isochronous with the heart.

Soreness of the abdomen, aggravated by motion and relieved by compressing it with the hands.

Abdomen tender on pressure for three weeks after the proving.

° Ascites, probably from hepatic disease. (*Miller.*)

### Stool and Rectum.

Sudden and unexpected urging to go to stool, which was diarrhœic, with slight tenesmus, accompanied by sweat on the forehead and head.

Urging before stool, with straining during diarrhœic stool.

Constipation, with a continual urging in the rectum.

Constant urging to stool, with rumbling in the bowels all day.

*Small, hard stool,* with much straining.

Hard and difficult stool, followed by smarting of the rectum.

Stools of usual consistence, with slimy coating, accompanied with straining and vertigo.

Involuntary discharge of flatus, with ineffectual urging to stool.

Urging to stool, with difficult passage of small, hard balls.

Constant, ineffectual urging to stool; a continual pressure in the rectum.

Pressure in the rectum all day, resulting in the discharge of a small stool of indurated fæces, with slight relief, apparently a true torpor of the rectum.

Pressure in the rectum, with qualmishness, aggravated by motion.

Violent urging, followed by a stool of fluid consistence and fœtid smell ; the passage accompanied with chilliness and straining; and after this, renewed tenesmus.

Urging to stool, and sudden copious discharge of thin diar-

rhœic fæces of a cadaverous smell, with smarting of the
    rectum.
Pressure in the rectum, as in dysentery, not relieved by a
    stool.
Two stools in succession, of fæces coated with mucus, fol-
    lowed by tenesmus; during stool, shuddering and chil-
    liness of sacral region ; after stool, smarting of the
    rectum, with itching.
Copious stool of fluid consistence and bilious smell; with it
    was a very copious expulsion of ascarides.
Diarrhœic stools of a dark color and sulphurous smell.
Distress in the small intestines before stool.
Mushy stools; dark-colored, lumpy stools.
° Chronic intestinal catarrh.

### Generative Organs.

*Male.*—Intense throbbing pain in the glans penis, extending
    into the pubic region, when retiring.
Increase of sexual desire at night.
Lascivious dreams in the morning.
*Female.*—Catamenia two days too early, and quite copious.

### Urinary Organs.

Urine of a deep color, and scalding slightly during passage.
Urine high colored; the yellowish-red of Neubauer and Vogel.
Urine scanty, and of a deep-reddish or reddish-yellow tint,
    during the whole proving.
Urine less, with a reddish, cloudy sediment.
Urine profuse and of a light color; the quantity decreased
    and then increased during the proving.
A deposit of muddy sediment in the urine ; afterwards
    whitish, with increase in quantity.
Pain in the region of the bladder, with headache intermitting.
Uneasiness in the bladder and prostate gland, obliged to rise
    in the night to urinate.
Tickling and uneasiness in the urethra after urinating.
Smarting and burning sensation in the urethra while urinating.
The quantity of urine increased each day, and afterwards
    slightly decreased. The condition of the kidneys im-
    proved by the proving.

### Respiratory Organs.

Aching pain, with occasional stitches in region of diaphragm.

Stitches in the diaphragm, arising from continued speaking.

Stitching pains in the upper part of the posterior medastinum, aggravated by breathing or a recumbent position, and accompanied with soreness of the trapezius muscles.

\* Pressure on the lungs, with a sense of suffocation.

Uneasiness and difficulty of breathing, coming on as the gastric and hepatic symptoms declined; with dull pain, especially in the right infra-clavicular region, accompanied by hacking cough, without expectoration. This has approached very insidiously, and now the right lung is dull on percussion at the apex.

During a full inspiration, sharp pains shoot from the sternum toward the nipples; worse on the left.

Pressure on the intercostal spaces, close to the sternum, causes a dull, aching pain.

These thoracic symptoms are better in the house and aggravated in the keen air.

Cough, with bursting headache, in the morning.

A sharp, darting pain through the upper part of left lung; frequently returning, and aggravated by stepping down.

Pain in the lower part of each lung, in the evening.

Stitches through the right lung, which is sound.

Pain back of the left breast, near the axilla.

Cramp-like pain in the cardiac region.

\* Dyspnœa; the walls of the chest feel as though they would sink in.

° Asthma (from retrocession of erysipelas). (*Hale, Miller.*)

° Phthisis; with purulent expectoration of sweetish taste, and hectic fever (probably a bronchial catarrh). (*Miller.*)

### Back and Neck.

Severe aching in the lumbar and sacral regions, in morning.

Pains in the left scapula, aggravated by the exertion of writing.

Bruised sensation in all the limbs and back; worse on pressure.

Drawing, aching pains in left scapula and shoulder joint.

Dull, aching pain in small of the back, aggravated by motion.

Severe aching pains in the back, worse in dorsal region.

Hard backache the whole length of spine and back of the neck, also through the right shoulder.

Walking arrested by a cramp-like pain in left sacral region.

Lameness in muscles of the neck, right side.

The whole neck feels swollen.

Dull, heavy pain and soreness in lumbar region.

### Upper Extremities.

A tingling prickling in the hands and fingers.

Dry heat over the whole body, especially the palms of the hands and the face, with a feeling as if the prover had been up all night; feels worse when the pains are worse.

### Sleep.

Sleep sound, but haunted by frightful dreams.

Sleep deep and heavy, awaking with racking frontal headache, aggravated by rolling the eyes upward.

The sleep is broken and restless, and disturbed by frightful and annoying dreams, waking in a profuse perspiration.

Sleep restless, and disturbed by dreams and by drooling of saliva.

Languid on awaking and unrefreshed.

Nightmare; of killing snakes; of seeing soldiers; of food.

Sleep restless, dream-haunted, with pain in the liver on awaking.

Sleeplessness, almost total, from harrassing pain in the back; worse in early morning.

Languid and drowsy, by day, and bitter taste in mouth.

Attacked with a kind of nightmare, on being awakened at quarter-past nine P. M.; quite conscious, but unable to stir, on account of a pressing weight on the stomach and whole front of body.

### Fever, Pulse.

Flashes of heat, mingled with chilliness, all day. Pulse 88.

Cold chills running up and down the spine.

Feverish heat, lasting all day, with pains in limbs, and nausea.

Hot, dry feeling on the body, with cold feet.

Dry heat over the whole body, with sweat on the forehead

° Tertian ague, with profuse vomiting of bilious matters.

$^c$Attacks of quotidian ague, continuing for two years, resisting many remedies. (*Miller*.)

Chilliness and shivering over the whole body, in a warm room; inability to keep warm at the stove (from 500 drops).

Pulse 104; and increase of 32 beats in fifteen minutes.

Shivering in a warm room, with heat of the head.

Shivering over the legs from the hips downwards.

Pulse 126, small and thready, seventy minutes after the large dose; shivering, with chattering of the teeth.

Scarcely comfortable near a large fire; but all the symptoms ameliorated in the open air.

Aching distress in all the joints, with great languor.

Very languid and faint, with flushed face and feverishness.

Pulse increased 12 beats, soft, weak and intermittent.

Pulse slow, strong and irregular.

Hot breath, which seems to burn the nostrils.

Hot flashes, with pain in the top of the head and in the eyes.

Profuse night sweats.

### Generalities.

Great lassitude and weariness, with a disposition to hurry through duties.

Extreme weakness of limbs, brain, memory, thought and will; as if from a powerful and all-pervading disease.

Aching of the limbs, especially of the flexor muscles.

A fine, violent agitation of all the muscles of the body and limbs.

Great languor and indifference to duties.

Soreness of the whole body.

Frontal headache during the whole proving.

Rheumatic, drawing, or wandering pains throughout the body.

Flighty, nervous pains, in different parts of the body.

Loss of energy, languor and depression of spirits. (*p.*)

Unusual aches and pains all over the body, especially in the abdomen and head.

Singing increases the nausea and aggravates the headache, causing shooting pains from within outwards.

Soreness and swelling of lymphatic glands under the right ear.

Great restlessness and despondency.

The symptoms assume the form of a severe bilious attack.

All the symptoms suddenly disappear after eating sour things

All the symptoms are better in the cool, open air.  (*p.*)

The thoracic symptoms are worse in the keen air.  (*s.*)

The symptoms are all aggravated in the warm room.

The gastric and hepatic symptoms are aggravated by pressure after meals, toward morning and after eating cheese, rich pudding, butter, or any fatty food; but relieved by motion in the open air.

The nausea is aggravated by lying down or by noise.

The pains in the head press from within outwards.

The headache is *worse* after eating or from mental exertion, moving the eyes, noise, walking, going up stairs, stooping, or warmth, or during the night, while in bed; but alleviated in the cool open air, or by pressure.

*Predominantly aggravated* in the warm room, after eating fatty food, when lying down, or early in the morning, from noise, or when stooping.

*Predominantly alleviated* in the cool, open air, when rising from bed, or during continued motion, and by the use of vegetable acids.

From above, downwards, from within, outwards, mainly in the right side, or from right to left.

---

## PROTOSULPHIDE OF MERCURY.

### (*Mercurius Protosulphide.*)

PHARMACOLOGY.—This is known as the Black sulphide of mercury, Black Sulphuret of mercury, and the Subsulphuret of mercury.

It is a black, impalpable powder, having none of the metallic lustre of mercury, and in its combination loses the characteristic appearance of the mercurial particles.

It may be prepared by triturating mercury and sublimed sulphur together in their atomic proportions. Thus: carefully weigh out one hundred grains pure mercury (quicksilver), and thirty-two grains sublimed sulphur, mix very thoroughly in a mortar which has been carefully washed and thoroughly dried, and then triturate with force from two and one-half to three hours.

OFFICINAL PREPARATIONS.—Triturations to the 6 × ; dilutions.

ANALOGUES.—*Arsenicum, Baptisia, Rhus, Terbinthina.*

## Characteristic Symptoms.

*Febrile heat*, pungent; pulse small, weak, 120–130; great weakness; paleness or flushing of the *face* in the middle and after part of the day.

*Drowsiness* or wakefulness, with restlessness; unconsciousness, with muttering delirium.

*Headache* in the forehead. *Eyes* with dark circles under them; *lips* dry and shrunken; tongue shrunken, covered with a dark brown crust; stiff, dry and black.

*Abdomen* tender, particularly in the coecal and epigastric region, distended (tympanitic). *Urination* frequent, scanty.

*Diarrhœa* bilious, dark yellow, watery, preceded by colic; followed by fainting; not profuse or frequent, only two or three evacuations a day.

° In the second stage of *typhoid fever*, with local lesion in the solitary and aggregated glands of the ilium, without much ulceration of the mucous membrane.

---

# PULSATILLA NUTTALLIANA.

### (*American Pulsatilla.*)

BOTANICAL DESCRIPTION.—Villous with long silken hairs. *Stem* erect; in flower, very short; in fruit, eight to twelve inches high. *Leaves* long stalked, ternately divided, the lateral divisions two-parted, the middle one stalked and three-parted, the segments once or twice-cleft into narrowly linear and acute lobes. *Involucres* below the stem, lobed like the leaves, sessile sabulately dissected, concave or cup-shaped in position. *Sepals* five to seven, purplish, spreading, about one inch long, silky outside. *Flower* single, appearing before the leaves, pale-purple, cup-shaped. *Carpels* (fruit) 50 to 75, with long plumous tails, one to two inches in length, collected into a roundish head.

BOTANICAL HISTORY.—This plant when first discovered by Nuttall, was called by him the *Anemone Ludoviciana.* It was afterwards called A. pratensis, by Hooker.

Gray, (Genera of plants of U. S.,) gives a minute description, illustrated by a beautiful plate. He calls it the Pulsatilla *pratensis.* In the later editions of his Botany, he applies the name Pulsatilla Nuttalliana. Wood places it in the genus *Anemone*, as the *A. Nuttalliana.* King (Dispensatory) calls it *A. Ludoviciana.*

Although it is well that the botanist, Nuttall, should be honored, I should prefer the name Pulsatilla *Americana* as the fittest designation for the only species of the *genus* growing in America. All botanists agree in giving it the common name of *Pasque-flower*, which is the popular name given the Pulsatilla in Europe, because the blossoms appear at Easter.

Nuttall states that this plant is to be found near the confluence of the Missouri and Platte rivers, and thence west to the Rocky Mountains. It is also met with in considerable abundance in the States of Wisconsin and Minnesota, especially on the dry and sandy bluffs forming the bed of the Mississippi. It has also been found in the most northern counties of the State of Illinois.

Gray says it does not extend down the Mississippi as far as Louisiana, probably no farther than the lower boundary of Iowa. Along the Rocky Mountains, however, it does extend as far southward as latitude 35°, Mr. Fendler having gathered specimens at Santa Fe.

It is a plant of peculiar appearance. The large cup-shaped flowers of a purple hue, appear before the leaves, almost immediately after the melting of the snow has shown that the long and dreary winter of the north is approaching its close. Hence these blossoms are eagerly sought for as the first offerings of the long desired spring.

The leaves and stalks of the plant are covered with long delicate silken hairs. It is from this appearance that it got the name of " Goslin Flower," which probably originated with children. The odor of the *dried* plant is rather faint, being slightly camphoraceous, the taste of the dried flowers simply sweetish and herbaceous, that of the leaves being more astringent with very slight acrimony.

The *taste* and, to some extent, the *odor* of the fresh plant are both acrid and irritating.

When the seeds are ripe, each one is surmounted by a long silken tail, giving the plant, at a distance, an appearance somewhat similar to the ripe Taraxacum. These seeds, with their comet-like tails, are borne by the winds which sweep over our prairies, to great distances, there to propagate themselves in new situations.

Gray is correct in stating that the American Pulsatilla is more like Pulsatilla Vulgaris, than the Pulsatilla Pratensis of Europe, as will be seen by a comparison given below.

Jahr, in his Pharmacopœia, gives the following description of the *Pulsatilla nigricans, or pratensis* used in homœopathic practice.

" Stems simple, erect, rounded, three to five inches high; leaves radical bipinnatified, downy; flowers solitary, terminal, having folioles of calyx campanulate, bent at the point, the odor of the herb but slightly evident, taste acrid and pungent. The fresh plant contains an acrid and vesicating principle, and furnishes a corrosive oil, as well as a kind of tannin which colors iron green; in the dry state it is entirely deprived of this acrid quality. Grows in sandy pasture grounds, on hills and declivities, exposed to the sun."

Jahr further says: " We must be careful not to mistake this plant for the common Pulsatilla. (Anemone Pulsatilla) " (Pulsatilla Vulgaris). " This last plant, of which homœopathy *makes no use whatever*, only grows on dry and sterile hills, and flowers in the spring-time alone, whilst the black-colored Pulsatilla flowers a second time again in the months of August and September. Besides, the Anemone Pulsatilla, is in all its parts, much less downy than the black-colored pulsatilla: its stem six to twenty-four centremetres high; flowers of clear violet or pale red, straight and not hanging like those of the black-colored pulsatilla; seeds surmounted by a long silky tail."

From this it would seem that the American Pulsatilla partook of the character of *both* the European varieties. Since the following pathogenesis was first published, the *American Pulsatilla* has been extensively used in this country, and its curative powers have been found equal to the foreign. I find no difference in their qualities. (*Hale.*)

OFFICINAL PREPARATIONS.—Tincture of the whole plant; dilutions.

ANALOGUES.—*Arnica, Clematis, Cimicifuga, Cyclamen, Euphrasia, Ferrum, Ignatia, Mitchella, Eupatorium purpureum, Platina, Pulsatilla nig., Senecio, Sepia.*

### Mental Sphere.

Gloomy state of mind, with eructations of sour air.

She feels very irritable, "cross," could not bear to be spoken to; noise vexed her; she felt like weeping at trifling annoyances.

Confusion of mind; impossible to study.

### Head.

Hard pain in the upper portion of the forehead, passing to the back of the head like a wave, affecting the whole brain.

Feeling as if a nail were being driven into the brain just above the left eye, a number of times.

Severe frontal headache all night, caused by a sour stomach.

Dull, heavy pains in the right temple; frequent, sharp, cutting.

Feverish, hot feeling of the head; severe headache: dull, heavy feeling in the head in the morning.

° Migraine—intense pain in one side of head and one eye, with chilliness; lowness of spirits and vomiting.

### Eyes.

Burning, smarting sensation in the eyelids

Agglutination of the lids in the morning.

Neuralgic pains in the eyeballs, while walking in the open air.

Hot feeling of the inside of the lids, in the evening; burning and smarting of the eyelids.

° Catarrhal affections of the eyes, acute and chronic. (*Hale.*)

° Opacity of the cornea, when the loss of sight was nearly complete. (*Miller.*)

## Ears.

Fluttering noise in the right ear (first symptom of the ear in the proving).

Drawing pains in the ears, from within outward, frequently.

Feeling as if the ears were closed.

° Catarrhal affections of the inner ear. (*Hale.*)

## Face.

Face hot and red at 4 P. M. till bedtime; with cold feet.

° Complexion becomes clear and good (previously rough).

## Mouth and Throat.

Yellowish coating on the tongue, along the centre.

Sensation of a lump in the throat, recurring frequently.

* Slimy coating on tongue, with offensive breath.

## Stomach.

* Prickling, burning sensation in the pit of the stomach.

Severe cutting pains in the stomach, with feeling of distension in the abdomen, and dull headache.

Sour eructations, with gloominess.

* Intense nausea, without vomiting, all the time.

Distress in the whole epigastrium, with sharp, cutting pain in the stomach, passing toward the spine.

Feeling as if fine needles were being pressed into the stomach.

* Weak, faint, fluttering sensation in the pit of stomach, even after eating. (*Wesselhœft.*)

* Vomiting of bitter, bilious slime, with chronic cough. (*Ib.*)

° Indigestion; dyspepsia. Vomiting of pregnancy. (*Hale.*)

## Abdomen.

Drawing, cutting pains in the lower part of the epigastrium, with constant colicky pains in epigastrium, after midnight.

Sharp pains in the epigastrium and right hypochondrium.

Rumbling in the bowels.

Aching pain in left groin, just above the crest of the ilium, on moving or bending.

## Stool.

* Hard, dry, lumpy stools. (*Wesselhœft.*)

Mushy stools, succeeded by cutting pains in the epigastrium.

Severe cutting pains in the umbilicus, followed by a dark colored stool.

Desire for stool all the afternoon and evening, followed by dark, lumpy stool.

Loose, papescent stools, with chilliness.

* Catarrhal diarrhœa; also from indigestion. (*Burt.*)

### Urine.

Frequent desire to urinate, desire soon passing off.

*Frequent urination, too profuse; light colored.*

Passed a large quantity of "skunky" smelling urine at midnight.

Dark brown sediment; (urate of ammonia).

Pain in the kidneys; tenesmus and strangury.

Pain in the end of the penis, after urinating.

### Generative Organs.

* *Female.---Sharp pains in the uterus, from side to side, accompanied with chilliness*, trembling weakness of the legs, urging to urinate and diarrhœa.

Premature and profuse menses.

° Amenorrhœa, with constant chilliness; coldness of the hands and feet; loss of appetite, sour eructations, melancholy and general malaise. (*Hale, Small.*)

° Retarded menses; irregular menses; leucorrhœa.

° Suppression of the menses; several cases. (*Small.*)

* *Male.*—Dull distress in the testicles, with drawing pain along the left spermatic cord to the testicles.

* Sharp, sticking pain in left spermatic cord and testicles.

Seminal emission for three consecutive nights.

### Cough.

Coughs a good deal.

° Constant loose cough, day and night, with fullness under the sternum.

° Chronic dry cough becomes loosened.

### Chest.

Sharp, stabbing pain in the left pectoralis-major muscle, followed by burning sensation when the pains occur.

° Aching pain in the pleura or lungs. (*Wesselhœft.*)

### Back.

Some distress in the lumbar region during a rain storm.

## Arms.

The flexor muscles of the arms ache severely, and are stiff.

Frequent drawing, flexing pains in the wrists and fingers.

Stiffness of the fingers, with drawing pain in the left meta-carpal bones.

° Hands hot and dry. (*Causland.*)

## Lower Extremities.

Drawing pains in the left sartorius muscle, when walking.

Sharp, neuralgic pains, passing from the hip joint down to the middle of the thigh, along the course of the ischiatic nerve.

Frequent dull pains in both ankles.

Severe, dull pains in the right knee joint, for two hours in the morning, while in bed, during a rain storm.

Trembling weakness in the legs, with a sensation of great weariness and heaviness.

° Rheumatic pains, which are wandering.

Restlessness in the feet, with constant desire to move them.

## Skin.

Eruption on the back, legs and ankles, of a dark, bluish-red color, with more or less itching during the day, but at night, in a warm bed, the itching is most intolerable.

Eruption stands out prominently from the skin, looking like measles.

\* Itching erythema; urticaria (nodules of irregular form, round, elongated, annular; turning white on scratching, with red base and white skin between).

## Fever.

Pale, weak, with a feverish feeling, and great debility.

Chilliness over the whole body, with frequent yawning.

\* Hands hot and dry.

Face hot and flushed, after four P. M., with dull headache.

## Sleep.

Sleep is often disturbed by awaking with headaches or frequent inclination to pass water; seminal emissions occur; but the most troublesome symptom is itching of the skin, the fore part of the night, caused by a species of urticaria or scalp erythema. ( *Wesselhœft.*)

# RHUS GLABRUM.

*(Common Sumach.)*

BOTANICAL DESCRIPTION. — Rhus glabrum (or smooth sumach), is a shrub from six to fifteen feet high, consisting of many straggling, glabrous branches, covered with a pale, gray bark, having often a reddish tint.

The *leaves* are alternate, odd-pinnate, and consisting of from six to fifteen leaflets, about three inches long and one-fourth as wide, lanceolate, acuminate, acutely serrate, shining and green above, whitish beneath, sessile, except sometimes the terminal odd one; during the fall they become red.

The *flowers* are greenish-red, and arranged in terminal, thyrsoid, dense panicles. *Calyx* of three sepals united at base; *petals* five; *stamens* five; inserted into the edge or between the lobes of a flattened disk in the bottom of the calyx; *styles* three; *stigmas* capitate.

*Fruit*, a small red drupe, hanging in clusters, and when ripe covered with a crimson down, which is extremely sour to the taste, owing to the presence of malic acid in combination with lime.

OFFICIAL PREPARATIONS. — Tincture of the bark or leaves; dilutions. [A tincture of the berries should be proven. (*Hale.*)]

ANALOGUES. — *Acidum gallicum, Acidum tannicum, Alnus, Baptisia, Borax, China, Geranium, Galium, Hamamelis, Hydrastis, Myrica.*

## Mental Sphere.

Weakness of memory, with much indifference to surrounding objects.

## Head.

Dull, aching pain in the frontal and upper portion of the head.

Fullness and pain in the top of the head.

° *Occipital headache,* usually of a rheumatic character. (Dr. Lilienthal says he has verified, over and over again, the recommendation of Dr. Burdick, as to its use in occipital headache. He cures with the 1st, the 200th and 1,000th; and says, "It differs materially in its symptoms from *Silicia* and *Gelseminum.*")

## Nose.

Hemorrhage from the left nostril.

Bloody scabs in the left nostril.

° Epistaxis.

## Mouth and Throat.

* Hemorrhage from the mouth.

* On waking, clots of blood are expelled from the throat.

* Small ulcers in the mouth.

° Nursing sore mouth; aphthous stomatitis.

35

° Sea-scurvy, and scorbutic affections generally.

### Stomach and Abdomen.

Distressing pain in the stomach, worse by eating or drinking.

Tenderness on pressure in the umbilical region.

Sharp, cutting pains in the abdomen.

° Diarrhœa.   ° Dysentery.   ° Bleeding piles.

° Diarrhœa, with spongy gums, vitiated appetite and swollen
abdomen.

### Respiratory Organs.

° Chronic hoarseness, with asthmatic troubles.   (*Hale.*)

° "Heaves"—in horses.   (A popular domestic remedy.)

### Urinary Organs.

Scanty, high-colored urine.

### Fever.

Skin hot and dry, with thirst.

\* Profuse night sweats.

Feeling of coldness, while there is an actual increase of heat
in the skin.

° Some of the conditions of *typhoid fever*, diarrhœa, scurvy,
etc.

° Hectic fever, with night sweats.

---

# RHUS VENENATA.

### (*Poison-Sumach.*)

BOTANICAL DESCRIPTION.—*The Rhus Venenata or Poison Sumach* is also
known as *Poison-wood, Poison-ash,* and inappropriately as Poison-elder and
Poison-dog-wood.  This has been compounded with the *Rhus vernix* of
Linnæus, a species which grows in Japan.  It is a shrub or small tree,
from ten to twenty, and even thirty feet in height, with the trunk from one
to five inches in diameter, branching at the top, and covered with a pale-
grayish bark, which is reddish on the leaf-stalks and ground-shoots.

"Rhus Venenata grows in low meadows and swamps, from Canada to
the Gulf of Mexico, flowering from May to August.  The milky juice which
flows when the plant is wounded, is similar in its action to that of the
Rhus toxicodendron, and may, according to Bigelow, be made into a beautiful shining and permanent varnish, by boiling, very analogous to that
obtained in Japan from the *Rhus vernix.*  It is more poisonous than the
R. toxicodendron, and its volatile principle taints the air for some distance
around with its pernicious influence, producing in many persons severe
swellings of an erysipelatous nature; sometimes the body becomes greatly

swollen, and the persons unable to move. Some persons are hardly, or not at all affected, even by handling it. The affection caused by it, generally abates after several days, and may be treated in the same manner as named for the poisonous effects of the Rhus toxicodendron."—*King.*

OFFICINAL PREPARATIONS.—Tincture of the bark or leaves; dilutions

ANALOGUES.—*Anacardium, Clematis, Comocladia, Croton tig, Ranunculus, Rhus tox., rad and vernix.*

[From provings by *Oeheme, Hoyt, and Burt.*]

### Mental Sphere.

Great sadness, no desire to live; everything seems gloomy.

Absence of mind; cannot concentrate the mind on any particular subject.

Mental labor increased the pain.

### Head.

* Dull, heavy, frontal headache, aggravated by walking and stooping.

* Dizzy sensations, worse in evenings; intolerable heaviness of the head.

* Great swelling of the head, face, and hands, with sharp, irritating fever.

* Erysipelas of the head and face.

° Vesicular erysipelas of the face and scalp. (*Hale.*)

### Eyes.

* Eyes closed from the great swelling of the cellular tissue around them.

* Profuse lachrymation; constant dull aching pains in the eye balls.

Smarting and burning of the eyes.

Œdema of the eyelids.

Constant irritation of the eyes.

° Chronic inflammation of the eyes.

### Ears.

Deafness that is quite troublesome.

* Vesicular inflammation of the ears, exuding a yellow, watery serum.

### Nose.

Great dryness of the nostrils—obstruction of the nostrils.

° Erysipelatous redness of the nose.

### Face.

* Face very red, swollen, and covered with vesicles, itching and burning.

\* Nose and right side of the face much swollen, especially
     under right eye.
\* Face hot, itching and burning in different parts of the face,
     especially the left cheek.

### Mouth.

\* Scalded feeling of the tongue, salty, flat, rough taste. (*Hale*.)
\* The centre and base coated white, the sides are very red. (*Ib*.)
\* Vesicles on the under side of the tongue with a scalded
     feeling.
\* Mucous membrane of the mouth is very red. (*Ib*.)
° Red vesicular eruption on the gums of the upper incisors.

### Throat.

Constant dry irritative feeling in the fauces.
Tonsils red and congested, with dull aching distress in them.
Throat very sore, red and swollen.

### Stomach.

Distress and pain in the stomach and umbilicus.
Loss of appetite, wants to drink a great deal.
° Dyspepsia, with red tongue, and tendency to erysipelas.

### Abdomen and Stool.

Abdomen much bloated and exceeding painful to pressure.
Constant rumbling and griping in the bowels.
Constant dull pains in the umbilicus, with rumbling in the
     bowels, followed by a soft diarrhœic stool.
Pains always worse before a stool, but an evacuation does not
     stop the pain.
Stool almost white, thin, papescent.
Pains in the umbilicus, with dry, lumpy, dark-colored stools.
Diarrhœic stools (stopped by tinc. juniperus vir. *Hoyt*).
Intolerable itching and burning of the anus; neuralgic pains
     in the anus.
Pains in the bowels worse in the morning.

### Urinary Organs.

(No notice taken of any urinary symptoms).

### Generative Organs.

Intense itching and burning of the scrotum and penis.
Glans penis swollen and very sore.
Cuticle of the penis and scrotum peels off in patches.

\* Scrotum much swollen, deep red color, covered with vesicles.

### Back.

\* Stiff neck, or "crick in the neck," and rheumatic pains between the shoulders.

Constant dull pains in the cervical dorsal and lumbar regions. Back is very stiff.

Itching at night on the back, but in the daytime on the face, neck and hands.

° Lumbago, from a strain or a cold.

### Upper Extremities.

Severe pains in the left elbow joint.

Drawing pains in the fore-arms.

Rheumatic pains in the shoulders and elbow joints, worse during motion.

Wrists and fingers are very stiff, constant aching distress.

Constant desquamation of the cuticle of the palms of the hands and fingers.

Violent itching of the palms of the hands, with watery vesicles on them.

Groups of watery vesicles on the fingers.

Œdema of the back of the hand.

### Lower Extremities.

Knees and ankles ache constantly, with great weakness.

Dull, drawing pains and distress in the knees.

Ankles very red and swollen, with watery vesicles all over the ankles, feet and toes, dischargeing large quantities of water.

Large watery blisters on the sides of the feet.

Intolerable itching of the ankles, feet and toes, worse from warmth.

Joints are very stiff in the morning, relieved by exercise.

Pains in the ankles are worse in the afternoons and evenings.

The itching and burning subdued by bathing in cold water.

### Fever.

Chills up and down the back, when warm and in a warm room, and in bed.

Great restlessness, with a dry, burning hot skin at night.

Skin becomes tense, hot, swollen, shining and very painful.

Increased temperature of the inflamed parts.

° Erysipelatous inflammations.

° Typhoid fever (indications the same as Rhus tox., and rad.)

### Skin.

Large fissures on the ends of the fingers, that bleed easily.

Fine vesicular eruptions on the fore-arms, wrists, back of the hands, between and on the fingers, scrotum and ankles.

Large watery vesicles on the ankles.

Upper lip and ears much swollen, covered with vesicles.

Boils on the forehead, neck and arms, and right thigh.

° Vesicular and erysipelatous eruptions of all kinds.

° Phlegmonous erysipelas.

### Generalities.

The symptoms all aggravated before a *rain*.

The joints all stiff in the mornings.

The itching and burning of the skin aggravated by **warmth**

*After* exercise the stiffness passes away.

### Sleep.

Great restlessness at night, with a dry, hot **skin.**

---

# RICINUS COMMUNIS.

## (*Castor Oil Plant.*)

BOTANICAL DESCRIPTION.—Ricinus Communis, the *Castor Oil bush*, in the United States, is a herbaceous annual, with a white, frosted or glaucous hollow, smooth stem, of a purplish-red color upward. The *leaves* are large, alternate, deeply divided into seven or nine lanceolate segments, peltate, palmate, serrate, from four to twelve lines in diameter, and on long, tapering, purplish petioles. The *flowers* in long, green, and glaucous spikes, springing from the divisions of the branches; the males from the lower part of the spike, the females from the upper. The *capsule* is *prickly*, three celled, three seeded. The *seeds* are ovate, shining black, dotted with gray.

HISTORY.—Ricinus Communis, or *Palma Christi*, is an East Indian plant, in which country it attains the size of a tree. In the United States, where it has become naturalized, it seldom grows higher than eight or ten feet; flowers in July and August, and matures its seeds in August and September. The fixed oil of the seeds is the Castor Oil of the shops.

OFFICINAL PREPARATIONS.—Tincture of the leaves; Fl. Extract of the .eaves.

ANALOGUES.—*Calc. carb* (?)   *Coriander* (?)   *Urtica* (?)   *Pulsatilla* (?) (*No provings.*)

The application of a poultice of the leaves of the plant to the breasts of women, even those who have never borne children, *causes a secretion of milk*.

° *Scanty*, or *suppressed* secretion of milk, in nursing women.

(*See Therapeutics.*)

---

# ROBINIA PSEUDO-ACACIA.

### (*False Locust.*)

BOTANICAL DESCRIPTION.—This tree is also known as *Black Locust* and *Yellow Locust*, found in several parts of the United States, principally west of the mountains, being seldom found north of Pennsylvania, or in the Atlantic Southern States; blossoming in May. It grows from fifty to eighty feet high, and from one to four feet thick; the bark is rough and dark. The numerous branches are smooth and armed with prickles. The *leaves* are unequally pinnate, the *leaflets* are from eight to twelve pairs, ovate and oblong-ovate, thin, nearly sessile, and very smooth; *stipules* minute, bristle-form, partial. Flowers white, fragrant, showy, in numerous, axilary, pendulous racemes. *Calyx* fine, cleft, short, slightly two-lipped; *standard* large and rounded, turned back, scarcely longer than the wings and keel; *stamens*, diadelphous; *style*, bearded inside; *legume, or pod*, linear, compressed, two to four inches in length, and about six lines wide, margined on the seed bearing edge; *seeds*, several, small, brown, reniform. When young, the tree is armed with thorns, which disappear in its maturity.

OFFICINAL PREPARATIONS.—Tincture of the bark and flowers; dilutions.

ANALOGUES.—*Calcarea carb., Iris ver., Pulsatilla, Magnesia carb., Rheum.*

[The fragmentary proving of Burt, may be considered reliable, and a few of the symptoms from Houatt. The pathogenesis of the latter, however, is too extensive, too tragic, and too much like his other provings to be true.]

### Mind.

Low-spirited, with great irritability. (*Burt.*)

### Head.

Dull, frontal headache, much aggravated by motion, with neuralgic pains in the temples.

° Sick headache with acidity of the stomach and some eructateous vomiting. (*Burt.*)

### Stomach.

Excessive acidity of the stomach.

Vomiting of intensely sour fluid, setting the teeth on edge.

Frequent eructations of sour fluid. (*Burt.*)

Great distension of the stomach and bowels, with flatulence;

the intestines distended almost to the point of rupturing, with severe colic.

Dull, heavy, squeezing pains in the stomach, especially after every meal.

Water, taken before eating, at night, returned in the morning, green and sour.

° *Dyspepsia,* "I have seen it helpful in dyspepsia manifesting itself at night and preventing sleep." (*Massy.*)

° Heartburn, and acidity of the stomach, *at night on lying down.* (Solanum has "heartburn at night."),

Sour regurgitations of infants.

Sour vomiting of infants; the whole child smells sour.

Desire for stool, but only flatulence passes off; finally constipated stools.

° Sour stools of infants, with sour smell from the body. (*Burt.*)

(See *Houatt's Pathogenesis, N. A. Jour. of Hom.* )

## RUMEX CRISPUS.
### (*Yellow Dock.*)

BOTANICAL DESCRIPTION.—This plant was introduced into this country from Europe, but may now be considered indigenous to this continent. It has a deep, spindle-shaped, yellow *root,* with a *stem* two or three feet high, angular, furrowed, somewhat zigzag, smooth to the touch, panicled, and leafy.

The *leaves* are lanceolate, acute, strongly undulated, and crisped at the edges, of a light-green color; the radical ones are long petioled, truncate or sub-cordate at the base; the uppermost are narrower and nearly sessile. *Flowers* numerous, pale-green, drooping, disposed in a large panicle, consisting of many wand-like racemes, of half whorls, interspersed with leaves below. The root, as found in the shops, is in slices, cut transversely and dried; and occasionally the root is divided longitudinally into halves and quarters. This species is sometimes called *Sour-dock, Narrow-dock, or Curled-dock.* The root is the officinal portion.

There are thirteen species of Dock growing in this country, about half of which are indigenous.

OFFICIAL PREPARATIONS.—Tincture of the root; dilutions.

ANALOGUES.—*Belladonna, Calcarea carb., Causticum, Cistus, Dulcamara, Eryngium, Hepar sulph., Iris, Juglans, Jodium, Lachesis, Lycopodium, Lobelia, Mercurius, Nuphar, Rheum, Sanguinaria, Spongia, Sulphur.*

### Head.

Headache after awaking in the morning, preceded by a disagreeable dream.

Dull pains on the right side; pain in the left temple.

Darting pain, or sharp piercing pain in the left side of the head.

Headache worse from motion.

Dull aching pain in the occiput.

### Eyes.

Sore feeling in the eyes, but without inflammation.

### Ears.

Ringing in the ears, itching in the ears.

Constant roaring in the ears, they feel as if obstructed.

### Nose.

Obstruction of the nose; with sensation of dryness, even in the posterior nares. (*p*.)

* Fluent coryza, with sneezing; mucous discharge from the *posterior* nares. (*s*.)

* Epistaxis—with violent sneezing, and painful irritation of the nostrils.

° Influenza with violent catarrh, followed by bronchitis.

### Face.

Heat and redness of the face in the evening; with dull headache.

### Mouth.

Sensation as of a burn or scald on the tongue.

Dryness of the mouth and tongue, tongue feels as if burnt.

° Ulceration of the mouth and throat.

### Throat.

* Excoriated feeling in the throat, with secretion of mucus in the upper part of the throat.

Sensation as if of a lump in the throat, not relieved by hawking or swallowing.

Aching sensation in the throat, as if a lump were sticking fast in the œsophagus.

* Aching in the pharynx, with collection of tough mucus in the fauces.

° Catarrhal affections of the throat and fauces.

### Stomach.

Heaviness in the stomach or epigastrium, soon after a meal.

Flatulency after meals, and nausea with eructations.

Stitching, cutting pain in the pit of the stomach, worse on movement.

* Shootings from the pit of the stomach into the chest; sharp pains in the left chest; dull aching in the forehead, and slight nausea. (*Joslin.*)

Pain in the pit of the stomach, aching in the left breast, flatulency, eructations, pressure and distension in the stomach after meals.

* Sensation of fullness and pressure in the pit of the stomach, extending up to the throat, and then back to the stomach (cured by the 200th). (*Ib.*)

Hypochondrium pained by coughing, rapid walking, or deep inspiration.

° Aching and shooting in the pit of the stomach, and above it, on each side of the sternum.

° Dyspeptic ailments, of various kinds. (*Hale.*)

### Abdomen.

Sensation of hardness, and fullness in the abdomen, with rumbling in the bowels.

Pain in the abdomen, occurring or increasing during deep inspiration.

Flatulent colic near the umbilicus soon after a meal, mitigated by a discharge of flatus.

* Pain in the abdomen in the morning, followed by a stool.

Griping pains near the umbilicus, partially relieved by discharge of very offensive flatus.

° Colic from a cold, with cough.

### Stool and Anus.

* Dark-colored fæces; stool brown or black.

* Liquid diarrhœic stool in the morning.

* Diarrhœic stool in the morning, preceded by pain in the abdomen.

Sensation as if from the pressure of a stick in the rectum.

Itching in the anus with discharge of offensive flatus.

° *Brown, watery diarrhœa*, chiefly in the morning. (*Small.*)

ᵒ *Diarrhœa in the morning with the rumex-cough.* (*Dunham, Joslin, et al.*)

## Urinary Organs.

Copious discharge of colorless urine in the afternoon.

Very sudden and urgent desire to urinate.

## Larynx.

\* Pain in the larynx, with excoriating cough. (*Joslin, Dunham, and others.*)

\* *Much tough mucus in the larynx, with a constant desire to hawk and raise it, but without relief.*

Cough excited by tickling or irritation behind the sternum.

° Acute catarrhal affections of the larynx, trachea and bronchi.

° Cough which is dry, harsh, loud, shaking, worse at night, excited instantly by pressure on the trachea.

° Dry cough, tickling in the throat pit; excoriation in the larynx, and behind the upper portion of the sternum.

[*Rumex* diminishes the secretions, and at the same time exalts in a very marked manner the sensibility of the larynx and trachea; the cough is frequent and continuous; it is dry and occurs in long paroxysms; *aggravated* by respiration more rapid or deeper than usual, and by cold air; attended by rawness and soreness in the trachea and bronchia, especially the left, where the tickling is very annoying and persistent; *worse* in the evening after retiring, or upon talking, or irregular respiration. (*Dr. C. Dunham*, in Amer. Homœop. Review, Vol. II, page 530.)]

## Chest.

Aching pain over the anterior portion of both lungs.

Raw pain under the clavicles while hawking mucus out of the throat.

Sharp pain near the left axilla.

Burning and shooting pain in the right chest.

Shooting in the left side, sometimes sticking pains.

Burning, sticking, or burning stinging pain in the left chest.

Dull pain, also burning pain, in the region of the heart.

Sensation as if the heart had suddenly ceased beating, followed by a heavy throbbing through the chest.

° Stinging pain near the heart, increased by lying down, and by breathing deeply. (*Dr. Rhees.*)

° Violent aching pain in the heart, with throbbing of the carotids, and throughout the body, visible to the eye, and shaking the bed, pulse 120; great dyspnœa especially when lying; had to sit up in bed; face red and puffed, especially about the eyes, which were red and lustre-less. (*Ib.*)

" It is a most useful remedy in that protean symptom, ' cough.'

" It greatly relieved a dry cough, in a medical friend, commenc-ing at 2 A. M.

" A useful indication for Rumex is 'clavicular pain.' This is borne out by the proving: 'Raw pain just under each clavicle while hawking mucus out of the throat.' " *Dr. Massy, " Notes on New Remedies."*

### Back.

Sore or burning pain near the sacro-iliac symphysis.

Pressing aching pain in the back, at the lower border of the scapula.

### Upper Extremities.

Pains in the shoulder, down to elbow, arms feel as if strained.

Dull aching pain in the left upper arm.

Pains in the wrist: (character of the pains undefined.)

### Lower Extremities.

Aching of the lower extremities.

Itching of lower extremities when exposed to cool air.

Stitch like pain in the knee joint when standing.

Rending like pains in the lower limbs.

* Legs densely covered with a rash, small red pimples.

Feet cold in the forenoons.

### Skin.

* Itching in various parts of the body, especially the surface of lower extremities, while undressing.

* Stinging, itching, or prickling itching of the skin.

* Itching of the vesicles when uncovered and exposed to cool air.

Eruption on the limbs, of small red pimples.

The eruption is produced by scratching.

° Vesicular eruption; " psoric itch," eruption from wearing flannel. (*Hale.*)

### Sleep.

Desire to sleep before the proper time.

Unquiet sleep with dreams of danger and trouble.

### Fever.

\* Increased frequency of pulse, and afternoon fever.
Sensation of heat, followed by that of cold, without shivering.

---

# SANGUINARIA CANADENSIS.

### (Blood-root.)

BOTANICAL DESCRIPTION. — Sanguinaria is a spring plant, found in Canada, and all parts of the United States, excepting southward to Florida and westward to Mexico and Oregon. It generally grows in rich lands, covered with forests and shaded in summer, avoiding the sea coast and high mountains.

The *root* is perennial, horizontal, oblong, and, when green, nearly of the length of the finger, from one-fourth to one-half an inch in diameter, knotty, fleshy, with numerous radicles. Its præmorse or abrupt form is occasioned by its making off-sets from its sides, which off-sets separate as the root decays. Its color, externally, is reddish-brown; but internally it is paler. It is succulent, and, when cut or broken, it emits, from numerous points on the tranverse surface, a bright orange, or rather dark vermillion colored juice, which has a bitterish, acrid, but peculiar taste, which remains long in the mouth, and leaves a persistent burning in the throat. The juice of the stem is between a red color and a yellow, as that from the stem of Chelidonium majus is pure yellow, and that from Papaver is white.

The chemical analysis shows it to contain an alkaloid called Sanguinarina. Dr. James Schiel, of St. Louis, claims to have determined the identity of Sanguinarina with Chelrythrin, obtained from Celandine. It also contains chelidonic acid.

OFFICINAL PREPARATIONS.—Tincture of the root, with strong alcohol; dilutions; triturations of the dried root, and of the Sulphate and Nitrate of Sanguinarina.

ANALOGUES.—*Arsenicum, Asclepias tub, Ammonium caust, Arum, Asarum, Belladonna, Bromine, Bryonia, Calcarea carb., Causticum, Chelidonium, Drosera, Hepar sulph., Iris, Lachesis, Lycopodium, Mercurius, Phosphorus, Rumex, Senega, Spongia, Stannum, Sulphur, Tart. emet.*

### Mental Sphere.

Mind confused, relieved by eructations. (*p.*)

Anxiety followed by delirium.

Delirium with hot skin.

Stupor, heaviness, sleepiness.

Extreme moroseness, with nausea, cannot bear to hear a person walk in the room.

Hopefulness, sanguine of recovery from illness. (*s.*)

### Head.

\* Vertigo with singing in the ears.

* Vertigo with diminished vision before vomiting.
* Vertigo with nausea and headache, followed by spasmodic vomiting.
* Vertigo on quickly turning the head, and looking upwards.
* Determination of the blood to the head, with whizzing in the ears, and flashes of heat.

Pressing drawing in the forehead, with heaviness of the head, better while walking.
* Headache as if the forehead would split, with chill, and with burning in the stomach.

Periodic stitches in the left temple and forehead, worse in evening.
* Painful soreness in small spots, especially on the temples.

Headache with rheumatic pains and stiffness in the limbs and neck.
* Pain in the head in rays, drawing upward from the neck.
* Beating headache with throbbing in the temporal arteries and bitter vomiting.

A feeling as if the head is drawing forward.

Sensation of looseness in the scalp, on raising the eyes.

Headache with a nausea and chill, then flying heat from the head to the stomach.
° Migraine with bilious vomiting, pains begin in the morning, last till evening; eyes feel as if they would be pushed out, aggravated by motion.
° Headache relieved only by pressing on the back of his head.
° Headache which occurs paroxysmally, once a week or longer, the pains begin in morning, increase all day, and last till evening; the head seems as if it must burst; the pain is digging, piercing, or throbbing, lancinating through the brain, on the forehead and top of head, worse on the *right* side, followed by chills, nausea, vomiting, and only relieved by sleep. (*Hering.*)
° Frightfully severe headache, the only relief obtained was from pressing the back of his head against the head-board of the bed. (*Hering.*)
° One of the most important indications for Sang. in headache

is, "Pain like a flash of lightning on the back of the head." (*Neidhard.*)

° Myalgic headaches; ° Rheumatic headaches; ° Congestive headaches; ° Headaches at the "change of life;" ° Headache from suppressed menses ; ° Dyspeptic headache; ° Migraines. (*Hale.*)

° Sanguineous apoplexy, with vertigo, dimness of sight, vomiting, burning in the stomach, and distension of the temporal veins. (*Hale.*)

° "North American sick headaches." (*Hering.*)

### Face.

* Distension of the veins of the face and temples, with excessive redness; a feeling of stiffness.
* Stitches in the left side of face, with pains in the forehead.

Severe burning, heat and redness of the face.

* Paleness of the face, with disposition to vomit.
° Red cheek, with burning of the ears.
° Redness of the cheeks, with cough.
° Cheeks and hands livid in typhoid pneumonia.

### Nose.

* Fluid coryza, with frequent sneezing; worse in right nostril.
* Watery, acrid coryza, rendering the nose sore, with copious watering of the right eye.

(The coryza disappears when diarrhœa sets in.)

° Acute and chronic coryzas, with loss of smell.
° Influenza, with rawness in the throat, pain in the breast, cough, and finally diarrhœa.
° *Nasal polypi*, or fungous growths in the nostrils (use the tincture or powder topically).
° Nasal catarrhs, chronic, with offensive discharges; (use 2 trit. as a "snuff.")
° Ulcerative ozæna, with epistaxis. (*Hale.*)

### Eyes.

Watering and burning of the right eye, which is painful on being touched, then coryza.

Feeling as if hairs were in the eyes, or as if smoke was in them.

Glimmering before the eyes, diminished power of vision, worse in the afternoon.

Dilatation of the pupils with vertigo (from the seeds).

° Catarrhal ophthalmia, granular lids. (*Hale.*)

° Ophthalmia followed by ulceration of the cornea. (*Hale.*)

° Is useful as a collyria in chronic conjunctivitis (2 × aqueous dil).

### Ears.

Beating under the ears, at irregular intervals, only a couple of strokes.

* Burning of the ears, with redness of the cheeks.

* Earache, with headache, with singing in the ears and vertigo.

Humming in the ears, with determination of blood.

Painful sensitiveness to sudden sounds.

° Acute internal otitis (also perhaps myringitis).

° Catarrhal affections of the inner ear. (*Woodyat.*)

### Mouth and Teeth.

Stiffness of the jaws, and pain in the upper teeth.

* Toothache from picking the teeth.

° Grumbling toothache, with pain in same side of the head.

Toothache worse from drinking cold water, better from warm drinks (*coffea* the reverse).

Looseness of the teeth and salivation.

Shooting and thrilling pain in a carious tooth.

* Spongy, bleeding, and fungoid condition of the gums.

Loss of *taste* and smell, with a burnt feeling on the tongue.

Prickling sensation on the tongue and roof of the mouth.

Feeling of dryness begins on the right side, spreading over the whole tongue.

Tongue sore, stitches on left side of the tongue.

Sugar tastes bitter, followed by burning in the fauces.

White coated tongue, with slimy, fatty taste in mouth.

### Throat.

Dryness, sensation of, not diminished by drinking.

Heat in the throat alleviated by inspiration of cool air.

Burning in the throat after eating sweet things.

° Throat feels swollen as if to suffocation, with **pain when** swallowing, and aphonia.

Pain, with feeling of swelling most on the right side, most perceptible when swallowing.

° Ulcerated sore throat, following quinsy.

° Tonsillitis, chronic, recurring frequently; prevents the recurrence. (*Hale.*)

### Stomach and Gastric Symptoms.

\* Soreness and pressure in the epigastrium, worse after eating.

\* Burning in the stomach, with headache.

\* Great weakness of digestion, with loss of appetite.

\* Strengthens the stomach, excites the appetite, and stimulates digestion.

\* Inflammation of the stomach, with burning, vomiting, headache, etc.

° Acute gastritis; ° chronic gastritis; ° atonic gastritis.

° Ulceration of the stomach.

° Nausea not diminished by vomiting.

\* Loss of appetite and great weakness of digestion.

Extreme nausea, with profuse water-brash.

° Vomiting, with severe painful burning in the stomach, and intense thirst.

° Pyrosis; a rising of burning, corrosive fluid from the stomach, for twenty years. (*Fairbanks.*)

Soon after eating, a feeling of emptiness in the stomach.

Jerking in the stomach, as if from something alive.

\* *Nausea,* intense, in paroxysms, *worse* when stooping, with flow of saliva; followed by nettle-rash; with heartburn; spasmodic eructations of flatus of unpleasant odor; with headache, chills, followed by vomiting, and sometimes diarrhœa.

\* *Vomiting;* *before* vomiting, great anxiety; pressure to stool; very disagreeable nausea; *during* vomiting, headache, burning in the stomach, with craving to eat; with prostration; *after* vomiting, relief of the headache.

\* *Vomiting of bitter water;* of sour, acrid fluids, and ingesta.

° In almost every form of indigestion, for many years, it has given me satisfactory results. (*F. W. Hunt.*)

° Especially useful in deficient gastric secretion, with loss of appetite, and periodic nausea.

36

° Offensive eructations, spasmodic, from constricted cardia, from congested mucous membrane and fermentation of food. (*Ib.*)

### Abdomen.

Severe and continued pain in the hypochondria, with vertigo and debility.

° Pain in left hypochondrium, worse on coughing, better by pressure and lying on the left side. (° Splenitis?)

Beating and cramps in the abdomen, moving from one place to another.

Sensation as if hot water poured itself from the breast into the abdomen, followed by diarrhœa.

Paroxysmal cutting and drawing pains in the abdomen.

Colic-like pains in the morning, followed by diarrhœic stool.

Twisting pain on the left side, above the groin; worse when sitting, standing, or bending toward the right side, increased by pressure, better when walking erect.

° Jaundice.   ° Hepatic torpor.   ° Biliary concretions.

° Atony of the liver. (*Allopathic and Eclectic.*)

° Cough from affections of the liver. (*Hale.*)

Pain in the top of the *right* shoulder.

### Stool.

* Pressure to stool, without evacuation, with the sensation of a mass in lower part of rectum, and discharge of offensive flatus only.

* Diarrhœic stools, watery, with great flatulence, preceded by cutting pain.

* Diarrhœa in the evening, with disturbance of the coryza and catarrh, and pain in the chest.

Food passes away undigested.

° Dysentery.   ° Hæmorrhoids.

### Urine.

* Frequent urination, also at night, which is copious and clear as water.

° Very copious urine at night, with pain in left hypochondrium; *worse* from coughing; better from pressure and lying on left side. (*Bates.*)

## Generative Organs.

*Women.*—* Pain in the loins, extending through the hypogastric and uterine region, and down the thighs, followed by the appearance of the menses (in cases of suppression).

* Abdominal pains (at night) as if the menses would appear.

Menses are much too early, too profuse, with a discharge of black blood.

Uterine hemorrhage, followed by amenorrhœa.

° Threatened abortion, characterized by nausea, pains in the loins, extending through the hypogastric and iliac regions, and down the thighs.

° Flushes of heat, at the change of life.

° Distension of the abdomen in the evening and flatulent discharges per vagina, from the os uteri, which was constantly open, and at the same time a pain passing in rays, passing from the nape of neck to the head.

° Burning of the palms of the hands and soles of the feet, at the climacteric period, compelling her to throw the bed clothes off, in order to cool them.

° Ulcerations of the os uteri; corrosive and fœtid leucorrhœa.

° *Polypi of the uterus.* ° Cancer of the uterus.

° *Dysmenorrhœa* in feeble, torpid subjects, with tendency to congestion of lungs, liver or head.

° Amenorrhœa, with disease of the lungs.

*Breasts:* Stitches in both breasts; soreness to the touch, under the right nipple, and painful soreness of the nipples.

## Larynx and Bronchia.

* Tickling in the throat in the evening, with slight cough and headache.

* Dry cough, awakening him from sleep, which did not cease until he sat upright in bed, and flatus was discharged upwards and downwards.

* Tormenting cough, with expectoration and circumscribed redness of the cheeks. (*Bute.*)

° Continued severe cough, without expectoration; pain in breast, and circumscribed redness of the cheeks.

° Feels stronger and freer in the breast, mornings, and in the afternoon and evening the customary dyspnœa does not appear.

° Whooping-cough.    ° Hydrothorax.  ° Asthma.  ° Pneumonia.

° Cough, with coryza, then diarrhœa, which cures both.

* Chronic dryness in the throat and sensation of swelling in the larynx, and expectoration of thick mucus.

° Chronic laryngitis, bronchitis and trachitis.

* Continued severe cough, without expectoration, pain in the head, and circumscribed redness of cheeks.

* Croup; catarrhal, with spasmodic, crowing, painful cough, and stridulous breathing. (*Hale.*)

° *Pseudo-membranous croup;* many severe and dangerous cases. (*Nichol, Helmuth.*)

[The *primary* action of Sanguinaria is like that of Tartar emetic. A loose, rattling cough, followed *secondarily* by a dry, painful, spasmodic, croupy cough, with scanty, tenacious expectoration. (*Hale.*)]

### Chest.

* Pain in the breast, with cough and expectoration.

* Pain in the breast, with dry, periodic cough.

* Burning and pressing in the breast, heat through the abdomen, with diarrhœa.

Stitches from the lower part of left breast to the shoulder.

* Slowly shooting pain in right chest, about the seventh rib; and *acute stitches in right breast.*

Shooting pain under the sternum, and the region of the heart.

° *Pneumonia,* with extreme dyspnœa, short, accelerated, constrained breathing, difficulty of speech, sputa becomes tenacious, rust-colored, and expectorated with much difficulty.

° *Hœmoptysis,* during phthisis pulmonalis.

* Continued pressure and heaviness of the whole upper part of the chest, with difficulty of breathing.

° *Typhoid pneumonia,* with very difficult respiration; cheeks and hands livid; pulse feels soft, vibrating, and easily compressed.

› *Pneumonia in second and third stages;* with dullness on percussion; bronchial respiration, with red or gray hepatization; and infiltration of the parenchyma. (*Hale.*)

° "Syphilitic pulmonary inflammation." (*Wolff, with the* 200*th.*)

° *Chronic pneumonia,* where it rivals *Sulphur* or *Phosphorus*

° Hydrothorax. ° Asthma. ° Pleurisy. ° Intercostal myalgia

[Sanguinaria, in affections of the lungs, occupies a place mid-way between Phosphorus and Tartar emetic; it has many symptoms common to both, and some possessed by neither. It closely resembles Sulphur and Lycopodium, and in chronic diseases rivals them in its curative powers. *Hale.*)]

### Heart.

Painful stitches in the region of the heart.

Pressing pain in the region of the heart.

Palpitation of the heart (before the vomiting), with great weakness.

Irregularity of the hearts action, and of the pulse, with coldness, insensibility, etc.

### Back.

Pain, stiffness, and soreness of the nape of the neck, left side, on being touched.

* Pain in the sacrum, from lifting. (*Bute.*)

Pain in the sacrum, alleviated by bending forward.

Rheumatic pains in the neck, shoulders and arms.

° *Lumbago,* from lifting; or myalgia of the great muscles of the back.

### Upper Extremities.

Sudden rheumatic pains in the shoulder joints.

* Rheumatic pain in the right arm and shoulder; worse at night, in bed; (sometimes in the forenoon;) cannot raise the arm. (*Bute.*)

* Pain in the right shoulder, and in the upper part of the right arm, more at night, on turning in bed. (*Jeanes.*)

Pain in the *left* shoulder, in the evening.

Rheumatic pains in the arms and hands.

Severe pain in the hand, with aching in the arm, when lying quiet and warm in bed.

* Burning of the palms, redness of the hands, and severe burning lividity of the hands, in pneumonia.

Stiffness of the finger-joints, also cutting and stitching pains.

Pain as if from a boil at the root of the nails on all the
fingers.

° Ulceration of the roots of all the nails on both hands. (*Bute.*)

### Lower Extremities.

Rheumatic-like pains in the left hip.

Pain as from a bruise in the left hip joint, whilst walking, but
worse on rising from a seat.

Rheumatic pain in inside of right thigh, alternating with pain
in the chest.

* Burning in the soles of the feet; worse at night.

Stiffness and tightness in the knees and under the knees.

* Acute swelling of the joints of the extremities.

° Acute, inflammatory, and arthritic rheumatism.

On touching the painful part, the pain vanishes, and appears
elsewhere.

* Paralysis of the right side.

° Pains in those places where the bones are least covered with
flesh.

### Fever.

Chill with headache, nausea and shivering in the back in the
evening in bed.

Shaking pain, with chill under the shoulder-blade on motion.

Heat flying from head to stomach.

Burning heat, rapidly alternating with chill and shivering.

Gradual increase in the force, and frequency of the pulse.

Slow pulse, with extreme nausea.

° Coldness of the feet in the afternoons, with painful and sore
tongue; stiffness of the knee, and finger joints (*Bute.*)

° *Hectic fever*, with cough, circumscribed redness of the cheeks.

° *Fevers* from *pulmonary*, hepatic or gastric inflammation.

### Sleep.

Sleeplessness at night, waking with fright as if he would *fall.*

Dreams of a frightful and disagreeable character.

Dreams of sailing on the sea.

### Skin.

Heat and dryness.

Itching and a nettle-rash before the nausea.

° Fungous growths.   ° Scaly eruptions; carbuncles.

° Old indolent ulcers, with callous border, and ichorous discharge.

### Generalities.

A quickly diffused, and transient, but at the same time a very peculiar thrill, often extended to the minutest extremity.

General torpor and languor; dilatation of the pupils.

---

# SANTONINE.

### (*The active principle of Wormseed.*)

BOTANICAL DESCRIPTION.—Santoninum. *Santonin*, or *Santoninic* acid, is a crystalline principle, obtained from *Levant Wormseed*, or *Artemisia contra*, which is the same as the "Cina" of our Materia Medica. It occurs in colorless, pearly, four-sided orthorhombic tables, soluble in from four to five thousand parts of cold and two hundred and fifty parts of boiling water; freely soluble in alcohol and chloroform; moderately so in cold ether; insoluble, or nearly so, in glycerine. It has a neutral reaction, but unites with alkalies to form salts, and hence is freely soluble in alkaline solutions. On exposure to light, the colorless crystals of Santonin acquire a golden-yellow tint. If this change is a chemical, and not a mechanical one, the alteration must be very slight, since, according to Kruss, the yellow crystals conduct themselves in their chemical relation precisely as do the colorless crystals, aad are precipitated by the addition of acids to their alkaline solutions, as colorless crystals.

OFFICINAL PREPARATIONS.—Triturations.

ANALOGUES.—*Artemisia, Chenopodium, Curcubita, Cina, Felix mas., Gelseminum, Kousso, Spigelia, Teucrium.*

### Mental Sphere.

* Light febrile paroxysms, with delirium.
* Wandering delirium, with great agitation.
* Depression of spirits, and inability to follow his work.
* Epileptiform convulsions.

Confused state of the mind.

Dizzy feeling, lassitude, prostration.

### Head.

Violent headache, with vomiting.

Intense headache, in its most aggravating form.

Numbness in the head.

Dull aching in the right temple.

Severe pains in front of the head.

Hot perspiration on the occiput; more clammy in front; head very hot.

Abnormal feelings and pains in the head.

° Brain symptoms, simulating hydrocephalus, when caused by
worms. (*Hale.*)

### Eyes.

Yellow appears *red;* yellow-sight in all; violet-sight in all;
visions, like shadows.

Sunken eyes, with pallor around the nose and lips.

Eyes glowing, and convulsive movements of the eyelids.

Loss of vision; dimness of the eyes; giddy feeling.

Dilatations of the pupils, and troubles of sight.

Convulsive twitching of the eyes.

Men appear like ghosts walking.

[The phenomena of visual illusion in persons *poisoned* by it, are reduc-
able to distinct classes. Every one, however small the quantity taken
could not recognize violet light  Some the spectrum, as if curtailed at the
violet end, overlooked everything of a pure violet color, whilst in all mix-
tures containing violet and yellow, the complimentary yellow appeared to
predominate. This has been called yellow-sight. (*Gelbachen.*)]

Quite different is the next higher degree of intoxication. The subject
of it is then unable to distinguish colors which in the healthy make a
different, even an opposite impression, such as lilac and dark gray, or
violet and black; he not only confounds these colors with one another,
but a great many dissimilar seem all alike to him. The colors which are
mistaken for each other had always a different degree of purity and
strength, which, however, continues unalterably the same for each color,
so that when one has exactly determined by measurement the purity and
strength of two colors that are thus mistaken, one can with perfect certainty and precision determine, *a priori*, by calculation with which two
of all the other colors these two may be confounded. There is hardly a
single color which can with certainty be distinguished from the rest; each
one resembles an endless number of others; and thus the infinite host of
colors which a healthy person can appreciate is reduced to an extremely
small number. This stage manifests itself in the fact that all colors, the
darker they really are, so much the more resemble a tint between violet
and ultramarine, with the determination of which tints all other changes
of color are determined alike. The yellow-sighted cannot at all perceive
certain impressions of light; violet rays are no more to him than the invisible thermic and actinic rays; he is color-blind. The violet-sighted, on
the contrary, sees every color, is susceptible to every stimulus of light;
but ever so many of them invariably make the very same impression. He
is not color-*blind;* he merely *confounds* the colors. In one of my early
experiments, when I knew nothing beyond yellow-sight, my colleague
went, when the narcotism seemed to have disappeared (*i. e., when he had got
used to it*), to dine at a restaurant. The experiment was over and forgotten;

during lively conversation in a friendly circle, in comes the waiter with yellow egg soup. It smelt peculiar to *him*, and looked *quite red*. Perfectly shocked, he sent the soup back as entirely spoilt. To the amusement of his friends, he persisted obstinately in asseverations which to them were inexplicable. They came to words, and my hot-headed colleague left the good-for-nothing eating house in a pet. No doubt the waiter thought he was "not all there." Now we know that in this delusion the first symptoms of olfactory hallucination and violet-sight were setting in, of which, then, no one as yet dreamed.

It is the opinion of Dr. Roce, of Berlin, who has made the most extensive experiments with Santonine, that the various colors which cover the field of vision is "not due to any actual change in the color of the media, by which the rays of light reach the retina, but to an *altered perceptivity in the nervous organ of vision itself*." If such is the case, the Santonine ought to prove curative in some internal disorders of the eye, when such disorders show similar symptoms. As might have been expected, it *has* been found curative in some cases of defective vision and weakness of sight. Dr. ——, in the reports of an English hospital, records its curative action in

° "*Nervous failure of sight.*"

It appears that the discovery of its curative power was accidental. An old man, quite blind, was given Santonine for worms. Under its influence his sight partially returned. This led to its administration in 36 cases of weakness of vision—or, as the writer terms it, "nervous failure of sight," a kind of paralysis of the optic nerve. Of the 36 cases, 27 recovered more or less perfectly, the rest were not much benefitted.

It was also used in *nine* cases of

° *Cataract.*

Of these nine cases, *four* were cured, and the rest not benefitted.

### Nose.

Very offensive smell experienced; hallucinations of smell.

Bluish pallor around the nose; pinched expression of nose.

\* Intense itching of the nose; the child rubs and bores into the nostrils.

### Face.

Face puffy and congested; convulsive movements of the face and lips; twitching in the facial muscles.

Heat and flushed face.

Pinched and distorted countenance.

### Mouth and Lips.

Pinched expression of the mouth.

Lips very much swollen.

Bitter taste; foaming at the mouth.

Burning and stinging sensation of the mouth and **lips.**
Bluish pallor around the mouth and nose.
Drawing in of the lips over the teeth.
Hallucinations of taste.

### Throat.

\* Choking feeling in the throat, very severe at times; **complete**
    loss of appetite.
\* Dry, hacking cough, tickling in the larynx and **windpipe.**
Continual thirst.

### Nausea, Vomiting, etc.

Gastric oppression, nausea, with vomiting.
Vomiting of yellowish, slimy mucus.
Vomiting, with intense headache, vertigo, dilated **pupils and**
    abnormal vision.
° Vomiting from worms—lumbrici, etc.

### Stomach.

\* Nausea, which disappears after eating.
Severe pain in the stomach and side, with **vomiting.**
Nausea, increased after eating; gastric derangement.
Dull, throbbing pains, worse on stooping.
Pressure in pit of stomach, with distension and **tenderness.**
Vomiting, purging and prostration.
Dull pain in the pit of the stomach.
° *Bloated stomach*, in worm affections.

### Bowels and Abdomen.

The bowels constipated and require gentle **purgatives.**
Dull, throbbing pains in the abdomen.
Abdomen very sensitive; tumid, but soft.
Intense abdominal pains, with profuse *diarrhœa.*
Purging of watery, flaky, foul-smelling stools.
° Bloated abdomen, hard or soft, especially when **occurring in**
    worm affections.
° *Verminous affections*, (worms in the intestines, etc.)

[Santonine is one of the most powerful *parasiticides*, and will destroy
the life of almost any species of intestinal parasite. It seems to have the
most decided power over *lumbrici*, (long, round worm,) less on *oxyuris*,
(pin worm,) and least on *tænia*, (tape worm.)

For the destruction of *lumbrici*, no better remedy is known. It should
be given in two or three grains of the 1-10*th* trituration, in a spoonful of

sweetened milk, at a time when the stomach is empty, as before each meal, or, in infants, before nursing. In young infants the 2d and 3d triturations should be prescribed. A few days of this treatment will remove the worm symptoms. It must not be expected that the worms will be seen in the evacuations, for when they die in the stomach, they are *digested*. If the child has diarrhœa, then the worms, or portions of them, may be discovered in the alvine evacuations.

In some cases of *oxyuris*, Santonine will prove useful, but it should be injected into the rectum, as well as given by the mouth. It is a late discovery that if injections of warm lard are used, for a few nights, the pin worms disappear—their propagation is arrested. If a few grains of Santonine in the lowest trituration is added to each injection of lard (one-half or one ounce,) the destruction of these parasites is rendered still more certain. I do not know that this medicine has ever destroyed a *tapeworm*, although instances may have been placed on record.

### Urinary Organs.

The urine is always colored a peculiar green or orange-green.
° Waking up suddenly with urgent desire to urinate; a few drops voided each time.
° *Chronic cystitis:*(chronic catarrh of the bladder.) It causes an immediate increase in the volume of the urine; and an amelioration of the worst symptoms; the bladder loses its sensitiveness and sense of fullness; the urine flows free and easy, and a cure is soon effected. Dose, half a grain, three times a day. (*Dr. E. C. Davis.*)
° *Suppression of urine.* ° *Incontinence of urine.* (*Berger.*)
° *Dysuria.* ° Scanty urine, with brick-dust sediment. (*Ib.*)
° Wetting the bed at night. (*Ib.*) ° Milky urine. (*Hale.*)
° Burning, scalding, tenesmus, and other unpleasant sensations in the urinary passages. (*Scudder.*)
° *Vibriones in the urine.* (In some cases these organic forms are found in urine just voided. It denotes a bad state of vitality in the patient. In such cases Santonine removes this condition, and prevents their formation. (*Hale.*)

### Skin.

Burning of the skin.
Rash-like eruptions appear on the body.
Skin of a corpse-like hue.

### Chills and Fever.

° Violent fever, with great frequency of the pulse, and dry, burning heat of the skin.

Lowering of the pulse.

° *Worm fever.*  ° Remittent fever, from worms.  (*Hale.*)

[All the fevers of children are liable to be aggravated by intestinal para sites.  In such cases a few doses of *Santonine* 1-10*th* removes the cause of irritation, after which, other remedies act better, and the fever is now easily combatted.]

### Sleep.

Very restless, sleeping only a few moments at a time.

Unnatural wakefulness; sleep disturbed by colic.

During restless sleep, light delirium manifested itself.

Abnormal sleep, when caused by worms; also such symptoms at night as grinding the teeth, wetting the bed, crying out in affright, etc.

### Tongue.

Loaded tongue.

* Tongue deep red, without coating.

### Teeth.

* Grinding and clenching of the teeth together during sleep.

### Upper Extremities.

Convulsive movements of the hands and arms.

Jerking of the upper limbs.

Coldness of the hands.

### Lower Extremities.

Extremities cold, with great restlessness.

Body nearly curved, with the legs set back (opisthotonos).

### Generalities.

The following is what happened in thirty cases in which Santonine was given.

Yellow sight in all,....................................30
Violet sight, ..........................................19
Nausea and vomiting, ..................................14
Dizzy feelings, lassitude, prostration, ..................  9
Visions, ..............................................  8
Hallucinations of smell, ..............................  6
Hallucinations of taste,...............................  5
Abnormal feelings and pains in the head,...............  8
Lowering of the pulse, ................................  2

(1.) Santonine produces a sort of parlysis, accompanied by rigidity of the muscles.

(2.) Its effects are produced in a manner analogous to the mode of action of Atropine and Physostigmine (Calabar bean).

(3.) It entirely destroys the irritability of muscles, rendering them completely rigid.

(4.) Its therapeutical properties deserve more fully to be inquired into.

In doses of more than three grains, Santonine sometimes occasions nausea and vomiting, with abdominal pains, great thirst, giddiness, and profuse diarrhœa. Decidedly poisonous effects sometimes arise from doses which are quite insignificant in comparison with those some experimenters have taken without serious inconvenience. In one case it is stated that a child six months old and convalescent from small-pox, took five grains of Santonic acid, instead of three, which had been prescribed. It became amaurotic, and did not recover its sight for two months. In another case, two grains of this substance were taken at a dose, by a healthy child of two years. In a quarter of an hour it was seized with convulsions, and within one hour it lay unconscious, with a hot head and congested face, the eyes twitching convulsively, the pupils largely dilated and insensible, the mouth foaming, the teeth clenched, the breathing stertorous, and the upper limbs occasionally jerking. On the morrow, recovery was complete. This resembles two cases in which Hoffmann witnessed such alarming cerebral symptoms, after the administration of Santonica, that he was obliged to apply leeches to the temples and cold compresses to the head. These examples are sufficient to illustrate the somewhat uncertain operation of Santonic acid, both in degree and in kind, and to suggest caution in its administration.

° Convulsions, when caused by worms.

[It may be found useful in cerebro-spinal convulsions.—*Hale.*]

---

# SARRACENIA PURPUREA.

### (*Huntsman's Cup, Pitcher Plant.*)

BOTANICAL DESCRIPTION.—This plant, also known as *side-saddle flower*, fly-trap and pitcher plant, is an indigenous perennial, and "owes its strange appearance to a curious pitcher-shaped metamorphosis of the leaf, which resembles very much an old-fashioned side-saddle. Six of these generally belong to each plant. The leaf, which springs from the root, is formed by a large hollow tube, swelling out in the middle, curved and diminishing downward, until it ends in a stem, contracted at the mouth, and furnished with a large, spreading, heart-shaped appendage at the top, which is hairy within, the hairs pointing downward, so as to cause everything which falls upon the leaf to be carried toward the petiole. A broad, wavy wing extends the whole length, on the inside. These lie upon the ground, with their mouths turned upward, so as to catch the water when it falls. They hold nearly a wineglassful, and are generally filled with water and aquatic insects, which undergo decomposition, or a sort of diges-tion, and serve as a nutriment to the plant. The stem rises direct from the root; it is round, quite smooth, and bears an elegant, deeply reddish purple, terminal flower, having two flower-cups; the external consisting of three small leaves, the internal of five egg-shaped, obtuse leaves, shining, and of a brownish purple. The blossoms are five, guitar-shaped, obtuse repeat-edly curved inward and outward, and finally inflected over the stigma, which is broad and spreading, divided at its margin into five bifid lobes, alternating with the petals, and supported on a short cylindrical style; this is surmounted by the stamens, which are numerous, having short threads, and large, two-celled, oblong, yellow anthers attached to them, on the under surface. In the yellow-flowered species of the Southern States, the bottle is very long, resembling a trumpet, by which name it is often called.—*King.*

The whole species are water plants, and are found only in wet meadows, wet, boggy places, marshes, mud-lakes, etc., and grow from Labrador to Florida, flowering in June. There are several *species.*

OFFICINAL PREPARATIONS.—Tincture of the root; infusion of the whole plant.

ANALOGUES.—(?) (Perhaps *Thuja.*)

° *Small-pox in its worst forms.*

° Dyspeptic and gastric difficulties. **(?)**

° Uterine disorders. (?)

° Psoric diseases. (?)

° Scrofulous eruptions.

[Those who care to consult Houatt's provings and pathogenesis, will find it in Vol. 18, page 70, of the North American Journal of Homœopathy.]

---

# SCUTELLARIA LATERIFLORA.

## *(Scull-Cap.)*

BOTANICAL DESCRIPTION.—Scutellaria lateriflora has a small fibrous perennial *root,* with an erect, very branching, diffuse, quadrangular, nearly glabrous *stem,* from one to three feet in height; the *branches* are opposite. The *leaves* are on petioles about an inch long, opposite, thin, entire, nearly membranous, subcordate on the stem, ovate on the branches, acuminate or acute, coarsely serrate and slightly rugose. The *flowers* are small, of a pale blue color, and are disposed in long, lateral, axillary racemes, with ovate, acute, entire, subsessile, distichous bracts, each flower axillary to a bract, and pedunculated. The *calyx* has an entire margin, which, after the corolla has fallen, is closed with a helmet-shaped lid. The *tube* of the *corolla* is about a quarter of an inch long, the upper lip concave and entire, the lower three-lobed. *Seeds*, four in the closed calyx, oval, verrucose.

Scull-cap is an indigenous herb, growing in damp places, meadows, ditches, and by the side of ponds, flowering in July and August. It is known by the names of *Blue scull-cap, Side-flowering scull-cap, Mad-dog weed* and *Woodwort*. The whole plant is officinal; it should be gathered while in flower, dried in the shade, and kept in well-closed tin vessels. It is inodorous, but has a bitterish taste; alcohol or boiling water extracts its properties. Scull-cap is said to contain an essential oil; a fixed oil, yellowish-green, and soluble in ether, a bitter principle soluble in water, alcohol, or ether; chlorophyll, a peculiar volatile matter, albumen, a sweet mucous substance; a peculiar astringent principle; lignin, Chloride of Soda, and other salts.

Scutellarin, the concentrated preparation, is of a light greenish-brown color, with a faint tea-like odor, and a peculiar, herbaceous, somewhat gritty, resinous, tea-like taste, is insoluble in water, partially soluble in alcohol, and more so in ether.

OFFICINAL PREPARATIONS.—Tincture of the plant; dilutions. [Scutellarin and its triturations are preferable.]

ANALOGUES.—*Ambergris, Coffea, Chamomilla, Cypripedium, Coca, Eupatorium aromaticum, Ignatia, Paullinia, Valerian, Thea, Zincum, Senecio.*

## Mental Sphere.

Great inability to confine the mind to study.

Exhilaration, with copious flow of ideas.

Happy, contented, and quiet mind, with a feeling of calmness and strength.

° Causeless depression of spirits.

° *Delirium tremens*, of a mild character. (*Hale.*)

## Head.

Great fullness and oppression of the head; sensation as if the entire contents were confined within a place too small.

* Hemicrania, worse over the right eye, relieved by moving about in the open air.

Vertigo, with a sensation of lightness of the head.

° Nervous headache; brought on by grief, joy, or any emotional excitement. (*Hale.*)

## Eyes.

Eyes feel as if protruding from the orbits.

Photophobia, in nervous, irritable subjects.

Pupils dilated slightly. (?)

### Chest.

A dull pain extending vertically beneath the sternum.

Oppression of the chest, with a sticking pain in the region of the heart.

Sensation of throbbing about the heart, with flushed face.

° Nervous disorder of the heart, such as irregular action, palpitation, tremor, and strange sensations, from emotional excitements (even in organic diseases is palliative). (*Hale.*)

Pulse slow and intermitting.

### Urinary Organs.

Difficulty in urinating and sharp pains in region of left kidney

* Scanty urine, before the headache; profuse clear urine after.

### Sleep.

* Sudden waking up from disagreeable dreams.

* Nightly restlessness; wakefulness from frightful dreams.

* Sleeplessness from pleasant thoughts crowding on the mind.

### Nervous System.

* Tremulousness and twitching of the muscles in various parts of the body.

° *Chorea*, of a purely nervous origin.

* Nervous jactitations and tremors (in typhoid fever). (*Hale.*)

° *Pseudo-hydrophobia.* (Drs. Vandemar and Rafinesque claim that real hydrophobia has been cured or prevented by the free use of an infusion of Scull-cap. (*Ib.*)

° *Hysteria* and hysterical spasmodic affections. (*Ib.*)

° Spasms and nervous irritation in teething children, or when the nervous system is irritated from disordered bowels.

° Reflex nervous irritation from uterine ovarian disease.

° Chronic symptoms arising from sunstroke. (?) (*Coe.*)

General uneasiness, with twitching of the muscles, and sticking pains in various parts of the body, occasionally extending up along each side of the forehead.

---

## SEMPERVIVUM TECTORUM.

### (*Common House-Leek.*)

BOTANICAL DESCRIPTION.—House-leek has a fibrous *root*, crowned with several rosaceous tufts of numerous, oblong, acute, keeled, fringed, extremely succulent leaves. The stem, from the centre of one of these

tufts, is about a foot high, erect, round, ? ·vny, clothed with several more
narrow, sessile, alternate leaves, and ter. : ating in a sort of many-flowered
cyme, with spiked branches. *Flowers* large, pale rose-colored, without
scent. Segments of the calyx, twelve or more, with a similar number of
petals, stamens and pistils. Offsets spreading.—*L.*

OFFICINAL PREPARATIONS.—Tinctures, triturations, and cerate.

ANALOGUES.—*Calendula, Symphytum, Pæonia (?).*

### Mouth.

° A sickly woman had, about the "change of life," a swelling
on right margin of tongue, scirrhus, size of a small bean,
with burning pain after shutting her mouth, occasionally
bleeding, invariably at night; the swelling was not hard,
but like a cyst; had two small knots, each size of a lentil.
Over the swelling were three varicose veins. Two drops
of the 2d, daily, reduced the tumor to one-third the size,
in ten days: menstruation reappeared, continuing five
days. Tumor diminished to the size of a small pea, and
became gradually less sensitive.

° Ulcer on the tongue, three-quarters to one-half inch deep,
oval, sharp edges, hard foundation, of a bluish color, with
four knots, size of lentils, two large veins, sensitive to
touch and while eating. Local application reduced the
size in a few days.

° A married woman, aged twenty-seven years, with a child of
six months, had for ten days a pain under the tongue,.
impeding eating and talking. On the lower surface, near
the root, was a bluish-white swelling, size of half a bean,.
smooth, but hard, on either side a large vein. At one
point a membranous exudation. Two doses of the 6×,.
one every other day, for four days; no pain. At the
expiration of eight days, much smaller; producing menstruation in three weeks; remains only a somewhat
enlarged vein.

### Shoulder.

° After removal of a fatty tumor from the shoulder, the wound
did not heal. The ulcer was a perfect circle, shallow, as
large as a silver half dollar; no pain, edges a little raised
and rounded; pus greenish, scanty and thick. The whole
sore was filled up with immense granulations, that hung

37

away over the edges.  Was cured in three weeks by a
cerate of the Sempervivum.

### Generative Organs.

*Women:*—Appearance of the menses, lasting five days, having
passed the climacteric.

Appearance of the menses in a nursing woman.

### Skin.

° *Erysipelatous affections, burns,* stings, and other inflammatory conditions.  (?)

° Said to be a perfect cure for warts and corns, (the leaf was
used.)

° *Ringworm and shingles* have been cured by it, (the juice
applied locally.)

---

## SENECIO AUREUS—(*et Gracilis.*)
### (*Life-Root.*)

BOTANICAL DESCRIPTION.—This plant is known by several other names,
as Ragwort, False Valerian, Golden Senecio, Squaw-weed, and Female
Regulator.  It was known to the Indians as "Uncum," the meaning of
which I have been unable to ascertain.

It has an erect, smoothish, striate *stem,* one or two feet high, flocose-
woolly when young, simple or branched above, terminating in a kind of
umbellate, simple or compound corymb.  The *radical leaves* are simple
and rounded, the larger mostly cordate, crenate-serrate, and long-petioled;
the *lower cauline leaves,* lyre-shaped; the upper ones, few, slender, cut-
pinnatifid, dentate, sessile or partly clasping; the terminal segments,
lanceolate; *peduncles* sub-umbellate, and thick upwards; corymbs, umbel-
like.  *Rays* from eight to twelve, four or five lines long, spreading.
*Flowers* golden yellow.  *Scales* linear, acute, and purplish at the apex.

The S. *gracilis* is merely a taller, slenderer variety.

OFFICINAL PREPARATIONS.—Tincture of the whole plant; dilutions.
*Senecin;* triturations.

ANALOGUES.—*Asarum, Cannabis sativa, Caulophyllum, Copaiva, Calcarea
carbonica,* **Cypripedium, Erigeron,** *Eupatorium purpureum, Helonias,
Pulsatilla, Sanguinaria, Sepia, Trillum.*

### Mental Sphere.

*Inability to fix the mind on any one object for any length of
time.*

Depression of spirits alternating with very cheerful moods.

Sad, desponding, meditative mood, in the evening.

A feeling like homesickness.

### Head.

Giddiness and pressing forward in the head.

Dizziness, feeling like a wave from occiput to the sinciput.

Shooting and cutting pains in frontal region, *from within outward.*

Sharp, lancinating pain in the left temple and over the eye.

Dull, stupefying headache, with fullness of the head.

° Catarrhal headache, or from suppressed secretions.

### Eyes.

Sharp, lancinating pain in the left eye, shooting from within outward.

Sharp, sticking pains in both eyes and forehead, from within outwards.

Sharp, lancinating pains *in the left temple*, upper part of left eye and inside of the left half of the lower jaw.

° Catarrhal ophthalmia from suppressed secretions.

### Nose.

Sneezing, and sense of burning and fullness in the nostrils, relieved by a copious flow of mucus.

Dryness of the nostrils, with inclination to sneeze.

° Coryza, with *bleeding* from the nose.

### Face.

Darting pain in the left side of the face.

Sharp, cutting pain inside of the left angle of the lower jaw.

Sharp, sticking pain in the face in common with other parts of the body.

Pale face, with depressed appearance.

### Mouth.

Lips and gums pale.

Dryness of the mouth, fauces and throat.

*Teeth very tender* and sensitive.

Digging or beating pain in a carious molar tooth.

### Gastric Symptoms.

Nausea on rising in the morning.

Eructations of sour gas and sour ingesta.

° Nausea from renal derangements.

° Morning nausea of pregnant women.

### Abdomen.

*Stitches* in both hypochondriac regions.

Sharp pain in the epigastrium.

Colic and diarrhœa, with fever, in the afternoon.

Pain seems to have a centre about the umbilicus, and spreads out in all directions; relieved by a stool.

Griping, colic-like pains, relieved by bending forward.

Griping, pinching pain in the abdomen.

Rumbling of wind in the abdomen.

### Stool.

Thin, watery stool, containing hard lumps.

Dark-colored stool, with much straining.

Fæces in hard lumps, mixed with mucus of a yellow color.

Copious diarrhœa in the morning, attended with great debility and prostration.

° Catarrhal diarrhœa and dysentery.

Thin, dark-colored, or bloody stools, with tenesmus.

### Urinary Organs.

Clear, limpid urine, frequent and profuse.

Urine scanty and high-colored, and tinged with blood.

Mucous sediment in the urine.

° Tenesmus of the bladder, with heat and urging.

° Ascites and œdema of the lower extremities in a young woman. (*Dr. Small.*)

° Intense pain over the right kidney, severe pain during urination, the urine is red, hot and acrid; bowels costive. (*Ib.*)

° Irritation of the bladder in children, preceded by heat in head and headache. (*Hale.*)

° Renal colic, with or without nausea. (*Ib.*)

° Chronic inflammation of the neck of the bladder, with bloody urine, and tenesmus of the bladder (three cases). (*Ib.*)

° Chronic inflammation of the kidneys. (*Hale.*)

° Will *palliate*, if not cure, Bright's disease. (*Ib.*)

### Generative Organs.

*Female:*—[No proving on women, but a large amount of clinical experience.]

° Amenorrhœa in young girls, with dropsical conditions.

° Suppression of the menses, from a cold.

° Dysmenorrhœa, with urinary sufferings, and scanty or profuse flow. (*Hale.*)

° Premature and profuse menses, (it rivals Calcarea carb.)

° Retarded and scanty (or profuse) menses, (rivaling Sepia.)

° Irregular menses, at times too soon, at times retarded.

° Leucorrhœa, instead of the menses, or with urinary troubles.

° Chlorosis, in scrofulous girls, with dropsy.

° Some of the ailments at the critical age. When given to a lady of 48, for great *sleeplessness*, it brought on the menses and restored sleep.

"Senecio gracilis is useful in anæmic dysmenorrhœa, especially when the strumous habit is present. Senecio symptoms, like those of Sulphur and Mercury, are aggravated during the night. (*Massy.*)

*Male:*—Dull, heavy pain in left spermatic cord, moving along the cord to the testicle.

* Prostate gland enlarged and feels hard to the touch.

* Lascivious dreams, with pollutions.

° Gonorrhœa and gleet.   ° Chronic prostatitis.

### Respiratory Organs.

Increased secretion from bronchial mucous membrane.

Labored respiration, with loose cough and mucous rales.

° Mucous, catarrhal cough (especially when attended with suppressed menses).

° Chronic hæmorrhage from the lung, with dry, hacking cough, hectic fever, emaciation and sleeplessness. (*Dr. Irish.*)

' Cough (after a cold), first dry, then loose, with copious expectoration of a yellow, thick, sweet mucus, often streaked with blood, with rawness and soreness in the chest, with debility; flashes of heat, red cheeks in P. M., night sweats, and irregular menses. Cured in two weeks by Senecio, 1-10 dil., gtts. 10, every three hours. (*Hale.*)

" Palliated the cough and bloody sputa in a woman far gone with consumption, and brought back her menses absent four months. (*Hale.*)

### Back and Extremities.

Pain in back and loins; in small of back, with soreness and rheumatic pains in the joints.

### Generalities.

Stitches and sharp pains in various parts of the body.

* Nervousness, sleeplessness, and hysterical moods.

Sensation as of a ball in the stomach, rising up into the throat.
° Affections of mucous membranes (catarrhal).
° Hæmorrhage from the uterus, kidneys, bowels, lungs, etc.
* Great sleeplessness, with vivid, unpleasant dreams.
Feverish heat and thirst, especially in the afternoon.

---

## SILPHIUM LACINIATUM.
### (*Resin-weed, Compass-plant.*)

BOTANICAL DESCRIPTION.—This plant is found growing on the prairies of Illinois and Wisconsin, from thence southward and westward. Flowers in July. On the wide, open prairies, the lower leaves are said to present their edges uniformly northward and southward. It is very rough and bristly throughout, with a stout *stem*, pinnate *leaves*, petioled and clasping at the base. *Heads*, few, and somewhat racemed.

OFFICINAL PREPARATIONS.—Tincture of the leaves; dilutions.

ANALOGUES.—*Cubeba, Copaiva, Terebinthina*, etc.

° Catarrhal affections, and diseases of the mucous membranes.
° Chronic catarrh of the nasal passages.
° Chronic laryngitis and bronchitis.
° *Asthma*, humid, with concomitant catarrhal affections of the bronchial mucous surfaces.
° *Horses* that eat of the leaves mixed in hay, are cured or relieved of the " *heaves*," and chronic loose coughs.
* Catarrh of the bladder. Gonorrhœa and gleet.

---

## SOLANUM NIGRUM.
### (*Black Nightshade.*)

BOTANICAL DESCRIPTION.—Solanum Nigrum belongs to the natural order *Solanaceæ* (Night-shade Family). It has a low stem, much branched, spreading, angular, nearly smooth, with ovate, wavy-toothed or sinuate leaves, and perforated, the edges erased, as if gnawed by insects. Flowers white, small, with yellow anthers, lateral umbels, drooping, five parted, on bractless pedicles. The berries are black when mature, globose, and of a sweetish taste. The flowers begin to appear in June, and September and in October we find ripe berries, green berries, and flowers appearing on the same plant. The whole plant has a disagreeable narcotic odor, resembling in some degree the tomato; the root is white and has little taste.

It seems to prefer a shady locality, though I have seen specimens growing in the sun, but always of a dwarfy, unhealthy appearance. Owing to the fact that this is often mistaken for the Belladonna, and used by many physicians under the impression that it is the Belladonna plant, I here give the botanical difference:

BELLADONNA.—Stems strong, branched, purple colored, from three to five feet high—hairy. Leaves of an equal size, oval, pointed, in pairs, on short foot stalks. Flowers, dark or brownish-purple color, large, pendant, bell-shaped, furrowed, cut in five segments. Berries ripe in September, of a shining black.

SOLANUM NIGRUM.—Stem low, much branched, spreading, rough on the angles. Leaves, ovate, many-toothed, almost always perforated by insects. Flowers white, very small, in small and umbel-like lateral clusters, drooping, five parted. Berries small, globular, black, ripe in September; ripe berries, green berries and flowers found on the same plant at the same time.

OFFICINAL PREPARATIONS.—Tincture from equal parts of the fresh leaves and berries, with strong alcohol; dilutions.

ANALOGUES.—*Agaricus, Æthusa, Belladonna, Cicuta, Hyoscyamus, Helonias, Lachnanthes, Stramonium, Lachesis, Cimicifuga, Cuprum, Gelseminum.*

### Sensorium.

Vertigo, with headache, nausea, colic and tenesmus.

Moaning as in hydrocephalus.

Fullness in the head accompanied with vertigo.

Vertigo on rising and moving about, with dimness of sight.

Vertigo after retiring; as if the bed was turning in a circle

Vertigo on stooping; everything seemed moving in a circle.

Great weariness and vertigo from bodily exertion.

When standing a feeling as if the body would fall backward.

While sitting the body seems to rock in different directions.

### Mental Sphere.

Confused and anxious expression of the countenance.

Complete cessation of the mental faculties.

Drowsy all day with indisposition to study.

Rage, imbecility, delirious raving.

° Sadness and anguish; ° absence of mind.

° Restlessness, inducing one to roam about without sense or object.

### Head.

Horrible headache, with red, bloated face.

Severe pain in supraorbital region, in the morning on waking, aggravated by the slightest motion.

Severe pain over the eyes, aggravated by motion or stooping.

A misstep sends violent pains through the temples.

Sensation in forehead after headache, as if it had been bruised

Sensation in the forehead as if from a blow.

Severe pains through the temples, as if the head would split.

On moving the head, the brain feels as if moving about.

Pain in a small circumscribed spot on top of the head.

Headache with throbbing of the carotid arteries, and swimming sensation in the brain.

Sensation of heat in the head, and of lightness in the head.

Sharp gnawing pain in the right temple, causing him to grasp his head and shut his eyes.

Stitches in the temple, and then in the ear.

Headache with throbbing of the temporal and carotid arteries; increased heat and redness of the face; countenance looks as though he had been intoxicated.

Violent, throbbing pain in the left temple, aggravated by the least misstep, or on stooping.

Violent, throbbing pain in the fore part of the head.

On the least motion, after sitting quietly, a feeling as if the brain would burst from the forehead.

Scalp feels sore on moving the hands through the hair.

Pressure in the centre of the forehead.

Forehead heavy; pressure in the forehead and dullness; gait staggering, heavy and uncertain. The head feels very dull and heavy (after three hours and a quarter).

Pressure in the vertex and forehead; dullness when walking; body inclined to the left side.

Head feels as if expanded, heavy and hot.

Pressure through the temples, drawing toward the forehead through the depth of the brain (several times).

Pressing, aching pain in the depression behind the right ear; head dull, pulse slower, weakness of the thighs, and contracted pupils.

* Very severe headache, of years standing.

[The cerebral symptoms are fully as important as those of belladonna. It is certainly homœopathic to congestion of the brain, incipient meningitis, acute hydrocephalus, basilar meningitis, cerebro-spinal meningitis, and irritation of the brain from teething, or during cholera morbus, and, finally, in sick and nervous headaches.—*Hale.*]

### Eyes.

Pupils dilated more than usual, and general heaviness in the body very soon after taking it and disappearing after one hour.

Very marked dilatation of the pupils, preceded by dullness of the head; pulse slow and small; trembling of the legs, especially of the muscles of the thighs, like short jerks following in quick succession.

Alternate contraction and dilatation of the pupils. (*vv.*)

Black rings before the eyes with dilated pupils.

Pupils somewhat widened next day, with uncertainty in walking.

Pupils very much contracted; many black spots and strips floating before the eyes when reading; alternately very wide pupils, which finally remain dilated.

Pupils more contracted than usual; everything appears too bright.

Contracted pupils, head feeling dull, and weakness in the thighs.

Darkness before the eyes with white spots and strips; also black rings around the eyes; pupils very large after three fourths of an hour.

Mistiness and dimness before the eyes, with vertigo.

Sparks before the right eye; with nausea.

Black spots and a network (gauze) before the eyes.

The amaurotic symptoms are attended by dullness and heaviness of the head.

Ordinary light seems too bright.

Pressure above and in the depths of the eyes, especially when looking at an object by daylight.

Things at a distance look blurred; pressure in the forehead.

Photophobia, with pressure above and in the eyelids.

After a quarter of an hour the pupils much dilated. The inner rim of the iris appears a bright yellow, as if illuminated; bright spots and black network float before the eyes; sometimes a fog before the eyes.

Black rings before the eyes and dilated pupils.

Flickering before the eyes; ° before the headache.

Great weakness of sight, aggravated by bright sunlight; watery eyes.

° Erethic amaurosis.

Eyes very sensitive to the light, and while reading [all day].
Sensation as if too much light shining in the eyes; biting sensation in the borders of the eyelids; pressure above the eyes and in the depths of the eye, especially when looking at an object by daylight; things at a distance look blurred; pressure in the forehead, lasting half an hour.
Staring, humid and glistening eyes.
Pain over the left eye, with pain in the bowels.
Shooting pains over the right eye.
Pain in the inner canthus of the left eye.
Severe pain over the eyes, almost unbearable when looking at a bright object.
Eyes feel dull and heavy.
Burning in the eyes and nose, also redness of the eyes.
Sensation as if there was sand in the eyes.
Biting sensation in the edges of the eyelids.
Stinging in the inner angle of the right eye, lasting one hour.
Muscæ volitantes.
Fullness and extension in the eyes.
Burning sensation in the eyelids, and redness of the eyes.

[These symptoms are notable and important. Its action on the pupils is peculiar; the rule appears to be dilatation, but contraction sometimes occurs, and an alternate contraction and dilatation is frequent. With the dilated pupil occurs the majority of the amaurotic symptoms, the dimness of sight, black spots, etc. In this respect it resembles belladonna. With the contracted pupils we find photophobia, light spots, sparks, etc. It would seem that a condition of cerebral congestion was present with the contraction of the pupils. With nearly all the eye symptoms there occurs dullness and heaviness of the head, or severe pains over the eyes. The homœopathic occulist will doubtless find this remedy a valuable one in internal affections of the eyes, especially in amaurosis.—*Hale.*]

### Nose.

Discharge during the day of thin, watery fluid, with considerable sneezing.
Copious, watery discharge from the right nostril and obstruction of the left.

### Face.

Red, bloated face, with a look of fatigue.
Feverish flashes across the face.

Shooting pains from the lower jaw up into the left ear, coming suddenly and going as suddenly.

\* Erysipelas of the face.

Face hot, congested, with heat in the hands and along the back.

### Ears.

Stitches in the ears; buzzing before the ears.

Every sound he hears seems as if coming from a great distance.

### Mouth and Teeth.

Insipid taste in the mouth.

Mouth very dry; lips dry and blistered. (*v.*)

Tongue sore, as if burned.

Dryness of back part of tongue and roof of the mouth.

Constant stinging in the fauces when swallowing.

### Throat.

Left tonsil feels swollen, with soreness on swallowing.

Stitches in right side of the throat.

Sensation as of a splinter in the right tonsil.

Raw sensation in the throat, painful on swallowing.

Dryness of the throat and fauces.

Stitches from the fauces to the internal right ear.

### Pharynx and Œsophagus.

Burning in the œsophagus, arising from the stomach.

Cramp-like sensation in the œsophagus.

### Gastric Symptoms.

Loathing, vomiting of ingesta.

Copious vomiting of a greenish colored matter, accompanied by thirst, dilated pupils, stertorous respiration, convulsions and tetanic stiffness of the limbs.

Frequent vomiting, first of mucus, afterward of a bluish or grey blackish fluid.

Empty eructations, with burning in the stomach.

Violent heartburn, after eating and after retiring.

Nausea with sparks before the eyes.

### Stomach.

Severe burning in the stomach, with vomiting.

Sharp, cutting pains in and across the stomach, better on pressure or on bending over.

Burning in the stomach (*vv*), with yellow, watery diarrhœa.

Severe pain in the region of the stomach, extending to the region of the heart and left shoulder.

Severe cramps in the pit of the stomach, aggravated by walking, relieved by eating.

Pains in the region of the stomach, accompanied by madness, delirium and convulsions of the limbs.

Great pressure in the stomach, by spells.

Continued pain in the scrobiculus.

° Inflammation of the stomach and bowels.

### Abdomen.

Sharp pains in the intestines, as if cut with knives; relieved by eating.

Violent cutting in the umbilical region.

### Stool and Anus.

Diarrhœa next day after the dose.

Stools loose, semi-solid.

Loose evacuations, of a yellow color, somewhat watery, followed by burning pain in the stomach, accompanied with nausea.

Constipation, dry, hard stools, small in quantity. (*secondary effect.*)

Frequent, ineffectual urging to stool; at last nothing but wind escapes.

Tenesmus of the anus.

### Urinary Organs.

It has great diuretic power. (*secondary action.*)

The quantity of urine increased.

Sudden urging to urinate every ten minutes. (*Bute.*)

° Dropsy, from suppression of intermittent fever. (*Ruckert.*)

° Ardor urinæ. (*Eberle.*)

° Dropsy, with previous obstruction of absorbent system. (*Hahnemann.*)

### Respiratory Organs.

Difficulty in breathing; constriction of the chest.

Tickling sensation in throat, causing him to cough frequently.

Yellow, thick expectoration.

Beating pain in the left chest, in which there is a pain, as if sore, when touched.

Pressure on the sternum and tenth vertebra.

Anxious feeling in the region of the heart.

### Back and Extremities.

Dull, heavy pain in the right arm extending to the fingers.

Pain in the right knee, extending upward toward the hip.

Lancinating pain extending down the left arm.

Bruised feeling in the back and limbs; the neck feels stiff and sore, as if it had been bruised. (*vv.*)

Wandering pain; first in the shoulder, then down the arm, then in the lower extremities.

Cutting pain in the left side.

Legs feel sore, as if bruised, from walking.

Stiffness of the limbs.

Extraordinary convulsions of the limbs (in poisoning).

Great weakness in both knees, which scarcely allows walking.

Tearing on the dorsum of left foot, with creeping sensation in left calf.

Pain in left shoulder and right wrist joint.

Arms heavy as if beaten, especially the left.

Crampy convulsions in the left calf.

Painful drawing in the arms and feet.

Painful and itching sensation in the ulcers on the feet.

### Skin.

° Obstinate herpetic eruptions.

Copious perspiration.

Red, scarlet-like spots on the skin of irregular form, nearly over the whole skin.

Great sensitiveness of the cutaneous surface.

Spasms excited by touching the skin (in poisoning).

Eruptions of small red pimples on the forehead, sore to the touch and very hard.

A few small pimples on the back of the hand, itching violently.

Pustular eruptions. Ulcers. Desquamation of the skin.

° Foul and painful chronic ulcers. (*Eberle.*) *

° Scorbutic eruptions and ulcers of a cancerous nature.

° Syphilitic eruptions and nocturnal pains.

° Erysipelas (when the swelling is in small spots).

[* Eberle used for the cure of the above conditions doses of two grains of dried leaves, night and morning.—*Hale.*]

## Sleep.

Coma, alternating with convulsions and moaning.
Sleep disturbed by dreams of falling from a great height.
Dreams of snakes; frequently awaking in fright.
A feeling in the morning on waking as of great loss of sleep
Deep apoplectic stupor; coma and torpor, attended with fever
Lassitude of the whole body without inclination to sleep.
° Night terrors in children.

## Fever.

Dry, burning heat, with small frequent pulse.
Heat in the face, hands, and down the back.
Hot skin covered with sweat.
Excessive thirst.
Slightly feverish, with flashes of heat in the face.
High fever on retiring, lasting half an hour, followed by very
profuse perspiration of short duration.
Great thirst, causing him to drink often and in large quanti-
ties, accompanied with feverish heat and redness of the
face.
High fever, with great pain in back of the neck, shoulders and
lower extremities.
Flashes of heat running up and down the back.
Fever all the afternoon, with violent beating of the carotid
arteries, headache, pulse ninety-five.

## Circulatory System.

Small frequent pulse; quick, irregular pulse; pulse 90 to 95.
Circulation generally excited, violent throbbing in the head.
Pulse full and irregular; pulse small and slow.
Anxious feeling in the region of the heart.
Increased distension and prominence of the varicose veins.

## Spasmodic Symptoms.

Convulsions and spasms; they stretch their hands during the
spasms, as if they would grasp something. After this
the hands are carried to the mouth, and the boys (of two
or three years) chew and swallow (in poisoning).
Tetanic rigidity of the whole body.
Great restlessness; violent, convulsive restlessness. (*Hahnemann.*)

° Tremor; trismus; violent subsultus tendinum. (*H.*)

° [Raphania.] Characterized by painful creeping in the limbs, with distortion of the hands, convulsions, tonic spasms, occasional attacks of tetanus, epilepsy, imbecility, rage.

° Convulsions, with moaning and coma.

° Tingling in the extremities; preceding the convulsions.

° Contractions of the flexor tendons as though they would hop about.

° Spasmodic contortion of the extremities.

° Tonic spasms; epileptic attacks; rage.

° Imbecility, risus sardonicus; contraction of the hands.

° Drawing in the fingers; cramps in the calves; inversion of the feet.

### Generalities.

Violent pain in every muscle and joint of the body, on waking in the morning.

Severe pains, apparently in the muscles of the neck and between the shoulders. (*vv.*)

Shooting pain in left arm and wrist.

General muscular soreness.

Whole surface of body tender to the touch. (*vv.*)

General torpor of the whole system.

General inflammatory swellings.

External swelling, from external application.

Heat diffused in a few hours over the whole body; a profuse sweat succeeding this heat, and a purging next day (from three grains of the leaves).

If a sweat does not follow the heat, profuse urination occurs, followed by purging.

Tremors with great debility.

Complete insensibility, with relaxed muscles, flushed face; free, irregular pulse.

General, violent, convulsive restlessness.

Great sensitiveness to cold air.

Increased distension and prominence of the varicose veins.

Excessive fatigue from bodily exertion, with vertigo.

# STICTA PULMONARIA.
### (Lung-wort.)

BOTANICAL DESCRIPTION.—Thrallous, coriaceous, lax, lacunose, reticu.
late, dark green, and olive colored on the upper side; the under side
tomentose, with naked white spots; lobes elongated, separate, sinuate-
lobed, retuse truncate; apothecia (fruit-caps) submarginal, reddish. This
lichen is common, fertile, on trunks, in mountains and forests, also on
rocks, where it varies and is oftener sterile. It is found in New England,
New York, and Pennsylvania.

OFFICINAL PREPARATIONS.—Tincture of the lichen; dilutions.

ANALOGUES.—*Asclepias tuberosa, Calcarea carb., Causticum, Copaiva.
Dulcamara, Eryngium aq., Gelseminum, Hepar sulphur, Mercurius, Rumex,
Sanguinaria, Sulphur.*

### Mind.

\* General confusion of ideas—inability to concentrate them
on any subject.

\* Her legs felt as if floating in the air; she felt light and airy,
without any sensation of resting on the bed.

° Hysteria, after loss of blood; as soon as it came night her
feet and legs would dance and jump round in spite of
her; she had to hold them or have them held down.
(*Burdick.*)

° Strange sensation about the heart, after which she felt as if
floating in the air. (*Ib.*)

### Head.

\* Dull sensation in the head, with sharp pains in the vertex,
side of the face and lower jaw.

\* Dull, heavy pressure in the forehead and root of the nose.

° Migraine—a kind of sick headache. She has to lie down;
light and noise aggravate; nausea and vomiting nearly to
faintness. (*Lilienthal.*)

° Catarrhal headache before the discharge sets in; a very successful remedy.

### Eyes.

\* Burning in the eyelids, with soreness of the ball in closing
the lids, or turning the eyes.

° Catarrhal conjunctivitis, with profuse but mild discharge.

### Face.

Darting pains in the side of the face.

### Jaws.

Darting pains in the lower jaw.

## Nose.

* Feeling of fullness and heavy pressure at root of the nose; with tingling in right side of nose. (*Burdick.*)
° Acute catarrh of the nasal passages. (*Ib.*)
° Chronic catarrh of the head. (*Ib.*)
° Acute coryza with fever. (many cases.) (*Ib.*)
° Epidemic influenza, after the usual remedies failed. (*Petitt.*)
° Influenza: excessive and painful dryness of mucous membrane; the secretions rapidly dried and formed scabby concretions, requiring great effort to discharge them; the soft palate felt like dried leather, making deglutition painful; irritation in the chest, more in evening and night. Sticta was the only remedy that relieved. (*Boyce.*)

## Throat.

° Excessive dryness of the soft palate, with painful deglutition.
° Dropping of mucus down the posterior nares, and the throat feels and looks raw.

## Respiratory Organs.

° Catarrhal affections of the respiratory tract. (*Hale.*)
° Loose cough in mornings, less free during the day; pain in the left side below the scapula; tickling in the larynx and bronchia. (*Dr. Silas Jones.*)

[It relieves continuous racking cough—in consumption—which lasts for hours, and causes great exhaustion; also, "incessant wearing cough."]

° Whooping cough in the early stages. (*Ib.*)
° Croupy coughs—during catarrh or influenza. (*Ib.*)
° Bronchial catarrh with oppression of the chest; hard racking coughs, excited by inspiration. (*Ib.*)
° Pain reaching through the chest, from sternum to spinal column; arms powerless from extreme pain; difficult breathing and speaking. Cured in three days. (*Chase.*)

## Rheumatism.

* Darting pains in the arms, legs, shoulders, fingers, joints, thighs, knees, toes, etc.
* General feeling of dullness and malaise, as when a catarrh is coming on.
° Rheumatism of all the large and small joints, with swelling and pain. [Cured by Sticta 1st.]

38

° Rheumatism of the wrist joints, with pain and swelling. (*Ib.*)

° Swelling and stiffness of the hands and feet.

° Rheumatism in right shoulder joint, deltoid and biceps muscles, extending into the forearm; worse in the morning, better during the day. (*Chase.*)

° Rheumatism in the right ankle joint. (*Ib.*)

**Sleep.**

° Sleeplessness—one of the most efficient remedies. (*Burdick.*)

**Nerves.**

° It ought to cure hysterical chorea. [See Mind.]

---

# STILLINGIA SYLVATICA.

### (*Queen's-root.*)

BOTANICAL DESCRIPTION.—This plant is known also by the name of *Queen's-delight, yaw-root* and *silver-leaf;* it is an indigenous perennial, with herbaceous stems, two or three feet high. The leaves are alternate, sessile, oblong or lanceolate oblong, obtuse, serrulate, tapering at the base, and accompanied with stipules. The male and female flowers are distinct upon the same plant; they are yellow, and arranged in the form of a spike, of which the upper part is occupied by the male, and the lower by the female. The male florets are scarcely longer than the bracteal scales.

This plant is found growing in pine-barrens and sandy soils from Virginia to Florida, and in Mississippi and Louisiana, flowering from April to July. When wounded, the plant emits a milky juice.

The *root*, which is the officinal portion, is large, thick and woody, in long cylindrical pieces, from one-third of an inch to more than an inch thick, wrinkled when dried, externally of a dirty yellowish-brown color, and exhibiting, when cut across, an interior soft, yellowish, ligneous portion, surrounded by a pinkish-colored bark. It has a slight, peculiar, somewhat oleaginous odor, which is strong and acrimonious in the recent root, and the taste is bitterish and pungent, leaving an impression of disagreeable acrimony in the mouth and fauces. It imparts its virtues to water or alcohol, and deteriorates in activity by age. Its properties appear to be owing to a very acrid oil.

OFFICINAL PREPARATIONS.—Tincture of the root with strong alcohol; dilutions. Stillingia; triturations.

ANALOGUES.—*Aurum, Ammonium mur., Argentum, Corydalis, Hepar sulphur, Guaco, Iodide of potassium, Phytolacca, Mercurius, Rhus tox., Sulphur.*

### Mind and Disposition.

Intellect dull and stupid.

Unusually dull and sleepy, with headache.

Depression of spirits, with gloomy forebodings.

## Head.

Slight headache, extending from anterior portion of the temples,—pain is dull and constant; slight frontal headache, with high-colored and frothy urine.

Headache in the evening. A constant flowing pain as if there was a current running from the median line of the forehead over the vertex to the occipital process and left cerebellum (this continued three days).

A slight, constant, dull headache, with depression of spirits and with spells of neuralgic toothache.

A stupid headache through the temples, with slight nausea and white-coated tongue.

A slight but persistent, dull headache in the vertex.

A dull, heavy pain in the right side of the head.

A feeling as of a heavy substance pressing upon the brain (frontal region). After a time the pain becomes sharp and darting,—in fact, almost unendurable.

Pains in the head, with inflamed and watery eyes, and general soreness of the muscles.

Violent frontal headache, with stinging, darting pains in the face.

° Bony swellings on the head and forehead—on the latter as large as a hen's egg.

° Mercurial periostitis of the skull.

## Sensorium.

Dizziness, with throbbing in the head.

## Eyes.

Eyes inflamed and watery, with severe headache and general muscular soreness, as though he had taken cold.

## Ears.

Burning sensation in the left ear (in the evening), on which in the morning there was a vesicular eruption.

## Face.

Stinging, darting pains in the face.

Pain under malar-bone, extending transversely across the face.

° Periostitis of the facial bones.

## Nose.

Catarrhal discharge from the nose, at first watery, then muco-purulent, with soreness of mucous membrane, followed by a small abscess on the inside of the right nostril.

° Influenza (compare Phos., Merc., Kali iod., Arum tri.).

° Inflammation and necrosis of the bones of the nose.

### Mouth and Tongue.

Yellowish-white, heavily-coated tongue; white-coated tongue.

Slightly coated tongue, in the morning.

Scalded sensation on the tongue, with soreness in the region of the larynx.

### Jaws and Teeth.

Paroxysms of neuralgic toothache.

### Throat.

Dryness, rawness, and smarting of the fauces.

Constriction of the throat.

Stinging pains in the fauces.

Slight inflammation of the left tonsil, lasting several days.

Burning in the throat with painful deglutition.

### Taste and Appetite.

Bitter taste in the morning.

Increase of appetite.

### Gastric Derangements.

Slight nausea, with white coated tongue, stupid headache and lowness of spirits.

Nausea and vomiting.

Pyrosis, coming on about three o'clock P. M., each day, lasting until he went to sleep at night. (The prover not subject to this affection.)

Pyrosis commenced about two P. M., and continued until bedtime.

### Stomach and Abdomen.

Griping in the region of the epigastrium, soon followed by a diarrhœic evacuation, and an abundant and explosive discharge of flatus.

Sensations as if diarrhœa would set in.

Pains in the umbilical region.

A heavy pain in the hypogastric region.

Burning in the stomach and alimentary canal.

Peculiar disagreeable burning in the stomach and bowels.

° Colic, periodical; (?) (used as a preventive.) (*Eclectic.*)

### Stool and Anus.

Stool nineteen hours after the regular time, attended with considerable pain, which was confined to the rectum and sphincter ani.

Pain in the sphincter ani, as though it had been bruised.

Stool delayed four or five hours after the usual time.

### Urinary and Sexual Organs.

A short but severe pain in the region of the right kidney.

Dull pain across the region of the kidneys, and sharp pains in the penis, commencing in the morning and lasting all day.

Dull pains in the region of the kidneys.

Urine colorless; sp. gr., 1026, depositing, the next day, a white, flocculent, mucous sediment.

Urine increased from 33 to 45 ounces, and high colored, with brick-dust sediment.

Urine high colored, and inclined to foam and form bubbles.

Urine thick and milky — containing much chloride of sodium.

Abundant white sediment deposited soon after being voided.

All through the proving a peculiar, copious, brownish-red, mottled-looking sediment or cloud, looking like sausage meat macerating in water.

Violent, smarting, burning pains throughout the entire course of the urethra, aggravated by micturition, with difficulty in passing urine; and dull pain in the region of the kidneys. The pains in the urethra were so severe that it was impossible to remain quiet; but can detect no discharge.

While urinating, has a sharp pain in the glans penis, extending up the urethra.

The pains in the urethra were so severe as to cause the perspiration to start.

Urethral irritation and chordee.

* Gonorrhœa.   ° Gleet.   ° Leucorrhœa.

° Syphilis — primary, secondary, tertiary and mercurial.

### Respiratory Organs.

Slight uneasiness and tickling in the trachea and bronchi — worse on rising in the morning.

* Tickling sensation in the trachea toward evening, which caused a dry, spasmodic cough.
* A sensation of lameness, seemingly in the cartilages of the trachea.
* Constriction in the region of the larynx, with stinging and burning in the fauces.
* A bruised, sore feeling of the cartilages of the trachea when pressed.
* Cough deep and loose.

Dryness and soreness in the region of the larynx.

Oppression of the chest.

Short, hacking cough, with some inflammation of the fauces.

Darting pains through the thorax, with tickling in the throat, and short, hacking cough.

Sharp, darting pains through the chest and shoulders, quite marked.

° Incipient phthisis, in strumous habits.

° Bronchitis.  ° Laryngitis.

ᶜ Hoarseness and chronic laryngeal affections of public speakers.

° Croup.  (See the above laryngeal and tracheal symptoms.)

### Heart and Pulse.

Boring pains about the region of the heart, with irregular pulse and a feeling of distress.

Pulse about ninety; weak and very irregular, except at times during the day, when he would have spells as if the room was too warm, and the pulse would become regular with general perspiration.

Pulse irregular in the morning, more regular at noon, and at evening again becoming irregular.

Slow and irregular pulse on lying down.

Pulse full and very irregular.

### Back and Extremities.

Dull pains across the region of the kidneys on waking.

Sharp, darting pains through the shoulder and chest.

[In a recent proving by Dr. Preston, it developed "*aching* pains in the *feet*, on the instep, in the *hips, legs*, left lumbar region; stiffness of the joints; pains in the toes and external malleoli; in *elbow, forearm* and *wrist;* aching pains in the back, extending down the thighs and legs. Another prover, M. O. G., experienced sharp, shooting pains in the arms, legs and hands. It seems, says Dr. P., to act *first* upon the *right* side, then on the left, the pain following the direction of the long bones.—*Hahnemannian Monthly, Oct.* 1870, *page* 127.]

Aching of the lower extremities in the evening.

Excessive itching of the legs below the knees, continuing six or eight weeks, but no eruption; this itching occurred only upon the exposure of the parts to the atmosphere or cold — relieved by warmth and in bed.

° A pustular eruption on the arm, that had persistently remained a month, rapidly healed.

° Very large node upon the olecranon.

° Chronic eruptions on the hands and fingers.

° Enlargement of the tibia to such a degree as to deprive the child of all power of motion; her limbs were contracted and swollen.

° Ulcers on the legs — venereal, chronic, and indolent.

° Periostitis and nodes of the tibia.

### Skin.

Vesicular eruption on the ear.

° Pustular eruption on the arm.

Itching of the skin below the knees upon exposure to the atmosphere or cold; relieved by warmth or covering.

° Various chronic eruptions.

° Lepra and elephantiasis.

° Ulcers, with unhealthy skin.

° Scrofulous, venereal, and other skin diseases.

### Fever.

Cold on going to bed; immediately afterward, broke out in perspiration, but with excessive warmth all night.

Feverish heat in the evening.

### Sleep.

Unusual drowsiness all day, with general malaise and headache.

Very sleepy after eating. Dull and sleepy.

### General Symptoms.

Malaise and general drowsiness.

General feeling of distress.

° *Secondary syphilis;* in a case which had resisted all the usual homœopathic remedies. The man suffered extreme torture from *bone pains.* "It had a wonderful, and I might almost say, an instantaneous effect."

He has slept well ever since he had it. The immense *nodes* have gone from the head and legs; and from the most deplorably down-hearted, (sometimes almost raving, from derangement,) miserable, thin-looking object, he is changed into a buoyant, joking, rotund-looking fellow.— *Dr. Mahlon Preston, of Norristown, Pa.*

### Conditions.

Aggravated morning and evening (heart); on lying down (respiration); exposure to air (skin).

Ameliorated in the middle of the day (heart), by warmth and covering (skin).

Direction of pains: — From before backward (head, chest and penis).

Character of pains: — Dull, heavy, stitching, boring, stinging and neuralgic.

Sensations: — Scalding (throat); burning, smarting, dryness and constriction (throat).

---

# STRYCHNIA.

*Strychnia.*—An alkaloid obtained from the Nux Vomica and the Ignatia Bean.

It is a white or grayish-white powder. When rapidly crystalized from its alcoholic solution, it has the form of a white granular powder; when slowly crystalized, that of elongated octahedra, or quadrilateral prisms, with quadrilateral terminations.

It is permanent in the air, inodorous, but excessively bitter, with a metallic after-taste.

This bitterness is so intense that one part of it will impart a sensible taste to 600,000 parts of water.

It is soluble in 6667 parts of water at 50°, in 2000 parts at boiling point. In absolute alcohol and ether it is very sparingly soluble. Boiling officinal alcohol dissolves it without difficulty, and deposits it on cooling.

The *Sulphate* occurs in colorless prismatic crystals, efflorescent on exposure, inodorous, extremely bitter, fully soluble in water, sparingly soluble in alcohol.

*Phosphate of Strychnia* occurs in a white, amorphous powder, almost entirely insoluble in water, sparsely soluble in alcohol.

OFFICINAL PREPARATIONS.—Triturations (centesimal).

*Citrate of Iron and Strychnia* occurs in garnet red amorphous scales. Is soluble in water, insoluble in alcohol. It has an acid and ferriginous, and persistently bitter taste, and is deliquescent. It contains 1% strychnine.

OFFICINAL PREPARATIONS.—Triturations (decimal).

(*See Therapeutics, Vol. II.*)

# SULPHATE OF NICKEL.

*(Niccoli Sulphas.)*

PHARMACOLOGY.—Formed by dissolving Carbonate of Nickel in dilute Sulphuric acid, concentrating the solution and setting it aside to crystalize.

It is in the form of **emerald**-green crystals, efflorescent in the air, soluble in three parts **water**, **insoluble** in alcohol or ether; has a sweet, astringent taste.

OFFICINAL PREPARATIONS.—Triturations; aqueous solutions.

ANALOGUES.—*Arsenicum, Atropine, China, Quinine, Gelseminum, Kali brom., Zincum.*

*(No Provings.)*

° Violent periodical headaches. *(J. Y. Simpson.)*

[This eminent physician found it useful in periodical headaches of various kinds, after Arsenic and Quinine had failed to prevent their recurrence.]

° Periodical headache of many years standing. *(Hale.)*

[In two cases where I gave it for this affection it omitted the paroxysms, which did not return for nearly a year. The remedy omitted them again. It was prescribed in the 2d × trit. A grain three times a day.]

° Neuralgia.

["Mrs. B. had suffered with Neuralgia for more than three years. During the last two months the paroxysms had been very violent and frequent, occurring every few minutes. She had taken Iron, Quinine, Strychnine, Colchicum, Aconite, Morphine, Chloroform, Valerian, Zinc, Mercury and Electricity, with only temporary relief. I began by giving half grain doses three times a day. In less than a week the paroxysms were reduced to only one within twenty-four hours; then the paroxysms appeared later every day, and finally disappeared. It seems to act like Bromide of Potassium. It reduced the pulse and produced sleep. It soothed pain quicker than Morphine (in this case)."—*Dr. ——, Richmond Medical News.*]

° Periodical headaches, every two weeks, lasting three or four days. *(Dr. A. E. Small.)*

[In this case the pain seemed to be most acute at the root of the nose, extending to the vertex and through the temples. She had some nausea, but no vomiting. She was unable to raise her head from the pillow when the attack was on her. The distress was so great that she lay and groaned in anguish. Cuprum, Ignatia, Sepia, Calcarea and Sulphur did not relieve. Two-grain doses of the 3d × trit. every day suspended the paroxysms four months — a respite she had not enjoyed for ten years.—*U. S. Medical and Surgical Journal, Oct., 1871.*]

[The pathogenesis of *Carbonate of Nickel*—from Hartlaub & Trink's Annual — see Symptomen Codex — is quite suggestive in this connection, and contains some notable headache symptoms; but it seems to be a neglected remedy, as are some other apparently well proven medicines.--*Hale.*]

# SUMBUL.

### (*Musk-Root.*)

DESCRIPTION.—The Sumbul is a native of Central Asia; supposed to be an aquatic plant of the order of *Umbelliferæ.* The odor is that of musk; the taste an aromatic bitter.

OFFICINAL PREPARATIONS. —Tincture and triturations of the bark of the root; dilutions.

[From provings in Vol. ix., No. xxxvi., of the *British Journal of Homœopathy,* by Dr. Cattell.]

ANALOGUES.—*Arnica, Asafœtida, Castoreum, Coffea, Cactus, Camphor, Digitalis, Iberis, Ignatia, Lachesis, Naja, Nux moschata, Pulsatilla, Spigelia, Sulphur, Scutellaria.*

## Mental Sphere.

Very mirthful disposition; inclined to be gay, witty and smiling. (*p.*)

Fits of hysterical laughter and tears.

Frequent mistakes of writing or summing; one letter or figure is written for another.

Depression of spirits; provoked and enraged by the least irritation. (*s.*)

## Head.

Dull pain and tension; fullness of the head.

Round, sore elevations of the cuticle, on left parietal bone; painful when touched; dry, and coming off in dry scabs.

Vertigo on stooping, and from using warm water, moving about, or on rising from a seat; feeling a want of security.

Pains in the head relieved by the warmth of the fire.

## Face.

Reddish spots on the face, forehead, chin and cheeks, that contain either water or white, thick, curdy matter.

Numerous black pores on the face.

## Eyes and Ears.

Sudden sensation of foreign body in left eye, like dust, obscuring the sight.

Intolerance to light, with aching pain in left eye; worse when moving it.

Swimming before the eyes.

Loud ringing and hissing in both ears.

## Nose.

Skin peels off the nose in dry patches.

*Tenacious yellow mucus in the nose; worse in left nostril.*

[This symptom was prominent and persistent, and resembles the Sambucus catarrh. It ought to prove curative in the worst form of nasal catarrh. —*Hale.*]

## Mouth and Throat.

Erosion, burning heat and rawness in the throat, with tenacious mucus.

Brown coating on the tongue in the morning.

Tongue feels rough, as if scraped, with heat in the throat.

*Tenacious mucus in the throat.*

[The same catarrhal condition of the nasal passages extends into the throat and posterior nares. I would advise a trial of it in the *catarrhs of children, with great nervous irritation, sleeplessness and even spasms.—Hale.*]

## Stomach.

Burning, dry heat in the stomach.

Shooting pains in cardiac end of the stomach, with nausea.

Increased appetite. (*p.*) Loss of appetite. (*s.*)

Eructations of wind, with taste of food.

Pain as if a knife was cutting the stomach.

Aching in the stomach, increased by pressure.

## Abdomen.

Tensive pain and gnawing in right hypogastrium.

*Abdomen full, distended and painful.*

## Rectum and Stool.

Constipation for eleven days.

Stool, with great expulsive efforts, preceded by sickliness, commotion of intestines and sickly pain in left inguinal region; rather soft, very long and thin, with sensations as if rectum protruded and anus was not closed.

Frequent inclination to stool, which is likely to be loose.

Liquid and small stool, followed by burning and cutting in the anus.

Thin stools, scanty, with much tenesmus.

° *Ascarides*, with bloated, drum-like abdomen and constipation; picking at the nostrils. (Two cases cured by the fifteenth dilution.)

## Urinary Organs.

Urine clear, when passed, with white, small threads; after

some hours, a white cloud forms, in which the threads look like white spots.

White sediment; the urine passes freely and painless.

Urine clear, yellowish-red, cloud in the bottom, and an *oily pellicle on the surface.*

Urine deposits a rosy sediment.

Frequent desire to urinate.

### Sexual Organs.

*Male.*—Heat and burning sensation in the genitals.

Increased sexual desire, with frequent erections.

Tingling in glans penis; the left scrotum hot and inflamed.

Phimosis; excretion of whitish curdy matter abundantly between glans and prepuce; glans and prepuce bluish-red and swollen; testes on left side dark red, excoriated.

Saltish-smelling semen from genitals, with exudation of greenish-yellow pus from excoriated surface of scrotum.

Violent preputial gonorrhœa, oozing pains, feeling as if drops were passing from the end of penis.

Pains in penis when pendant; relieved by being kept up.

Dreams of an emission, at first with, then without, an emission (Dioscorea).

*Female.*—During catamenia, pains around the head, from cerebellum to frontal region.

Leucorrhœa (whites), especially after sitting, which continues.

° "Cork-screw" pains in the *left* region of the uterus and its appendages. (*Cattell.*)

### Larynx.

Cough from tickling in the throat.

Cough, hacking, detaching sweet mucus into the throat.

### Chest.

Dull pains through the left chest, worse on moving the left arm or leaning forward.

A jerking, inspiratory murmur, very distinct, below left nipple, over seat of pain; not so on right side.

Prickings in left chest, in a line with nipple, externally.

*Tensive* pain, like a string pulling, in right breast.

*Tightness, tensive, stretched* feeling across chest, between left breast and sternum, and in left breast, worse on inspiration.

[It corresponds to the symptoms of spasmodic and hysterical asthma. It is used as a "patent medicine specific" for asthma, and with some popularity. A Dr. Weaver, in *Investigator*, says it works like a charm in asthma, and that it arrested the paroxysm in an "old case." I think it will prove useful in cardiac-asthma.—*Hale*.]

### Heart and Circulation.

[In the *North American Journal of Homœopathy*, May, 1872, I published the following "Heart Symptoms of Sumbul," as a study, illustrative of the best plan of studying the cardiac symptoms of our medicines.—*Hale*.]

### Motor Symptoms.

*Palpitation of the heart*, with transient flushes of heat, irregular and weak pulse.

The heart beats softly, *as if in water*, with "sinking" of the heart, sickliness and faintness all over.

Palpitation of the heart, from the least exertion; going up stairs; increased by paying attention to it.

Violent and irregular palpitation, with bellows sounds.

Palpitation and jerking of the heart, at intervals, worse during the flushes of heat, after drinking "stout," and in the evening.

Intermittent palpitation, uneasiness over the heart, jerking whilst lying down or sitting.

Pulse: *irregular pulse;* at times *weak*, at other times *strong*, ranging from 100 to 70 per minute; always *compressible*, and attended with transient flushes of feverish heat; skin moist.

Pulse very irregular, strong, then "narrow," or weak, low, with occasional full, quick beats, 100 to 60, compressible; with coldness of the body.

### Physical Signs.

The action of the heart full and sharp, strokes at times irregular, beating rapidly eight or ten times, then slowly, (like Arnica and Spigelia.)

Heart's impulse strong, *jerking*, especially after exertion, or when ascending stairs, and during digestion.

Posteriorly, over left scapular region, an indistinct viscid murmur and purring sound, similar to that which has been supposed to depend on muscular contraction, and often associated with rheumatism (like Spigelia); this sound is not heard at all, anteriorly.

Bellows sound of the heart, with violent and irregular palpitations, and flushes of heat in floods from the back.

[These last two symptoms were removed by Spigelia 3d.]

### Sensory Symptoms.

Lancinations and biting pains in left breast, increased by a deep inspiration.

Sharp pains, like a knife, in the left chest, every day.

*Tightness* — a tensive, stretched feeling across the chest, between left breast and sternum, and in left breast; worse on inspiration.

*Oppression* in left chest, clogged sensation, as if it were difficult to force the blood through that lung; (s.) worse on stooping.

Chest on left side feels loaded and oppressed, with choking constriction (in chest). (?)

Dull, tensive pains and pricking in left chest, under armpit and near nipple, in a line with it externally.

Dull pains through the left chest, worse on moving the left arm or leaning forward.

Dull, tightened pain in left chest, on blowing the nose.

Pain like a knife darting through left chest, from a spot a little below the breast, with flashes of heat; worse after meals; with irregular pulse.

Pricking as of needles in left chest.

### Concomitant Symptoms.

*Near.*—Aching, bruised, beaten sensation in the muscles of the left arm.

The hand (left) was ruddy, with distended veins, flushes of heat, and very irregular pulse.

The left hand red, with painfully distended veins; the veins become empty when raising the arm, but painfully distended on depressing it.

*Left* arm numb, heavy, and weary, with sharp, wiry, shooting of the fingers, laterally, and in the joints of second and fourth fingers.

The left arm easily numbed by the slightest cold, or by resting it on anything; causing tingling, pricking numbness; the lateral surfaces of the fingers felt sore, and the arm felt bruised. The left arm and hand is easily chilled and numbed in the cold, despite gloves and friction; the fingers, especially the third and fourth, are then bluish-white; the nails blue, with a sensation as if they were being rooted up; when brought into the warmth, this hand is slow in recovering itself, and held near a fire, or in a heated room, its vessels become distended much more than those of the right, and in a cool temperature this is some time in disappearing. (The left suspender is inclined to slide off the shoulder.)

The whole *left side* of the body is similarly affected, easily benumbed, with loss of elasticity in the blood vessels.

*Flushes of heat*, with dry or moist skin; palpitation of the heart, and irregular compressible pulse; sensation of throbbing in neck, head, (left side most.)

*Remote.*—Vertigo on stooping, or using warm water; fainting, swimming before the eyes, loud singing and hissing in both ears, weakness and trembling; worse in evening.

Faint feeling, and tendency to faint on slightest exertion, after excitement, and on hearing music.

*Hysterical* mood (even in men); alternate laughter and tears; easily excited; emotional; irritable; fidgety; at first the spirits are exalted, then depressed.

Dreams of falling from a great height.

An oily pellicle on the urine, and a tenacious, ropy, rose-colored sediment.

Rheumatic pains in various parts of the body, joints, muscles, especially of the *left* side.

### Neck.

Pressive feeling on nape of neck, left side, which is swollen and hot.

Sensation of throbbing in neck and nape of neck, on left side, increased by heat.

### Back.

Aching pain across the lumbar region of the back.

Pains in left lumbar region of back, and pricking in right side
  under the ribs.
Frequent chills through the back, with debility.
Frequent feeling as if hot water passed through the lumbar
  vertebræ.
Tensive pains and pulsations in swelling, extending down left
  side of spinal column, not tender to touch or pressure.

### Extremities.

Aching, beating sensation in muscles, chiefly triceps of left
  arm.
Rheumatic pain from right knee to ankle, when walking.
Tensive pain in left shoulder.
Aching pain down left arm, and in knuckle joint of the fore
  finger.
Debilitated muscular power.
Jerking in the limbs and starts in the muscles, even to contor-
  tion of the whole body.
Aching in knee joints, worse from heat.
Sensation (painful) as if internal ligaments of right knee were
  loosened, on stepping.
Shooting pain from back of ring finger to wrist of left hand,
  (ulnar nerve).
Twitching pain in left iliac region.
Numbness of left arm.

### Sleep.

Sleep, with prolonged amorous dreams.
Unpleasant dreams, not frightful.
Sleeplessness, from nervous excitation.

### Fever.

Dry, transient heat over the body, increased by exertion.
All the symptoms accompanied by heat.
Flushes of heat in the throat, mouth and head.
Sensation of cold wind blowing on the lumbar region.
Heat and profuse sweat at night in bed.
Coldness of the body; pulse 66.
° Marked benefit in low and nervous fevers succeeding typhus.
* Typhoid fever, with cerebral excitement.
Numbness and coldness of the tips of the fingers.

### Skin.

Itching in the skin; miliary spots on back, especially right shoulder blade and hip, which provokes scratching till they bleed.

Skin dry, as if washed in acid water.

Coldness, and dry, white shrunken skin.

* Porrigo in infant, on the left scalp; spots round and dry, slightly raised and reddened at the edges, with bran-like scales in the centre. (*Dr. Cattell.*)

### Generalities.

° Dropsy, dependent on impaired nervous vitality.

° Hysteria and hysterical spasms.

° Epilepsy; she falls suddenly forward, foaming at the mouth; unconsciousness. (*Dr. Cattell.*)

° Chorea, with ravenous appetite, constant jerking of limbs and head, with protrusion of the tongue; happy disposition, with continued and inappropriate smiling; constipated bowels; vomiting of food; idiotic expression; fears she shall go mad. (*Ib.*)

* Tendency to faint from the slightest cause. (*Ib.*)

A want of elasticity in the blood vessels.

---

# TANACETUM VULGARE.

### (*Tansy.*)

DESCRIPTION.—Tansy has a perennial, moderately creeping root, and an erect, herbaceous, somewhat six-sided, leafy, solid, striated, smooth *stem* one to three feet in height, and branched above into a handsome corymb of flowers. The *leaves* are smoothish, dark green, doubly and deeply pinnatifid. The *flowers* are golden-yellow, and arranged in dense, terminal, many-headed, fastigiate corymbs. There is a variety called *Double Tansy*, *Tanacetum Crispum*, with crisped and dense leaves.—*L. W. G.*

HISTORY.—Tansy is indigenous to Europe, but has been introduced into this country; it is cultivated by many, and also grows spontaneously in old grounds, along roads etc., flowering in the latter part of summer. The whole plant is official; it has an unpleasant, aromatic odor, and a strong, rather pungent and bitter taste, which properties it owes to a yellow or greenish volatile oil, which possesses in a strong degree the taste and odor of the plant, a sp. gr. of 0.952, and ultimately deposits a camphor. Its medicinal properties are extracted by alcohol, ether, chloroform, and by water in infusion. Drying impairs much of its activity.

(Symptoms *not* marked, came from tincture.)

39

## Mind.

Inability to think coherently.

Confusion of thought. (*oil.*)

Mind *unusually clear*, seemed able to accomplish **anything** intellectually. (*secondary.*)

Sadness. with desire to be let entirely alone. (*P. M.*)

Fatigue of the mind after the least exertion. (*oil.*)

Gay and ambitious. (*secondary.*)

Wants to stand on his head, stretches and draws up his feet, and says "it does me good." Irritable and lazy, very nervous and low spirited, annoyed by trifles; noise of the children almost unbearable.

Extremely sensitive to noise.

Dullness of all the senses. (*oil.*)

Coma and *violent convulsions.* (*Poisoning.*)

## Head.

Sensation of fullness. (15 *minutes.*)

Sense of uneasiness, but no pain in the head.

Dull, heavy, confused sensation in the head.

Slight giddiness. (½ *hour.*)

Headache and depression of spirits.

Headache with *nausea* and *dizziness.*

Nervous headache and *nausea*, from excitement; 4 P. M. headache and nausea, especially in *warm room;* the nausea partially relieved by eating.

Dull pain in temples, particularly right, also in forehead; rest of head unusually clear.

Dull pain over whole head, especially temples and forehead, with excessive sleepiness.

Lameness and soreness in base of brain.

Aggravation of headache in the close room.

Sensation as if something closed the ears very **suddenly. (*oil.*)**

## Ears.

Ringing in the ears, dizziness. (20 *minutes.*)

Stitches in the internal ear. (*oil.*)

Roaring in the ears. (*oil.*)

## Eyes.

Agglutination of the lids in the morning. (*oil.*)

Dull, aching pains in the eyeballs. (*oil.*)

## Nose.

Dryness of the nostrils. (*oil.*)

Profuse secretion of mucus in nose, with frequent coryza. (*oil.*)

## Face.

Sense of fullness. (15 *minutes.*)

Burning sensation, flushed.

Twitching in the face over left molar bone at intervals during the day.

Lips dry, parched, must be frequently moistened by tongue.

## Mouth, Tongue and Teeth.

Sore mouth, not quite apthous.

Flat, insipid taste. (*oil.*)

Bad taste in the mouth.

Frothing at the mouth. (*oil.*)

Mouth and tongue very dry upon awakening.

Tongue feels rough. (*oil.*)

Tongue coated white and looks frothy.

Toothache, dull, in the right lower molar.

Soreness of upper teeth, right side, on closing the mouth.

## Throat.

Roughness of the throat. (*oil.*)

Feeling in the throat as if would cough all the time, without being able to cough, during whole proving. (*oil.*)

## Stomach.

*No appetite*, thoughts of eating unpleasant, but not while eating, except sweet things or soft food, like oat-meal, etc., which increases the *nausea*. Food has no relish, directly after eating little, but *thirsty*. Sweets and soft food are very *nauseating*.

*After eating, pain in the bowels*, urgent stool relieves; *intense thirst*, especially for cold water; *intense nausea* all day, with increased watery menses, or with suppression of the menses.

*Excessive nausea* soon after rising, continuing severe all day, with temporary relief from eating; weight at the stomach.

Drawing, cutting pains in the epigastrium many times. (*oil.*)

Nausea greatly increased by eating *sweet things* or *soft food*, like oat meal, etc.

Nausea and bilious vomiting.

Eructations tasting of tansy ($\frac{1}{2}$ hour); of sour air. (*oil.*)

Eructations with relief; sense of heat in stomach (immediate),

Sharp, stitching pain in whole umbilical region. (*oil.*)

### Abdomen.

Sensation of warmth over whole abdomen. (15 *minutes.*)

Dull pains in right hypochondria, sharp pains in left. (*oil.*)

*Pains in bowels after eating*, and within an hour soft stool with relief.

On awaking in the morning, dull pain in hypogastric and iliac regions as if menses would appear; this pain continues all through the morning with slight nausea, pain around the waist and from thence down to the knees.

Pain in region of liver while sitting.

Constant dull pain in liver, which seemed sometives to prevent lying on the right side.

Feeling of weakness in abdomen, with disinclination to stand erect and intense sleepiness, especially between 11 A. M. and 2 or 3 P. M.

Weakness of abdominal muscles, also tension, causing inclination to stoop forward.

Hard, dull, aching pain in the whole of the bowels, constant symptom. (*oil.*)

Frequent colicky pains in the umbilical region, through the day, and especially at 4 A. M., for two weeks. (*oil.*)

Constant, hard, drawing pains in left groin. (*oil.*)

### Stool, etc.

*Pain in the bowels relieved by stool.*

*Desire for stool almost immediately after eating.*

Constant urging in rectum, with pain while passing stool, relief after; stools soft and painless during the day, but oftener than usual; constipation, yet urging quite frequent after eating, particularly morning; diarrhœa from large doses. (*oil.*)

Soft papescent stools, preceded by sharp, cutting pains in the umbilicus. (*oil.*)

### Urine.

Constant inclination to urinate, with dull, heavy pain in the small of the back. (*secondary.*) (*oil.*)

At first suppression, followed by profuse flow. (*oil.*)

Urine very scanty and cloudy.

Urine thick, pinkish and cloudy.

Frequent desire to urinate — three times in four hours — not strangury.

Emission of large quantities of normal urine; urine fetid. (*oil.*)

Urine light-colored, pale, increased.

Urine strongly impregnated with the odor of tansy.

Urine slightly scalding.

Urine high colored. (*oil.*)

### Female Genitals.

Scanty menstruation.

Suppression of the menses, with *intense nausea*, and scanty urine with cloudy deposit.

Menses three days too soon and scanty, with little pain.

Increased watery menses with *nausea*.

Menses *very scanty and pale*, almost ceasing at times.

Menses appeared at right time, but very pale and watery, with soreness and swelling of abdomen.

Severe pain in uterine region, back and limbs, with *nausea*.

On awaking in the morning, dull pain in hypogastric and iliac regions, as if menses would appear; the pain continues all through the morning, with slight nausea, pain around the waist and from thence down to the knees.

*Abortion*, with spasms and hæmorrhage. (*oil.*)

Very much interferes with the development of the fœtus.

Labia excoriated and slight leucorrhœa.

### Chest.

Constant tickling sensation in larynx and fauces, that produces a constant inclination to cough, but no coughing. (*oil.*)

Difficult respiration, with irregular pulse and frothing at the mouth. (*oil.*)

Strong desire to draw a full breath, which did not relieve the oppression of the chest.

Dull pain through right lung, *from front to shoulder blade.*

Feeling of numbness in right lung, shoulder and arm.

Constant pain under right shoulder blade.

Swelling of left axillary glands.

Respiration disturbed, laborious. (*Poisoning.*) (*oil.*)

Heart gradually becomes weaker until death; pulse irregular (*Poisoning*); pulse 98, temperature 99, 5, F.

Pulse 115, temperature 100, 5, F. (*after* 2¾ *hours.*)

### Back.

Severe, dull pain in lumbar region.

Constant, dull pain in back and in region of liver.

Constant, dull, aching pain in lumbar region for ten days. (*oil.*)

Severe attack of lumbago, all one evening. (*oil.*)

### Neck.

Left sub-maxillary glands swollen and sore.

Pain and stiffness in right sterno-mastoid, when turning head to the left.

Dull darting pain in back of neck simultaneous with pain in both shoulders and arms.

Stiffness of the muscles of the neck.

### Extremities.

Left wrist very lame and sore in the morning. (*oil.*)

### Upper.

Dull, darting pain through both shoulders, arms and in back of neck, rheumatic in character.

Pain in muscles of left arm from elbow to shoulder.

Stiffness of muscles of right shoulder and neck, extending later down right side.

### Lower.

Soreness and lameness in right leg from inguinal region to knee.

Great weakness of the legs with general prostration of strength.

Spasmodic contractions of legs. (*oil.*)

### Sleep.

Went to bed drowsy, but not restless.

Intense sleepiness, especially between 11 A. M. and 2 to 3 P. M.

Sleepy all the afternoon, could not apply herself to anything; 2 A. M. awoke with hiccough, lasting an hour.

Uneasy sleep, awaking with sharp, darting, stitching pain low in uterine region, lasting until dressed.

Restless, sleepy, but cannot sleep.

Very sleepy, especially in a close, warm room.

Dreaming of ridiculously unnatural things in early morning sleep.

### Generalities.

Great mobility; extraordinary motions and strange gesticulations. (*Lippe.*)

St. Vitus dance. (*Ib.*)

Slight rheumatic shooting pains in different parts of the body, particularly in left arm.

" Laziness " all through; not a stupor, but an uneasy desire to do something, yet nothing was the right thing.

Intense feverish heat throughout the body.

Tired feeling when walking.

Excitement causes nervous headache and *nausea.*

A tired, nervous feeling all the time.

Dull pain in limbs and back; uneasiness, compelling frequent changes of position, most comfortable on the *left* side.

Feeling of numbness in right lung, shoulder and arm.

Neuralgic pain in muscles of various parts of the body, and in muscles of hips and neck a stiffness with every motion, which commenced in morning and continued all day. Frequent and violent clonic spasms, with disturbed respiration. (*Poisoning.*)

Prickling sensation coming and going in the extremities and along the spine, with flashes of heat.

### Conditions.

*Aggravation* in general, in a close room.

Evening exhaustion.

*Amelioration* when walking out doors.

Feel better generally in the evening than in middle of the day.

---

# TARANTULA.

OFFICINAL PREPARATIONS.—Triturations of the whole spider.

ANALOGUES.—*Agaricus* (?), *Cimicifuga* (?), *Crotalus* (?), *Naja* (?), *Lachesis* (?), *Mygale* (?), *Stramonium* (?).

[The extraordinary pathogenesis of this remedy, published in the *No.* *American Journal of Homœopathy,* is one of the creations which I am no ready to accept. I would call attention to the criticism of Dr. S. A. Jones, in the *American Homœopathic Observer,* which I fully endorse.—*Hale.*]

° Chorea, according to the testimony of several physicians, who assert it has been useful in some of the more aggravated forms.

# THASPIUM AUREUM.
### (*Meadow Parsnip.*)

BOTANICAL DESCRIPTION.—This is a perennial herb, growing by moist river banks, flowering in June. *Stem* branched, one to two ternately divided or parted (or rarely some of the root-leaves simple and heart-shaped), the divisions or leaflets oblong-lanceolate, very sharply cut, serrate, with a wedge-shaped, entire base. *Flowers* deep yellow; fruit oblong, oval, with ten-winged ridges. The whole plant is glabrous. The *root* is from two to four inches long, not larger than the little finger, distinctly and rather deeply yellow internally; externally brown. It has, when fresh, a strong, unpleasant, and rather nauseating odor, not unlike that of Conium. It has an aromatic, pungent taste, remaining long in the mouth, and is disagreeable and loathsome to the stomach.

In the Transactions of the New York State Hom. Soc. is a careful comparison of the botanical differences of the Zizea and Thaspium, which prove quite conclusively that the pathogenesis published under Zizea really belongs to Thaspium aureum. Dr. J. S. Douglas, the author of the paper, contends that the Z. integerima could not have caused the symptoms said to belong to Zizea. Moreover, the plant once known to botanists as Z. aureum, is now removed to the genus Thaspium. I have, therefore, taken the liberty to place the pathogenesis under that name.

OFFICINAL PREPARATIONS.—Tincture of the fresh root with strong alcohol; dilutions.

ANALOGUES.—*Agaricus, Æthusa, Belladonna, Cicuta, Œnanthe, Stramonium, Solanum.*

### Mental Sphere.

Depression of spirits, with disgust of life.

Depression of spirits, followed by great exhilaration.

Laughing and weeping moods in alternation.

### Head.

Sensation of tightness around the head.

Acute aching pain in the whole left side of the head.

Rush of blood to the head and face, with feeling of fullness.

Pressure upon the top of the head.

Severe pain in the right temple with nausea.

Headache, with nausea; inclination to bilious vomiting.

Light, noise and jarring aggravate.

*Pain permanent on the right side*, associated with back-ache.

° Migraine with acid and bitter vomiting. (*Marcy.*)

° Neuralgia of the head. (*Ib.*)

### Eyes.

Redness of both eyes, which are sensitive to light.

Sharp pains in the right orbit, increased by moving the balls, stooping and stepping.

° Shooting pains through both orbits.

Yellowish, muco-purulent secretion, glueing the lids together.

Right eye is more particularly affected.

### Nose.

Burning and smarting sensation in the nostrils and eyes.

Discharge of mucus.

Obstruction and soreness of the right nostril, which is painful to the touch.

° Cold in the head, with sneezing and watery discharge.

° Chronic catarrh, with yellow and fœtid discharge.

### Face.

Face pale and puffy.

Redness and heat of the cheeks.

Boring pains in the cheek bones.

### Appetite and Taste.

Craving for acids and stimulants.

Tongue covered with a whitish fur in the middle, and reddened at the tips and sides.

Unusual sensitiveness to cold or warm drinks.

### Stomach.

Nausea; acid and bilious vomiting.

Pressure occasions nausea and faintness.

### Generative Organs.

*Male;* Sexual power increased.

° Great lassitude following coitus.

*Women:* Acrid leucorrhœa; profuse leucorrhœa.

Sudden suppression of the menses.

Profuse menstruation for one day, followed by acrid leucorrhœa.

° Leucorrhœa, with retarded and suppressed menses.

° Intermittent neuralgia of left ovary.

### Chest.

Dry cough, with shooting pains in the chest.

Pleuritic stitches in the right side, increased by coughing, or taking a long breath.

Pressure excites pain in intercostal muscles.

Sharp pains extending from the sides of the chest to both shoulder blades.

Asthmatic respiration with inability to retain a recumbent position.

° Cough which is tight, with stitches in chest, worse in the evening and during the night.

### Back.

Dull, aching pains under the right scapula.

Severe shooting pain extending from front part of the thorax to the scapula.

Smarting, burning pain in small of back.

Dull pains in loins, increased by movement.

### Upper Extremities.

Lameness in the muscles of both arms.

### Lower Extremities.

Dragging sensation in both hips.

Unusual tired feeling of the legs after the slightest muscular exertion.

### Nervous System.

Convulsions.

° Epilepsy.

### Sleep.

Exhilaration of all the faculties, followed by strong desire to sleep.

Spasmodic twitching during sleep.

### Fever.

Feverish symptoms, accompanying severe stitching pains in the chest.

Fever, with headache, pain in back, thirst, dryness of the mouth.

Chilliness and heat alternating with faintness, nausea, and pain in right temple.

Redness of the eye-balls, dry and red tongue, and thirst for cold water.

Hot flushes in face and head, followed by perspirations.

Chilliness, accompanied with spasmodic twitchings of the muscles of the face and upper extremities, followed by fever.

Flushed cheeks, hot head, visible pulsations of the carotid and temporal arteries.

**Skin.**

Itching pimples on forehead, wrists and legs.

Redness of one cheek and paleness of the other.

White and puffy appearance of the whole body.

---

# THERIDION CURASSAVICUM.

*(A small Spider found on orange trees in the West Indies.)*

OFFICINAL PREPARATIONS.—Triturations.

ANALOGUES.—*Aconite, Belladonna, Calcarea, Graphites, Ignatia, Lycopodium, Spigelia, Sepia, Solanum.*

**Mental Sphere.**

Despair; want of self-confidence.

Very joyous; he sings, although the head is internally hot.

Aversion to professional labor.

Thinking is hard for him when it is of a comparative nature, but not when it is creative; he can easily write out a case or problem, but finds it difficult to select remedies; writes a treatise with facility, but finds it hard to classify and determine places in systems.

**Head.**

Much vertigo on every occasion, particularly on stooping.

Vertigo and nausea increased to vomiting.

Vertigo increased by every noise and sound.

* Attacks of vertigo and vomiting, with cold sweat, were changed in such a manner by Theridion, that the nausea, always occasioned by closing the eyes, now appears on opening them, so that she must keep her eyes constantly closed. (*Hering.*)

* Vertigo, together with blindness, caused by pain in the eyes.

* The headache is such that she cannot describe it, and cannot make it clear to herself.

Headache like a pressing band in the root of the nose, and over and around the ears.

* Pains principally in region of eyes, with starting in right eye. (*Neidhard.*)

* Suddenly in the morning, pressing pain over left eye, aggra-

vated by the slightest motion, talking; at the same time, sickness of stomach, with retching; better from drinking warm water; bowels open, with colic and flatulency, after which the head is worse.

\* Throbbing over left eye, and across the forehead, also in a slight degree in the right eye, with sick stomach, particularly on rising from a reclining position — like sea-sickness — the pain was at first aggravated from the medicine, but disappears entirely in one hour.

Headache is the beginning of every motion.

ᶜ Violent frontal headache, with throbbing extending into occiput.

° The least motion of the head while lying increased headache and nausea.

ᵓ The walking of persons over the floor increases the headache.

ᵓ The least noise aggravates the headache.

ᵓ Headache of the worst kind, with nausea and vomiting, like sea-sickness, and with shaking chills. In several cases of women in the climacteric year. (*Neidhard.*)

° Sunstroke. (*Hering.*)

## Eyes.

\* Hard, heavy, dull pressure behind the eyeballs. (*Wells.*)

She lost her vision; everything seemed very far, as a veil was drawn before her; it blazed and flickered before her eyes; she was obliged to lie down. Even when closing the eyes flickering continued. Thereupon she became very weak, and the head was much affected.

ᶜ For many years, flickering before the eyes, in frequent paroxysms.

° Flickering before the eyes in hysterical subjects.

° Sensitiveness to light; when she is in the light she experiences a "dark sparkling" before her eyes; everything appears double, and through this "fluttering" nausea is created, accompanied by cold hands. Long afterwards she dare not stoop.

° On closing the eyes, nausea and vomiting. (*Hering.*)

When her eyes closed (with weariness or sleep) the dizziness and nausea reappeared.

### Ears.

* Rushing like a waterfall in both ears.
° The least noise aggravates the headache.
° Itching behind the ears, so that she would like to scratch them off.

### Face.

In the morning, on awakening, and sometimes at other times of the day, the lower jaw is immovable; but then opens, as it were, of its own account.

Froth before the mouth, with shaking chill.

Tetanus (with trismus).

Paroxysm of frequent, violent sneezing, and frequent necessity of blowing the nose; thereupon heaviness deep above in the nose.

### Mouth.

Tongue seems as if burnt; it is so numb that she can tell nothing properly.

Mouth so impure, as if the teeth were full of slime, must rinse the mouth frequently.

Salty taste, and hawking up of salty mucus.

Every sound penetrates the teeth.

Teeth, gums and palate affected by burning and tensive pain.

### Appetite.

Appetite for acidulous fruits.

Constant desire for food and drink, he knows not what.

Much thirst; after drinking, sweat.

Thirstless, with coldness.

### Stomach.

* Nausea and vomiting, like sea-sickness, with headache. (*Neidhard.*)
* Nausea called forth by the sparkling before the eyes.
* Nausea and vomiting when closing the eyes, and on motion "feels thick in the head." (*Hering.*)
° A woman having had (in childbed) a violent spell of sickness at the end of the first week, and apparently recovered, was, in the third week, after washing clothes, suddenly attacked by nausea and vomiting; after it, very pale, and sick at the stomach as soon as she closed her eyes, with

vanishing of her thoughts. She recovered completely. (From olfaction of the 30th.)

° Nausea always increased when he closed his eyes.

° Nausea increased when he gazed steadfastly at an object.

Nausea on moving.

° Talking creates nausea and vomiting.

° Nausea created by fast riding in a carriage, in hepatic diseases.

° Sensitiveness of the region of the stomach and epigastrium.

### Hypochondria.

* Violent burning pain in hepatic region, which grows still more painful when being touched; during the pains, retching, vomiting, finally bringing up bile.

° In abscess of the liver, Theridion relieves vertigo and nausea.

° Anthrax of sheep, with great tumefaction of hypogastrium and with great thirst. The adipose skin of the whole posterior belly suddenly swelled, became hot, tense, sooner or later it was red, blue, and finally gangrenous. As soon as it became red the appetite vanished. Immediately an appearance of swelling, great thirst, constantly increasing. If the sheep could reach a puddle of manure water, they would lie down in it as well as in the water-trough; sheep never do this when in health. Theridion cured all cases when the swelling had not turned blue. (*Braun.*)

° A cow was tied to a stake, in the heat of summer, suddenly became restless, wild, and her whole body swelled visibly; and bellowing, she tried to break the chain; after a dose of Theridion, she recovered within one hour. (?!) (*Ib.*)

### Stool and Anus.

Scanty discharge, with much urging (tenesmus).

Diarrhœa, without colic, with the vomiting and vertigo at night.

° Bowels open twice, with colic and flatulency, after which the headache is worse.

The anus protrudes and is painful, especially while sitting, without hemorrhoidal bunches, which he usually has frequently; this passes off, returns again later, and the hemorrhoidal tumors appear.

(A spasmodic contraction of rectum and anus returns again.)

### Urine.

Much urination with a young man disposed to it.

Increased urination in an elderly woman not disposed to it.

### Generative Organs.

*Male.*—(Upon the glans little red spots.)

Scrotum very much shrivelled.

The excessive sexual desire is immediately lessened, but the usual morning erections appear.

Sexual desire appears to have vanished, nor will erections take place.

Strong erections in the morning, without desire.

While at sleep after dinner, a seminal emission, very violent and profuse.

*Women.*—Menses omitted after the proving more than ten weeks, in a woman in the climacteric years, but who in the following year gave birth to a son.

° Hysterical affections during puberty. (*Hering.*)

° Hysterical affections in climacteric years. (*Ib.*)

° Affections in climacteric years; headache of the worst kind.

° From washing in third week after confinement, attack of fainting.

### Chest.

Night cough.

Violent stitches up high in the chest, beneath the left shoulder, even up into the throat.

### Heart.

\* Anxiety about the heart. (*Braun.*)

° Slow pulse, with vertigo. (*Wells.*)

### Upper Limbs.

Stinging pain from elbow to shoulder.

Violent burning, itching on inner and upper part of left ring finger; the spot becomes very red; soon disappears.

### Lower Limbs.

Itching and knots on the nates.

Swelling of the feet. (Secondary effect of the bite.)

Pains in all bones as if broken; as if they were about to fall asunder.

Heaviness in all limbs before the chill

She is so weak that she cannot stand long; she becomes **trem-ulous** and perspires.

° Weakness, that all the limbs tremble.

Great inclination to be startled, with many provers.

° Hysteria.

### Sleep.

Sleepy after breakfast, before the chill; sleeps throughout the whole day.

Long and dreamful mid-day sleep; dreams of journeys in distant regions, and riding on horses; a person who scarcely ever sat upon a horse.

While sleeping he often bites into the point of his tongue, so that it is sore the following day; occurs frequently, even after the lapse of weeks.

* *Paroxysm.*—She awakes after a short sleep, at 11 o'clock; already in sleeping she felt the vertigo, and was awakened thereby; could not remain lying; tried to reach the chamber-pot, but fell down as if in a swoon; cold sweat broke out; she strains to vomit, till this takes place and is repeated every quarter of an hour; during which icy perspiration breaks out all over her; at the same time she has several attacks of diarrhœa, without abdominal pain. At first she vomited acid, slimy water, almost preventing her from regaining her breath. At length she felt entirely empty at the stomach. The least motion again brought on vertigo and vomiting; she dares not to stir, and, when her eyes dozed, the lids feeling as it were from being tired, vertigo and nausea immediately returned. In the morning, on rising, the nausea came again, and she vomited bile.

### Chill Fever and Sweat.

Violent shaking chill, during which foam appears at the mouth, after the bite.

Shaking chill during headache, with vomiting.

After breakfast, heaviness in every limb; he must lie down, grows sleepy; he is attacked by a severe internal chill, so that he trembles (from the 30c).

Pain in all the bones, as if every part would fall asunder.

feels as if broken from head to foot; thereupon violent coldness, so that nothing would warm her; without thirst, after the bite.

Being internally cold, it draws from the hip to below the knee, without external coldness; warmth is agreeable.

Cold hands, with flickering of the eyes, and nausea.

Icy sweat covers the body, with faintness and vertigo, and vomiting at night.

### Skin.

Itching on the head, behind the ears, on the nose, on the back of the neck, on the edge of the shoulders, on the back, on the nates, on the calf.

° Phthisis florida. (Cures if given in the beginning.) (*Baruch.*)

° Scrofulosis. (A dose arouses the latent reacting powers.) (*Ib.*)

° Rhachitis, caries, necrosis. (Great success from it.) (*Ib.*)

---

# THLASPI BURSA PASTORIS.

*(Shepherd's purse.)*

BOTANICAL DESCRIPTION.—This plant belongs to the Cruciferæ, or mustard family. It is now known as the Capsella Bursa Pastoris. It is an annual, growing in waste places, bearing small white flowers; is not indigenous, but naturalized from Europe, and is become one of our commonest weeds. The root-leaves are clustered and toothed; the stem leaves are arrow-shaped and sessile.

OFFICINAL PREPARATIONS.—Tincture of the plant.

ANALOGUES.—*Trillium, Sabina, Crocus, Millefolium, Ledum, Hamamelis, Ipecac.*

### Head.

° Frequent occurring epistaxis, of a passive nature.

### Urinary Organs.

° Passive hæmaturia.

### Generative Organs.

*Women:* ° Passive metrorrhagia with too copious and frequent menses

° Delaying menses caused by inertia of the uterus.

° Hæmorrhages, with violent uterine colic; with cramps consequent upon abortion at the critical age, and even when there was cancer of the cervix.

° Menorrhagia of three years standing, every menstruation

40

with hemorrhage; the first day barely shows, the second, profuse flooding, severe colic, vomiting and expulsion of clots; the flow continues ten to fifteen days.

° Menses three days too soon, very profuse, uterine colic and discharge of clots.

° Hemorrhage, from cancer of the neck of the uterus.

° Hemorrhage after abortion.

---

# TRIFOLIUM PRATENSE.

### (*Red Clover.*)

DESCRIPTION.—Red Clover is a biennial plant with several *stems* arising from the same root, ascending, somewhat hairy, and varying much in its height. The *leaves* are ternate; the *leaflets* oval or obovate, entire, nearly smooth, often notched at the end, and lighter colored in the centre. The *stipules* are ovate, mucranate; the *flowers* are red, fragrant, and disposed in short, dense, ovate, sessile *spikes* or *heads*; the *corollas* unequal, mono-pelatous; the *lower tooth of the calyx* longer than the four others, which are equal, and all shorter than the rose-red corolla.—*W. G.* This plant is common to the United States, being extensively cultivated in grass lands, with herds-grass (*Phleum Pratense*) and other grasses, and often alone; it flowers throughout the summer.

OFFICINAL PREPARATIONS.—Tincture of the ripe flowers; triturations, and dilutions.

ANALOGUES.—*Ipecac, Hepar sulphur, Mercurius, Spongia, Sanguinaria,* etc.

### Mental Sphere.

Dullness of intellect; confused; memory feeble.

### Head.

Intermittent headache for half an hour; fullness of the head.
Dull aching in the anterior lobes of the brain.
Brain feels large.
Headache in the morning.
Headache all day, but worse in the evening.

### Eyes.

The eyes feel dull and sore.

### Nose.

Nasal mucous membrane dry.
Discharge of thin mucus; with much irritation.
Increased flow of mucus.
Coryza — like that which precedes hay-asthma.

## Mouth.

Increased flow of saliva in men.

*Salivation* in horses.

° Suppressed drooling in children.

## Stomach.

Hiccough for half an hour.

Great thirst.

## Abdomen.

Griping pain on rising A. M.

Severe pain in the bowels.

Colicky pains all day.

## Stool.

Very costive, with hemorrhage from the rectum, while at stool, for two weeks.

Slight tenesmus.

Stool hard and covered with mucus.

Stool loose and slimy.

## Urine.

Quantity increased; bladder feels too full; clear; copious.

Great urging to urinate. Urates decreased.

Phosphates increased.

Urine diminished in quantity.

## Pharynx and Throat.

Sharp pain through the uvula, causing tears to start; throat feels dry.

Irritation of the bronchi, causing a short, hacking cough.

Irritation of the pharynx and trachea, with dry, hacking cough.

Accumulation and expectoration of mucus.

Great irritation of the throat.

Throat dry; then increased flow of mucus.

Throat feels raw, as if a foreign body was stuck in it.

Sore throat, as if scalded all the way down.

Sore throat, with hoarseness.

## Chest.

Oppression of the chest, with a feeling as if the air were loaded with impurities.

Oppression of chest on lying down.

Asthmatic oppression of the chest in a close room; relieved in open air.

Cough on coming into the open air.

Feeling as if breathing hot air.

Faint feeling when in a close room.

Continual short, dry cough.

° Hooping-cough; paroxysms worse at night.

° Hay-asthma; hay fever.

### Back.

Constant uneasiness in region of the kidneys.

### Extremities.

Tingling in the palm of the left hand and in left arm.

Feet and hands cold.

### Fever.

Pulse 72 (second day); 68 (third day); 64 (fourth day).

Pulse weak, intermitting one or two beats, if stopped for a few seconds, and this was followed by a full, bounding pulse.

### Generalities.

Better in the open air and cool room.

Worse when in a close, hot room.

Headache worse in the evening.

[Extract of red clover is the sole ingredient of Dr. Thompson's Cancer plasters, and it is the principle ingredient of Dr. Howard's celebrated Cancer Salve. Many cases of cancer have been reported cured by the extract, and supported by proof which appears trustworthy. It is taken internally, 5 or 10 grains daily, and applied externally. (*Hale.*)]

---

# TRILLIUM PENDULUM.

## (*White Beth-Root.*)

BOTANICAL DESCRIPTION.—*Root* oblong, tuberous, from which arises a slender *stem*, from ten to fifteen inches in height. *Leaves*, three, whorled at the top of the stem, sub-orbicular rhomboidal, abruptly acuminate, from three to five inches in diameter, on petioles about a line in length. *Flowers*, white, solitary, terminal, cernuous, on a recurved peduncle, from one to two and a half inches long. *Sepals*, green, oblong-lanceolate, acuminate, an inch long. *Petals*, white, oblong-ovate, acute, one and a quarter inches in length, by half an inch broad. *Styles*, three, erect, with curved stigma.

This plant is common to the Middle and Western States, growing in rich soils, in damp, rocky, and shady woods, and flowering in May and June. Wood enumerates nine species indigenous to this country. King says "nearly all the species are medicinal, and possess analogous properties; among them the T. Erythrocarpum, T. Grandiflorum, T. Sessile, T. Erectum, and T. Nivale are the most common, and consequently the most frequently collected and employed. These may be known by their three verticillate, net-veined leaves, and their solitary terminal flower, which varies in color in the different species, being white, red, purple, whitish yellow, or reddish-white. Some have the peduncle erect, others recurved." The common names of the species are Wake-Robin, Birth-root, Indian-balm, Lamb's quarter and Ground-lily.

PHARMACOLOGICAL OBSERVATIONS.—From the remarks of King, quoted above, from the Eclectic Dispensatory, we learn that it is a matter of indifference which, or how many species of Trillium go to make up the preparations in use in that school. It is my conviction that no reliable knowledge can be gained by using a preparation made in this loose manner. For use in disease, some definite, reliable tincture, made from a single species should be used. I am satisfied, however, from my inquiries, that none of the tinctures or triturations now in use by homœopathists is prepared from the Trillium pendulum alone. We must adopt one of two methods — either one species exclusively, or several combined.

If the T. pendulum is scarce, not sufficient to meet the demands, several species may be used in definite, equal proportions, not varying after once fixed upon.

The *roots* of these plants are oblong or terate, somewhat tuberous, dark or brownish externally, white internally, from one to five inches in length, and from half an inch to an inch and a half in diameter, beset with a few branching fibres, laterally. They have a faint, slightly terebinthinate odor, and a peculiar aromatic and sweetish taste; when chewed, they impart an acrid, astringent impression in the mouth, causing a flow of saliva, and a sensation of heat in the throat and fauces. The rootlets have but little of the acrimony of the root.

OFFICINAL PREPARATIONS.—Tincture of the root; dilutions; triturations of the root. Trillin: triturations.

ANALOGUES.—*Asarum, Crocus, Copaiva, Chimaphila, Erigeron, Erechthites, Hamamelis, Pulsatilla, Sanguinaria, Senecio, Sabina, Terebinthina, Thlaspi.*

(*No provings.*)

### Nose.

° *Epistaxis* —"A solution of Trillium, or the dry powder snuffed up the nostrils will immediately check epistaxis. (*Eclectic.*)

° *Nose-bleed* may be easily checked by smelling the broken end of a fresh root of the *red* beth root. (*Merrill.*)

### Mouth.

° Hemorrhage from the gums and mouth; the diluted tincture to be used as a wash.

° Useful in cancrum-oris.

° Putrid sore throat.

° Bleeding from the cavity after extraction of a tooth.

### Stomach.

Heat and burning in the stomach; rising up into the œsophagus.

° Hæmatemesis, with erosion of the mucous coat of the stomach.

### Abdomen and Stool.

Constipation; hard, dry stool. (*p.*)

° Chronic diarrhœa; discharges, bloody mucus. (3.)

° Dysentery, when the passages are almost pure blood. (*Hale.*)

### Urinary Organs.

° Hæmaturia, passive. (*Hale.*)

° Chronic catarrh of the bladder, etc.

° *Diabetes*, (which kind?) "I have used it frequently in
diabetes, and from the advantages derived from its use,
we think much reliance can be placed upon it in that
disease. (*Dr. Jones, Eclectic.*)

### Generative Organs.

*Female:* ° Hemorrhage from the uterus, with pain in the
back, etc.

° Hemorrhage after abortion. (*Dr. Peterson.*)

° Threatened miscarriage, with excessive flooding.

° Menorrhagia, with profuse yellowish leucorrhœa during the
period.

° Metrorrhagia at the climacteric. (*Hale, Peterson.*)

° Post-partem hemorrhage.

° Facilitates labor, and prevents hemorrhage.

° Vaginal and uterine leucorrhœa.

° Profuse lochial discharge. (*Hale.*)

### Bronchi.

° Cough of catarrhal nature dependent upon chronic bronchitis
or laryngitis. (*Scudder.*)

° Copious, purulent expectoration, troublesome cough in
phthisis. (*Ib.*)

° Cough with spitting of blood. (*Coe.*)

ᵗ Hæmoptysis from any cause. (*Eclectic.*)

# TRIOSTEUM PERFOLIATUM
## (*Fever Root.*)

BOTANICAL DESCRIPTION.—Indigenous, with a perennial, thick and fleshy *root*, subdivided into numerous, horizontal branches. *Stems*, several from the same root, simple, stout, erect, hollow, soft, pubescent, from two to four feet high. *Leaves* opposite, oval, acuminate, mostly crenate, entire, abruptly contracted at the base, nearly smooth above, pubescent beneath, prominently veined, six inches long by three broad; in some plants the upper leaves are almost amplexicaul. *Flowers*, of a dull purple color, axillary, sessile, mostly in clusters of from three to five, in the form of whorls, rarely solitary. *Fruit*, an oval berry, about nine lines long, and six thick; of an orange-red or purple color, when ripe; hairy, somewhat three-sided, crowned with the persistent calyx; three-celled, each cell containing a hard, bony, furrowed seed.

The root is the officinal part. It is of a dirty, yellowish-brown color, externally; about a foot and a half long, and about nine lines in diameter; whitish internally; sends out fibres, has a nauseous smell and a disagreeable amarous taste. When dried, it is readily reduced to powder.

Its virtues are imparted to water, alcohol and ether. The *T. angustifolium* is a smaller species, and considered to have the same medicinal action.

OFFICINAL PREPARATIONS.—Tincture of the root and berries; dilutions.

ANALOGUES.—*Æsculus, Arnica, Bryonia, Chilidonium, Chamomilla, Arsenicum, Ipecac, Nux vomica.*

## Mental Sphere.
Extreme nervous irritability; fear of death.

## Head.
Headache, which is worse in the right side of the head.

Pain in the occiput, with sensation of weight there; coldness and stiffness of the feet.

Head aches worse on sitting up.

Boring pain in the left temple.

° Bilious headache, with vomiting.

## Throat.
Soreness, as if from swelling of the pharynx, and pain in the œsophagus on swallowing.

° Sore throat from influenza. (*Matthews.*)

## Stomach.
Feeling of a load and oppression in the epigastrium.

Pain in the epigastrium increased by drinking water and by turning in bed

\* Nausea on rising, followed by copious vomiting and cramps in the stomach.

### Abdomen.

Copious evacuations of thin stools, without pain.

\* Stools watery and frothy, without pain, followed by exhaustion.

Evacuation from the bowels *at 7 a. m.*

Evacuations most frequent in the evening.

° Bilious colic. (*Tallmadge.*)

° Diarrhœa, with severe colic pains. (*Neidhard.*)

### Chest.

Audible beating of the heart, and slight pain under the left breast.

° Asthmatic troubles. (*Dr. Tallmadge.*)

### Back.

Pain in the neck and back.

Rheumatic pain in the back from stooping.

Pain and stiffness in the loins (left side).

### Extremities.

Stiffness of all the joints (upper and lower).

Stiffness of the knees when attempting to rise.

Drawing and shrinking sensation in the legs.

Coldness and stiffness of the feet.

° Rheumatism of the extremities. (*Matthews.*)

### Skin.

Vesicular eruption on the forehead, over left eye, middle of the chest, and on the right arm.

Violent itching eruption of the skin.

° Urticaria, from gastric derangement.

### Fever.

Fever, with hot skin and increased thirst.

Aching pains in every part of the body.

° Typhoid and gastric fevers. (*Dr. Tallmadge.*)

° Violent attacks of bilious fever, with pain in the limbs, headache and vomiting. (*Dr. Matthews.*)

# URTICA URENS. *(Dioica.)*

*(Stinging Nettle.)*

BOTANICAL DESCRIPTION.—A well-known perennial herbaceous plant, growing both in Europe and the United States, by the roadsides, in hedges and gardens. The stinging, or irritating property, is caused by the free formic acid, which is found in the little hairs, which are very sharp.

OFFICINAL PREPARATIONS.—Tincture of the plant; dilutions.

ANALOGUES.—*Arsenicum, Apis mellifica, Belladonna, Clematis, Copaiva, Comocladia, Dulcamara, Petroleum, Rhus.*

## Head.

Dull aching pain in right sinciput; right side of the face, extending to malar bone.

Neuralgic pain in right face and forehead.

Fullness, dullness, and dizziness, like rush of blood to the head.

Dull aching in head, with stitches in region of the spleen.

Dull aching in occiput and over the eyes.

° Urticaria of the scalp — suddenly appearing and determining internally.

## Face and Eyes.

Pain in right eye and right parietal bone — a stinging pain, compelling one to rub and press it.

Pressing pain over right eye and in the eyeball.

Pressing pain in left eye.

Pressing pain over both eyes; they feel weak and sore.

Pain in eyeballs as if from a blow, and a sensation as of sand in eyes.

Fever blisters on lips, itching.

Lips, nose and ears swollen; eyelids closed and œdematous — followed by small transparent vesicles, filled with serum, afterwards desquamation.

° Urticaria appears, after being suppressed.

° Vesicular erysipelas appears, after suppression.

## Mouth and Throat.

Burning in throat, with frequent throwing up of frothy mucus, with cough and frothy expectoration.

Burning in throat, with nausea.

## Gastric and Intestinal.

Nausea, with burning in throat.

\* Vomiting from suppression of nettle rash.

\* Constipation.   (*p.*)

Pain around the umbilicus, with severe dysenteric stools of
  whitish slime.

White and yellow stools, with slimy mucus, tenesmus and
  colic-like pains.

Small dysenteric stools of greenish-brown slime, with urging
  and tenesmus.

Soreness in the bowels, and on pressure a sound as if they
  were full of water.

Dysenteric stools during the greater part of the proving.

Stools, small and painful, mixed with white matter, like the
  boiled white of an egg, with much pain over the whole
  abdomen.

° Dysentery, if accompanied or preceded by nettle rash; during and after passage of stool, a sensation of rawness and
  burning in anus.

A small hæmorrhoidal tumor, itching and burning, at times
  quite severe.

### Urinary Organs.

Complete suppression of urine for twelve days, with œdematous swelling of the whole upper body down to the umbilicus.

° Strangury.   ° Gravel.   ° Disease of bladder and kidneys.

° Hemorrhage from the bladder.

### Generative Organs.

*Women.*—The breasts of a woman who had had twelve children, but never nursed any, became swollen and filled
  with a serous, and afterwards milky fluid — (in the case
  of œdema of the upper body).

Menorrhagia after confinement, and at the critical period.

° Sudden suppression of milk.

### Chest.

Soreness and bruised feeling in sides of the chest.

° Hæmoptysis — from violent exertion of the lungs.

### Extremities.

Pain in right deltoid muscle, worse at 9 P. M., could not put
  on his coat without assistance.

Pain in both arms, right the worst, and in ankles; cramp-like pain in right arm, the deltoid feeling sore to the touch; worse on rotating the arms inward; worse in evening.

Rheumatic pains in right arm; worse when lying on it.

A sharp stitch darting through the arm.

Muscles of right arm sore, as if bruised.

Inability to stretch or raise the right arm, on account of a pain in the right hypochondriac region.

*⋅Urticaria nodosa on hands and fingers.

Rheumatic pains in right wrist and ankles.

* Blotches, "hives," on the hands and fingers, itching.

Soreness on inside of right knee joint.

Rheumatic pains, attended with urticaria.

### Skin.

The skin of the face, arms and chest burnt frightfully; she complained of itching and burning as if the skin was scorched; the lips, nose and ears were swollen; the eyelids œdematous, as if full of water, and closed; (in morning, after drinking an infusion of Urtica at night;) at noon the whole upper part of body, down to the umbilicus, was enormously swollen, but rather pale and dropsical than inflamed, and covered with confluent, small, transparent vesicles filled with serum (sudamina). In other respects the patient was free from pain; the breathing and circulation were undisturbed. On the third day there was violent itching; on the sixth, desquamation.

* Raised, red, itching blotches on the skin of the hands and fingers.

* *Urticaria nodosa*, with stinging itching.

° *Urticaria* attending or preceding rheumatism.

° *Burns*, when the integuments and subjacent tissues are not destroyed, and when the injury is confined to the skin.

° Vesicular erysipelas, of a not very severe character.

° Erythema, with burning and itching.

The skin-symptoms tended to return every year at the same date.

### Generalities.

General œdema of the upper half of body.

The *seeds* induce lethargic sleep.

° Hæmorrhages from various organs.

° Results of retrocession of urticaria, and other eruptions.

° Affections attended by urticaria.

The rheumatic pains worse in evening.

° The seeds are said to have cured *Goitre.*

° Intermittent fever. (?)

° Insufficiency or entire want of milk after parturition. (?)

° Nettle rash, which affects the patient every year at the same season.

---

## USTILAGO MAYDIS.

### (*Maize-Smut.*)

DESCRIPTION.—The smut of Maize (*Zea Maize*), or Indian corn, is a fungus produced on the stems, germens, etc. It often attains a large size, larger than an orange. It is covered with a dark gray or brown epidermis, which bursts when ripe. The *spores* are spherical, minute, their surface covered with echinulate warts, like prickles; they are deep-seated, nearly black and pulverulent, having the appearance of soot, under the naked eye. This species must not be confounded with the "Corn-Smut" of English botanists (*U. segetum*), found on wheat, rye, oats and barley.

It is interesting to know that an analysis of this fungus shows it to contain *Ergotin*, the supposed active principle of Secale.

OFFICINAL PREPARATIONS.—*Triturations* of the fungus, gathered when it has turned black, but before the frosts have affected it. *Tincture* made from the *fresh,* just ripe fungus.

ANALOGUES.—*Secale, Sepia, Sabina, Tanacetum, Gossipium, Borax, Platina, etc.*

### Moral Symptoms.

Great depression of spirits during the whole proving. (See sexual group.)

### Head.

Feeling of fullness of head, dull, pressive, frontal headache.

Violent frontal headache, as if the forehead would burst open.

Sharp flying pains in the forehead.

° Nervous headache from menstrual irregularities. (*Burt.*)

### Eyes.

Aching of the eyeballs, with profuse secretion of tears.

Smarting of the eyes, with profuse secretion of tears in the open air.

### Ears.

Constant dull pain in the left ear, caused by extension of inflammation of the tonsil along the eustachian tube.

### Nose.

Dryness of the nostrils, as if I had taken cold.

### Face.

Burning sensation of the face and scalp.

### Mouth.

Slimy, coppery taste is a prominent symptom.

Constant dull, aching pain in the first and second upper molars; they are decayed, and have ached before.

Shedding of the teeth in animals. (*Roulin.*)

Pricking sensation in the tongue, with a feeling as if something was under the roots of the tongue pressing it upwards.

Dryness of the fauces, with difficult deglutition.

Congestion and inflammation of the tonsils, left one greatly enlarged, of a dark color, accompanied with dull pain, much aggravated by swallowing.

### Throat.

Dryness of the fauces, with a burning distress in the stomach.

Dryness and roughness of the fauces, with difficult deglutition.

Feeling as if there was a lump behind the larynx, which produces constant inclination to swallow.

### Appetite and Thirst.

Loss of appetite, followed by canine hunger.

### Gastric Symptoms.

Eructations of the ingesta, with strongly acid taste.

Very faint feeling a number of times in the epigastrium, with pain in the region of the liver and bowels.

### Stomach.

Constant distress in the region of stomach.

Burning distress in the sternum and stomach, accompanied with fine neuralgic pains in the same region.

Fine, sharp, cutting pains in the epigastrium, lasting about three minutes at a time, came on every ten or fifteen minutes for a number of hours.

### Abdomen.

Grumbling pains in the abdomen all the afternoon, followed by dry, hard stool.

Fine, cutting, colicky pains every few minutes all day, relieved by a hard, constipated stool, followed by dull pains in the bowels.

### Liver.

Good deal of pain for two days in the region of the right lobe of the liver.

Dull pains in the right hypochondrium, with distress in the small intestines.

### Stool.

Constipation, (where the Ustilago is indicated the stools are generally papescent or constipated.)

Black, lumpy stool.

### Urinary Organs.

Urine diminished one-half, and very red and scanty. (*p.*)

Great increase of colorless urine. (*s.*)

### Genital Organs of Man.

Sexual dreams every night, with no emissions.

Great depression of the sexual system for weeks, with great relaxation of the scrotum.

Constant aching pains in the testicles for a number of days.

Sharp, neuralgic pains in the testicles, more in the right.

Constant aching distress in the right testicle for days.

Spells of violent pains in the testicles, more in the right.

Every five minutes, sharp pains in testicles, causing faintness.

Two nights had a profuse cold sweat upon the scrotum, which was greatly relaxed.

\* Spermatorrhœa, with erotic ideas and amorous dreams.

° Seminal emissions, and irresistible tendency to masturbation, erotic fancies, melancholy, etc. (*Burt.*)

° One to four emissions, with sexual dreams, every week, followed the next day with great prostration of strength, dull pain in the lumbar region, with great despondency and irritability of mind. (*Ib.*)

### Organs of Generation of Women.

Constant aching distress in the uterus, referred by the patient to the mouth of the womb.

In a cow house, where cows were fed on Indian corn infested
with this parasite (Ustilago), eleven of their number
aborted in eight days; after their food was changed none
of the animals aborted. (*Anl. Med. Vetr. Belge. and
Rep. de Ph.*)

Six drachms given to two pregnant bitch dogs, soon caused
them to abort. (*Burt.*)

Fowls fed on this fungus lay eggs without shells. (*Roulin.*)

* Menorrhagia, with menses too frequent. (*Hale.*)

* Metrorrhagia, after confinement and after miscarriage.

* Tendency to miscarriage, with or without hemorrhage.

* Menstruation too frequent, too profuse and too long. (*Burt.*)

° Suppressio-mensium, from ovarian irritation, with much pain
in the ovarian region, and flatulence and soreness of
the bowels.

° Vicarious menstruation from the lungs or bowels.

° Scanty menstruations from ovarian irritation.

° Menorrhagia at the climacteric period, with much pain on the
top and side of the head; with burning distress in right
ovary; goneness in the epigastrium; the flooding lasts for
weeks; blood dark colored, with many clots, and vertigo.

° Active and constant flooding, with frequent clots of bright
red blood, with bearing-down pains. (*Burt.*)

° Passive hemorrhage; blood dark colored, lasting many days,
with anæmia, and dull, heavy headache. (*Ib.*)

° Abortion, with bearing-down pains, as if everything would
come from her. (*Ib.*)

° Deficient labor-pains, when the os is soft, pliable, and dila-
table. (*Hale.*)

° Dysmenorrhœa of a congestive character, with much ovarian
irritation; severe pain in the ovaries, uterus, and back,
every few minutes.

Spasmodic pains in the left ovary, which is very sore and
tender.

° Ovaritis; constant pain in the ovary, with sharp pains passing down the legs with great rapidity; ovary much
swollen and very tender. (*Burt.*)

° Intermittent neuralgia of the left ovary, which is large as a hen's egg, and very tender to the touch.

° Between the menses, constant misery under left breast at the margin of the ribs.

° Hypertrophy of the uterus. (*Burt.*)

° Vertigo at the climacteric period, with too frequent and too profuse menstruation.

° Slow, persistent oozing of dark blood, with small black coagulæ, lasting many days. (*Woodbury.*)

° Passive congestion of the uterus, which is enlarged, the cervix tumefied, and somewhat dilated.

° Menorrhagia after abortion. (*Bennett.*)

° Profuse menstruation, the flow lasting ten days or two weeks, at first very abundant, gradually wearing off; always worse from motion; discharge dark, and quite painless.

° Menorrhagia; the flow usually lasted three weeks; very profuse, dark, painless; given from the commencement Ustilago 1 × ; shortened it to five days. (*Hale.*)

---

# VIBURNUM OPULUS.

### (*High Cranberry.*)

BOTANICAL DESCRIPTION.—This is a shrub, growing from three to ten feet high, with smooth, gray, spreading branches. *Leaves* three to five inches in diameter, the lobe often somewhat falcate, nearly smooth above, sparsely hairy underneath; *petiole* about an inch long, with four to six glands on the upper part; stipular appendages, one or two pairs at or near the base of the petiole, subulate, often tipped, with a gland; *cyme*, three to four inches in diameter; the sterile flowers few or numerous, nearly an inch in diameter; *calyx*, teeth nearly obsolete; *drupes*, nearly half an inch long, juicy, intensely acid, and slightly bitter—translucent when dry. The common snow-ball bush of our gardens is a cultivated variety of this species. The two plants do not differ sufficiently to be considered separate species; cultivation increases the number of sterile flowers. The bark contains *valerianic acid*, the odor of which is very distinct in the tincture.

OFFICIAL PREPARATIONS.—Tincture of the bark.

ANALOGUES.—*Cauloph llum* (*?*), *Viburnum prunifolium* (*?*). *Gossipium.*

### (*No proving.*)

° Hysterical convulsions, from uterine irritation.

° General irritation of the nervous system.

° Cramps and contractions of the extremities — especially during pregnancy.

° Paralytic conditions, coming on *after* cramps and convulsions.

° Amaurosis. (?)

° Dyspepsia, with constipation and incontinence of urine

° Cramp-like (?) difficulty of breathing.

° Cramps in the feet after long walking.

° Spasmodic dysuria in hysterical subjects. (*Woodbury*.)

° Spasmodic dysmenorrhœa. (*Ib.*)

° *Dysmenorrhœa* of a *spasmodic and neuralgic* character, with intense cramp-like pains in the uterus. (*Hale.*)

° *Pseudo-membranous* dysmenorrhœa.

° Very painful, scanty, but regular, menses. (*Dr. Ruddock.*)

° Cramp-like pains and spasms of the stomach, bowels, bladder, or other organs, when reflex from uterine irritation. Irritable ovaries with dysmenorrhœa. (*Ib.*)

*(See Therapeutics.)*

---

# VIBURNUM PRUNIFOLIUM.

*(Black Haw.)*

BOTANICAL DESCRIPTION.—This is a shrub or small tree, growing from eight to fifteen feet high, with numerous spreading branches, and short, lateral spurs, which are sometimes almost thorny; *leaves* usually from one to two inches long, and rounded, smooth on both sides: *petiole* about half an inch long; *cymes* are about three inches in diameter, terminating the short lateral branches or spurs, the primary divisions usually about four; fruit about one-third of an inch long, bluish-black, and slightly glaucose when mature, the nucleus much compressed.

Found in woods and thickets, flowering in May and June, and the fruit maturing in September and October.

OFFICIAL PREPARATIONS.—Tincture of the bark.

ANALOGUES.—*Pulsatilla* (?), *Caulophyllum* (?), *Gossipium* (?).

*(No proving.)*

° Aphthæ in the mouth and throat.

° Ulcerations of an obstinate character.

° Cancerous ulcerations.

° *A preventive in cases of habitual miscarriage.* (*Dr. Phares.*)

° Prevents miscarriages from any cause — especially when attended by severe pains. (*Ib.*)

41

° Completely neutralizes the effects of the Gossipium when that drug is taken to cause miscarriage. (*Ib.*)

° It has never failed to prevent a threatened miscarriage, as far as I can learn. (*Ib.*)

° *Renders the pains of confinement milder and more bearable.* (*Ib.*)

° *After pains*—of a severe character.

° Cramps in the limbs during pregnancy.

° Palpitation of the heart, especially in pregnant women.

(*See Therapeutics.*)

---

## VISCUM ALBUM.

(*Mistletoe.*)

BOTANICAL DESCRIPTION.—This is the *Viscum Flacceus* of MISTEL and the *Viscum Verticillatum* of NUTTALL. This parasitic shrub is found growing on various trees, but that which is found growing on the oak is preferable. The bark and leaves have an unpleasant odor and a mawkish, bitterish taste. The proper time for collecting is in November, when it should be gradually dried, pulverized, and kept in a well stopped bottle. It should never be kept more than a year, as age impairs its active qualities.

OFFICINAL PREPARATIONS.—Tincture with strong alcohol, from the green plant, gathered in November; triturations from the dried and powdered plant.

ANALOGUES.—*Agaricus, Cicuta, Stramonium, Œnanthe, Æthusa, etc.*

[The following symptoms were taken from clinical cases published in the *British Journal of Homœopathy*, vol. 22, pp 637, translated from Dr. Huber's article in the *Zeitschrift*.]

### Head.

° Constant vertigo, even when in bed.

° *Epilepsy.* (Many cases cured by large and small doses. Old authorities and recent writers.)

° Dull headache, with stitches in the temples.

' Sensation in the vertex as if the scalp was numb.

° Frequent flow of blood to the head, with heat and redness of the face.

° Great vertigo and shooting headache.

° Shooting, tearing, frequently recurring pains in the temples.

° Head confused, tearing pains in the left temporal region, extending over the forehead and hairy scalp.

° Feeling as if the whole vault of the skull would be raised up.

° Pains in the temples, coming on periodically, worse in the evening and at night.

### Eyes.

Redness of the conjunctiva.

° Blue rings around the deep lying eyes.

° Double vision.

### Ears.

° Catarrhal deafness.

° Drawing, tearing sensation in the left ear.

ᶜ Loud buzzing and stopped up feeling in the ear.

° Deafness, from a cold.

### Mouth.

Ulceration of the corners of the mouth.

Great soreness of the tongue, but clean; taste natural.

° Difficulty of protruding the tongue.

° Sore throat.

### Face.

° Muscles of face in constant agitation.

° Distressed look of the face; an almost idiotic expression of the face.

° Tearing, drawing pain in the left lower maxilla and teeth.

° Pale face, with blue rings around the sunken eyes.

° Heat and redness of the face, with metrorrhagia.

° Red, bloated face.

### Stomach.

° Constipation (with retention of placenta).

° Weight, fullness and contractive pain in the hypogastric region.

° Contractive, sometimes burning pains in the abdomen.

ᶜ Spleen larger than normal.

° Shooting pains through the spleen, sometimes extending to the heart.

### Thorax.

° Hydrothorax.

° Rigor with shooting in the left false ribs, with dry cough.

° Expectoration of a greenish mucus.

° Dyspnœa increased by lying on right side.

° Dyspnœa and aggravation of pain when coughing.

° Feeling of suffocation when lying on left side.

° Sensation as of a frightful stab with a lancet through the entire right thoracic cavity.

### Generative Organs.

° Metrorrhagia.

° Hæmorrhage accompanied by pain, the blood partly bright red, partly in dark clots.

° Hæmorrhage, with violent contractive labor-like pains.

° Hæmorrhage continually, at one time in a stream, at another in clots, of a blackish color.

° Pains, periodic, proceeding from the sacrum into the pelvis, worse in bed, accompanied with tearing, shooting pains from above downwards, in both thighs, as well as in the upper extremities, with sleeplessness and general prostration.

### Extremities.

° *Sciatica.* (many severe cases.)

° Metastasis of pain from nape of the neck to the buttock and outside of the thigh.

° Fearful, tearing, shooting, throbbing pains in left side of sacrum, extending to the thigh.

° Extremely violent pain in left sacro-ischiatic region, on the slightest motion of the thigh, the pain extending along the outside of the thigh in a strip about four fingers broad, to the knee joint, and is often throbbing as if suppuration would take place.

° Tearing, burning pain in right thigh, also when extending the whole length of the limb to the ankle joint.

° Sensation as if the flesh of the thigh was frequently torn away with hot pincers.

° Great sensitiveness of the thigh, the slightest touch causing pain.

° Painful tearing in the muscles of the calf and in the ankle, then going into the patella and knee joint.

° The right knee swelled around the patella, with a doughy feeling and sensitiveness to pressure.

° Tension in the patella, as if the tendons around it were contracted.

° Pains periodic, when at rest as well as when in motion.

° Pains alternating in the knee and ankle, with the shoulder and elbow.

° The right tibia very much swelled in the middle of the bone, where it is but slightly covered with skin.

° Digging, gnawing, distressing pain in the tibia and a metatarsal bone on the dorsum of the foot, especially aggravated at night.

° Swelling of a metatarsal bone on dorsum of foot.

### Generalities.

° Chorea from a fright, with perfect inability to remain still for the space of three minutes, and inability to walk without assistance.

° Choreic movements continuing during sleep.

° Sleep unquiet on account of general weakness and profuse sweats.

° Great debility from metrorrhagia.

° Weakness nearly amounting to faintness.

Usually the bowels and urinary organs are in a normal condition when this remedy is indicated.

[In Culpepper's English Physician, published in 1810, I find the following remarks by Matthiolus: "The mistletoe of the oak (that being the best), made into powder, and given in drink to those who have the falling sickness" (epilepsy) "doth assuredly heal them, provided it be taken forty days together."

Culpepper himself reports a case as follows: "A young lady, having been long troubled with the falling sickness, for which she had taken everything prescribed for her, by the most famous doctors, without effect, but growing rather worse, having eight or ten dreadful fits in a day, was cured only by the powder of the true mistletoe, given as much as would lie on a sixpence, early in the morning, for some days, near the full moon."

---

# VALERIANATE OF AMMONIA.

### (*Ammonia Valerianas.*)

Obtain, from the Muriate of Ammonia, placed in a suitable vessel, in coarse powder, and an equal weight of lime, previously slaked and in powder, gaseous ammonia, and cause it to pass, first through a bottle filled with pieces of lime, and afterward through four fluid ounces of Valerianic acid, contained in a tall, narrow, glass vessel, until the acid is neutralized: set the vessel aside that crystals may form. Break the salt in pieces, drain it in a glass funnel, dry on bibulous paper, and keep in a well stopped bottle. It is now white, pearly, four-sided crystals, perfectly dry, of an offensive odor, like Valerianic acid, and a sharp, sweetish taste. Effloresces in dry air, deliquesces in a moist atmosphere. Very soluble in water and alcohol.

OFFICINAL PREPARATIONS.—Triturations. Tincture; dilutions.

° Violent neuralgiæ with great nervous agitation.

*(See Therapeutics.)*

# VALERIANATE OF ZINC.

## (*Zinci Valerianas.*)

Take of Sulphate of Zinc, five ounces and three-quarters; Valerianate of Soda, five ounces; dissolve each in two pints distilled water, raise both solutions to near the boiling point, mix them, cool, and skim off the crystals which form. Evaporate the mother liquor at a heat not exceeding 200°, till it is reduced to four fluid ounces; cool again, remove the crystals which are formed, and add them to those already obtained. Drain the crystals on a paper filter, and wash them with a small quantity of cold distilled water, till the washings give but a very feeble precipitate with the Chloride of Barium. Again drain and dry on filter paper at ordinary temperature. It is in white, pearly scales, having a strong odor of Valerianic acid, and a metallic styptic taste. Dissolve in 160 parts cold water, and in 60 parts alcohol.

OFFICINAL PREPARATIONS—Triturations. Pills. (The triturations are of such an intensely disagreeable taste and smell, that it is best to use either a sugar-coated pill, of one-fourth or one-half grain crude; or pilules made from a trituration with gum arabic instead of sugar.)

ANALOGUES.—(?) Probably those of its two constituents.

### Mind.

° Insanity—recurring with the headache. (*Hale.*)

### Head.

° Neuralgic headaches of three weeks duration, cured in three days. (*Dr. Banks.*)

’ Terrible headache, involving the whole head, occurring once or twice a week for many years. She becomes insane; beside herself with pain; almost unconscious; screams; pulls her hair; eyes red; face pale and drawn; the pain is piercing and stabbing. She speaks of many other horrible sensations. It has injured her health; she looks pale and cadaverous, and her mind is not sound any of the time; loss of memory; melancholy. Gave one grain of the 1-10 trit. three times a day, for several weeks. In the meantime she had several attacks, but all lighter. In three months she wrote me that the attacks were very se_ dom and very slight. She had regained her health, and was quite clear in her mind. One of the finest cures I ever made. (*Hale.*)

° Uncontrollable sleeplessness from pain in the head in children with meningitis: it produces sleep, and the children seem better from its use. (*Ib.*)

° Facial neuralgia, for more than three years, nothing ever gave her any relief. (*Dr. Banks.*)

° Neuralgia of three months standing. Pain excessive in inferior maxillary and left temple. (*Ib.*)

° Many other cases of violent, obstinate facial neuralgia have been reported cured by Valerianate of Zinc, in the practice of several other homœopathic physicians.

° Neuralgia of the ovaries. (*Hall, Hale.*)

° Sciatic neuralgia, with great nervous erythema in a lady who had suffered for years. (*Hale.*)

° *Angina pectoris*, several cases. (*Ib.*)

° " *Spinal neuralgia* ": the patient was almost crippled; when a permanent cure was effected in one week; a dose (no mention of size) was given every six hours. (*Morrill.*)

° The severe pains in neck, spine and elsewhere, in the sequelæ of cerebro-spinal meningitis. (*Hale.*)

---

# VERATRUM VIRIDE.

### (*American Hellebore.*)

BOTANICAL DESCRIPTION.—*Root* perennial, thick, fleshy, its upper por. tion tunicated, its lower half solid, and sending forth a multitude of large whitish roots. *Stem* from three to five feet high, roundish, solid, pubes. cent, striated, closely invested with the sheathing hairs of the leaves. *Lower leaves* large, from six inches to a foot long, and half as wide, oval, acuminate, pubescent, strongly plaited, nerved, the lower parts of their edges meeting round the stem. *Upper leaves* gradually narrower; the *uppermost* or bracts, linear lanceolate; all alternate. *Flowers* numerous, green, in compound racemes, axillary from the upper leaves, terminal, the whole forming a sort of panicle. * * * * * A part of the flowers barren, so that the plant is strictly polygamous. *Seed vessels* of three capsules, uni*ed together, separating at top, opening on inner side. *Seeds* flat, winged, imbricated.

HISTORY.—This plant is indigenous to the United States, growing in swamps, low grounds and moist meadows, flowering in June and July. It is known by the common names of *Indian poke and Itch weed.* The officinal part is the *root*, which should be gathered in autumn, after the decay of the leaves. As it rapidly loses its virtues, it should be renewed annually, and kept in well-closed vessels. When fresh, it has a very unpleasant odor; when dried, it is nearly inodorous, and has a sweetish-bitter taste, succeeded by a persistent acridity. Its physical and therapeutical properties strongly resemble those of white hellebore, and contains *Veratria*, gallic acid, etc.—*King*.

Pharmaceutists assert that the Veratria obtained from *Veratrum viride*, and the alkaloid obtained from *Veratrum album*, are *identical*.

The root imparts its properties to alcohol, 835, *i. e.*, diluted with 165 parts water to 1,000.

There are three other species of Veratrum, indigenous to the United States, namely, the *V. pariflorum* and V. augustifolium (grass leaved veratrum). The latter is called by Gray "Stamantheum." These are probably medicinal and ought to be investigated. The third species, *V. Woodii*, or Indiana veratrum, found also in Illinois and Iowa; of this nothing is known concerning its medicinal powers.

OFFICINAL PREPARATIONS.—Tincture of the root; dilutions.

ANALOGUES.—*Aconitum, Colchicum, Calabar, Gelseminum, Helleborus niger, Ammonium bromidum, Lobelia, Phytolacca, Tabacum, Tartarus emeticus, Veratrum album, Kali bromidum*.

### Mental Sphere.

Depression of spirits, but not always the intense anxiety and fear of death as from Aconite.

° Cerebral congestion, causing insanity.

° Puerperal mania. (See generative organs.)

### Head.

\* Headache, with vertigo; dimness of vision, and dilated pupils.

\* *Headache, preceding from the nape of the neck,* with heaviness of the head.

Sharp, drawing pains over the left eye; with a contracted feeling of the skin of the forehead.

\* Dull, frontal headache, with neuralgic pains in the right temple, close to the eye.

\* Great pain, with fullness in the head; face much flushed; burning in the head; spots before the eyes; delirium or a kind of stupefaction.

\* Severe frontal headache, with vomiting.

° Active *cerebral congestions;* congestive headache in plethoric persons from suppression of the menses.

° Acute inflammatory meningitis.

° Fullness and heaviness of the head, with throbbing of carotids; booming in the ears; sensitiveness to noise.

° *Cerebro-spinal meningitis,* when ushered in by high fever, great congestion, etc., or without fever, but cold, haggard face, slow pulse, etc.

### Face and Nose.

\* Pale cold face; bluish, and covered with cold perspiration.

\* Convulsive twitching of the facial muscles; mouth drawn at one corner.

Nose looks pinched, cold and blue.

° *Chorea;* convulsive motions of the facial muscles.

### Ears.

Ringing in the ears; moving quickly produces complete deafness.

The ears are cold and pale.

### Eyes.

Profuse secretion of tears.

\* Dimness of vision, with dilated pupils.

Immense circles of a green color appeared around the candle, which as vertigo comes on, and I closed my eyes, turned to red.

\* Double vision.

Sudden change of position, and washing brings on blindness and faintness.

° Amaurosis from anæmia.

° Amaurosis from irritation or congestion of the optic nerves.

### Mouth, Fauces and Œsophagus.

*Tongue feels as if it had been scalded.*

\* Tongue coated yellow along the centre, with flat, bitter taste in the morning.

' Tongue *yellow* at the sides, (edges) and a *red* streak in the middle.

\* Intense burning in the fauces and œsophagus, with constant inclination to swallow.

\* Spasms of the œsophagus, with or without rising of frothy, bloody mucus into the mouth.

° Sensation as of a ball rising in the œsophagus.

° Œsophagitis (in one case where the inflammation was located at the cardiac orifice, prompt relief was obtained by Veratrum viride). (*Hale.*)

### Appetite.

Increase of appetite, and digestion (from small doses).

### Stomach.

\* *Excruciating pain in the* lower part of the stomach.

\* Constrictive pain, increased by warm drinks.

\* *Violent nausea and vomiting*, with collapse; very slow pulse, and cold sweat.

\* Painful, empty retching, with ejection of only a little bloody mucus.

Severe hiccough, with sensation of dryness and heat in the throat.

Violent vomiting, coming on every fifteen minutes.

\* *Smallest quantity of food or drink is immediately* rejected.

Pains in the stomach are drawing, twisting, pressing, aggravated by the least noise.

Stomach seems to press against the spine while lying upon the back.

Vomiting of bile and blood.

Sharp, flying pains in the epigastrium and umbilical region, pressing down to pelvis.

\* Gastritis, acute—(here the high dilutions are useful).

° Neuralgic or spasmodic affections of the stomach, accompanied by vomiting, retching and excessive irritation.

### Abdomen and Stool.

\* Neuralgic like pains at the right side of the umbilicus, passing down to the groin.

Dull, heavy aching pains in the umbilical region.

\* Cutting, aching pains in the umbilical region, with rumbling in the bowels, and desire for stool.

Soft, mushy stool, preceded by cutting pains in the bowels, and followed by cutting pains in rectum and anus.

Neuralgic and long-lasting pains in the rectum.

Neuralgic pains in the left groin.

Hæmorrhoids, half the tumor red and the other half purple.

* Cholera and cholera morbus.

° Acute enteritis with high fever, dark and bloody stools.

### Kidneys, Urine, etc.

Profuse urine, which is pale.

Specific gravity is decreased.

Increases the solid constituents of the urine.

It is said to eliminate lithic acid.

° Cystitis acutus, with fever.

### Generative Organs.

*Male:*  ° Orchitis (acute), the local application is especially useful.

*Female:*  ° Acute metritis. (Internally give the 1-10th and apply a lotion externally.)

° Congestions during uterine disorders—(reflex congestions to chest and brain).

° Menstrual colic (previous to the discharge, when the congestion is great).

° Puerperal fever (with bounding hard pulse; cerebral congestion; delirium, etc.)

° *Convulsions before, during and after labor;* (Hale, Ludlam, and many other authorities of all schools.)

° Vomiting during pregnancy. (?)

° Hysterical convulsions.

° Congestive dysmenorrhœa in plethoric subjects.

° Puerperal mania; she becomes silent, suspicious and distrustful; would not see her physician; his presence seemed to terrify her; she feared he would poison her; complete sleeplessness, could be with difficulty confined to her bedroom (cured in six hours).

### Chest.

* Active congestion and engorgement of the lungs.

* Anxious oppression of the chest.

* Sensation as of a heavy load on the chest.

* Constant, dull, burning pain in the region of the heart.

Oppression of the chest with nausea.

° Pneumonia, with high fever, *will arrest the inflammation
 in the first stage.* (*Hale.*)

° Pleurisy in the first stage; often superior to Aconite.

Respirations fall from 18 to 12 in the healthy.

Respirations fall from 40 to 12 in pneumonia.

### Heart.

Prickling pains in the region of the heart.

Dull, aching pains in the region of the heart.

*Constant burning distress in the cardiac region.*

° Faintness after rising from the recumbent position.

Syncope when walking, only relieved by lying down.

Pulsations reduced from 68 to 24 in health; and from 140 **to**
 33 in fever.

Beats of the heart low and feeble. (*p.*)

Palpitation of the heart. (*s.*)

Fluttering sensation in the region of the heart. (*s.*)

Palpitation on taking the least exercise. (*s.*)

Strong, loud beating of the heart, with quick pulse. (*s.*)

° Palpitation, with dyspnœa.

° Cardiac oppression, with passive congestion, and tendency to
 fainting and collapse [from the 3 × to the 6 × dilutions].

° *Carditis and pericarditis,* especially rheumatic, with strong
 forcible impulse, during the first stage [from the 1st to
 the 3d dilutions]. (*Hale.*)

### Back.

\* Very severe, and constant aching pains in the back of the
 neck and shoulders.

Neuralgic pains in the back.

° Cerebro-spinal congestion and cerebro-spinal meningitis.

### Extremities.

Drawing pains in the right elbow and calves of the legs.

\* Cramps of the legs and of the fingers and toes.

\* Galvanic-like shocks in the limbs, of great violence.

Coldness, blueness and dampness of the hands, feet and limbs,
 with cramps of extremities.

Paralysis of the lower limbs.

### Sleep.

Some sleep every night, but has frightful dreams of being on
 the water.

Restless nights, and frightful dreams of being drowned.

### Fever.

*Chilliness with nausea.*

\* Coldness of the whole body with cold perspiration on hands, feet and face.

\* Coldness, with pale skin, flabby muscles, and quick, weak pulse.

° Pulse reduced from 130 to 60 in fever.

Pulse 35, slow and soft, with nausea and vomiting.

Weak, scarcely perceptible pulse, reduced from 68 to 52.

Feeble, irregular, scarcely perceptible pulse.

° Ephemeral fevers, with vertigo, headache, dimness of sight, nausea and weakness.

° Remittent or bilious fevers, not dependent on miasmatic influences.

° Typhoid fever, commencing with violent arterial action; pulse 120 hard; violent pain in the back of the head; delirium and black diarrhœa. (*Dr. Henry.*)

° Typhus fever. (?) Fevers, with tongue yellow on the *edges*, and red in the centre.

° All fevers *with full, frequent, hard pulse*, and tendency to congestion of the head, spasms, etc. (*Hale.*)

° Yellow fever [was successfully used in Savannah].

° In certain typhoidal cases which the morbid action has continued for weeks, pulse at 130, under the use of Veratrum viride, the pulse sinks to 70 or 80, and rapid convalescence sets in.

° Cerebro-spinal fever ["spotted fever"] in the first stage. (*Ib.*)

### Generalities.

° Acute rheumatism with high fever, full, hard, rapid pulse, some pains in joints and muscles; very scanty red urine —use the lowest dilutions. (*Hale.*)

Sensation of prickling and tickling, particularly in the extremities.

° Violent pains attending the inflammations.

\* Contortions of the muscles of the face, neck, fingers and toes; head drawn to one side; mouth drawn down at one cor-ner, and the facial muscles affected with convulsive twitching; at turns these contortions would take the form of tonic spasms, while at other times the action would simulate a series of galvanic shocks, frequently of such violence as to precipitate the patient out of bed.

° Exerts a sedative influence over the nerves of motion.

° Hysterical, epileptiform and puerperal convulsions and convulsions of children.

Complete loss of power of the locomotive muscles.

° Trismus, opisthotonos and other convulsions.

° Convulsion coming on suddenly, frothing at the mouth and violent jactitations of all voluntary muscles.

° Chorea of two months' duration.

° Chorea in a girl aged 12, the muscular commotion was violent, universal and unaffected by sleep; the lips covered with foam, worked up by a continued champing of the teeth; had not taken nourishment for days—[cured in four days].

° Chorea, in a woman, childless, and subject to menorrhagia, with continual nodding of the head and violent convulsive action in one arm, and jactitation of one leg.

° Chorea of two months' duration; the entire muscular system was in a continuous and tumultuous motion, the face was worked into the most horrible and ludicrous contortions; head constantly jerking; writhing of the whole body, and no sleep.

° Chorea, in a lady of thirty, constant moving of the head, lower jaw, larynx and tongue, twitching of the head, jerking of the arms and lower extremities; when these symptoms would subside, she would be attacked with violent palpitation of the heart. Veratrum always relieved this cardiac chorea.

° Puerperal convulsions, with furious delirium, found curative in doses from ten to thirty drops every hour till the convulsions subsided.

° Cerebro-spinal disease; pulse quick and wiry; pupils dilated; muscles of the back and neck contracted, drawing head back on the shoulders; delirium; spasmodic cough; finally tetanic convulsions occurring every five or ten minutes for five days; opisthotonus; cold, clammy sweat over the body. Veratrum brought about a rapid recovery.

° Cerebro-spinal disease in a child; burning fever, frequent vomiting, cries out on any attempt to move him, draws the head backwards, rolls up the eyes, puts the hands back of his ears, rolls the head from side to side, pulse wiry, rapid, 150, spinal column pungently hot and dry with petechiæ; cured in five days. (2.) A child of three months, very much emaciated, head much enlarged and misshapen, drawn back, so much contraction of the spinal muscles is compelled to lie on side, eyes rolled upwards, rolling of the head, moaning and screaming, great heat in back of the head and spine, respiration feeble and sighing, pulse 160 and feeble, watery diarrhœa, urine scanty and high colored; all these alarming symptoms disappeared in a week.

° Epileptiform convulsions in a boy of four and a half, with high fever, pulse 190, rapid respirations, 76 in a minute, and much cerebro-spinal irritation.

### Skin.

Coldness of the skin, which is usually perspiring.

Tingling and prickling of the skin.

Cold, clammy and insensible skin.

Vesication of the skin when applied externally, also erythema.

Hot, burning and sensitive skin.

° Eruptions of the skin, with very high fever.

° The first, or inflammatory stage of scarlatina, small-pox, measles.

° *In scarlatina it wards off cerebro-spinal irritation.*

° *Erysipelas; phlegmonous or vesicular;* apply topically a lotion ʒ i to ℥ iv, and internally 1st × dilution.

---

# VERONICA BECCABUNGA.

*(Brook-lime.)*

BOTANICAL DESCRIPTION.—This plant is called by Grey, Veronica Americana. It is perennial, with opposite, usually serrate, leaves; flowers in axillary, opposite racemes; corolla wheel-shaped, pale blue, with purple stripes; pod rounded, notched, many-seeded. Flowers in June and August. Found in brooks and ditches, and grows from eight to fifteen inches high.

OFFICINAL PREPARATIONS.—Tincture; dilutions.

ANALOGUES.—(?).

° "Nursing sore mouth." — Stomatitis materna. (Dr. N. F. Prentice,) who gives it internally in the first decimal attenuation, and has an aqueous solution of the same strength applied to the mouth.

[*King's Dispensatory* says: "It is anti-scorbutic, diuretic, vermifuge, and emmenagogue — useful in scurvy, fever and cough."]

---

# VERBENA HASTATA.

### (*Blue Vervain.*)

OFFICINAL PREPARATIONS.—Tincture of the leaves or root; dilutions (Infusion for external application.)

ANALOGUES.—*Arnica* (?), *Bryonia* (?).

[The uses of this remedy are given in a paper contributed to the transactions of the New York State Homœopathic Society, by Dr. S. M. Griffin, accompanied by beautiful engravings of the plant. See Vol. VIII, 1870, page 324.]

° *Rhus poisoning.* Dr. Griffin reports many cases of persons who were suffering severely from poisoning by poison ivy, cured in a very short time by the external application of an infusion, or the tincture largely diluted. He says the swelling, itching and burning are relieved in a few hours.

° Promotes the absorption of blood effused in bruises, and allays the attendant pain. (*King.*)

Vesicular erysipelas. (?)

[The country people call this plant Ague-weed, from its supposed value in intermittents. It is as bitter as Quinine, and I have known many instances of old agues being arrested, not to return, by the use of the infusion.—*Hale.*]

---

# XANTHOXYLUM FRAXINEUM.

### (*Prickly Ash.*)

BOTANICAL DESCRIPTON.—A shrub, ten or twelve feet in height, with alternate *branches*, which are armed with strong, conical, brown *prickles*, with a broad base, scattered irregularly, though most frequently in pairs at the insertion of the young branches. The *leaves* are alternate and pinnate, the leaflets about five pairs, with an odd one, nearly sessile, ovate, acute, with slight vesicular serratures, somewhat downy underneath. The common petiole is round, usually prickly on the back, and sometimes unarmed. The *flowers* are in small, dense, sessile umbels, near the origin of the young branches; they are small, greenish, diœcious, or polygamous, appear before the leaves, and have a somewhat aromatic odor.

[The *X. Carolinianum* is the only other indigenous species. It is found only in the Southern States, and is a large tree, sometimes growing forty feet high, and having a diameter of ten or twelve inches.]

OFFICINAL PREPARATIONS.—Tincture of the berries and bark; dilutions.

ANALOGUES.—*Camphora, Ammonium carbonicum, Asarum, Veratrum album.*

### Mental Sphere.

Great despondency; irritability.

Anguish about the chest.

Fearfulness; terrible nervous frightened feeling.

### Head.

Head feels full and heavy.

Vertigo; bewildered feeling; insensibility.

Pain over both eyes, throbbing pressure above root of **nose.**

Grinding pain in the head, with nausea.

Severe pain in top of head, as if it would come off.

The head feels as if it was divided.

### Eyes.

Lachrymation; pain in the lid of right **eye.**

Dull heavy pain in the left eye.

° Ophthalmia. (*Dr. Cullis.*)

### Ears.

Dull pain in the left ear; ringing in the right **ear.**

### Nose.

Fluent coryza.

Discharge of bloody scales of mucus from the nose, **right side.**

### Face.

Pain in the right jaw-socket.

Dull pain in the left side of the lower **jaw.**

### Mouth.

*Ptyalism;* tongue coated yellow.

### Throat.

Throbbing in the throat, and sensation of swelling.

Soreness, with expectoration of tough mucus.

42

A "bunch" in left side of throat when swallowing.

Aphonia, from cold or general debility.

### Stomach.

Fluttering in the stomach; feeling of fullness.

### Abdomen and Stool.

Fullness and pressure at the epigastrium, with colic pain in right iliac region.

Rumbiing, with soreness on pressure.

° Epidemic dysentery, characterized by spasmodic tenesmus, intestinal spasms, tympanitis, etc.

Inodorous discharges, with tenesmus.

° *Cholera,* in the stage of collapse (when **Veratrum album fails**).

### Urinary Organs.

Profuse and light colored urine.

### Generative Organs.

*Women.*—Menses too soon.

Profuse menses, with violent pains.

° Leucorrhœa, with amenorrhœa.   ° After pains

° Menorrhagia, and threatened abortion.

° Amenorrhœa, recent.  (*Dr. Cullis.*)

° *Amenorrhœa of one year's standing.*  A girl æt. 18: paleness of face, lips, tongue, fauces and conjunctiva; face bloated, with dark rings round the eyes; appetite poor; abdomen bloated; urine cloudy, and deposits a brick-dust sediment, scanty; œdema of feet and limbs, great weakness, dyspnœa and a chlorotic condition. (The first dilution brought on the menses in four days, after other remedies had failed; cure completed by Calcarea and Ferrum. (*Dr. C. A. Williams.*)

° *Amenorrhœa for five months;* face and legs œdematous; very nervous, sensitive to the least noise, hysterical mood; voice tremulous; fears she is going to die; general chlorotic appearance, constipation, scanty, frequent and dark urine; (the 1st dil. cured this case in a few weeks.) (*Ib.*)

° *Amenorrhœa for five months;* with severe pains over right ovary; constant headache; bearing down and tension in hypogastric region, (the 1st, soon relieved the pain in the head, and restored the menses in a few days.) (*Ib.*)

° *Amenorrhœa* from getting the feet wet; lasting six months. Symptoms: emaciation, with cough; dirty-gray expectoration; pale face, night sweats, (cured in a short time by the 1st.) (*Ib.*)

° *Ovarian and sacral pains during pregnancy.* (*Ib.*)

° Ovarian pains, with scanty and retarded menses. (*Ib.*)

° *Dysmenorrhœa*, with agonizing pains, driving patients almost distracted. (*Dr. Cullis.*)

° Is indicated in *neuralgic dysmenorrhœa* by the presence of pain along the course of genito-crural nerve. Spare habit, nervous temperament, and delicate organization, seems more particularly to call for this remedy. (*Dr. Massey, of England. "Notes on New Remedies."*)

### Chest.

Oppression of the chest, with a desire to take deep inspiration.

Shortness of breath.

Tightness of the chest; difficulty to inflate the chest.

Pain in the left side, under the fourth rib.

### Arms.

Pain in the right shoulder and arm.

Pain and pricking feeling in the right arm, extending to the third finger.

Numbness of the left arm.

Pricking and throbbing sensation in the left arm and fingers.

### Legs.

Excessive weakness of the lower limbs.

Pain in the left leg, between hip and knee.

### Generalities.

Prickling sensations extending to the whole body and extremities.

Gentle shocks, like electricity, pouring through the body.

Numbness all through left side of the body.

° Paralysis of single members.

° Hemiplegia, after Nux vomica failed.

Fever, with flushed and hot face, followed by great depression

Flashes of heat from head to foot.

Nausea, followed by chills.

° Typhoid fever, in the stage of collapse.

## ZIZIA INTEGERIMA.

*(Golden Alexander.)*

BOTANICAL DESCRIPTION OF Z. INTEGERIMA.—*Stem* smooth, erect, glaucous, one to two feet high; *leaves,* bi or tri-ternate: *leaflets* entire, ovate, oblong, one inch or more in length, petiolate; *rays* of the umbels very slender, two or three inches long, about thirteen in number, with minute involucels or none; *seeds* terate or five-angled.

"The root of this plant is very large, sometimes the size of a small wrist or a large thumb, very soft and spongy, perfectly white internally, with a weak, not unpleasant odor, a weak, sweetish, aromatic taste, not very unlike that of sweet cicely; not pungent or disagreeable. Swine are very fond of it, and eat it eagerly." (*Dr. J. S. Douglas.*)

It is doubtful if *Z. integerima* is capable of causing poisonous symptoms in men.

The Zizia Aurea has been removed from that genus, and is now called the *Thaspium aureum.* I am satisfied that the symptoms recorded in the pathogenesis under that plant, belong to the Thaspium. I have therefore placed it under that name. (*Hale.*)

(*See* "*Thaspium aureum.*")

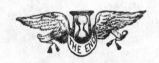

# APPENDIX

TO THE

# SYMPTOMATOLOGY OF NEW REMEDIES,

BY

## E. M. HALE, M.D.

---

THIS *Appendix* contains all the remedies mentioned in the last edition of *Therapeutics of New Remedies,* and not mentioned in the last edition of *Symptomatology.*

It gives the latest provings of such remedies, or the characteristic symptoms of their pathogeneses.

If no provings of the drug have been made, the curative or clinical symptoms are given.

The description, officinal preparation, etc., of each remedy is given, as in the body of this work.

The author has aimed to bring this volume, by means of this *Appendix,* fully up to the date of this writing.

E. M. H.

CHICAGO, January 1st, 1882.

## ALSTONIA CONSTRICTA.

### (*Bitter Bark.*)

DESCRIPTION.—A tall shrub or tree, belonging to the order of Apocynaceæ, indigenous to the colonies of New South Wales and Queensland.

PREPARATION.—Tincture of the bark.  Triturations of Alstonin.

Invariably produces great debility and general prostration.  Low fever often, with diarrhœa.  When pushed sufficiently far, rigors, sweats (usually cold), and other symptoms resembling fever and ague.  (*Cathcart.*)

° Intermittent fever, especially after the abuse of quinine.

° Great debility during convalescence from acute diseases of every kind.

° Summer diarrhœa in hot climates, with passage of undigested food.

° Malarial dysentery, or from bad water impregnated with decayed vegetable matter.

° Camp diarrhœa and dysentery of soldiers.

° Atonic diarrhœa.

° Typho-malarial fever?

---

## AMMONIUM IODATUM.

### (*Iodide of Ammonia.*)

DESCRIPTION.—The Iodide of ammonia is made by mixing the Iodide of potassium and the Sulphate of ammonia in boiling water, and cooling the mixture.  Alcohol is then added, and the mixture cooled to below 40° C. This is filtered and evaporated.  The crystals are granular, white, and deliquescent.  It dissolves freely in water and alcohol, the solutions becoming yellow on exposure.

PREPARATION.—Triturations.

### (° *No Provings.*)

° Chronic, persistent headache in young or full-fed persons.

° Headaches, caused by close rooms or confinement indoors.

° Headache in school children.

# AMYL NITRITE.

*(Nitrite of Amyl.)*

PHARMACOLOGY.—See page 42 of Symptomatology.

### Head.

\* *Beating, throbbing, bursting sensation in the head and ears, with constriction of the throat and heart.*

### Face.

° *Flushing and perspirations of the face and neck of women at the change of life.*
° Neuralgia of the fifth nerve.
° Supraorbital neuralgia.

### Eyes.

Under the ophthalmoscope *the veins of the disk were seen to become enlarged,* varicose and tortuous.

### Ears.

*Much throbbing in the ears.*
\* Tinnitus aurium.

### Nose.

\* Epistaxis.

### Throat.

*Choking feeling in the throat on each side of the trachea, along the carotids.* Feeling of constriction. *The collar seemed too tight, with desire to loosen it.*

### Stomach.

° Spasm of the stomach (Dr. Anstie), very successful in seasickness (by inhalation and internally).
° *Hiccough.*

### Generative Organs.

° Violent dysmenorrhœa with scanty menstruation.

### Chest and Respiration.

*A feeling of constriction in the throat extended to the chest, and produced dyspnœa and asthmatic feeling in the larynx and trachea with desire to eructate.*
° Asthma, it removes the dyspnœa immediately and prevents its return.

## Heart and Circulation.

* *Præcordial anxiety.*
* *The beating of the heart and of the carotids is in some persons very marked.*
* *Accelerated heart-action, with increased frequency of cardiac pulsations.*
* Great cardiac oppression and tumultuous heart-action.
* An aching pain and constriction around the heart.

It invariably quickens the pulse, sometimes doubling its pace.

° Angina pectoris with throbbing of the heart and carotids as high as the ears.

* Angina pectoris with great agony (Drs. Brunton, Anstie, and Talfourd Jones).

° Very successful in sun-stroke or heat-stroke.

° *Fainting*—from any cause.

## Extremities.

Tired feeling of the limbs.

## Generalities.

° A severe burning sensation over the loins, from whence a glow of heat spreads over the whole body, followed by perspiration.

---

# ANTIMONIUM ARSENITUM
### (*Arsenide of Antimony.*)

DESCRIPTION.—Antimony unites with most metals by fusion, forming alloys, which are generally brittle. The alloy with antimony is very hard, brittle, and fusible. It is completely decomposed by ignition at a moderate heat in an atmosphere of carbonic anhydride, the arsenic volatilizing and the antimony remaining It is found native in the Chalanche Mountains, Isère, Allemont, and a few other places. It then has the form of fine-grained, spherical or kidney-shaped masses with uneven fracture.

PREPARATIONS.—Triturations.

Congestion of the head.

Pain in the forehead. Pressure in the temples. General sick feeling. Sense of weakness. Pain in the orbits. Conjunctivitis. Œdema of the face. Loss of appetite. Nausea. Diarrhœa, slight without pain. Pulse, 90. Wandering pains along the sciatic nerve.

\* Cardiac dyspnœa, with cough.  (*Hale.*)

o Excessive dyspnœa in cases of emphysema.  (*Dr. Payr.*)

\* Great weakness of the heart (chronic).  (*Dr. Hale.*)

---

# ANTIMONIUM IODATUM.

### (*Teriodide of Antimony.*)

DESCRIPTION.—Iodine and antimony combine together directly, with the evolution of so much heat, that if large quantities are employed explosions may ensue.  It is a brownish-red crystalline mass, yielding a cinnabar-red powder.  On heating it melts to a garnet-red liquid and forms a violet-red vapor, which at a higher temperature becomes scarlet.  Water decomposes it, with the formation of a yellow iodide.

PREPARATION.—Triturations.

### *No Proving.*

o Bronchitis, humid asthma, and even cases simulating pulmonary phthisis.

o Frequent spells of coughing, with the expectoration of frothy, white, or yellowish mucus.

o Loss of appetite and strength.

o Moderate febrile action.

o Coated tongue, with nausea and disgust for food.

o Yellowish discoloration of the skin and conjunctiva.

o Chronic bronchitis, with or without asthma.

o Uterine areolar hyperplasia.

---

# ARUM DRACONTIUM.

### (*Green Dragon—Dragon Root.*)

DESCRIPTION.—A low perennial herb, with a tuberous root-stalk, sending up a single scape, sheathed with the petioles of the veiny leaves, as if caulescent.  Leaf usually solitary, pedately divided into 7–11 oblong, lanceolate pointed leaflets; spadix androgynous, tapering to a long and slender point beyond the oblong and convolute-pointed spathe.  Corus clustered.  Petiole 1° to 2° long, much longer than the peduncle; spathe greenish, rolled into a tube, with a short, erect point.  Found in low grounds along streams.  Flowers in May.

OFFICINAL PREPARATIONS.—Tincture and triturations from the root.

ANALOGUES.—*Arum triphyllum, Arum maculatum, Arum italicum, Ailantus, Argentum nit., Belladonna, Causticum, Carbo veg., Eryngium, Hepar sulph., Io-*

dine, *Kali bich.*, *Nitric acid*, *Merc. iod.*, *Phosphorus*, *Phytolacca*, *Rhus vernix*, *Sticta*, *Sulphur*, *Sanguinaria*, *Spongia*, *Wyethia*.

### Ears.

Shooting pains in the right ear, transient and frequent, and leave a *feeling of fulness and slight aching in the middle ear.*

A feeling of warmth and fulness in the ears.

Accumulation of mucus in the left Eustachian tube. (*See Throat Symptoms.*)

### Mouth and Fauces.

* There is a feeling of *dryness* and *smarting in the throat*, a feeling of *rawness*, with a sense of *fulness*, not really painful, but sufficiently annoying to attract constant attention.
* *Hawking; hoarseness;* expectorated a quantity of thick mucus.
* Produce a *continual disposition to clear the throat by swallowing and coughing.*
* *Throat raw and sore.*
* *Constant rawness of the throat.*
* *Constant coughing* with mucus in the morning.

Bad taste in the mouth :

Tongue and mouth coated with a foul, slimy mucus, having a putrid taste.

Expectoration consisting of thick, heavy, yellowish-white pus. (?)

Continuation of violent cough.

Rawness of throat and purulent expectoration.

### Larynx.

* *Soreness of the larynx* and great disposition to cough.
* *About midnight great oppression of breathing*, soon passing off, leaving considerable rattling of mucus in the larynx and upper part of the trachea.
* *Paroxysms of dyspnœa would sometimes occur, with much aching in the chest,* always associated with a considerable secretion of mucus in the larynx and trachea.

*Expectoration of thick, heavy, yellowish-white pus from larynx in large quantities.* (*Hart.*)

*Croupy cough, with hoarseness and rawness of the throat ;* during an epidemic influenza. (*Hale.*)

### Stomach.

Pain in the bowels, caused by incarceration of flatus.

Sinking feeling at the pit of the stomach.

Bilious passages from the bowels, attended with aching in the abdomen, and burning in the rectum.

### Urinary.

Irresistible desire to pass urine, which is diminished in quantity, very high-colored, and has a burning or smarting effect on the urethra. (*Primary.*)

Frequent, copious emissions of limpid urine; inclination to urinate every hour or so during the day.

Urine increased to four or five times the normal amount.

Tenderness and slight smarting or burning of the orifice of the urethra, especially during micturition. (*Secondary.*)

### Sexual.

During the proving a great diminution, and most of the time an entire absence of the sexual desire.

Penis flaccid and relaxed.

### Respiratory Organs.

* *Awoke about midnight with great oppression of breathing, a kind of asthmatic attack,* which, however, soon passed off.

* *Paroxysms of dyspnœa* would sometimes occur, with much aching in the chest, and always associated with a considerable secretion of mucus in the larynx and trachea.

### Heart.

Slight aching pain in præcordial region and down the left arm, flushing of hands and face, and increased heart's action

### Back.

Aching along the spine, particularly between the shoulder-blades and the lumbar region.

Great weakness across the loins.

Feeling of extreme prostration.

### Extremities.

Tingling, or slight stinging sensation in the fingers.

Tingling, or slight stinging sensation in the toes.

Preternatural heat in the palms of the hands.

Burning of the soles of the feet.

---

## AURUM ARSENIOSUM.

*(Sulph. Arsenate of Gold.)*

DESCRIPTION.—There are two salts of these elements, a tribasic and a dibasic salt.

The tribasic is formed by precipitation from a gold solution with the tribasic Arsenate of sodium. It is a dark-brown precipitate, soluble in water.

The dibasic salt is obtained by precipitation of a solution with the neutral salt arsenite of sodium. It dissolves in pure water, with a red-brown color.

PREPARATION.—Triturations, from $3^x$ to $6^x$.

° *Suicidal mania*, accompanied with great fear of death. ° *Chronic headaches*, due to syphilis, necrosis, periostitis, and ozæna.

° Cancer of the face, nose, stomach, and uterus.

° Malignant diseases of the intestinal tract.

° Lupus, depending upon scrofula, are rapidly ameliorated and ultimately cured.

° Rapid increase of appetite. The peristaltic contractions of the stomach and intestines are excited, and absorption occurs with greater rapidity. ° Functional cardiac diseases. (*Hale.*)

° Anæmia and chlorosis.

---

## AURI ET SODII CHLORIDUM.

*(Chloro-aurate of Sodium.)*

DESCRIPTION.—Crystals are long four-sided prisms, permanent in air.

PREPARATION.—Aqueous solutions, and triturations with granular sugar of milk.

Violent gastro-enteritis, accompanied by cramps, convulsive trembling, insomnia, priapism, insensibility.

Epigastric pains; nausea; loss of appetite; constipation; increased secretion of mucus from the intestinal glands.

° *Constipation*, with intestinal catarrh.

° *Nervous dyspepsia*, with melancholy, desire for death, with red glazed tongue. Pain in the stomach (left side), of a burn-

ing, drawing, pressing character, after eating, with tendency
to diarrhœa after eating.

○ *Gastric and duodenal catarrh,* and in some cases of *jaundice*
from catarrh of the gall-ducts, when the peculiar suicidal
melancholy is present.

○ *Syphilis,* after abuse of mercury, or when, during secondary or
tertiary stages, the bones of the nose are affected or the
throat is ulcerated.

### Sexual Organs.

* *Congestive irritation of the uterus and ovaries,* resulting in *sub-
acute metritis, ovaritis, profuse and premature menses, habitual
abortion, nymphomania,* and even *ulceration of the uterus, and
endo-cervicitis.* (*p.*)

○ *Puerperal mania,* with *sexual excitement, ovaritis, gastro-intestinal irritation, suicidal impulses?* (*p.*)

○ *Atonic amenorrhœa; scanty and delayed menses; deficient sexual desire; sterility from ovarian torpor; ovarian dropsy.* (*s.*)

○ Sexual erethism from plethora; seminal emissions with vivid
dreams; strong erections. (*p.*)

○ Decline of sexual power; diurnal seminal losses, or nightly
emissions, with feeble erections and no dreams; impotence
from weak, inefficient erections, irritability of the sexual
organs, and premature emission of semen. (*s.*)

○ Melancholy, suicidal mania, and hypochondria.

○ Cerebral anæmia; vertigo.

○ Dropsy, from chronic Bright's disease.

○ Cardiac diseases, from sexual disorders.

---

# BENZOATE OF LITHIA.

DESCRIPTION.—Prepared by heating Carbonate of lithia and water with
Benzoic acid until effervescence ceases, filter, and evaporate to dryness. It is
soluble in 3½ parts cold and 2½ parts hot water.

PREPARATION.—Aqueous solution or triturations.

○ Diminishes the uric acid deposits.
Consult the pathogeneses of Lithium and Benzoic acid.

# BERBERIS AQUIFOLIUM.

BOTANICAL DESCRIPTION.—This tree is a native of California and Oregon. It should not be confounded with Berberis vulgaris, the common Barberry.
PREPARATION.—Tincture of the root.

° Syphilis in all its stages. (?)

° Syphilitic psoriasis.

° Psoriasis diffusa.

° Terrible eruption, covering the scalp and extending downwards over the face and chest; exact species not stated, but probably eczema capitis.

° Eruption confined to the ears and back of the head and neck, of six months' standing.

° Roughness of the skin of the face in women.

° Dry, rough, and scaly skin.

° Cutaneous affections, especially squamous, such as psoriasis and pityriasis.

° Tumor of the breast, with sharp pain in it, worse at night; hard and circumscribed, like scirrhus.

---

# BISMUTHUM.

DESCRIPTION.—Bismuth is a grayish-white metal. The crystals are pyramidal cubes like common salt, and become coated with a film of the oxide when exposed to water. It expands when it solidifies, possesses the property of dimagnetism, and burns with bluish flame and yellow fumes. It is completely soluble in nitric acid.
PREPARATION.—Triturations (of oxide, or subnitrate).

### Mind.

He was morose and discontented with his condition, and complains about it.

### Head.

Vertigo. A sensation as if the anterior half of the brain were turning in a circle several times during the day, lasting several minutes.

* Pressure and sensation of heaviness in the forehead, more violent on motion.

\* Violent pressive heavy pain in the forehead. Pressure and sensation of heaviness in the occiput, more violent on motion.

### Stomach.

\* Nausea in the stomach; feels as if he would vomit, especially violent after eating.

\* Pressure in the stomach, especially after eating.

\* *Frequent empty eructations and feeling of discomfort in the stomach.*

\* Nausea with pressure in the stomach.

\* Uncomfortable feeling in the stomach.

\* Pressure in the stomach changes to burning.

\* Distressing pressure and burning in the region of the stomach.

\* Some pressure in the region of the stomach and empty eructations.

### Abdomen.

Pinching pressure in the lower abdomen, and rumbling with desire; a sensation as if he must go to stool.

### Urinary Organs.

\* Frequent urination, every time profuse. Urine is watery.

### Chest.

\* Pain in the chest and back, with burning, with boring and burning.

\* *Pinching-pressive pain in the region of the diaphragm, extending transversely through the chest.*

### Sleep.

In the morning, a few hours after rising, an excessive sleepiness, but after eating he was unable to take an accustomed nap.

At night, frequent waking in sleep as from fright.

At night, frequent wakings, with weariness. Restless sleep at night on account of voluptuous dreams, without, or frequently with, emission of semen.

# BRACHYGLOTTIS REPENS.

*(Puke-puké, New Zealand.)*

OFFICINAL PREPARATION.—Tincture of the green leaves and flowers.

### Head.

Confusion in the head and pain in the forehead.
Giddiness and flushed face.
Headache, pressive and throbbing in the forehead.

### Ears.

Itching and pricking in the ears.

### Nose.

Itching and burning in the nostrils.

### Face.

Faceache, left side, as if the submaxillary glands were affected, extending to the upper part of the face.

### Mouth.

Pricking and numbness in the tongue, evening.

### Throat.

Soreness and rawness in the throat, evening.

### Stomach.

Nausea and eructation of the taste of the ingesta, evening.
Fluttering in the stomach.

### Abdomen.

Fluttering sensation in the abdomen.
Soreness in the groins, as if in the spermatic cords, and a thrilling sensation through the penis and testes.
Almost constant pain in the groins and weariness in the limbs.
Throbbing in the left groin, morning.

### Stool.

Evacuations of dry fæces, with sore, constrictive pain in the anus, evening.

### Urinary Organs.

Soreness in the region of the kidneys.
Pressure and soreness in the neck of the bladder.

43

When passing urine, pain in the bladder and soreness in the urethra; feeling as if the urine could not be retained.

Urine abundant; sp. gr., .08; full of mucous filaments under the microscope, consisting of mucous corpuscles and epithelium.

Pain in the neck of the bladder.

A large quantity of pale-colored urine voided; sp. gr., .08; boiling and nitric acid test prove albumen.

Passed a large quantity of dark-colored urine, containing long threads, which, when examined microscopically, proved less mucus, but more transparent waxy casts.

Urinary secretion painful in the bladder and urethra, and distinct in the penis.

Passed about 56 ounces of urine in twenty-four hours; sp. gr., 20; full of white mucous sediment, containing epithelium, triple phosphates, and mucous casts from the kidneys.

### Sexual Organs.
Throbbing in the penis, and desire to pass urine.

### Respiratory Organs.
Oppressive breathing.

### Chest.
Pain in left side of chest, region of the heart, evening.

### Neck and Back.
Pain in the neck by moving the head from one side to the other.

Weariness in the back from coccyx upwards, and dull pain in the region of the kidney.

Soreness in the lower spine, violent and intense.

After riding, the pain in the lumbar region returned with great intensity, extending also to the pectoral muscles and anus.

Feeling as if the whole back would contract backward, and the muscles of the neck were affected.

Great prostration and pain in the lumbar region by walking.

### Extremities.
Prostration and weakness in the extremities.

Great inclination to stretch the limbs, and especially the arm, to give relief to the weariness between the shoulder-blades and trapeze muscles.

### Superior Extremities.

Weariness in the arms.

Pain of great intensity in the deltoid of the left arm.

Sensation of pain running along left upper arm, becoming stationary.

### Inferior Extremities.

Great lassitude and prostration.

Except in the spine, where the pain is not constant, it appears as if its action could be traced along the anterior branches of the saphenic nerves, and perhaps along the sciatic nerve.

The pain in the groin is unquestionably due to the crural nerve.

It was some time before the irritability of the bladder and urethra ceased.

The prostration and weakness lasted several days, and the isolated troubles through the arms, legs, and thighs continued several weeks.

---

# THE BROMIDES.

DESCRIPTION.—Bromine unites directly with most metals. The application of heat is necessary to induce the combustion of some of them.

Vapor of bromine passed over ignited. Calcium, potassium, or sodium forms a bromide of the metal. Mercury combines with the liquid bromide at ordinary temperatures. Bromide of ethyl is formed by distilling hydrobromic acid or bromide of phosphorus with alcohol. Nearly all the bromides are soluble in water. They strongly resemble the chlorides. Chlorine with the aid of heat readily drives off the bromine and converts them into chlorides. They are rather unstable, some of them giving off part of the bromine on exposure to the air.

---

# BROMIDE OF CALCIUM.

OFFICINAL PREPARATIONS.—Triturations.

*(No Provings.)*

° Congestion of the brain, with delirium and sleeplessness.

° Sleeplessness, with great nervous irritability.

° Controls the cerebral congestions and irritations of children, whether direct or reflex.

° In the incipient and first stages of cerebral diseases in nervous, irritable children.

# BROMIDE OF ETHYL.

DESCRIPTION.—Ethylic bromide is a transparent, colorless, neutral liquid, with a strong ethereal odor, and a disagreeable sweetish taste, with a somewhat burning after-taste. It is sparingly soluble in water, but mixes in all proportions with alcohol and ether. It burns with difficulty, giving a beautiful green flame, which does not smoke, but which evolves a strong odor of hydrobromic acid.

PREPARATIONS.—Never given except by inhalation.

The action of ethyl bromide has been observed by numerous experimenters, who give it the following physiological actions:

By inhalation or subcutaneously, it causes death by a toxic action on the centre of respiration.

An injection into the jugular toward the heart kills by cardiac arrest, probably due to an action on the cardiac muscles.

In toxic doses it diminishes the frequency of the heart, followed by a subsequent permanent rise to normal rate.

In toxic doses, it depresses the actual tension steadily, due in major part to the depressant action of the drug upon the heart, and in minor part to a partial loss of tone of either the spinal vaso-motor centres, or the peripheral vaso-motor system.

The inhibitory power of the pneumogastric is not paralyzed.

----

# BROMIDE OF MERCURY.

OFFICINAL PREPARATIONS.—Triturations.

### Mouth.

Increased salivation. Very nauseous tastes. Very disgusting metallic taste.

### Throat.

Disagreeable sensation in the pharynx. Very raw, scraping sensation in the pharynx, provoking cough.

### Stomach.

Eructations. Nausea. Vomiting with painful effort and most violent griping pain in the abdomen. Violent efforts to vomit and obstinate vomiting of tenacious, and afterwards of bloody mucus. Burning pains in the stomach and pharynx. *Pressure in the stomach.*

### Abdomen.

The abdomen is drawn back to the vertebral column, very sensitive to touch. Griping in the abdomen. Slight pressure and pains in the intestines. Colic-like pains. Most violent colic and painful tenesmus.

### Stool.

Frequent stools, with colic and rumbling in the bowels. Thin stools, repeated four times in a few hours, quite watery. Pasty stools.

### Urine.

Increased secretion of urine.

### Chest.

Difficult respiration. Heaviness in the chest. Small, slow pulse. Great weakness.

### Skin.

A large number of boils on various parts of the body, especially in the left axilla and left arm, where the drug had been rubbed in. They were very painful and would not heal. When one heals another appears in its place. Perspiration over the whole body, with great apprehensiveness during the violent pains.

° Diphtheritic sore throat. (*Hale.*)

---

# BROMIDE OF NICKEL.

PREPARATION.—Triturations.

(*No Proving.*)

° Congestive and neuralgic headaches. (*Hale.*)

---

# BROMIDE OF QUINIA.

PREPARATION.—Triturations.

(*No Proving.*)

° Intermittent fever, with cerebral congestion.

## BROMIDE OF SODIUM.

OFFICINAL PREPARATIONS.—Triturations.   Aqueous dilutions.

Melancholy.   Loss of will power.   Mental indolence.

Stupor on waking.

Vertigo; the ground seems to waver under his feet.

Lachrymation.   Sneezing.

Face pale.

Salivation, salty taste.   Loss of sensibility in the throat.   Thirst.

Cough.   Pulse small and rapid.   Ataxia.

Suppression of reflex sensibility.

Great desire to sleep.

° Cerebral hyperæmia, with nervousness and sleeplessness.

---

## BROMIDE OF ZINC.

PREPARATION.—Triturations.

(*No Provings.*)

° Pain in the nerves of face and head in teething children.

° Exhausted condition, due to teething, causing marked stupor, alternating with wakefulness.

° Symptoms simulating hydrocephalus.

° Periodical violent pain in the head, during brain-fag in business men.

° Chronic congestion of the brain, with a tendency to dementia or melancholy.

## BUFO.

OFFICINAL PREPARATION.—Trituration of the poison from the cutaneous glands, obtained by irritating the Rana Bufo.

### Head.

Inclination to be angry, to bite.   Stupor.   Giddiness, with heaviness of the head.   Headache in the forehead and on the vertex; the parts are tender to the touch, especially in the evening.   One-sided headache (right side), relieved by bleeding of the nose.   Headache after breakfast, aggravated by light and noise, accompanied by cold feet and palpitation of the heart.   Profuse perspiration on the head.

Eyes red, injected, itching, swollen. Appearance of objects as if there were a veil before the eyes. Sneezing in the evening when going to bed. Bleeding of the nose relieving the headache.

### Face.

Pimples on the upper lip, with coryza. Momentary hot flushes of the face. Erysipelas.

### Mouth.

Stuttering. Black tongue. Fetid odor from the mouth. Mucus descends from the nose into the posterior nares. Dryness in the throat, impeding deglutition (morning).

### Stomach.

Faintness from emptiness of the stomach. Eructations, as from rotten eggs. Vomiting after drinking. After eating, irresistible sleepiness. Colic pain after drinking milk and after smoking tobacco.

### Bowels.

Stools white. Constipation, with coldness of the body and hot head. Hæmorrhoidal tumors, with discharge of bright-red blood.

### Urinary Organs.

Frequent discharge of pale urine. Urine brown, of offensive odor. Burning pain in kidneys, with oppressed breathing and faintness.

### Sexual Organs.

*Men.* Inclination to touch the genitals.

*Women.* Menstruation too early, with headache.

### Chest.

Cough, with stitches in the larynx. Sensation as if the chest and the heart were constricted. Stitches in right side of chest. Palpitation of the heart after a meal, with nausea.

### Extremities.

*Upper.* Large blisters in the palms of the hands. Panaritium, swelling blue-black around the nail, followed by suppuration. After a slight contusion of the finger, tearing pain, with redness along the whole arm, following the lymphatic vessels into the armpit, causing there painful glandular swelling.

*Lower.* Cramps in the legs.   Great weakness of the legs.   Blisters on the soles of the feet.

### Skin.

Yellow color of the skin.   Small wounds suppurate much.   Carbuncles.   Ulcers, with burning pains.

### Generalities.

Great weakness, fainting.   Swelling of the whole body.   Twitching of the muscles.   Convulsions.   * Epilepsy (after fright).

---

## CADMIUM IODATUM.

### (*Iodide of Cadmium.*)

DESCRIPTION.—Prepared either in the dry way or by digesting Cadmium with Iodine and water.   It crystallizes in large, transparent, six-sided tables, which are not altered by exposure to air.   It melts easily, and solidifies again in the crystalline form.   It dissolves readily in water and in alcohol.

PREPARATION.—Triturations, and as an ointment.

### (*No Provings.*)

° Enlarged glands, of a scrofulous character.

° Nodes and chronic inflammation of the joints.

---

## CALCAREA IODATA.

### (*Iodide of Calcium.*)

DESCRIPTION.—Prepared by heating Calcium and Iodine vapor, or dissolving lime or the Carbonate of calcium in Hydriodic acid, evaporating, and fusing the residue in a closed vessel.   It resembles the chloride.   It melts below a red heat, and if in contact with the air is decomposed with the formation of lime and the separation of Iodine.   It is very soluble and deliquescent.

The provings of Calcarea iodata so far are of little value.   They do not afford any characteristic clue to its physiological effects.   It is better to consult the provings of Calcarea and Iodine for indications.

# CEANOTHUS VIRGINIANA.

*(New Jersey Tea—Red Root.)*

DESCRIPTION.—(See page 167, "Symptomatology.")

### Generalities.

" *Great nervous excitement, with chilliness, loss of appetite.*

" Feeling as if the nerves were shaken, and one day at dinner could scarcely hold knife and fork.

Chilliness, chiefly down the back.

*Shivered with cold chills (i. e., rigors).*

### Abdomen.

Bowels were relaxed.

\* *Menses appeared ten days too early, and were very profuse.*

### Spleen.

° Enormous enlargement of the spleen. *(Dunham.)*

° " Splenitis, with violent vomiting, pain all up the left side, cough, with expectoration, profuse perspirations, and fever.

Considerable fever, cough, pain in left side, and dulness on percussion of the same side.

° Chronic splenitis. Chronic swelling in the left side under the ribs, with considerable cutting pain in it.

Patient stated that it was worse in cold, damp weather, and always felt chilly.

Chilliness severe and lasting.

Spends most of the time by the fire.

Dreads winter.

In summer is nearly well, but the lump in spleen and chilliness and pain persisted, but are quite bearable in warm weather.

° Severe pain in the left side in the region of the spleen.

° Severe pain in the left side and a large swelling in the same position.

° Enormous spleen, occupying the entire left hypochondrium, and reaching inferiorly to about an inch above the crest of the ilium; it bulged toward the median line, and ran off to an angle laterally.

° Chronic hyprtrophy of the spleen.

° Considerable and very painful swelling in the left side under
  the ribs.
° Jaundice, characterized by very severe pain in the left side.
° *Metrorrhagia*, characterized by pain in the left hypochondrium.
° Chronic splenitis, chills, and leucorrhœa.
° Pain in the *left* side for several months, aud *right*-sided head-
  ache.
° Severe pain and fulness in the left side, with inability to lie
  on that side. (Cured symptoms, all from Dr. Burnet, of
  London, Eng.)

## CHIONANTHUS VIRGINICA.

DESCRIPTION.—(See page 209 of "Symptomatology.")

### Stomach and Bowels.

Sensations of contractions in the stomach, as if some living thing
  was moving in it. Uneasy sensations in the region of the
  liver, and occasionally in the region of the spleen. Unpleasant sensations in the stomach and hypochondria increase
  and become very annoying.

Sensations like spasms or palpitation of the heart in the stomach.
  Uneasy feeling in the region of the sigmoid flexure, as if
  caused by flatulence. Uneasiness in right hypochondrium,
  extending to left iliac region. Tongue coated yellow in the
  centre; previously clean. Evacuation of bowels at bedtime of black, tarry-like fæces. A feeling as if the bowels
  were about to move off violently from the action of a purgative, with the nausea usually associated with such an action, though there is no discharge from the bowels.

° *Jaundice*, with enlarged liver.

### Spine.

Pain for a short time in the spine, from seventh to tenth dorsal
  vertebræ.

### Head.

Head remarkably clear for a few hours, and all the symptoms of
  the previous aphasia (before proving) disappeared, but returned the next day not so severe.

# CUCURBITA PEPO SEMEN.

(*Pumpkin Seed.*)

PREPARATION.—The bruised seed, taken in doses from one to two ounces.

° *Tape-worms.*   (See " Therapeutics," page 212.)

---

# ERIODICTYON CALIFORNICUM.

(*Yerba Santa.*)

DESCRIPTION.—This plant is a native of California, somewhat branching, and attains a height of from two to four feet, presenting a most beautiful aspect to the eye.   The leaves are petiolate, finely serrated, and oblong, the upper surface being a dark, glistening green.

PREPARATION.—Tincture made from the leaves.

### Head.

Dizziness, like slight intoxication.

Head heavy and dull.   Sense of pressure outwards on all sides in the head, greatest at cerebellum.   Severe, oppressive headache.

Dull, frontal headache.

Sharp pain in right ear at intervals, or upon suddenly changing position of head to right or left.   Shooting pains about external ear.

Face flushed.   * Yellowish-green catarrhal discharge from the nose.   Coryza and sneezing.

### Throat.

Burning sensation in fauces and throat.

* Occasional small, jelly-like mucous discharge from posterior nares.   Dryness of posterior nares.   Irritation of posterior nares, sticky mucous discharge downward into throat, constant hawking, some irritation of fauces.

### Stomach.

Deathly sickness at stomach, lasting one hour.   Nausea, with looseness of bowels on taking the least food, followed by sense of repletion.   Feeling of great distension of stomach and bowels, though no real distension is perceptible.   Oppressive sensation in cardiac region.

## Abdomen.

Sensation of great distension of the abdomen, continuing for thirty-six hours.

Very disagreeable relaxation of anus and rectum—prolapsus ani.

## Sexual Organs.

Sore and tender feeling of left testis principally; could not bear any pressure upon it, and dreaded to move because of its tenderness; relieved by great pressure.

## Respiratory Organs.

* Wheezing voice; asthmatic symptoms. Constriction of larynx; sensation as if something pressed on the trachea near the supra-sternal notch. Constriction and dryness of larynx. Irritation of larynx and trachea. Increased sensitiveness of larynx and trachea to changes of the atmosphere, and also to the use of the vocal cords; either cause provokes a paroxysm of coughing. Expectoration of white mucus.

° Acute and chronic bronchial catarrh.

## Chest.

Constant heavy feeling in chest behind sternum. Sensation of heavy weight on chest. Heaviness of chest, which occasionally requires a deep breath to relieve it. Sharp pain in right lung, occurring at short intervals, or upon sudden change of position.

## Heart and Pulse.

Slight pain in the præcordial region.

Pulse accelerated 10 beats, accompanied with a peculiar nervous sensibility.

## Extremities.

Pains in left forearm.

Severe pain in left knee, with difficulty in using leg.

## Skin.

Covered with scarlet rash, which lasted four or five days.

## Fever.

Slight fever. Cheeks flushed and burning.

## Sleep.

Groaned much in sleep. Moaning during the night.

# EUONYMIN.

DESCRIPTION.—Euonymin is the active principle of Euonymus Atropurpureus, which is described in the "Symptomatology," page 293.

PREPARATION.—*Triturations.*

No systematic proving of Euonymin has yet been made, and in lieu of a proving I submit an article, which appeared in the New York *Medical Times,* for September, 1881.

A proving of Euonymus Europæus can be found in Volume X, of Allen's *Encyclopædia of Materia Medica.*

"Before entering upon the subject-matter of this paper, the writer desires to call attention to the valuable work recently issued, entitled ' An Experimental Research on the Physiological Action of Drugs on the Secretion of Bile,' by William Rutherford, M.D., F.R.S. Edinburgh: 1880. Dr. Rutherford, aided by his two pupils, Vignal and Dodds, entered upon the experiments which are detailed in this volume, with a determination to ascertain the exact value of certain drugs supposed to influence the secretion of bile. After showing that clinical experience is very untrustworthy, and previous experiments not wholly reliable, they decided to adopt the following improved plan of experimentation. Briefly, it was as follows:

"'The *dog* was selected. 1. Because the size of the common bile duct renders it possible to introduce a canula with an orifice sufficiently large to prevent its being blocked up by particles of inspissated mucus from the gall-bladder. 2. For the reason that its digestion resembles that of man, inasmuch as its stomach becomes empty when the process is completed. . . . .

"'The selection of the dog has proved fortunate, for the results of our experiments are in complete harmony with every perfectly ascertained fact regarding the action of medicinal agents on the human liver, and prove that the liver of this animal is affected in the same *sense*—although it may not be in the same *degree*—by substances that act on the human liver. All the experiments have been performed on animals of the same species, placed as nearly as possible under similar conditions; the results are fairly comparable; although it must be borne in mind that, just as no two members of the human species can, even in their normal condition, be regarded as equally susceptible to the influence of any medicinal agent, neither can any two members of the canine species be held to possess identical susceptibilities. All the animals had a full meal of lean meat at three or four o'clock in the afternoon, and the experiment was begun between nine and ten o'clock on the following morning, so that the digestion and absorption of the food was completed, and the animal was therefore in a fasting condition.

"'This was an essential preliminary; for, as is well known, the secretion of bile is accelerated during the process of digestion; and had we taken the amount of bile secreted per hour during digestion, as an index of the activity of the liver previous to the administration of a drug, our experiments would necessarily have been worthless. The disturbing effect of irregular muscular movements upon the biliary flow was prevented by injecting into a vein small doses of *Curare*, repeated at intervals, when the motor paralysis which it induces became too slight.　In consequence of the *Curare* palsy, artificial respiration was had recourse to, and maintained at regular intervals throughout the whole experiment.　*Chloroform* was used during the preliminary operation in two cases, but the stimulation of the liver which it induced rendered the experiments worthless.　On the other hand, we have abundantly proved that the doses of *Curare*, administered in the following experiments, have no influence on the biliary secretion, and do not interfere with the effects of hepatic stimulants.　It is therefore an exceedingly valuable auxiliary in a research of this nature.

"'The method of experiment we adopted was always that of a *temporary biliary fistula*.　Through an opening in the linea alba, a glass canula was inserted into the common bile duct, near its junction with the duodenum, and tied therein.　To the end of the canula projecting from the abdomen a short caoutchouc tube was attached, and to the free end of this a short glass tube, drawn to a narrow aperture, so that the bile might drop·from it, as Röhrig (Op. VI.) had recommended.　The gall-bladder was then compressed, in order to fill the whole tubing with bile, and the cystic duct was clamped to prevent its return to the gall-bladder, and so compel all the bile secreted by the liver to flow through the canula.　The wound in the abdominal wall was then carefully closed, and in all save the earliest experiments the animal was thoroughly covered with cotton-wool, in order to quickly restore it to its normal temperature; and, guided by a thermometer in the abdominal cavity, great care was taken to keep the temperature normal—a matter of no small importance; for if the temperature fall several degrees, the liver secretes more slowly.

"'The respiration requires to be maintained with regularity, otherwise the biliary flow is rendered somewhat unequal by irregular diaphragmatic compression of the liver.　Moreover, if the respiration be deficient, the secretion of bile is always diminished.　Some of the slight oscillations observable in the charts of the biliary secretion in these experiments are probably owing to variations 'n the respiration; for in the earlier experiments we were obliged to have the 'espiratory bellows moved by hand, and this is never so regular as a machine. Notwithstanding this, however, the main results of these experiments are perfectly clear.

"'Until it is attempted, one might suppose that this mode of experiment is extremely simple, but it is by no means so simple as it appears.　It is needful to manipulate the abdominal viscera with great care, and to avoid all dragging at the bile-duct; otherwise the secretion of bile becomes so irregular that the experiment may be useless.　The canula must be very carefully retained in a position which will permit its moving with the diaphragm, but will prevent it from twisting the duct, and thus impeding the exit of the bile by forming a valve at its orifice.

"'Röhrig estimated the velocity of the biliary secretion by counting the seconds·that elapsed between the fall of the drops from the orifice of the tube.　A single trial convinced us that this method is extremely laborious, and leads to inaccurate results, because it does not permit of continuous observations for any length of time. Variations in secretion often occur independently of the administration of any substance, and it is impossible to estimate their significance, and make due allowance for them, unless the method of continuous collection of the bile be adopted. Moreover, we soon found that the degree of viscosity of the bile caused a variation in the size of the drops, and, therefore, in the intervals between their fall. We therefore abandoned this for the more accurate method of allowing the bile to flow into a fine cubic centimeter measure and recording the quantity secreted every quarter of an hour. In addition to constant collection of the bile, this method has the great advantage of permitting a graphic representation of the results.'

"The experiments are illustrated by cuts showing the rise or fall of the bile current. They are similar to those cuts used to illustrate the rise and fall of human temperature in fevers. I append one of the cuts,—showing the tracings, —illustrating the action of *Euonymin* on the liver, also the text explaining the experiment.

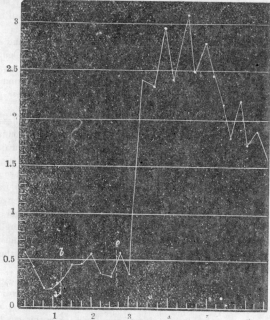

"Secretion of bile before and after 'Euonymin.' 1.1 cc. bile and 3 cc. water injected into the duodenum at *b*. The same five grains 'Euonymin' injected at *e*.

" ' *Experiment* 28.—Dog that had fasted twenty-four hours. Weight, 23.3 kilogrammes. The unusually long fast resulted from the animal having refused to take food on the afternoon of the day preceding the experiment. It was probably owing to this circumstance that the secretion of bile was so low at the beginning of the experiment.

"'*Autopsy.*—Stomach contracted, mucous membrane normal. The "Euonymin" had extended along about a third of the small intestine. The mucous membrane of the upper third was extremely vascular. Mucous flakes were scattered over the surface, and the whole appearance of the membrane reminded us of the effects of Podophyllin. But notwithstanding the very obvious irritation, the intestine at this part contained only a small quantity of watery fluid. The remainder of the intestine was dry and contracted, without any signs of irritation.

"'*Results of Experiments with* "*Euonymin.*"—1. Five grains of "Euonymin," when mixed with a small quantity of boiling water and placed in the duodenum, powerfully stimulated the liver. The analysis of the bile secreted before and after "Euonymin" was lost. 2. Coincident with the marked action of the liver there was only slight increase of intestinal secretion. Seeing that Mr. Clothier found "Euonymin" to be an active purgative in the human subject, these experiments suggest that the purgative effect may be chiefly due to increased secretion of bile. At any rate these experiments clearly show that this substance is worthy of receiving far greater attention in practical medicine than it has done hitherto.'

"These experiments, which were carried out with great labor and scientific exactness, will be of infinite value to physicians of all schools, but more especially to those who recognize the law of *Similia* as the universal law of cure. Those also who understand the true 'Law of Dose,' as deduced from the primary and secondary actions of drugs, will be greatly aided in their prescriptions of these hepatic remedies.

"Rutherford records some facts which prove conclusively that these hepatic drugs have a double action, the one exactly opposed to the other, namely: (1) That, whereas small, or medium doses always produced a physiological increase of bile-flow, massive doses decreased or completely arrested the secretion of bile. (2) That when a drug produced active *increase* of the intestinal secretions, it *decreased* the secretion of bile. (3) That the primary increase of bile was often followed by a corresponding suspension of the secretion for a longer or shorter period. These observations are in accordance with my teachings regarding the pathogenetic actions of medicines, and from which I deduce the following axiom relating to the selection of the dose: (1) When the symptoms of a disorder resemble the *primary* action of a drug, prescribe that drug in the smallest rational dose.

"*Illustration.*—The primary action of *Podophyllin* was found to cause an increase of the secretion and flow of bile of a thin character, with colic, nausea, and irritation of the intestinal mucous membrane, especially the colon and rectum, with congestion and inflammation of the liver. For this condition the dose should not be below the 3x trit. or dil., if we desire prompt curative action. The *secondary* action of *Podophyllin* causes constipation, with arrested or retarded secretion of bile, with jaundice, hepatic enlargement, etc., or profuse choleraic discharges, with suppressed biliary secretion. For this condition the drug must be prescribed in more appreciable, yet small doses, as the $\frac{1}{100}$, $\frac{1}{75}$, $\frac{1}{50}$, $\frac{1}{25}$, or $\frac{1}{10}$ of a grain (I mean enough of the 1x or 2x trit. to make either of the above-mentioned doses), repeated at suitable intervals.

"The law of dose will apply to all the hepatic remedies whose primary and secondary action is similar to that mentioned above. There are some drugs which cause hepatic symptoms in a reverse order.

"As regards the relative power of the drugs experimented with by Dr. Rutherford, it is exceedingly interesting to compare their action by consulting the following list of indigenous drugs, which I copy from the monograph. The drugs are mentioned in the order of their relative inherent power:

| "Podophyllin, | per cent. | of bile | above | normal, | . | . | . | 0.47 |
|---|---|---|---|---|---|---|---|---|
| Iridin, | " | " | " | " | . | . | . | 0.39 |
| Euonymin, | " | " | " | " | . | . | . | 0 30 |
| Sanguinarin, | " | " | " | " | . | . | . | 0.42 |
| Baptisin, | " | " | " | " | . | . | . | 0.33 |
| Phytolaccin, | " | " | " | " | . | . | . | 0.16 |
| Hydrastin, | " | " | " | " | . | . | . | 0.38 |
| Juglandin, | " | " | " | " | . | . | . | 0.40 |
| Leptandra, | " | " | " | " | . | . | . | 0.31 |

"The table shows that *Podophyllin* caused the greatest amount of bile discharged during a given time; but the doses were larger than the doses of *Euonymin*, although the former is a very much more powerful drug. So with other drugs; they seem to show a higher degree of power, but, considering the relative potency of all the drugs (I mean the inherent power per grain) as disturbers of the general system, the *Euonymin* may be considered the most powerful in its pure, specific action, and in its influence over the secretion and expulsion of bile from the liver.

"It is interesting to note the different behavior of the discharge of bile under the influence of these drugs. Some cause a steady, continuous flow; others a rapid powerful 'spurt,' or high rise in the tracing; while a few cause an intermittent discharge. The latter two peculiarities are especially noticeable in the case of *Euonymin*. The above tracing beautifully illustrates the effect of *Euonymin* on the secretion of bile. Note the sudden high rise, then the slight arrest, followed by the still higher rise, and the intermittent flow during the gradual decrease. Another interesting feature in this proving is, that, on postmortem, the *upper third* of the mucous membrane of the *small intestines*—in the two experiments—was found to be *highly vascular*, and covered with flakes of mucus, while the lower two-thirds was *dry*. In the experiments with *Podophyllin*, 'the mucous membrane of the stomach and whole length of the small intestines was intensely red, and contained a large quantity of fluid; in another case the mucous membrane of the duodenum was intensely vascular.' This is what we might deduce from the provings of that drug, judging from the symptoms in our Materia Medica.

### CLINICAL OBSERVATIONS.

"We have no provings of *Euonymin* made in the usual manner of our school. Eclectic authorities have recorded that in doses of one-half drachm (ʒss) it causes 'nausea, vomiting, and purging.' Dr. Payne says the same dose taken by him caused 'all the symptoms of cholera morbus.' In the *Encyclopædia of*

44

*Materia Medica* is a case reported of a man who took 18 seeds of the *Euonymus Europeus* one evening, and 18 the following morning. 'He was seized with frightful abdominal pains and profuse diarrhœa, eventually bloody. He was not seen till evening, when he was in a state of profound collapse, with involuntary evacuations of blood and mucus. On lifting him up, tetanic convulsions were induced, which immediately preceded death.' *King's Disp.* records that the seeds of the *Euonymus Americanus* are a violent emetic and purgative. The seeds are doubtless more powerful than the bark, but the crude tincture or infusion of the bark is a powerful drug, for the following symptoms are recorded in my *Symptomatology of New Remedies*, and were collected from various sources, namely: 'Deathly sickness of the stomach, with perspiration and heat in face; violent catharsis with deathlike nausea; excessive tormina, prostration and cold sweats; evacuations violent, profuse, with much flatus.' It is true that large doses of the *Euonymin* would cause all these violent symptoms, but I think that in the process of separating the so-called active principle, from the crude bark, much of the acrid and irritating property is eliminated. The same occurs with other drugs, *e. g.*, *Quinine*. The taste of *Euonymin* has nothing about it reminding one of the pungent, acrid, and burning taste of the mother tinctures or the powdered bark. Rutherford suggests that if *Euonymin* causes purgation, it does so by causing a *profuse flow of bile*, which is a powerful purgative. This may be true of *Euonymin*, but I believe the crude bark or tincture has, aside from its cholagogue effect, an irritant action on the small intestines of the same *nature* as *Podophyllum*, but not in the same *degree*. I have used the 2x and 3x dilution of tincture of *Euonymin* in profuse and painful diarrhœa and cholera morbus and cholera infantum, and find it equal to *Podoph.* or *Verat. alb.* Eclectic authorities claim that *Euonymin* is very useful and efficient in the same affection, but my experience with it in such conditions is limited to a few cases. In another class of disorders, however, I have, during the last few years, used the lower triturations of *Euonymin*, with unqualified success, and I have selected it homœopathically, basing my selection on its one physio-pathological symptom, namely, *a profuse and irregular flow of bile* (primary) followed by its natural sequence—*a scanty or suppressed secretion of bile*.

" *Biliousness.*—This condition, so well known to the laity as well as the physician, is characterized by such symptoms as general *malaise*, a yellow or brown tongue, bitter or coppery taste in the mouth, headache, generally frontal, worse in the morning, or sometimes occipital, vertigo, dark spots before the eyes, disinclination for mental or physical labor, dark urine, constipation, or loose fecal, offensive evacuations, and muddy complexion. These symptoms are usually treated by homœopathists with *Nux vom.*, *Bry.*, *Merc.*, or *Podoph.* By the allopathic school with *Blue Mass*, or *Calomel*, followed by bitter-water, or some saline purge. Both methods are palliative, but not completely curative. The former method is by far the best. But I have had better success with *Euonymin* than with any other remedy. I find a few grains of the 1x trit. three times a day amply sufficient. After forty-eight hours, if the bowels do not move normally and the tongue is cleaning, I advise two or three ounces of bitter-water in the morning before breakfast. I use the 1x trit. because this condition simulates the *secondary* effects of *Euonymin*. *Per contra*, if the patient has a yellow-ish-white tongue, some nausea and griping in the bowels, with loose yellow or greenish stools, which burn the rectum, the 5x or 6x is prescribed, because these symptoms show an increased secretion and expulsion of bile, thus simulating the *primary* effect of *Euonymin*. In children of all ages, who are especially prone to this form of biliousness, or bilious diarrhœa with congestion and irritation of the small intestines, *Euonymin* 6x trit. acts more promptly and happily than any other drug, unless some *special* symptoms indicate *Merc.*, *Dulc.*, *Iris*, or *Podoph*. It is a notable fact, which any physician can verify, that if he prescribes *Euonymin* to his bilious patients to whom he has usually given *Nux*, *Bry.*, *Merc.*, *Podoph.*, or *Iris*, he will find that nearly all\will testify that they prefer *Euonymin* to any of the above, for they soon recognize its prompt, happy action, and its excellent effect upon their condition, especially in its power of restoring normal appetite and digestion. Many of my readers will recollect the cases of *Albuminuria* reported by Dr. W. H. Holcombe, and incorporated in the last edition of *Therapeutics of New Remedies*. The curative effects were brilliant, and the drug selected solely on account of its power over the secretion of bile.

"Referring to the hepatic and intestinal disorders of children, it must be remembered that the liver is much larger and more irritable in the very young than at any other age. *Euonymin* is, *par excellence*, the panacea of these disorders in children. But it must be used intelligently and in accordance with my law of dose, when it will act most happily. There are three conditions characterized by peculiar symptoms in which it is indicated.

"1. In children, especially in summer, when the bowels are disordered—the passages green, yellow, or olive-colored, colic, nausea, vomiting of bile, or food mixed with bile, some fever, loss of appetite, indigestion, especially of milk, languor and stupor, with pale, yellow, or earthy complexion—no remedy with which I am acquainted acts so favorably on this state as *Euonymin*, from the 3x to the 6x trituration, frequently repeated. It is possible the higher triturations may be efficacious, but I have never tried them.

"2. Every one who has had much to do with gastro-intestinal diseases of children have observed the peculiarly variable appearance of the stools and vomit. 'No two passages are alike' is the common report of the nurse. At one time they are green, then white, then watery or yellow, and the vomit just the same. *Pulsatilla* is said to be indicated for this, but I have succeeded better with *Euonymin* 3x trit. I believe this variability to be due to an irregular secretion and expulsion of bile, and for this Rutherford's experiments show *Euonymin* to be the *similimum*. In very young children the 3x trit. repeated in one grain doses every three hours, changes the character of the stools to a normal color and consistency. In older patients the 2x is required.

"3. In children or adults there often occurs the following group of symptoms: After a sudden attack of vomiting and purging of bilious matters—sometimes, however, without this first stage—we find the stools clay-colored, white, gray or watery and colorless, and very offensive; there is some gagging or nausea, the urine is high-colored, strong-smelling and contains bile; the food is not digested;

there is great prostration ; the complexion is sallow or jaundiced, and the expression dull and listless. Here the hepatic cells fail to eliminate biliary matters from the blood, and it seeks outlets through the skin and kidneys. Often the brain is poisoned and we have marked bilæmia. *Benzoic acid* has often done me good service in these cases, but I have found the 1x trit. of *Euonymin* to act more satisfactorily. This condition is such a one as we might expect would arise from an overstimulation of the liver with large doses of *Euonymin,* a reaction or secondary effect. Consequently the law of dose calls for the lowest trituration or material doses. In the jaundice of adults due to

" 4. *Biliary Calculi or Concretions,* the solid constituents of the bile are in excess. If such constituents are crystallizable we have *Calculi,* if not, we have concretions in the form of tarry, tough balls, often in great numbers. The indications of treatment are to increase the fluid portion of the bile, making it thinner, and thus dissolving the solid mattters, or washing them out of the gallbladder. After they have formed, and obstruct the gall-duct, the use of large doses of *Olive Oil* will aid in their expulsion ; but we should at the same time give hepatic remedies which thin the bile. *Chelidonium* is the chief remedy for this condition, although Rutherford says *Podoph., Iridin,* and nearly all the drugs he experimented with have this effect. I believe *Euonymin* has this effect equally with *Chelid.,* although, unfortunately, the analysis of the bile, after the use of *Euonymin,* was lost. I think I have prevented the formation of biliary calculi in many cases, by the use of both *Chelid.,* and *Euonymin,* with greater certainty than any other medicine. But we do not get good effects with doses higher than the 1x or ¼ trituration in material quantities repeated every three hours.

" 5. *Malarious Diseases.*—In true malarious disorders, notably those which cause intermittents, the poison in the blood paralyzes the hepatic cells. It often primarily irritates them, causing them to secrete an abnormally acrid bile, which results in bilious vomiting and catharsis. After this always comes paresis, with a whole train of symptoms, such as occur under bilæmia. Careful observers are aware that so long as this 'bilious' condition exists it is impossible to cure the ague or fever, but as soon as the tongue clears, and the stools become normal, the fever is easily subdued or the paroxysm arrested. This fact accounts for the ill success of the unscientific treatment of both schools ; the *old* with their routine of *Quinine ;* the *new* with the fruitless chase for the specific in each case. While engaged in practice in the State of Michigan, when four-fifths of all my cases were malarious fever, I observed that the country people used an infusion or a maceration of the bark of the " Wahoo" (*Euonymus*) in whiskey as a remedy for ague. It certainly succeeded after all other drugs failed, especially after the abuse of *Quinine,* for *Quinine* injures the liver as seriously and in a similar manner to malaria. Taking the hint from this domestic practice I used to give the tincture of the bark in appreciable doses, in alternation with homœopathic anti-periodic remedies, and with satisfactory results. I would advise those who have to deal with miasmatic, intermittent, or remittent fevers, that they give *Euonymin* 1x trit. doses of 2 grs. every two hours, until the tongue cleans and the secretions become normal. *Then* and not till then, select the *similimum* for the paroxysms, namely: *Quinine, Arsenicum, Cedron.*

*Gelseminum, Alstonia,* or one of the few antiperiodic remedies in our Materia Medica.

"This plan will insure success, and we shall escape the opprobrium of allowing our patients to pass out of our hands into those of the Philistines, or their own resort to the abuse of *Quinine.*

"6. *Dyspepsia.*—This protean disorder, depending as it does upon a great many pathological conditions of the stomach, liver, and nervous system, needs for its successful treatment a host of medicines. When, however, it depends upon *hepatic disorders,* as it does in this country in very many cases, we find in *Euonymin* its most powerful remedy. The *symptoms* for which I have found it most useful, are those which usually accompany slow and imperfect digestion, namely: sense of unnatural satiety, bloat of the stomach, sour, acrid, or bitter eructations, vomiting or regurgitation of food, headache after eating, sluggish or irregular action of the bowels, foul coated tongue, and bad breath. I usually prescribe two or three grains of a low trituration one hour before each meal. Its curative action is often generally aided by giving a few grains of *Pepsin* just before meals. If the digestion is painful—a hard, pressing, aching pain soon after meals—*Bismuth* 1x, a few grains, instead of *Pepsin.* If the pain comes on three or four hours after eating give *Nux* or *Lycop.*

"Finally, I use *Euonymin* in many other affections due directly or indirectly to hepatic disorder, but the limits of this paper will not allow further experience."

---

# FUCUS VESICULOSUS.
## (*Seawrack.*)

DESCRIPTION.—A perennial seaweed found on the shores of Europe and this country. The frond or flat leaf is smooth and glossy, from one to four feet long, from a half to one inch and a half broad, furnished with a midrib throughout its length, dichotomous, entire upon the margin, and of a dark olive green color.

PREPARATION.—Tincture and trituration of the dried plant. (Infusion.)

### Head.
Intolerable headache; forehead felt as if compressed by an iron ring.

### Stomach.
\* The act of digestion is no longer accompanied by flushings of the face, fulness, weight in the epigastric region, and fits of heat towards the head. The stomach acts with more rapidity, and the hour of repast is more impatiently looked for. Qualmishness. Weight in the stomach.

° Dyspepsia.

### Abdomen.
\* Flatulency diminishes and then disappears in those who have been habitually accustomed to it. Obstinate constipation.

° Chronic diarrhœa.

## Urinary Organs.

Urine more abundant, colored, and odorous than usual. It is only after two or three septenaries that the urine becomes more abundant, and begins to present upon its surface a coating or black film.

° Chronic cystitis.

° Irritable bladder.

## Respiratory Organs.

Sense of suffocation, especially during menses.

° Palpitation of the heart, with great dyspnœa.

## Extremities.

Skin of legs and thighs soft and flabby.

## Sexual Organs.

° Amenorrhœa with dysmenorrhœa.

° Functional derangement of the menstrual function dependent upon some fault of nutrition, or from plethora or excessive obesity. (° Scanty menses.)

## Generalities.

Lost upwards of five pounds weight, without any change in habits or diet, or experiencing any inconvenience from the use of the remedy. Diminution of thirty pounds in weight. The resolvent properties are manifested, and the first intimations of becoming thinner are displayed from the period when the urine is affected.

The thinness is not always produced in a uniform manner. I have seen it limited to isolated parts, which are, then, almost always those where the fatty tissue accumulates in the greatest abundance, thus, with one it is in the chest, with another in the abdomen, with a third in the nape of the neck and upper part of the shoulders.

* Emaciation.

° Debility. Malnutrition. Enlarged glands.

° Not a reducer of adipose tissue in the healthy subject. For cold, torpid, individuals, with cold, clammy skin, loose and flabby rolls of fat, pendulous belly.

° The plant is beneficial for lean people to use to make them fat and plump.

# GENTIANA QUINQUEFLORA.

### (Gall-weed.)

DESCRIPTION.—A member of the order *Gentinaceæ*.  The plant grows in woods and pastures, flowers in September and October, is found from Vermont to Pennsylvania, and a variety of it is common through the Western States.

PREPARATION.—Tincture of the herb.

### (No Proving.)

° Chronic ague where there is debility, and a tendency to relapse.

° Obstinate intermittents where Quinine and other antiperiodics had failed.   Increasing the flow of gastric juice, it is a valuable remedy for

° Dyspepsia, either primary or secondary.

° Liver affections.   Jaundice.

° Headache, periodic.

# GRINDELIA ROBUSTA.

DESCRIPTION.—This is a small herbaceous plant, with perennial root.  It belongs to the order *Compositæ*.  This species and the *Grindelia squarrosa*, which is often mistaken for it by herb-gatherers and druggists, is found on the plains of the Pacific Slope.  The whole plant, like the *G. squarrosa*, is permeated with a peculiar resin, which is most abundant in the flower-heads.

PREPARATIONS.—Tincture of the plant; dilutions.

° Chronic bronchitis and asthma.

° Humid asthma.   Dyspnœa dependent on an accumulation of mucus in the smaller bronchi—tenacious and difficult to detach.

° Spasmodic asthma.   Spasms due to irritability of the respiratory nerves.

° Dyspnœa due to paresis of the respiratory nerves.

° *A fear of going to sleep on account of loss of breath, which awakes him.*

° Cardiac asthma, due to deficient spinal innervation.

° Dyspnœa from heart disease.

° Acute catarrhal asthma.

° Chronic bronchitis, and cough, with muco-purulent expectoration after pneumonia.

° In the catarrhal stage of pertussis with profuse mucous secretion.

° Many forms of renal and cystic diseases, when the mucous discharge is a prominent symptom.

° Gonorrhœa and gleet.    ° Irritating leucorrhœa (*locally*).

° Local application for itching and erythematous eruptions, and mosquito-bites.

° *Antidote for poisoning by Rhus toxic.*   Apply to the skin in the form of an infusion or dilute tincture.

---

## GRINDELIA SQUARROSA.

DESCRIPTION.—This plant belongs to the natural order of *Compositæ*, and is a small herbaceous plant, indigenous to California.

The whole plant is permeated with a peculiar resin, which is most abundant in the flower-heads.   This and *G. robusta* are very similar in appearance, and belonging to the same genus, their actions on the human organism are very much alike.

PREPARATION.—Tincture of the herb.

### Head.

Terrible fulness in the head, similar to the effect produced by a large dose of Quinine.   Pain in the left eye, and right knee-joint, precisely like acute rheumatism.   The pain in the knee did not last long.   The pain in the left eye became very intense, then the right eye was affected; simultaneously with the affection of the right eye was an unbearable pain in the region of the liver and spleen, so severe that it was impossible to lie still.   Pains like acute rheumatism.

The pain of the eyes was in the *eyeballs* and ran back to the brain; pain increased by motion of the eyes.   Characteristic of the pain wherever occurring was that of rheumatism; pain with soreness.

The conjunctiva was remarkably injected.   Eyes presented the appearance noticed in congestion of the brain.

### Nervous System.

Full doses act first on the optic nerve, and in a little time influence the par vagum and interrupt respiration.   The disturbed respiration prevents sleep.   The moment the prover fell asleep respiration ceased, and it would not resume until awakened by the suffocation that resulted from the suspension of respiration.

# GUARANA.

*(Paullinia Sorbilis.)*

DESCRIPTION.—See page 484 of "Symptomatology."

## Head.

Giddiness. Tinnitus aurium. Redness of face. Staring eyes. Slight irregularity of the pulse. Moisture of the skin. Delirium. Dulness of hearing.

After its use in neuralgic headache phenomena of its poisonous action may be observed from the appearance of a malaise more distressing than the headache which has disappeared.

Sensation of pricking and cold, extending to the whole cutaneous surface.

Gayety. Extravagant behavior. Mental hyperæsthesia. Intellectual excitement. Unusual humor for continued hard work. Head confused from 9 P.M. until bedtime. Awoke at midnight, and complained of a tightness across the forehead; fell asleep shortly, and had no return of pain in the head on waking the next morning.

Aggravation from large doses when taken for headache. The pain became almost unbearable, and nearly the whole night he suffered from delirium.

Persistent twitching of the eyelids.

Sleeplessness. ° Sick-headache. ° Hemicrania. ·

## Chest.

Aggravation when taken for asthma. The difficulty of breathing became so great that he was forced to grasp a support and struggle for breath. The face was flushed with blood, then purple and livid, the eyes bright and staring at first, and the struggle for breath almost agonizing.

## Heart and Pulse.

Diminution of the heart-beats.

## General Symptoms.

Unsettled, restless. Unable to work with vigor. Distressing fulness and throbbing in the head, chiefly in the temporal regions, afternoon and evening.

° Rheumatic-neuralgic lumbago.

# HYDROBROMIC ACID.

SQUIBB'S PREPARATION.—By weight—Sulphuric acid, sp. gr. 1.838, at 15.6° C., parts 7, add to water part 1, and allow to cool. Potassium bromide, parts 6 ; water, parts 6 ; dissolve the salt in the water and heat. Add the acid to the Pot. Bromide solution slowly and with constant stirring. Set aside for twenty-four hours and allow the resulting salt to crystallize out ($KBr + H_2SO_4 = HKSO_4 + HBr$). Pour the liquid off into a retort, break up the crystalline mass and wash with water, parts 2; add the washings to the liquid in the retort, and distil to dryness. The residue is assayed with a solution of normal soda and diluted.

PREPARATION.—In aqueous dilutions.

## Head and Nervous Sphere.

○ Sleeplessness from mental or emotional irritation.

○ Cerebral irritation from overwork and business worry.

○ Cerebral congestion.

○ Nervousness from reflex irritation.

○ Hebetude of mind, tendency to sleep. Semi-stupor, with rest-
     lessness. Red tongue and great weakness.

○ Nervous fretfulness of children, when teething or from heat,
     even when feverish, when Aconite and Coffea are not efficient.

○ Hysterical erethism of nervous women, who suffer from the
     effects of social dissipation.

○ Tinnitus aurium. "Surring" and throbbing in the ears.
     Flushed face. Heat and heaviness in the heads of plethoric
     people.

○ Prevents and antidotes the cerebral effects of quinine.

## Sexual Organs.

○ Headache of women with scanty menses.

○ Plethora from celibacy, with repressed sexual functions.

# HYDROPHYLLUM VIRGINIANUM.

DESCRIPTION.—See page 361 of "Symptomatology."

## Eyes.

Eyes water and burn, with slight itching. Eyelids swollen, and the sclerotica much injected, presenting a fiery redness, and there was some sensitiveness to light. In the morning my eyelids were agglutinated, and, on opening my eyes, they were quite sensitive to the light. The burning and smart-ing was less, still, my eyes discharged water for two or three days.

* Catarrhal inflammation of the eyes.
° Erysipelas produced by Rhus.
° Snake-bites.

# IRIDIN.

DESCRIPTION.—Iridin is the active principle of Iris versicolor.

PREPARATION.—Triturations. Its symptoms are incorporated in the provings of Iris.

There is no distinct proving of Iridin. So far as is known, its symptomatology is like that of Iris versicolor, and the indications for the one may be taken for those of the other, as a general rule.

---

# KUMYSS.

DESCRIPTION.—Originally, fermented mare's milk. It is now made from cow's milk.

It is a sparkling, milky fluid, of sweetish, acidulous taste, which reminds one of sour cream. It always appears curdled. There are three grades of Kumyss: *new*, from two to seven days old; *medium*, from seven to twenty days old, and *old*, from twenty to sixty days or more. It is equally good, new or old. It may be made on a small scale by nearly filling a strong champagne bottle with fresh cow's milk, add an ounce of sugar, and some yeast about the size of two peas; cork and tie the cork firmly down; shake the bottle repeatedly, and place in a cellar, where it should be turned up and down a few times each day for five days, when it is ready, and may be used the twentieth day.

Kumyss, being purely a dietetic remedy, has no pathogenesis, though some of the head symptoms of lactic acid have been noticed after the long-continued use of Kumyss.

---

# MELILOTUS.
### (*Sweet Clover.*)

DESCRIPTION.—There are two varieties of sweet clover, one having yellow flowers (*M. officinalis*), and the other having white flowers (*M. alba*). A tincture made from both varieties was used in making this proving, and either variety can be used in practice.

PREPARATION.—Tincture made from the flowers.

### Mind.

Furious; was obliged to lock the prover in his room. Loss of consciousness.

### Head.

* Headache lasting four days, with oppression of the chest.
* Severe headache, almost delirious with headache. Extremely nervous, and during the day the severe, heavy, throbbing headache returned, so much so that it was feared some

of the bloodvessels would burst and some lesion of the brain occur. The odor gives some people the characteristic oppressive headache. In the afternoon had a heavy oppressive headache, which towards night assumed a heavy throbbing nature.

\* A frightful, heavy oppressive headache for three days, which is easiest relieved by applying vinegar to the head. Headache began gradually, and was confined to the left supraorbital region ; it was aggravated by motion ; on lying down it was better; if I allowed myself to think hard, as there was a disposition to do, it would ache worse ; on talking it would disappear from the frontal region and settle in the occipital region ; when silent it would return to the forehead. On waking the whole head would be affected, but worse over the eye.

### Nose.

\* Epistaxis. Blood gushed from the nose with loss of consciousness.

### Face.

\* Very red, highly congested face, almost livid.

### Stomach.

Acrid eructations all day, of a burning and smarting nature.

### Rectum.

Had a heavy throbbing and fulness in the rectum, due to internal piles, which had never before caused trouble.

### Urinary Organs.

Obliged to leave business to evacuate the bladder.

### Respiratory Organs.

Terribly distressing cough, causing great anxiety. Harsh, spasmodic cough. Dry cough, spasmodic and distressing. Smothered or partially suppressed cough. Very harassing cough, throat and bronchi not relieved until evening, when it began to loosen ; could expectorate freely the next morning. Oppressed for breath.

### Chest.

Much oppression of the chest ;. there seemed to be a load on the chest; difficult breathing. Awoke after sleeping badly, with a great deal of soreness in my chest, internally, with an oppression as of a great weight.

Through the day much difficulty of breathing. Every respiration was labored, with a continued feeling of fulness of the chest and head. Awoke with a spasmodic cough, and yet with the same oppression and spasmodic breathing and fulness of the chest. A great deal of soreness of the chest, both externally and internally.

\* Hæmoptysis.

### General Symptoms.

Very nervous and easily annoyed. Quite weak. Symptoms only relieved by profuse bleeding from the nose. Suffered for three days with a terrible headache, a bad cough, and oppression of the chest, but was relieved when the nose began to bleed, which it did to a frightful degree.

### Sleep.

Poor sleep. Passed a miserable night. Slept better towards morning.

### Fever.

Cold extremities.

---

# MERCURIUS IODATUS CUM KALI IODATUM.

### (*Double Iodide of Mercury and Potassium.*)

DESCRIPTION.—It is a yellow salt, made by adding Potassium iodide to a hot concentrated solution of Mercuric iodide, and cooling. Long yellow crystals are deposited from the mother liquor. These crystals, when heated, first give off water, and then melt into a red liquid, from which some of the Mercuric iodide separates. It is soluble in alcohol and ether, but water decomposes it, separating about one-half the Mercuric iodide; then the liquid yields by evaporation a saline mass.

This salt is also readily made by boiling a solution of Potassium iodide with Mercuric oxide.

PREPARATIONS.—Triturations.

### (*No Provings.*)

It causes profuse, watery mucous discharge from the throat, nose, and deeper air-passages.

° Influenza, with profuse, irritating discharges.

° *Secondary and tertiary syphilis.*

## MYOSOTIS SYMPHYTIFOLIA.

DESCRIPTION.—It belongs to the Myosotis family, and resembles the *M. Arvensis* somewhat. The plant grows in low, marshy grounds, also in high ground among the trees, and on the hill-sides in rich ground. The stalks grow from one to two feet high, either single or in bushes of from five to six. The leaves are lanceolate, not slim ; distinct median vein ; smaller veins, running out to near the edge of the leaf, and branching from the median alternately, not anastomosing. Both sides of the leaf are hairy. Flowers are small, whitish, or tinged faintly red or blue.

The root is at the largest parts hollow, the pith seemingly having rotted ; the smaller ones are woody and tortuous.

PREPARATION.—Tincture of the root.

(*No Provings.*)

○ Cough, with purulent expectoration.

---

## PENTHORUM SEDOIDES.

DESCRIPTION.—A perennial herb found in wet places in Canada and the United States. The flower is symmetrical, having 5 sepals, 10 stamens, 5 pistils, uniting below into a 5-angled, 5-horned, 5-celled pod, the quinary order of the flower probably giving the plant its name.

PREPARATION.—Tincture of the plant.

### Mind.

Mind dull, exceeding discouraged and desponding, everything went wrong but dinner. Reading interfered, because of mental dulness.

### Head.

Vertigo. On closing the eyes, felt like floating, could not read. Much annoyed by little noises. Dull, heavy headache with heat and soreness in the sacrum. Catarrhal aching in forehead.

Ringing and singing in both ears.

### Nose.

* Discharges from nares, thick, pus-like, streaked with blood, and an odor as if from an open sore.

* A peculiar wet feeling in nares as though a violent coryza would set in, which did not. Wet feeling in trachea and bronchi, passing from above downward, as if coryza would set in, followed by a slight feeling of constriction, which passed from above down through the chest.

\* Catarrhal feeling repeated itself. Nose felt stuffed, as if swollen. Sense of fulness of the nose and ears. A secondary symptom, a drawing, or contractile feeling of the muscles of the side of the nose affected with catarrh. Itching in the nares.

### Mouth.

Prickling, burning sensation on the tongue, as if scalded. Increased flow of saliva. Bloody sputa.

### Throat.

Posterior nares feel raw as if denuded of epithelium.

### Stomach.

An unpleasant sensation of disgust and nausea, which lasted three hours, but did not interfere with the next meal, which was eaten with greater relish.

### Rectum.

A crawling sensation in lower rectum. Burning in the rectum at stool, continued during the afternoon. Itching of the anus. Hæmorrhoids with aching in the sacrum.
Semi-fluid evacuation of the bowels, after having been constipated.

### Urinary Organs.

Dull aching in kidneys. Bladder sore on pressure. Burning in the urethra when micturating, continued for a week. Urine clear, passed more frequently, actively acid. Sediment thrown down when boiled with sulph. acid, ammonia, nitrate of silver, and nitric acid. Next day the urine was alkaline, slightly cloudy and caloric. Increased in quantity.

### Sexual Organs.

Sexual orgasm. Erethismus of the sexual system, almost a satyriasis; a slight varicocele of long standing was apparently cured. This condition was succeeded by a corresponding depression of sexual function approaching impotence, returning to the normal condition only after months.

### Respiratory Organs.

In the morning a cough, seemed to come from deep in the chest, with soreness in chest.

### Neck and Back.

Aching through basilar region. Aching in the sacrum, with itching of anus, hæmorrhoids.

### Extremities.

Arm went to sleep. Hand felt swollen. A trembling of legs for several days, with soreness of knees. While on the lounge the muscles of the leg were suddenly contracted, jerking up the foot as in stepping.

### Skin.

A long-cured impetiginous eczema reappeared on both legs. A few hot prickings in the skin. Itching of face and forehead.

### Sleep.

Fantastic dreams. Voluptuous dreams and increased sexual desire, sympathetic and urinary excitement. A few cold chills rush in succession up the spinal column.

---

## PHORADENDRON FLAVESCENS.
### (*Mistletoe.*)

DESCRIPTION.—It belongs to the Loranthaceæ family. A shrubby plant, which has a parasitic growth on trees in the northern temperate zone. The American mistletoe prefers elms and hickories, and is found from New Jersey to Illinois and southward.

### (*No Provings.*)

° Prevents miscarriage.   ° Hastens labor.

---

## PILOCARPUS PINNATUS.
### (*Jaborandi.*)

DESCRIPTION.—The name Jaborandi is applied in South America to several plants possessing diaphoretic properties. The Pilocarpus jaborandi is a shrub growing in Brazil. It is about five feet high; the root is cylindrical and slender; the leaves alternate and resemble those of the cherry-laurel.

PREPARATION.—Tincture of the leaves. Triturations of the alkaloid pilocarpin.

### Head.

Confusion of mind. Vertigo slight. Headache almost every day just about noon, for over two weeks after taking. Headache returned about noon, dull aching pain same as before, hurried breathing, pressure on the chest, great anxiety, palpitation of the heart, and pain in the region of the heart. Throbbing pains in the forehead and top of the head; next came pains in chest and around the heart; pain in the forehead became less, but increased in severity in the chest and above the heart. Dull pain in the occiput, extending over left side of head to the forehead.

## Eye.

Eyelids stiff and heavy. Augmentation of the lachrymal secretion. Eyeballs feel sore on moving them. Contraction of the pupil. When the perspiration and flow of saliva were at their height, sight became so dim that objects held near the face were imperceptible. Sight became blurred; at a distance of four feet could see a person, but could not distinguish the eyes. Impaired vision continued but only affected the sight of **distant** objects, near objects were distinctly seen. **Swimming of** distant objects. During the sweating and **salivation, appearance** as of numerous white spots before the eyes like flakes of snow. Dimness of vision returns. The state of the vision is constantly changing, becoming suddenly more or less dim every few minutes.

## Nose.

Profuse, watery, bland discharge from the nose.

## Face.

Slight increase of color. Redness and heat of face. Throbbing of the temporal arteries, and increased warmth of face, but skin still dry. Flushing of the face, ears, and neck. In those instances in which sweating took place the face became flushed, and was most marked when the perspiration was greatest.

## Mouth.

*Primarily.* Increased secretion of saliva, for a time requiring constant ejection; the secretion of this from the glands in the cheeks caused a kind of collapsed feeling in them; saliva distinctly alkaline; measured sixteen ounces in addition to that which flowed on the pillow while asleep. Salivation commences, and in a few minutes the mouth is literally

45

flowing with water; this continues for four or five hours, during which period ten to sixteen ounces can be collected. Free salivation, with profuse sweating. Salivation and sweating continued to be profuse until the sight became blurred. The salivation, when it occurred to a marked extent, began simultaneously with the sweating, was greatest when the sweating was most profuse, and lasted as long as the sweating. Salivary secretion extremely active. Submaxillary gland especially enlarged; on pressing it there was a gush of saliva under the tongue. Sat with forehead resting on edge of table, and let saliva run into a vessel on the floor. Tried to sleep, but had to clear the mouth of saliva every two or three minutes.

*Secondarily.* Great dryness of the mouth. Speech so affected that articulation was both difficult and indistinct.

### Throat.

Throat dry and inflamed. Quite a sore throat, smarting pain. Moderate swelling of the submaxillary glands.

### Stomach and Bowels.

Eructations and vomiting. Hiccough. Was sick and vomited a quantity of saliva which was swallowed. Dull, heavy distress in the pyloric portion of the stomach, as though some hard, indigestible substance was lying there, relieved by eating a full meal. Empty, gone feeling in the bowels.

° Nausea, vomiting, with salivation of pregnant women. (*Hale.*)

*Primarily.* Diarrhœa for several days, very loose; came with a gush; thin, watery, and yellow. Gone, empty feeling from the diarrhœa, but no pain whatever. Eleven copious, watery, undigested stools since 7 A.M. Continues to have from five to ten yellow, watery, painless stools a day.

*Secondarily.* Constipation.

### Urinary Organs.

Buring in the urethra, with urging to urinate. When administered in fractional doses, Jaborandi does not produce either perspiration or salivation, but becomes a powerful diuretic.

## Respiratory Organs.

Augmentation of bronchial secretions. Hurried breathing.

## Chest.

Pains in the chest, around the heart. Pressure on the chest; great anxiety, with palpitation of the heart and pain in the cardiac region. Sense of heavy pressure on the chest, hurried breathing, and great prostration.

## Heart and Pulse.

Pains about the heart, very severe, accompanied with severe palpitation.

Sphygmographic tracings, taken at different stages of the administration of the drug, showed almost complete asystolia, with a very noticeable diminution of vascular tension during the sweating stage. In each experiment the pulse became rapidly quicker, the increase varying from 40 to 50 a minute.

Pulse rose from 88 to 120.

## General Symptoms.

Very soon the face becomes red; the temporal arteries throb more strongly; then there is a peculiar feeling of heat in the mouth and face, and the flow of saliva commences. In a little while the forehead becomes moist, and the face more red; then beads of perspiration appear on the forehead, cheeks, and temples. The flow of saliva increases, all the salivary glands successively contributing to this effect. The mouth is filled with immense quantities of fluid, and expectoration is incessant; at the same time perspiration covers the face and neck; then the whole body becomes red and moist, and a pleasant warmth is experienced; in a few minutes perspiration breaks out over the whole surface, and soon runs down on all sides. Meantime, other symptoms have supervened. The eyelids first become moist, then the lachrymal secretion gradually augments, and, after collecting in the canthi, rolls slowly over the cheeks; at the same time there is a copious discharge from the Schneiderian membrane, increased by the tears which escape through the nasal canal; moreover, there is a heightened activity of the mucous

glands of the back-throat, trachea, and bronchi.   All these
effects reach their maximum of intensity in about three-
quarters of an hour after taking the drug, continuing thus
for thirty or forty minutes.   Lying on one side, that the
saliva may run more freely, the patient spits ten or fifteen
times a minute; the flow is so rapid that he can scarcely
speak; the salivary glands are enlarged, and the mouth becomes hotter.   From time to time the mucous accumulations
in the bronchi are cleared away by a slight cough; the sight
is dimmed by the flow of tears.   The body is bathed in perspiration; a shirt is wet through in a few minutes.   Now a
feeling of comfort or of weakness, as the case may be, is
experienced.   Thirst is intense.   The pupils are slightly
contracted.   By degrees the excessive activity of the secre-
tory processes is diminished; in an hour and a quarter, or
an hour and three-quarters, the lachrymation, the nasal discharge, the bronchial expectoration, and, finally, the flow of
saliva and the perspiration are sensibly lessened, and the
parts involved gradually return to their normal condition.
When the perspiration and flow of saliva have ceased, the
subject is prostrated and drowsy.   The parts which secreted
so copiously are now very dry, especially the mouth and
back-throat.   There is also much thirst.

Tried to walk about the room, but felt very weak, his legs giving
way under him.

Prostration of strength, even a short walk causing weariness,
hurried breathing, and palpitation of the heart; these symptoms lasted four days.

### Sleep.

Sleeplessness at night from restlessness, and on account of a sensation of firm pressure on the chest, with hurried breathing.

Fell asleep at 9.30 P.M., and spent a most wretched night; a
smart fever; increased pain in the head; general malaise;
no thirst; very restless, talking, moving, with some delirium.

### Fever.

Chilliness.   A decided fall in temperature occurred.   At the
moment the sweat was produced, there was an increase of

the temperature and of the pulse; then, during the period of active sweating, it was sometimes noted that these elements remained at the same point as at the outset of the experiment; sometimes there was slight diminution, but after the sweating a very notable lowering of the temperature and of the pulse was observed, which sometimes lasted two days after the experiment. (This was true in thirty-two experiments.)

Sweat breaks out on the face and upper part of the chest, which have been quite red for five or six minutes.

Simultaneously with the flow of saliva, the perspiration breaks out on the forehead and over the whole body; it extends to the limbs, but is most marked on the trunk.

Sweat quite profuse. Excessive perspiration from all parts of the body. ° Nightsweat.

---

# PIPER METHYSTICUM.
## (*Kava-Kava.*)

DESCRIPTION.—A plant indigenous to the islands of the Pacific Ocean. It grows to a height of 6 feet, and has a slender stem. The leaves are large, and as broad as long. 10 or 12 prominent veins radiate from the petiole, the 3 central ones being very close together. The root is large and fibrous, but light and spongy in texture.

PREPARATION.—Tincture of the root.

## Mind.

When concentrated, drunkenness is almost instantaneous; with the ordinary dose, it occurs about twenty minutes after ingestion. In a small dose kava is a tonic, stimulating beverage, producing an agreeable excitement, and affording support against great fatigue. In increased doses, this root determines an intoxication of a sorrowful, silent and sleepy character, completely different from that produced by alcoholic drinks. The habitual drinkers of kava take it six or eight times a day, but then a nervous trembling seizes them, and they can scarcely raise the cup to their lips. The intoxication does not last longer than two hours, but if a person only takes it occasionally, the effects may continue twelve; when taken at intervals of some days, the intoxication continues for six hours. When made from the root grown in damp soils, the drinker remains plunged in a deep torpor, and becomes irritated by the least noise. Often when the dose is too great or too small, instead of the sleep an intoxication, accompanied by fantastic ideas and a strong desire to skip about, although one cannot for a moment hold himself on his legs. Felt all day unusual life, vigor, and exhilaration. Felt more lively than usual; in better spirits; inclined to work. Capable of doing more work, without fatigue or brain-fag.

### Head.

Dizziness and frontal pressure, even when lying in bed in the morning.

From 5 to 9 P.M. unusual dizziness, swimming sensation and faintness.

Pains, especially of the head, relieved temporarily by turning the mind to another topic.

Awoke with very worn feeling of the brain, decided brain-fag; getting on foot felt better.

Headache and sleepiness so great as to interfere with work. Head ached all night with fulness of frontal region. Feeling as if the frontal region was solid with pain. This ache, during the day, gradually moved backward to base of brain and along the medulla oblongata; relieved by slight motion, increased by large, continued, and more active motion. Slight mental effort, passing from topic to topic, for an instant relieves; sustained effort increases the pain.

Vessels of neck and base of brain full, as if circulation had been cut off by a cord; the whole back of head, neck, and cerebellum felt congested to the brain and cord-centre; sore inside and tender to outside pressure; all those parts of the nervous system felt as if double or treble their ordinary size.

### Eye.

A pain along the line of the optic nerve of the right eye when reading. Conjunctiva very red. While dressing, a dizzy blindness came upon me; dizziness less on closing the eyes;

directing attention to the head and exerting the will diminished the dizziness ; at same time, dizziness followed by rush of blood and fulness in the frontal region, soon followed by similar sensations in occipital and basilar regions, soon disappearing.

### Face.

A curious sensation of fulness in face, as of pressure from inside out.

### Mouth.

Teeth have been very sensitive to cold water, cold air, toothbrush, washing, etc.

Sensation as if the tongue was covered with fur or velvet. Abundant salivation.

### Stomach.

During some of the proving, noticeably a day or two previous, and succeeding to the ninth day, took in food with a sort of ravenous haste. Sour eructations, especially an hour before meals, at times rolling up and rumbling all the way from stomach to mouth, but for the most part breaking at the throat-pit with frequent succession.

### Abdomen.

Colic about 9 A.M., every morning. * Colic relieved by motion, or thinking of something else.

Sensation of going to have a stool every evening: Sensation of desiring a stool all day.

### Urinary Organs.

Burning in the urethra in passing water. Urine when first passed was hot, burned the urethra.

° Gonorrhœa, gleet.

### Sexual Organs.

More amorousness during the primary part of the proving than for years.

Large emissions in the morning. The emissions come on without dreams. Awakened by a large quantity of semen running over him.

### Generalities.

An agreeable languor alternates with a pleasant, youthful freshness and vigor of body and mind ; feeling of general tonicity comes on, as during the primary or actionary stage of the proving; voluntary muscular action, as then, so easy as to be almost involuntary ; muscular action increased, but power of involuntary unconscious co-ordination of muscular action impaired; find myself walking fast before I am conscious of it, legs and feet seem to be running away with or from me ; my will is called consciously into action to regulate my movements; feel otherwise unusually well and active.

Better in the open air and when moving.

## Skin.

The skin is covered, as in leprosy, with large scales, which fall off and leave lasting white spots, which often become ulcers. Skin dry, cracked, scaly and ulcerated, especially where it is thick, as on the hands and feet.

---

# POLYMNIA UVEDELIA.

### (Bearsfoot.)

DESCRIPTION.—Bearsfoot belongs to the genus *Compositæ*, of the tribe Helianthæ. It is an erect herb, roughish, hairy, stout, four to ten feet high, leaves broadly ovate, angled and toothed, nearly sessile, the lower palmately lobed, abruptly narrowed into a winged petiole, outer involucral scales very large; rays ten to fifteen, interlinear oblong, much larger than the inner scales of the involucre; flower yellow. Grows in rich soil west of New York to Illinois, and southward. The flower and whole plant exhale a strong odor ; they look like small sunflowers.

PREPARATION.—Tincture of the herb.

### (No Proving.)

° Enlarged spleen.    ° Uterine hypertrophy.

---

# PICRIC ACID.

### (Carbazotic acid; Welter's Bitter; Nitro-phenisic acid; Nitro-phenolic acid.)

DESCRIPTION.—Picric acid is a yellowish substance obtained by the action of Nitric acid  n Carbo    acid, Indigo, Salicin, and other substances. It forms in whitish yellow prisms, with rectangular bases, which in thin layers is almost colorless.  I    ddens vegetable blues, and has an exceedingly bitter taste. It is fusible and volatile, and burns with a yellow flame, leaving a residue of charcoal. It is nearly insoluble in cold water, but is soluble in hot water, alcohol, and ether.

PREPARATIONS.—Triturations and alcoholic dilutions.

## Head.

Heavy, throbbing pains in the head, extending from behind the ears forward to the supraorbital notch, thence downward to the eye.

All head-pains relieved by bandaging tightly.

Heavy pain in occipital region, extending down the neck and spine.

Heat and congestion of the head, with bleeding at the nose.

Severe, sharp, intermitting pains in the left temple.

Full, pressive sensation in the head, from within outward.

Pains in the head, aggravated from motion.

## Eyes.

Burning, throbbing pains, with dilated pupils, conjunctivitis, and lachrymation.

Everything seems blurred, as if looking through a fog or a thick veil.

Can read only with the book about five inches from the nose.

Great heaviness of the lids; can't keep them open.

Eyeballs sore to the touch, with photophobia.

Severe, sharp shooting pains in centre of eye, extending back to occipital region—seems to follow the course of the optic nerve.

Lids sore, and slightly swollen.

## Mouth, Throat, and Ears.

Ears burn, look puffy, with sensation as of worms crawling on them.

Bitter taste in the mouth.

Throat feels raw, scraped, stiff, and hot, as if burnt.

Collection of thick, white mucus on the tonsils.

Great difficulty of swallowing; sensation as if the throat would split open.

Dry cough, as from dust in the throat, followed by nausea.

## Stomach.

Nausea, bitter eructations after breakfast; sensation as of something in lower portion of œsophagus.

No appetite; bitter taste in mouth; aversion to food.

## Abdomen and Stool.

Stools light-colored, and passed with much burning and smarting in the anus.

Scanty, soft stools, with burning at the anus.

Crawling, stinging pain in the abdomen.

## Rectum and Anus.

Smarting, stinging burning of the anus after a passage from the bowels.

## Urinary Organs.

Urine profuse, very hot when passed; urethra feels as if burnt.

Urine dark, high-colored, sp. gr. 10.25 to 10.28.

## Generative Organs.

*Great sexual desire, and painful erections, with emissions.*

Lewd dreams, with emissions.

*Very hard erections; terrible erections.*

*Erections,* with severe pain in the left testicle, as if bruised, extending up the cord as far as the external abdominal ring.

## Chest.

Heavy, throbbing pain under tenth and eleventh ribs on left side.

Dull, stunning pain in the chest.

## Back.

Heavy, throbbing pain in the region of the kidneys, extending down the legs, especially the left.

Small of the back sensitive to pressure.

## Extremities.

*Legs feel heavy, and very weak.*
Legs below the knees feel very sore and tender to the touch.
Severe pain in the anterior portion of legs when touched.
*Legs heavy, like lead.*
*Great coldness of the feet.*
Great heaviness in the *arms* and *legs,* especially on exertion.
Shooting pain in the left arm, at elbow.

## Skin.

Small, painful, reddish elevations, like furuncles, around the
mouth and face; when opened they exude a thin, clear
serum, which soon dries into a transparent scab; they then
become pustular and very painful, and contain a thick,
opaque pus.

## Fever.

Great thirst for cold water; drank in large quantities, without
relief.
Fever; great chilliness; can't get warm; followed by cold,
clammy sweat; chilliness predominates; pulse 50, weak and
small.

## Sleep.

Sleep sound, but unrefreshing.
Restlessness.

## Generalities.

Throbbing and jerking of the muscles in the different parts of
the body, with severe chills and great pain between the hips.
Profuse cold, clammy sweats, with great chilliness.
Very tired on going upstairs.
*General lassitude.*
Rheumatic stitches in different parts of the body, with *great*
*muscular weakness.*

# PICRATE OF AMMONIA.

### (*Carbazotate of Ammonia.*)

DESCRIPTION.—The Picrate of Ammonia is a yellow crystalline salt, very soluble in water, but sparingly so in alcohol.   It is very bitter, and stains organic matters yellow.

PREPARATIONS.—Trituration, or alcoholic tinctures.

### (*No Proving.*)

° Intermittent fever.   ° Bilious headache.   ° Cerebro-spinal headache.

---

# QUEBRACHO.

DESCRIPTION.—This is a Brazilian plant, the Arpido-sperma Quebracho, a tree belonging to the Apocynaceæ, and is used as a febrifuge by Brazilian physicians.

### (*No Proving.*)

° Spasmodic asthma.   ° Emphysema.

---

# QUINIA SULPHATE.

### (*Chininum Sulphuricum.*)

DESCRIPTION.—There are two forms of the sulphate, a neutral and an acid salt.

The neutral salt is produced by neutralizing quinine with a dilute solution of Sulphuric acid, and adding a few drops of an alkali to determine the crystals. It dissolves in about 700 parts cold water, and 30 parts hot water.

The acid salt always separates from a solution of quinine in excess of sulphuric acid.   It is much more soluble in water than the neutral sulphate.   It will dissolve in 11 parts of water.

PREPARATIONS.—Triturations.

## Mind.

Feeling of intoxication, though the mental powers are perfect. Awoke at midnight with long-continued cries; knew that he was crying, but could not help it; was obliged to get out of bed; wrapped himself in his clothes and remained sitting; after a few moments he came to himself again, and soon fell asleep.   Delirium.

* Despondency.
* As if some evil were impending.
* *Feeling of impending evil,* in the afternoon.

### Head.

Vertigo, with palpitation.
* *Whirling in the head like a mill wheel.*
Rush of blood to the head, towards evening.
Heaviness and confusion of the head continue until going to sleep in the evening.
* Very severe headache, worse towards evening, with violent palpitation of the arteries of the head, as if the head would be torn asunder, with glowing heat of the face, vertigo, at times ringing and roaring in the ears.
Violent headache in the forenoon, especially in the left side, with frequent pulsation of the temporal arteries, with excitement through the whole body.
Pain in the forehead and temples appeared towards evening and gradually increased in intensity, with visible pulsation of the temporal arteries, heat of the head, and ringing in the ears.
Violent pains in the left temple; the pain extends to the eyebrow, and obliges him to lie down, with which he seeks a cool place on the sofa in order to relieve the pain. Meningitis; symptoms like delirium tremens.

### Eye.

With some the eyes become red, and there is swelling of the lids, with the appearance of pimples. Peculiar dryness of the eyes. All day, eyes feel as if they had been in a glare, or as if the atmosphere were too dry, as if parched. * Pain in the left infra-orbital, malar and superior maxillary nerves; aching and boring, worse in cold air, but nearly constant, even involving the eye at times, with tumefaction adjacent to upper molars. Lachrymation in the open air.
* Disk and retina both very anæmic. Disk looks dry, with the vessels smaller than usual.

* Dilatation of the pupil.
* Dimness of vision, as from a net before the eyes, and once as from a dark fog.

More or less complete, or even incurable amaurosis of one or both eyes. Blindness.

* Great sensitiveness of the eye to the light, with lachrymation in the full glare of light.
* Bright lights and sparks before the eyes.
* Black spot, size of pin's head, about eighteen inches from right eye, and moving with eye for some weeks. Blackness before the eyes, with pain in the forehead, so violent that the head seemed as though it would burst.

### Ear.

Deafness of both ears on account of loud ringing in them. Intolerance of noise.

* *Ringing in the ears, especially noticed in the left,* seldom in the right. Frequent transient ringing in the ears. Constant ringing in the ears. Roaring in the ears and head, so that the patient was almost completely deaf.

### Nose.

° Hay fever.

Epistaxis, with cerebral congestion; flushed face.

### Face.

Suddenly seized with œdema of the face and limbs, accompanied by an unusual erythematous rash.

* Face flushed and hot.
* Face pale and suffering.
* Aching about left malar bone in the evening.
* While writing, sudden ache above left zygoma, while inclining head to that side, also at temporal ridge.
* Neuralgia of the supra-orbital branch of the fifth nerve, especially when periodic.

### Mouth.

Tongue coated with a thick yellow fur, which cannot be scraped off, except the tip, which is red. Mouth full of mucus. Great hunger, compelling him to eat.

° Quinia acts best after the tongue has been cleaned by the use of Mercurius or Euonymin. Dryness of the mouth and fauces. Mouth tastes as if its secretions were unhealthy.

* Articulation seems impaired. Have to repeat words to make them understood. Disturbance of the organ of speech; occasionally entire loss of voice for a longer or shorter period.

### Throat.

Throat feels a little full; clogging of the upper pharynx by mucus; slowly detached by repeated swallowing in the afternoon. Constant scraping in the throat, with irritation to cough, and slimy expectoration, difficult to loosen, in afternoon.

Catarrhal secretion descended the pharynx in considerable amounts; again some hawked up the windpipe; and all the afternoon there remained a tenacious coating of the same on the back of the palate, causing efforts to swallow it.

### Stomach.

Ravenous hunger after a hearty meal, becoming a qualmishness and nausea when continuing a long time.

Anorexia, aversion to food.

Thirst, with unusual appetite and sensation of fasting. Thirst, eructation, and nausea, with great appetite.

Eructations and heartburn. Nausea and vomiting during a meal.

Frequent vomiting of an insipid taste in the afternoon. Cardialgia.

A feeling as if the stomach were too full, and something had failed to go down and lodged in the chest; better by eructation, but fulness still felt.

* After eating, pressure in the stomach, followed by cutting in the upper and middle abdominal region.

* Even slightest food causes pressure in the stomach and a return of the usual symptoms.

### Abdomen.

* Pain in the region of the liver shortly before going to bed.

\* Dull, painful sensation in the region of the spleen, disappearing on pressure. Pressive pain in the region of the spleen.

\* Stitches in the left side, below the short ribs. Much distension of the abdomen, followed by diarrhœa.

Great distension of the abdomen without passage of flatus. Profuse passage of flatus upward and downward.

Colic in the transverse and left colon. Colic immediately after rising, followed by stool, at first mushy, like diarrhœa, with cadaverous odor, with gradual relief of the colic.

### Rectum.

Increased hæmorrhoidal troubles.

Discharge of bright blood from the anus, without previous pain in the back.

Diarrhœa, with violent colic-like pains across the abdomen. Stool at first mushy, then like diarrhœa, preceded by exceeding offensive flatus at 9 A.M.

Stool difficult, fæces of ordinary consistence. Obstinate costiveness, with distension of the abdomen.

### Urinary Organs.

Urine copious, high-colored and turbid. Secretion of urine increased; urine deposited a large quantity of orange-colored crystals, shown under the microscope to be right-angled prisms, with rhomboidal fragments. Increased secretion of urine, preceded by distension of the upper and lower abdomen and oppressed respiration. Hæmorrhage of the urinary passages. Urine deposited a rose-red sediment, which under the glass showed rhomboidal flat crystals, with here and there double pyramids. These crystals consisted of Urate of ammonia and phosphates and traces of Quinine. Brick-dust sediment in the urine. After taking 6 grammes of Quinia, over 4 grammes were found in the urine within 48 hours.

### Sexual Organs.

Decided depression of the sexual sphere during the proving. An emission during the night without waking. Uterine epistaxis.\*

---

\* This is neither a hæmorrhage nor a menorrhagia but a steady flow, drop by drop, from the uterus.

F.45

* Menses too soon and too profuse, or too scanty.
° Deficient labor pains from exhaustion.
° Irregular menses.   (*Hale.*)

### Respiratory Organs.

On rising in the morning scraping soreness of larynx and trachea
when swallowing, with raising and coughing of considerable mucus, accumulated during the night, relieving the
laryngeal scraping by degrees, but causing rawness in bronchi
and lungs of left side; later in the day the cough affected rather
the fauces, with rending sensation.  Hoarseness at 4 P.M.,
with a deep tone to the voice.  Aphonia.  The attack of
hoarseness, without anginal symptoms, recurred every afternoon for a long time.  Cough and tickling in windpipe.
* Respiration increased.  Slow and irregular breathing.  Respiration slow, interrupted by sighs.
* Oppression of the chest.
Pressive pain in the left half of chest, which was very sensitive to
deep inspiration, most sensitive when the left arm was thrown
forcibly backward.  Sticking in the right half of the chest,
extending up the shoulder; during the afternoon impeding
respiration, relieved by bending the body forward.  Stitches
in the left side of the chest, preventing deep breathing, continuing uninterruptedly until the next day, and very gradually disappearing.

### Heart and Pulse.

Extreme præcordial anxiety.  Sticking in the region of the apex
of the heart, disappearing after a few minutes.  Sitting, the
heart's action subjectively felt, extending to head.  Palpitation of the heart.
Pulse full and rapid.
Action on circulation was constant; it usually occurred half an
hour after taking, and proportionate to the size of the dose,
producing slowness of the pulse.
Pulse irregular, weak, and small.  When the pulse was at its
quickest it became irregular and intermittent.

46

### Back.

* *Sensitiveness of the last cervical and first dorsal vertebræ to pressure.*
* The dorsal vertebræ are painful to pressure with the fingers or on leaning against any hard substance.
* Pain in the first and second dorsal vertebræ on pressure.
* Third dorsal vertebra very painful to touch, *with oppression of the chest;* it was not noticed on pressing on the other vertebræ.

### Extremities.

* Weakness in the limbs. Great weakness and weariness of arms and legs.
* Trembling in the extremities; the power of the will over them seemed very much hampered.
* Hemiplegia.

Fingers blue and cold.

### General Symptoms.

General excitement of the arterial system, similar to that produced by strong wine. An internal trembling, wherewith the face became pale, with some urging to urinate, followed by pale urine.

Twitchings, in the evening. Convulsions.

* General weakness, especially of the feet, so as to interfere with walking.
* Collapse, with feeble pulse and colliquative sweats.

Disturbance of nervous system and of the heart's action, producing general prostration and feebleness of cardiac movements.

° Nearly all neuralgic pains when periodical and malarial.

Exhaustion as from hunger.

Very restless at night.

Excessive great sensitiveness of the body during the proving.

### Skin.

Rash all over the body, vivid as scarlatina and attended with intolerable and incessant itching. The rash and irritation were persistent for several days; and then gradually and slowly subsided, followed by univeral exfoliation of the cuticle. Scarlatina-like eruption, with extremely violent itching over the whole body, followed by desquamation, lasting fully three months.

With some, pimples appear over the whole body, accompanied with an intolerable itching, and which eventually discharge a matter, somewhat thicker than serum, though not exactly of the consistence of pus; having reached the suppurative stage, the eruption gives place to squamous scabs.

* Skin cold, pale, moist, and shrunken. Sudden, long, pricking stitches, as with needles, in the skin of the chest, back, and thighs, followed by moderate sweat on the chest and back, in the evening, while walking slowly in the open air.

### Sleep.

Constant inclination to yawn. with decided **weakness.** Coma.

Sleep very uneasy, interrupted by wonderful **dreams**; constant tossing about the bed.

* Sweat, especially on the back and neck when sleeping.

Frightful dreams, with restless sleep.

### Fever.

Decided shaking chill at 3 P.M.; at 6½ P.M., heat of the face, lasting until 9 P.M., but no sweat followed. Chilliness, with paleness of the face, pain in the forehead and temples, and ringing in the ears at 11 A.M.

The fever shows itself at one time by an effervescence of the blood, causing great pulsation (or "snapping") of the veins, at another by an icy coldness of the whole body, insomuch that it has been compared to the action of an intermittent fever; this fever seems to terminate by a sharp spontaneous accession.

Extremities, hands, feet, chin, and nose cold from noon until evening.

Heat over the whole body, which gradually breaks into sweats.

Sweat breaks out over the whole body from time to time, even during perfect quiet. Sweat during the morning sleep so profuse that the bed was soaked with it.

° *Intermittent fever, quotidian, with well-developed chill, fever, and sweat.*

° Congestive or pernicious ague, quotidian, **rarely** good for quartan fever.

--------

# RHUS AROMATICA.

DESCRIPTION.—It is a shrub, growing from two to six feet high, inhabiting high rocky soil; stems straight, branching near the top; flowers yellow, fruit clustered, red, seedy, and acid. When the bush is broken it emits a strong odor, from whence it takes its common name.

PREPARATION.—Tincture from the bark of the root.

*(No Provings.)*

° *Diabetes Insipidus.*—Large quantities of urine of low specific gravity. Emaciated and haggard.

° *Diabetes Mellitus.*—Great lassitude and languor. Pain in the back, considerable thirst, appetite variable, sometimes ravenous, and sometimes deficient; skin sallow and doughy; temperature, 101½°; slight cough and occasional nightsweats; loss of flesh; sugar in the urine.

° *Incontinence of urine,* whether from atony of the muscular, or irritation of the nervous fibre, which prevent normal distension.

° Constant dribbling of the urine.

° Enuresis nocturna.

° *Hæmorrhage of the kidneys,* resulting from a diseased state of the whole system, or that which commonly precedes Bright's disease.

° Hæmorrhage from the bladder.

° Uterine hæmorrhage.

° Menorrhagia.

° Summer diseases of children.

° *Chronic Diarrhœa and Dysentery.*—Stools sometimes copious or scanty, with pain; discharge blood and mucus, or clear blood.

° Patient thin, anxious, sallow; bowels flabby.

# SALICYLIC ACID.

DESCRIPTION.—It is prepared from flowers of Spiræa Ulmaria, Oil of Gaultheria (Wintergreen), Salicin, Indigo, and Phenol.

It has a sweetish-sour taste, and produces irritation of the throat. Slightly soluble in cold water, much more so in hot water. Alcohol dissolves it more readily than water, and either take up a considerable quantity.

PREPARATION.—Triturations.

## Head.

Delirium; the patient's mind became very stupid; it was difficult for him to collect his ideas, then he laughed without cause, talked incessantly and disconnectedly, frequently looked about him, with apparent hallucinations.

Vertigo,—dulness of the head.

Rush of blood to the head. Headache.

Diminished acuteness of vision.

Roaring in the ears, with difficult hearing.

° Menière's disease,—aural vertigo.

## Throat.

Hæmorrhagic pharyngitis, with difficulty of swallowing. Great dryness of the pharynx. Violent efforts to swallow, with difficulty in swallowing, woke him from sleep; the pain and difficulty in swallowing became confined to the right side of the throat, with sticking pain, extending along the Eustachian tube to within the ear; swelling of the right tonsil, so that it was noticed externally below the angle of the jaw, with sensitiveness when touched, and with increased temperature in the vicinity; examination revealed redness and swelling of the mucous membrane of the throat and posterior fauces, with ulcers the size of a pin-head; after a time a small lump of cheesy matter of a strong odor was expectorated, with some bluish-red blood; this was followed by a gradual return of the throat to its normal condition.

° Diphtheria (but inferior to Eucalyptol).

## Stomach.

Erosions and ulcers in the stomach and bowels.

## Generalities.

Immediately after the first powder he began to sweat profusely. The perspiration increased and his strength diminished so visibly, that his wife was unwilling to give him the fourth

powder.   He insisted, however, and after taking it, vomiting
and an agonizing headache set in, which continued all night.
In the morning he seemed unconscious and simply groaned
loudly.   Only for a moment did his mind seem clear, when
he cried out, " My head, my head ! " to the physicians who
were present.   All treatment was futile, and he died in forty
hours after taking the first powder.   No post-mortem examination was permitted.   The course of the case was too
rapid to be explained on the theory of a complicating cerebral inflammation ; all the symptoms seem to point to poisoning (10-grain doses).

### Fever.

Increased warmth of skin.   Profuse sweat.   Sweat at times more
or less profuse.

## SALICYLATE OF SODA.

DESCRIPTION.—Salicylate of soda is a white granular salt, very soluble in
water.   Some of the salts in the market have a leaden look or reddish tinge.
The redness is always present when it is evaporated from an alkaline solution.

It is prepared by putting one part of salicylic acid in two parts of hot distilled water, and gradually adding bicarbonate of soda, until the salicylic acid
is dissolved and the liquid has but a slight *acid reaction*.   Filter this solution
and evaporate to dryness.

PREPARATIONS.—Triturations, or in syrups and elixirs.

### (No Proving.)

o Menière's disease.   Vertigo from disease of the ear.

o Ringing in the ears from the abuse of quinine.

o Rheumatism, rheumatalgia.

o Neuralgia.   o Sciatica.

## SANGUINARINA NITRATE.

DESCRIPTION.—This preparation is a very fine brownish-red powder, pungent, acrid, bitter, and inodorous.   Soluble in alcohol, ether, and water and
oils, but not in all proportions.   Alcohol and water separately will dissolve
about half a grain to each one hundred minims, while dilute alcohol (equal
parts of alcohol and water) will dissolve about one-fourth of a grain more.

PREPARATION.—Triturations up to the third centesimal; then it may be
carried higher in alcohol.

### Head and Neck.

Pain in the supra-orbital region, proceeding from pain in the
right eyeball, of a sore, aching character.   It soon extended

across the forehead, and seemed to be deep in above the root of the nose. Burning pain in the forehead and the root of the nose, with aching and soreness in eyeballs, worse on pressure; *the pain became more severe on the left side of the head, through the left temple.* Slight aching sensation, with soreness all over the head and scalp. Slight dizziness through all of the proving. The pain in the left side extended to the parietal ridge and back to the mastoid process, attended with sensation of stiffness in the muscles of left side of neck and top of left shoulder, as if from exposure to a draft of cold, or damp, raw air. *Sensation of obstruction and fulness in head,* which was relieved by a discharge of a large quantity of thick, yellow, sweet-tasting mucus. Heat in the forehead; bathed in warm water gave some relief. Uncomfortable feeling about the head all day; worse at night. ° Catarrhal and sick-headaches.

### Eyes.

*Pain in right eyeball,* extending to the supra-orbital region; pain of a sore, aching character. *Profuse lachrymation;* the tears gush from the eyes. *Dimness of sight,* as if looking through gauze or mist, as if a thin film of mucus was spread over the sight. Redness and soreness of the inner corners of the eyes, which feel as if swollen. *Pain in the left eyeball,* extending over the orbit and left side of the head. Redness of lids and conjunctiva. *Heat and burning of the eyes,* which was quite severe. Burning, pressing, aching, and sore pains in the eyes.

### Ears.

\* Obstruction of the Eustachian tube; difficulty in distinguishing sounds; roaring in the right ear.

### Nose.

fifteen minutes after taking first dose, observed water trickling from right nostril. \* *Watery mucus flowed freely from both nostrils,* attended by a violent *sneezing,* repeated every few minutes, with profuse lachrymation. Sensation arising to nostrils as if he had taken strong horseradish. *Burning pain in both nostrils. Accumulation of mucus, obstructing* *nose* and bronchial tubes. Dry, sore, and raw feeling in nostrils. * *Free discharge from posterior nares, tinged with blood,* especially from left side.

### Mouth and Fauces.

Bitter taste, extending back to the root of the tongue. Slight acrid burning sensation on the tongue. Roughness and dryness in the mouth and throat, with sensation of constriction in the throat, which passed off in fifteen or twenty minutes. Increased flow of mucus and saliva, with sneezing and burning in the forehead.

*Soreness, rawness, and roughness on right tonsil, with difficulty in swallowing,* as if the throat indicated diphtheria, but on examination there was only a red and irritable spot.

In the morning *raised large quantities of thick, yellow, sweet-tasting mucus.* This continued all day. Heat in the mouth, as if pepper had been taken. *Great accumulation of mucus in the throat and bronchi.* Awoke frequently with dry mouth and throat, from breathing with mouth open, the nose being obstructed. Everything tasted dry, like chips. Coffee did not taste natural; wanted something succulent, not pungent, but soothing to the mouth and throat, which was hot, dry, parched, and raw. ° Catarrh of fauces and pharynx.

### Chest.

* *Heat and tension behind centre of sternum; sensation of tightness in the chest, inducing a short hacking cough;* the cough became harsh, leaving soreness and rawness in the throat and chest, with scraping, raw sensation in the pharynx. Coughing up large quantities of thick, yellow, sweet-tasting mucus several times during the day.

Tension, burning, and accumulation of mucus behind centre of sternum.

In forty minutes after taking, the tension and heat behind the sternum had increased, with desire to cough,—a short hacking cough; raised a clear mucus; the cough became deeper and rattling; the pressure extended to both lungs, greatly increasing the sense of suffocation, feeling as if the air-passages were lined with thick, stiff mucus or pus.

### Stomach.

*Sensation of burning in stomach and œsophagus.* Belching up of putrid-smelling gas, though she had eaten nothing since morning. Little appetite.

### Urinary Organs.

Passed urine nearly every hour during the night, which, on standing until morning, weighed twenty-eight ounces, and deposited a white sediment.

### Abdomen.

*Borborygmus and pains in abdomen, as if diarrhœa would set in,* with sharp cutting pains.

---

# STRYCHNIA ARSENATE.

DESCRIPTION.—Acids easily dissolve Strychnia, forming neutral solutions, having an intensely bitter taste, and being virulently poisonous. The Arsenate is a salt, forming in monoclinic prisms, soluble in fifteen parts cold and five parts hot water.

The Arsenite is in the form of dull white cubes, efflorescing in air.

PREPARATION.—Triturations.

*(No Proving.)*

° Chronic diarrhœa in a child with paralytic conditions of bladder, rectum, and lower extremities.

° Certain forms of paralysis where Arsenic and Strychnia both appear to be indicated.

---

# SULPHUR IODATUM.

(*Iodide of Sulphur.*)

DESCRIPTION.—Iodine and Sulphur combine when heated together, even under water. The Iodide is a blackish-gray radio-crystalline mass, resembling native Sulphide of antimony. It decomposes at higher temperatures, gives off Iodine on exposure to air, and is insoluble in water.

PREPARATION.—Triturations.

### Head.

Sides of the head ached, with a sensation as if the head were pressed in a vise.

Inclination to close the eyes, as if to press out tears.

° Cataract cured. (*Burnett.*)

Singing in the ears.

Nasal coryza. Flow of "acrid serum" from the nose. Excoriation of the nostrils.

Erythematous breaking out in the upper lip, with yellowish pustules, painful, sore, and tender, quickly disappearing in dry scales.

### Mouth and Throat.

* Tongue dry and hard, furred at the root, red at the point.

Throat dry and painful to touch, feeling as if swelled.

* Sore throat in the morning. (*Burnett*.)

Constant disposition to swallow saliva; throat and gullet parched; the saliva did not allay the dryness.

### Stomach.

Anorexia; desire for acids, pickles, lemonade, etc. Soreness and sinking in the epigastrium.

### Respiratory Organs.

Accumulation of dark purulent mucus in the windpipe, causing constant inclination to swallow saliva, which does not moisten it. Sensation of dryness in the trachea. Much troubled with cough during the early part of the night, accompanied by a nasty taste in the mouth and a fetid breath.

### Chest.

Difficulty of expanding the chest on inspiration, with prostration of strength.

Boring pain, as if in the heart, with some difficulty of respiration.

### Back.

Pain in the loins, as if bruised, with weakness of the spinal column.

### Generalities.

Prostration of strength, with difficulty of expanding the chest on inspiration.

Faintness, much worse on waking in the morning, when stooping or leaning forward, when running or ascending the stairs.

### Skin.

Pustules on the upper lip. Erythema on the chin. Arms covered with an itching rash, like nettlerash.

° Barbers' itch.   ° **Acne.**   (*Hale.*)

### Sleep.

Unrefreshed by sleep at night; confused dreams.

---

## THYMOL.

DESCRIPTION.—Thymol is obtained from Thyme oil by fractional distillation, at 225°. It forms about one-half of Thyme oil. The more volatile parts of Thyme oil (Thymene and Cymene) likewise contain a considerable quantity of Thymol, which may be obtained by agitating the liquid with soda-lye, separating the undissolved oil, diluting the alkaline solution with water. Supersaturate this with Hydrochloric acid and Thymol will be precipitated. Thymol is purified by crystallization from an alcoholic solution. The crystals are transparent rhomboid tables. It has a mild odor and an aromatic, peppery taste. Somewhat heavier than water. It dissolves in about 300 parts water, and is easily soluble in alcohol and ether. Water does not precipitate it from the alcoholic solution.

PREPARATION.—Thymol, 1 part; alcohol, 10 parts; glycerin, 20 parts; water, 1000 parts. Used as an antiseptic.

See " Therapeutics of New Remedies."

---

## TRIFOLIUM PRATENSE.
### (*Red Clover.*)

PREPARATION.—Tincture of the flower-heads.

### Head

Head and perceptions very dull. Brain feels very dull. Has been dull all day; cannot think nor remember.

Head is hot and feels very large.

Intermittent headache; the attacks last but half an hour.

Eyes feel dull, sore, and heavy.

Mucus secreted in large quantities in the nose. Nasal mucous membrane feels dry.

### Throat.

Throat feels dry and hard in the forenoon. Feels raw, as if something were in it. I continually try to clear it. Throat feels much irritated. Throat all the way down feels as if scalded.

Great dryness of the trachea, causing me to clear the throat of some foreign substance. While in a close room, feel as if I could not get air enough; feel much better while out of doors.

Throat dry in the afternoon, then after two hours it became quite moist, and there was great expectoration.

Have had continued irritation of the pharynx and trachea, causing a continued short hacking cough, with an accumulation of mucus, which I must expectorate.

A sharp pain through the uvula, causing the tears to start.

### Abdomen.

Griping pains in the abdomen, continuous and severe.

Very costive. Bowels afterwards were very costive, and each defecation was followed by several drops of dark blood, attended by a bearing-down sensation, not a griping nor a true tenesmus, but more as if the bowel would prolapse from its own weight; this lasted about two weeks, after which the bowels became regular.

### Urinary Organs.

*Primary.* Kidneys very sore; an increase in the quantity of urine. Great urging to urinate; the bladder feels full to overflowing. Whole mucous membrane of the urinary tract feels irritated.

*Secondary.* Urine scanty.

### Respiratory Organs.

Some irritation in the bronchi, causing a short hacking cough. Felt oppressed in breathing, or rather that I was breathing air loaded with impurities after retiring; pulse slow and irregular. Some dyspnœa, disappearing on going into the fresh air.

Lungs feel as if full of blood, at 2 P.M. At 10 P.M., had to leave a close room on account of the oppressed feeling in my chest; on coming into the fresh air I was obliged to cough much; this was followed by hiccough and profuse expectoration.

On reclining or lying down my chest feels distressed as from deficient aeration of blood in the lungs.

Pulse slow and irregular; very weak, intermitting one or two beats; once it stopped for a few seconds, then followed a bounding pulse.

### Sleep.

Felt as if I had not been asleep, on waking in the morning.

### Fever.

In a few minutes after retiring, I began to feel cold; pulse at the wrist very weak, intermitting one or two beats; once it stopped for a few seconds; this was followed by a bounding pulse; I became very warm, and my breathing stopped; my lungs felt as if I were breathing in hot air. Feet and hands cold; head hot.

---

## TRIFOLIUM REPENS.

( *White Clover.* )

PREPARATION.—Tincture of the flower heads. Dr. Douglass took a trituration of the flowers, one part to six of sac. lactis; the effects were so speedy and marked that six other persons took it, with substantially the same results in a few minutes.

A feeling of fulness and congestion of all the salivary glands; in some instances amounting to decided discomfort, and even pain, quickly followed by increased, sometimes copious flow of saliva. One of the provers placed her hands on the parotid gland and said she felt just as if an attack of mumps were coming on.

---

## TURNERA APHRODISIACA.

( *Damiana.* )

DESCRIPTION.—It belongs to the natural order of Turneraceæ. The genus Turnera is a small family of chiefly tropical American plants allied to the Passifloraceæ. The flowers are small, yellow, subsessile near the end of the small branches. Turnera aphrodisiaca, as found in the market, consists of broken leaves mixed with fragments of the branches, and sometimes with seedpods. The branches have a reddish-brown bark, and are covered, when young, with white, cottony hairs. The leaves are less than an inch long, obovate, wedge-shape, and taper at the base to a short, slender leaf-stalk; when young they are covered with a slight pubescence, but become smooth when old.

PREPARATION.—Tincture of the plant.

( *No Proving.* )

° Paresis of the genital organs of both sexes.

° Partial impotence. Sexual debility, chiefly from nervous prostration.

° Sexual neurasthenia.

° Incontinence of urine **in old people**.

° Atonic spermatorrhœa.

° Chronic prostatic discharges.

It seems to be an analogue of Helonias Aletris, Strychnia, Phosphoric acid and the Hypophosphites.

---

## VIBURNUM OPULUS.

### (*Cranberry tree, Cramp bark.*)

DESCRIPTION.—This shrub grows from five to fifteen feet high, on low ground along streams; common in Canada and the Northern and Western States, extending south as far as Virginia; very abundant in the Catskill and Alleghany mountains. Flowers in June and July. The acid fruit is a substitute for cranberries, whence the name, *High cranberry bush.* The common, well-known *Snowball tree,* or *Guelder rose* of our gardens is a cultivated variety of this species, with the whole cyme turned by cultivation into showy, sterile flowers.

The Viburnum prunifolium (Black Haw), which is found in **dry copses** from New England, Canada, and Illinois on the north, to Tennessee and Virginia on the south, is a much larger shrub, and should not be confounded with Viburnum Opulus.

PREPARATION.—Tincture from inner bark of shrub, and bark of root.

### Mind.

Confused, and unable to concentrate the mind on usual mental labor. Stupid feeling, as if I could not tell where I was or what to do on awaking in the morning. Inability to study to such an extent that he abandoned the proving.

### Head.

*Dull frontal headache,* extending to the eyeballs, aggravated by mental exertion, and relieved by moving about. Dull, aching pain over left eye. Dull, confusing frontal headache, extending to both temporal regions, as after night watching or loss of sleep, so severe as to compel cessation of mental exertion. Headache beginning about 3 P.M., worse at night.

Vertigo with inclination to turn to the left. Vertigo on rising from a seat; feel as though would fall forward. Vertigo on **closing eyes**. Severe pressive pain in right supraorbital **region**. Dull, supraorbital and frontal headache, with **profuse flow** of clear, watery urine.

Severe pain in head just over the eyes on opening them; the soreness extending back into the head.

*Severe left-sided headache*, aggravated by a sudden jar, bending over, false step movement. Eyes heavy; feel almost sick enough to go to bed. *Severe pain in left parietal region;* the pain is sharp and penetrates into the brain, aggravated by every cough, moving the head, when the bowels move. *Every cough hurts the head.*

### Eyes.

Sore feeling in eyeballs. Heaviness over the eyes and in the eyeballs, so severe that at times would have to look twice to be sure of seeing an object. Eyes burn; can hardly see on account of profuse flow of tears.

### Ears.

Sharp, jerking pains in ears as if stabbing with a sharp knife, lasting nearly an hour, with more or less severity. Would awaken during the night with great pain in ears; *deep in the bone.* External ear sore as if bruised; could not lie on affected side. Compelled to change position several times during the night in consequence of pain, first in one ear and then in the other.

### Stomach.

*Deathly sickness at the stomach at night*, not relieved by any position. When lying perfectly quiet had no unpleasant feeling, but on moving, a deathly nausea in pit of stomach came on; would faint on attempting to get up. *Constant nausea* (but no inclination to vomit), *relieved by eating.*

Nausea and faintness, at times very distressing, relieved by eating, but felt immediately afterwards. Aching pain in stomach in the afternoon, relieved by stretching the body and throwing the stomach forwards.

° Nausea and vomiting of pregnant women.

### Hypochondria.

Severe sticking, darting pain in left hypochondrium, deepseated as if in spleen, with a sensation as if some hot fluid were running through the splenic vessels; relieved by walking about the room, or by hard pressure, aggravated by lying on left side; could not lie on the left side at all. Intense pain in region of spleen, producing fainting, relieved by perspiration. Most intense pain in left lumbar region between floating ribs and wing of ilium.

### Abdomen.

Whole abdomen tender and sensitive to pressure, especially about the umbilicus. Rumbling, darting pain in bowels. Cramping colic pains in lower bowels. Bearing down pains in abdomen as during menstruation, with heavy aching pain over pubes. Severe, heavy, aching, bearing down pain, accompanied by drawing pains in anterior muscles of the thighs, and occasionally by sharp shooting pains in ovarian regions. *Crampy colic pains in lower abdomen almost unbearable, the pains coming on suddenly and with terrible severity,* as if going to be "unwell," mostly or wholly at night.

### Stool.

Constipation. Great inactivity of rectum; no inclination for stool. Stool dry, hard, scanty, painful, and difficult of expulsion. Obstinate constipation; desire for stool, with much straining. Stool large, hard, and when passed attended with a cutting sensation in rectum and anus. During and immediately after stool, profuse hæmorrhage of dark-red blood.

One prover had profuse, watery diarrhœa, accompanied by terrible chills and cold sweat on the forehead.

### Urinary Organs.

Profuse flow of clear, watery urine; compelled to urinate every hour. A constant sensation as if the urine continued to flow, followed each urination. Profuse and frequent flow of clear, watery urine, accompanying frontal headache.

### Sexual Organs.

*Male.*—Severe pain and swelling of epididymis and testicle of left side. Epididymis of right side so painful and swollen that a suspensory bandage was necessary. (This prover was subject to attacks of epididymitis from exposure to cold or violent exercise, but in this case he had not been exposed to either.)  Involuntary seminal emissions without dreams. ·

*Female.*—Uneasy sensation in pelvic region and slight bearing-down pains.  Pain in back, loins and lower abdomen, as if the menses were coming on, aggravated· in early part of evening and in a close room; ameliorated in open air and by moving about.

° **Was "unwell"** during second week while taking the remedy, but felt so perfectly free from pain and uneasiness so peculiar to that period, that I attributed my freedom from pain to the action of the remedy.  Severe bearing-down pains as during menstruation, accompanied by drawing pains in anterior muscles of thigh and occasional sharp shooting pains over ovaries.  Three days after discontinuing the drug the above pains were repeated in the morning, with *great nervousness;* could not sit or lie still but for a few minutes at a time, on account of the pain.  Ten days after commencing the proving—which was at mid-menstrual period, regular menstruation recurring two weeks before—a flow began which lasted two days, *in all respects like normal menstruation,* but with much cramping pain and great nervous restlessness.  Menses delayed ten days; when flow appeared was scanty, thin, light-colored, and continued but a few hours, and attended with a sensation of light-headedness; must lie down; faintness when attempting to sit up.  During menses, nauseated all the time.

*Leucorrhœa,* thin, yellowish-white for two days following menstruation.  Leucorrhœa, thin and colorless, except with evacuation of the bowels, when it was thick, white, inodorous, blood-streaked mucus from the vagina.

° Excruciating colicky pain through womb and lower abdomen, coming on quite suddenly just preceding the menstrual flow, relieved by 1ˣ dilution.

° Pains, beginning in the back and going around to the loins (?) and across to the pubic bones, like labor-pains; have been promptly relieved.

47

—° *Prevents miscarriage,* and premature labor.    ° *Dysmenorrhœa.*
    *Dystocia.*    ° *False pains.*

## Chest.

Sharp shooting pains in left chest over sixth rib near the sternum.
    During the proving an old heart trouble (remission every
    third beat) returned.    Felt as if the breath would leave her
    body and her heart would cease beating.

## Back and Neck.

Tired, bruised pain in muscles of the back, extending from scap-
    ula to wing of ilium on each side of spine, relieved by firm
    pressure.    Wandering, tired pains in muscles of back, worse
    on left side.    Severe pain in back (region of kidney), ren-
    dering ordinary work difficult; relieved by pressing across
    the back.    Stiff, sore feeling in nape of neck.    Neck stiff
    for several days, and attended with pain in occiput.

## Extremities.

Strange buzzing feeling in hands as if they would burst.    Wan-
    dering tired pains, extending to hips and knees, with dis-
    inclination to move about.
° Cramps of the legs—in pregnant women.

## Sleep.

Restless and unrefreshing sleep.    Sleepy after dinner.

## Generalities.

Could not lie on affected side.    The muscles of entire left side of
    body sore, as if bruised or strained by over-lifting.
Muscles of back lame and bruised, as after severe physical exer-
    tion.    Inability to lie on left side during entire proving.
    Tired in the morning on rising.

## Modalities.

Aggravation.—In a warm room; evening or at night; lying on
    affected side.
Amelioration.—In open air; *pressure;* motion, walking about.

# WYETHIA HELENOIDES.

PREPARATION.—Tincture of the root.

### Head.

Dizziness. Rush of blood to the head.

Severe headache. Pain in the forehead over the right eye, at first sharp, followed by a feeling of fulness.

Itching in the right ear.

### Mouth and Throat.

Mouth feels as if it had been scalded.

Increased flow of tough, ropy saliva.

* Throat feels swollen ; epiglottis dry, and has a burning sensation; constant desire to swallow saliva to relieve the dryness, yet affords no comfort.

Swallows with difficulty.

* Prickling dry sensation in posterior nares ; sensation as if something were in the nasal passages ; an effort to clear them through the throat affords no relief.

The uvula feels elongated.

* Dryness of the fauces; constant desire to clear the throat by hemming.

Sensation of heat down the œsophagus into the stomach, worse on eating.

### Stomach.

Belching of wind, alternating with hiccough.

Nausea and vomiting. Sense of weight in the stomach, as if something indigestible had been eaten.

### Abdomen.

Pain and bearing down in the right side. Itching of the anus.

Passages diarrhœic, loose, of a dark-brown color, came on in the night, and lasted five days. Passage small and dark-brown ; look burned. Passages previously light-colored, irregular, and constipated, became dark-colored, regular and soft.

Great constipation accompanied with hæmorrhoids, not bleeding ; never had them before or since.

### Sexual Organs.

Pain in left ovary, shooting down to knee. Leucorrhœa. Menses appear for the first time in over a year since birth of last child ; color purple and scanty, with great pain.

### Respiratory Organs.

Burning sensation in the bronchial tubes.

Dry hacking cough, caused by tickling in the epiglottis.

Sharp pain just below the ribs on the right side, deepseated, followed by soreness.

Slowness of pulse; decreased in ten hours from 72 to 58 per minute.

Cold sweat over the whole body, which soon dries off, and again comes and goes as if by flashes.

### Generalities.

Feels weak and nervous, uneasy; is apprehensive that some calamity is about to occur. Feels very weak, as a person feels after a severe illness.

Unable to make much exertion; the least exercise causes perspiration.

All the symptoms worse in the afternoon.

# INDEX OF REMEDIES

### Upper Extremities.

Both wrists are lame and ache severely.

Pain in the left shoulder and arm.

Chilly sensation at the shoulder and down the arm.

### Lower Extremities.

Feet and legs cold and numb.

### General Symptoms.

Languid, tired feeling, with great prostration.

Physical and mental depression, with vertigo and drowsiness.

---

# LILIUM TIGRINUM.*

### (The Spotted Lily.)

DESCRIPTION.—The Tiger Lily is a well-known, showy, orange-colored coarse-flowered garden plant, very abundant in cultivation, and is a native of China and Japan. The *stem* is from four to six feet high, unbranched and woolly. *Leaves* scattered, sessile, three-veined, the upper cordate-ovate. The *axils* bulbiferous. *Flowers* large, in a pyramid at the summit of the stem, dark orange-colored, with black, or very deep crimson, somewhat raised spots, which give the flower the appearance of the skin of the tiger. It blooms in July and August.

OFFICINAL PREPARATIONS.—Tincture of the flowers and pollen; dilutions.

ANALOGUES.—*Aquicea, Belladonna, Cimicifuga, Cactus, Helonias, Mater, Podophyllum, Platina, Sepia.*

### Mind and Disposition.

*Females.*—Great depression of spirits, with fearfulness and apprehension of an impending fatal internal disease, or that it was already preying upon her; constant inclination to weep (very marked). Blurred vision, all objects appearing very indistinct.

Despondent and gloomy, with loss of memory and great difficulty in expressing her thoughts; often selecting wrong words, but in making the correction would as often take other words quite as inappropriate; great fear and dread of insanity.

Does not want to be pleased, and don't want to talk, but wants to sleep, and, during sleep, very unpleasant dreams.

* From the exhaustive resume of Dr. Paine, in *American Observer* and N. Y. Transactions for 1872. (*Hale.*)

*Scalp.*—Fine, rash-like eruption about the forehead, and around the border of the hair, with much itching.

### Eyes and Sight.

*Eyes.*—Intense pain in both eyes, extending backward into the head, with great dimness of sight.

Right eye very sensitive to gaslight, with intolerable burning pain subsequently extending to the left eye, and continuing for several days.

Burning in the eyes after reading or writing, and feeling of great general weakness.

*Sight.*—Blur before the eyes after a night made restless by lascivious dreams and seminal emissions toward morning, attended by difficulty in keeping the mind fixed upon the subject under consideration; selecting wrong words with which to express his ideas.

Blurred vision, cannot see objects distinctly, with loss of appetite, aversion to coffee, nausea when thinking about it; frequent desire to pass urine, but in small quantities; faint in a warm room and when standing, with cold perspiration on the back of the hands and feet; fearfulness and apprehension of some impending evil.

Dimness of sight, with intense pain in both eyes, extending into the head; shooting pain in the right temple, passing over to the left; crampy pains in the left mamma and fingers, and pressing pain in the right arm and wrist, beginning at seven o'clock p. m. and continuing through the night.

*Muscæ volitantes* at various times.

Eyesight, which was always weak, hypermetropic, wearing 1-14 glasses, is now much worse; this aggravation continued for more than four weeks, when the eyes had returned to their natural condition with this improvement; whereas, formerly she had a habit of turning the head toward the left when reading, in order to see the whole of a letter, for example, s p d and f y, when looking straight forward, could see only the straight part of the letter and not the curve; now can see the whole letter distinctly without looking sideways.

### Ears.

Rushing sound in both ears.

### Nose.

Frequent sneezing at ten o'clock P. M., relieving a severe, ...
ing headache, and pain in the eyes.

Sensation as if blood would issue from the nose when ...
it, with feeling of fullness and heaviness of the ...

Heat and fullness of the face and head.

The left cheek bright and red hot in the morning on ...

### Mouth and Throat.

Hawking mucus from the throat, with constant disposi...
vomit.

* Hawking of mucus, with constant nausea.

### Taste and Appetite.

*Taste.*—Taste of blood in the mouth, with severe ...
of the chest; weak beating of the heart.

Great craving for meat, and the more pronounced ...
toms the greater the desire.

Voracious hunger, seemingly in the back, extending ...
vertebral column, and up to the occiput, not ...
eating.

Loss of appetite, and aversion to bread particularly, ...
for three weeks after the last dose of the ...
depression of spirits; disposition to weep; pressing ...
rectum from *prolapsus uteri?*; cold chills, ...
particularly after going to bed, with hot flushes ...
morning.

* *Loss of appetite cured.*

*Thirst.*—Great thirst, drinking often and much.

### Gastric Symptoms.

Frequent eructations, with great distention of the stoma...
and escape of flatus from the rectum (constant during ...
proving).

Constant nausea, with the sensation as of a lump in the st...
ach, which moved down at every attempt to swallow ...
immediately returned.

Nausea, with pain in the back; aversion to food; depre...
of spirits, and disposition to weep.

F.47